Clara Barton

Professional Angel

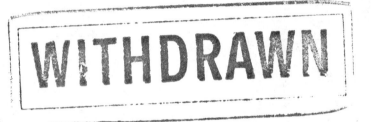

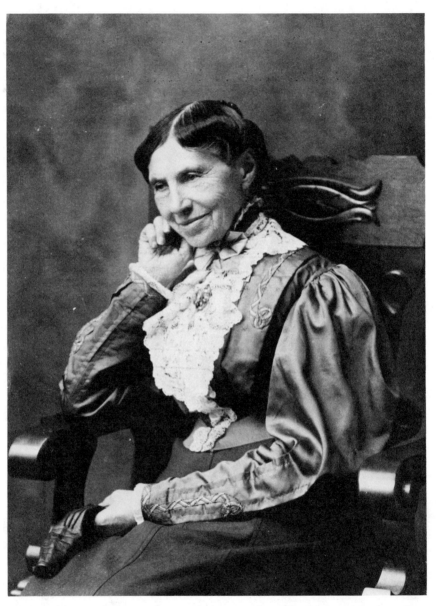

Clara Barton at eighty-five. This sympathetic portrait was taken in Washington, D.C. Library of Congress.

Clara Barton
Professional Angel

Elizabeth Brown Pryor

upp   University of Pennsylvania Press   Philadelphia

Permission is acknowledged to quote material from the following sources.
Manuscript Department, William H. Perkins Library, Duke University, Durham, NC (Clarissa
Harlowe Barton Papers and Mary Norton Papers); Dun & Bradstreet Credit Services (R. G. Dun
& Co. Collection, Baker Library, Harvard University Graduate School of Business Administra-
tion); Western Reserve Historical Society, Cleveland, OH (John J. Elwell Papers); American
Antiquarian Society, Worcester, MA (Clara Barton Papers and Ira Moore Barton Papers); Hunt-
ington Library, San Marino, CA (HM 26917, 26921, 26922, 26933, 26943); American Red Cross,
Washington, DC; Minnesota Historical Society, St. Paul, MN (Austin Craig and Family Papers,
Marion Louisa Sloan Papers); National Park Service, McLean, VA (Clara Barton Papers, Clara
Barton National Historic Site, Glen Echo, MD)

Library of Congress Cataloging-in-Publication Data

Pryor, Elizabeth Brown.
  Clara Barton: professional angel.

  Bibliography: p.
  Includes index.
  1. Barton, Clara, 1821–1912. 2. Nurses—United
States—Biography. I. Title.
HV569.B3P78 1987   361.7′634′0924 [B]   87-13868
ISBN 0-8122-8060-1 (cloth)
ISBN 0-8122-1273-8 (pbk)

Reprinted 1988
First paperback printing 1988

Design: Adrianne Onderdonk Dudden

For my mother and father,
who in so many ways made this book possible

contents

preface

Among the handful of heroines in America, Clara Barton has stood foremost in the field of philanthropy for more than a century. Small girls are taught to revere her early contributions to the field of nursing; her bravery on the battlefields of the Civil War has taken on the quality of legend; the whole nation is indebted to her for the establishment of the American Red Cross. Lesser known, but of equal importance, are her achievements as a feminist, her role as the first female American diplomat, and her notable successes in the fields of education, foreign aid, and black rights. She participated in an astonishing number of the nineteenth century's major events and was a personal friend of figures as varied as Susan B. Anthony, Frederick Douglass, Benjamin Butler, and Kaiser Wilhelm.

Yet in a curious way Barton's splendid achievements seem to have obscured her intriguing and complex personality. Whereas all know of her courage, most would be surprised that she could "remember nothing but fear" about her childhood. For every characteristic that gave force to Barton's crusades there seemed to be a weak link that prevented her attaining personal happiness. What is found, in short, is a personality often at odds with itself. The qualities of courage, empathy, and determination so often ascribed to the beloved heroine undoubtedly existed, but just as evident were a merciless driving force, a shattering insecurity, a demanding and erratic ego. For when Barton wrote that her work had been accomplished "against the fearful odds," she did not refer solely to the difficulties of pursuing a career in the male-dominated Victorian world. She was speaking of the many battles waged internally; the long fight against crippling depression and fear of insanity that grew out of her need to excel, and her belief that she had never done enough to secure a place in the world. It is an understanding of this darker side of Barton's nature that makes the story of her accomplishments so poignant, and so very interesting.

"I have lived my life, well and ill," Clara Barton wrote a few years before her death, "always less well than I wanted it to be but it is, *as* it is, and as it has been; *so small* a thing to have had so much said about it." A modest statement, especially from a person whose name had been a household word for more than forty years. Modest, and disingenuous, for like so many other noble pronouncements made by Miss Barton, one suspects that this philosophical acceptance of her own actions was written with an eye to the fitting word and quotable phrase. In reality her whole life had been spent in a search for the public acclaim that served as a salve for the indifference of her family. Whatever the importance of her work for all of humanity, whatever its role in the larger scope of philanthropy, it certainly had significance for her. There were, in fact, few subjects on which she was less acquiescent.

There were times when Barton admitted her shortcomings or the disappointments of her life, but they were rare, and never public. She was certain of her abilities, yet always unsure whether others shared her high regard. Thus she made an early determination that if she were to be a public figure she would create a public image. It did not particularly concern her that that image was somewhat at odds with reality. Hence she began to write a series of statements and letters, cleverly crafted to be appropriate for publication, which portrayed her personality and achievements in an idealized light. The pupils she taught as a young woman were always the greatest rogues or the most accomplished scholars; titles were invented if not earned. Even her movements were falsified to show that she was continually at the center of the action. To some extent these measures were necessary to offset those who would question what, for example, a woman was doing following an army in wartime. (If through no fault of her own she was doing nothing, the worst was assumed.) Yet, it was not only major undertakings she sought to justify, but personal traits and family matters about which she need not have commented at all. Though she dyed her hair (and why not if she chose to do so) she told friends and public that her "raven locks had never turned gray." Desiring to appear robust, she cosmetically lowered her age when the press inquired or the census taker came round. Barton's obsession with obscuring even the smallest details of her life reflected a sad lack of self-esteem and a need to project an image of perfection.

During periods of great stress Barton often expressed the desire to confide the whole convoluted story to some sympathetic ear—to impress upon someone how difficult the struggle against emotional instability, sexual prejudice, and family scandal had really been. On rare occasions she did give candid glimpses of her life, but always to physicians with whom she sought an alliance against the nervous breakdowns which plagued her. And if the world at large was to see the strong image of a dedicated, unflappable, and compassionate woman, if she built a brick wall around the facts of her life, a wall so high that the most dedicated biographer could chip away for years before here and there dislodging a bit of the shining facade, she also kept a scrupulous and frank diary in which she recorded all the small triumphs and ugly thoughts, the petty details which make up every life. She did not destroy these diaries, nor the mass of vividly written correspondence which so illuminates her character. These papers, some hundred thousand pieces, give lie to the idea that Miss Barton lacked a sense of the value of her life.

Barton's outrage at criticism, and the half-truths she told, were symptoms of a broad and terrible insecurity that stemmed partly from her unusual childhood, when she had been outside the nuclear family, and partly from her position as a childless, spouseless, intelligent, and hard-driving woman in a world that chose to glorify only the homemaking female. Barton saw herself, perhaps accurately, as an anomalous person in society. She occasionally took pleasure in viewing herself as a maverick, and genuinely enjoyed her role as a pioneer among working women. But the lack of an established niche clearly made her uncomfortable, and she vacillated between self-righteous conformity and rebellion. She traveled thus, without authority, unwilling to accept the mores of her day, improvising as she went. Unable to blame herself for the discomfort she felt, she lashed out at the world at large. Times of depression nearly always caused her to condemn the world as nothing more than a set of drear and confining societal standards. She often spoke of suicide, of the pleasure of leaving behind this "world of strife and bickering and lies." Periodically her nerves gave way under the constant strain of building the law as well as the substance of her life. Then for a time she would drop out of sight, and demand a coddling attention before she would rejoin the race for praise.

Fostering as she did a kind of self-imposed exile from the normal bonds of family and friends, Barton came to rely on herself for loyalty and approbation. In her eyes, she was the best candidate for every job, the ideal housekeeper, the most affectionate friend. Never did she learn to take criticism, and under its yoke she felt either persecution or smug superiority. To her mind there was little difference between observation, comment, suggestion, and censorship—and censorship was always the fault of the censor. Even the closest of nephews was accused of betrayal when he wisely tried to reshape his aunt's disastrous Spanish-American War policy. She could never bring herself to delegate authority; she was simply unable to believe that anyone else could do the job as she could. Worse yet, they might succeed as well as she, and threaten to rival her for glory or authority. Of course this made both personal and professional relationships difficult. Fealty to Barton was the one common characteristic of those who chose to work and live in her shadow. Sometimes she inspired great loyalty; always she demanded it. One of her most prized aides called her "the Queen."

We are all creatures of contrast, now confident, now hindered and terrorized by the prospect of a new day. But in Barton the normal toss and pitch of life was exaggerated, so that she felt always the need to compensate for some heightened emotion. Depression was countermanded by excessive work or a zealous crusade for some cause, and the frantic activity did not stop until nervous collapse or increased depression made it a necessity. Balance and serenity, the very traits she peddled to the press, were flighty visitors to her life. Chaos came to form such a semblance of normality for Barton that she fought the few periods of calm that came to her. Finding the tranquility boring, if not downright disconcerting, she hastened to take on the burden of more troubled souls. The celebrated incident of her childhood, during which she nursed her adult brother for nearly two years, was little more than an exercise to fill—with emotional tension and hard work—a stretch of time that, at the age of twelve, she already thought wasted in play. Moreover, in aiding her brother David she found (as she would with the myriad others who came under her care) that she could change the direction of a life, or alleviate the terrible distress of physical suffering, a sharp contrast with her own life, in which she was powerless to check the pain or lessen the sorrow. For Barton every fresh wound was bound up on another human being. She never learned to administer first aid to herself.

Hence it was achievement that lent definition to Clara Barton's life. Her identity was completely tied to her career, and work itself held a deep significance for her. More than an activity, it became a kind of creed. "You have never known me without work and you never will," she once declared. "It has always been a part of the best religion I had." It was while working, especially under stress, that the quick intelligence, the undaunted bravery, the brilliant timing, came to the fore. With work she gained purpose, a justification for her existence, independence, and praise. Only when her career lagged did the greatest despondency come.

It is the nature of Barton's work that has most interested the world; there is something perennially fascinating about those who trade in the misfortunes of others. Of course for her purposes only the most noble of causes could suffice. Even the most hostile world could hardly dare to criticize a woman working for humanity, and in a crisis she could always be the center of attention. No altruist, she craved the teary-eyed thanks, the clinging hands, and the eternal gratitude of those she helped. The love and adoration missing from her home life were found here, as well as the larger praise of the world. Until well into her eighties she never hesitated to rush to the scene of disaster, where she would be needed and revered, no matter what pressing business should have kept her in Washington.

Yet it would be wrong to treat Barton's lifework cynically, for she was filled with honest qualities which lent it integrity. She bore dreadful shocks of exposure, and faced hideous scenes, with equanimity and always with unflinching valor. A strong current of philanthropy ran in her family's blood; she honored charity because her father had encouraged her to do so, and she lived what he had taught. She had true compassion for the weak or disadvantaged and ever sought to supplement their dignity as well as their material possessions. If she was quick to grasp the dramatic possibilities of a relief mission, she did not ignore the little kindnesses which in aggregate made up so much of her work. Unable to be brave for herself, anxious over every irreverent tweak of fate, Barton was a miracle of sustenance for others.

Thus the paradox exists; the woman frightened by life, but confident in the face of terror; the driven achiever who worrried that she had failed to do enough; the beloved heroine who died alone. Her long list of accomplishments, un-equalled in the annals of American women, must be placed in this perspective: that she dared to offend a society whose acceptance she treasured, and to patch up the lives around her when her own was rent and frayed.

acknowledgments

I was home not long ago and one of my friends said to me, "But what will we do without Clara? She is the only continuity in our lives." And indeed, the writing of this book has spanned my entire adult life, with all of its friendships, false starts, high times and low moments. I feel, thus, that just about everyone I know has lived through—some would say survived—this exercise with me. My debt for their support and patience is correspondingly large.

The dedication of this book to my mother and late father was not made idly. I owe everything I have, or have achieved, to them. And in these acknowledgments I would expand this to include my two wonderful sisters, Beverly Louise Brown and Peggy Ann Brown.

I would also specially note the assistance I received from Charles Rosenberg and Drew Faust of the University of Pennsylvania. Not only did they stretch my thinking and encourage me, they read and reread the manuscript, offered significant critical advice, and in the end virtually acted as agents for the book. All of this strikes me as considerably above and beyond their duties as graduate advisors.

Mention should also be made of the fine help given to me over a ten-year period from the staffs of the Clara Barton National Historic Site, the National Archives, the American National Red Cross, and, particularly, the Library of Congress Manuscript Division. Their willingness to share their resources and offer information and assistance were invaluable.

And for all of those who suffered through tales of Miss Barton at cocktail parties and dinners, who prodded me when I most needed it, who typed, read, proofread, listened to my frustration or exhilaration: there is nothing I can do to repay you. To those listed below I can only offer my love, and a most heartfelt thank you.

George Beuchert, Ed and Agnes Chatelain, Elizabeth David, Pepe Garcia, Robert Grogg, John and Julie Hamre, Frank Parker, Barbara Pryor, Tony Pryor, Cheryl Russell, Dean Sagar, Janet Tighe, Sandy Weber.

Clara Barton

Professional Angel

one

On a cheerless Christmas Day in 1821 Captain Stephen Barton finished his round of chores and wearily entered the house to sit by the fire. The small Massachusetts town in which the Bartons lived had not yet given up the austere customs of Puritan times, and he looked forward to a quiet evening rather than a gay holiday celebration. He leaned back in his chair and stretched out his legs, only mildly disturbed by the voices of his wife and a female cousin in the adjoining bedroom. But the commotion increased, and the cousin finally emerged in a flutter to ask him to fetch the doctor; his wife Sarah was about to give birth. Tired and a little blasé—for this was his fifth child—Stephen Barton did not hurry, and a new daughter arrived before he could return.[1]

They named her Clarissa Harlowe Barton after a paternal aunt, who in turn had been named for the fashionable and romantic heroine of a Samuel Richardson novel.[2] But whether inappropriate to the middle-class household or lengthy and cumbersome to pronounce, the name never stuck. The Barton family liked nicknames and the new baby had her share. A brother, walking home from the strict New Oxford school, which held classes even on Christmas Day, met a neighbor who encouraged him to get home quickly, saying, "there's a little tot at your house"; he dubbed his new sister "Tot," a nickname that held on until she was well into her eighties.[3] Others called her "Tabatha" or "Clary," and "Baby" was the inevitable appellation for the youngest family member.[4] But her name was shortened most consistently to "Clara," and it was with this name that she identified closely throughout her life. Some early school papers have the careful signature "Clarissa H. Barton," and until the Civil War she signed herself "Clara H. Barton." After that time, however, the middle initial disappeared altogether, and she used only the name by which she became known to the world—Clara Barton.

"I am told there was great family jubilation on the occasion," Clara Barton wrote of her birth.[5] Jubilation, but also expectancy and a sense of novelty, for the family had thought itself complete long before 1821. Stephen Barton and Sarah Stone had married hastily in 1804, and a daughter, Dorothea, was born to them five months later. Two sons, Stephen and David, and another daughter, Sally, had made their appearance by 1810. Sally, closest in age to Clara, was nearly eleven years her senior. Since all of the Bartons were old enough to anticipate the important occasion, the family dignified it with the purchase of a set of Blue Willow china and a pink and white tea service, relatively extravagant purchases for their middle-class household. The china was handed down in the family, a symbol of this happy event and the many later celebrations at which it was used.[6]

They were shaped strongly of New England, these Bartons, reflecting the hard work and hard principles needed to earn a living in the rocky countryside and the individualism that gave fire to town meetings and church councils. Their village of North Oxford, Massachusetts, was well established in 1821, not very different from the other towns of the countryside fifty miles west of Boston, but with a strong local gentry and a bit of romantic history to call its own. The Bartons, Learneds, and Stones—the rootstock of Clara's family—had not been among the original Huguenot settlers of North Oxford, but they had very early seen the possibilities in its location along the swiftly moving French River and by 1713 had become prominent in the town's farming and milling industries. A hundred years later, their hopes for the town had been fulfilled. It was then a place of clapboard houses and steepled churches, surrounded by self-sufficient farms. Both saw and grist mills dotted the banks of the French River, providing a prosperous sideline for some of the area's farming families. A "handsome village on a large plain" is how one gazetteer described it.[7]

Clara learned of the history of her family and town on long winter evenings while sitting by the fire. Throughout her life she recalled the thrill she felt in hearing of the Bartons' part in the English Wars of the Roses and how the family had come to Massachusetts to begin a new life. There were scores of colorful relatives to take pride in: Samuel Barton, the first to come to North Oxford, who had fled from Salem after unsuccessfully defending an accused woman during the witch trials;[8] Ebenezer Learned, an early and successful industrialist, a leader of the Massachusetts General Court, but a taciturn and flinty man, the legends of whose stingy ways were overshadowed only by the spectacular exploits of his enormous-footed black slave, Mingo;[9] and Dr. Stephen Barton, a romantic rebel during the American Revolution, a delegate to the Committees of Correspondence and Safety, and a noted philanthropist, whose independent wife flew in the face of his authority and brewed tea even after the imposition of the hated tax in 1774.[10] ("I have been entertained hours and hours by your interesting, precise and intelligent grandmother Barton, telling us of the tea parties she and her sister Aunt Ballard held in the cellar when grandfather was out or *up* and didn't know what was going on in his own disloyal and rebellious home," Clara told a nephew years later, "and how they hung blankets inside the cellar door to prevent the savory fumes of the tea from reaching the loyal and official olfactories of 'Pater familias.'"[11]) Added to these major figures was a list of tantalizing characters that included French and Indian War soldiers, tireless midwives, and bear-wrestling cousins.[12]

It was from her father that Clara Barton heard most of this family lore. Born in 1774, son of the Revolutionary Dr. Stephen, he had grown up with the heroes of the struggling United States. As a young man he found his own military adventure in the army of General "Mad" Anthony Wayne, a troop that fought numerous Indian wars in the wilderness of the Northwest Territory. The elements of this experience—the three years of privation in uncivilized regions, the expanse and promise he saw in the newly formed United States, the regimen and hardiness required in military life—were the definitive influences of his youth. He spoke often and forcefully of these campaigns, and the tone of his language was one of patriotic loyalty. "His soldier habits and tastes never left him," his daughter Clara wrote. To the end of his life he delighted in military jargon and the comradeship of fellow veterans.[13]

Tall, lean, sharp-eyed Stephen Barton returned to North Oxford and took up his ancestors' occupations of farming and milling. He kept to himself, gaining a reputation for minding his own business, which came to be a watchword of the Barton clan. His stately bearing and well-respected family connections, however, made it natural that he should serve as moderator of the town meeting, as selectman, as captain of the militia, and later, in 1836, as representative to the Massachusetts General Court. Local citizens noted his sound judgment, stubbornness, wit, and integrity. He was liberal in his political views, a lifelong democrat and admirer of Andrew Jackson, and he fostered notions of progress for North Oxford in the forms of mechanization of the milling industry, improved education, and religious tolerance. But, in contrast to the intellect that readily embraced technical innovation, his personal inclinations were old-fashioned. He maintained a conservative stance against dancing, gambling, or drinking, and one neighbor recalled that he was the last man in North Oxford to stop tying his hair back in a queue.[14]

Leadership often implies high social standing, but Stephen Barton undoubtedly exemplified the middle class. Clara always regarded her background as a "humble life," lived out in "small environments."[15] Barton provided well for his family, but their way of life was modest. His accounts with local merchants show that he bought more molasses than sugar, and that calico, not silk, clothed the family's women. Any available opportunity was seized to make a little extra money, and ends were met by selling excess hay, renting out land or equipment, and boarding the neighbors' livestock.[16] Like his father he was a versatile worker; he built not only the home in which his youngest daughter was born but many simple pieces of furniture and household equipment. The house was cleverly designed, with a convenient indoor well, but far less imposing than his grandfather's home.[17] Barns and meadows, an orchard, and a kitchen garden completed the homestead. There were lilac bushes to beautify the place, and Captain Barton was not ashamed to open his house to all who visited the town.

Barton's democratic tendencies were also fostered by an early association with the Universalist church. Unlike the traditional New England churches with their aristocratic God, the Universalists believed that God encouraged all men and women to accept him and charged them to grasp the opportunity to earn salvation—an opportunity open to all. The Universalists were socially aware, interested in abolition, education, and charity. As a young man Stephen Barton had been present at the North Oxford ordination of Hosea Ballou, a zealous and influential early leader of Universalism. The experience had affected him strongly, causing him to leave his family's Baptist church. He was not a consistent churchgoer—Clara wrote that although she "could not say that he worshipped in that church, he surely always saw that his family worshipped in it"—yet he worked consistently to build and maintain the church and three years after Clara's birth was elected an officer.[18]

Universalism and his own father's charity encouraged a strong commitment to philanthropy in Stephen Barton. Between 1826 and 1836 he annually donated $574 toward caring for the community's poor, and in 1831 he used his own funds to establish a house in which destitute families could be maintained.[19] These acts were gratefully remembered by many Oxford citizens. "I never new [sic] a Barton much stuck up," stated a neighbor who had benefited from Stephen Barton's benevolence. "I well recolect [sic] the time I was sick at your house and how you doctored me and wated [sic] on me a Poor Boy I never shall forget it."[20]

Stephen Barton exercised his influence at home as well as in the community, though there he had considerable competition from his strong-willed wife. Sarah Stone was ten years younger than her husband. She may once have been the "fine looking" woman of Clara's memory, but she came to have a rotund, featureless face. She was the daughter of a well-respected North Oxford family, middle-class and with few pretensions. Sarah shared her husband's Baptist background and his more recently developed interest in Universalist principles.[21] She seems to have been a homebody, indulging in few activities outside the domestic circle, but she had strong opinions on political and social topics. In the 1830s, well before the abolitionist movement gained a foothold in New England, she signed several antislavery petitions that were sent to the United States House of Representatives.[22] Sarah Barton was also outspoken on the subject of women's rights. Her youngest daughter recalled that she was so early exposed to feminist ideals that she believed she "must have been born believing in the full right of woman to all privileges and positions which nature and justice accord her. . . . When as a young woman I heard the subject discussed it seemed simply ridiculous that any sensible rational person should question it."[23]

Stephen and Sarah Barton shared liberal sentiments, but they were of entirely different temperaments. Clara described her father as a "calm, sound, reasonable high-tuned moral man"; she remembered her mother as ambitious and of "extreme vigor, always did two days work in one, never slept after 3 o'clock, both

6

nervy and *nervous.*"[24] Industrious and ingenious, she carried on the multitude of daily chores expected of a New England housewife. Her eccentricities and thriftiness were legendary in the town. A daughter-in-law reported to her family that Sarah fed the Bartons on fruits and vegetables that were not fresh, curiously waiting until they were beginning to decay before she served them. She diligently inspected the vegetable bins, picked out the half-spoiled produce, and spent hours paring and cutting away the decayed portions. Sarah also had the habit of baking a great number of mince or apple pies, then carefully storing them in the cellar pantry. She protected this hoard jealously and was highly displeased if the family requested a slice. The pies, like her fresh produce, inevitably became moldy and unfit to eat. Once in a burst of anger her son Stephen slipped down to the cellar and threw the pies into a pail for hog feed. When confronted by his mother he told her that only pigs would eat moldy pies. The protest did not cure her.[25]

Sarah Barton coupled this peculiarity with a short and fiery temper. Difficult to please, she exhibited her dissatisfaction with color and gusto. She once dismantled a new iron cookstove, the gift of her husband, and threw it piece by piece into the farm pond because she thought it less functional than her old fireplace oven. She muttered and swore whenever anything displeased her and had little patience with the people around her, who she believed did not work up to her expectations. A story is told that when Sarah Barton died, one of her young granddaughters was brought to see her as she lay in her coffin. A few minutes later someone asked the child if she had seen her grandmother. "Yes," the little girl replied, "I saw grandma and she never swored once."[26]

Stephen and Sarah Barton's strong personalities made for a stormy relationship. While Stephen's word was the rule, Sarah loudly protested any interference in her domestic work. Frequently they quarreled violently. In one case Sarah, exasperated with her task of changing the bedding, threw a feather tick down the stairs, catching her husband full in the face and scattering feathers over the entire room. Stephen's anger knew no bounds for some time. He ordered Sarah to recapture every feather, but she complied with such a vigor, "muttering imprecations so vengeful," that Stephen left home for several days. It was with such scenes that domestic issues were reconciled, and with which Clara grew up.[27]

The eldest child of this tempestuous union was Dorothea, called Dolly after a paternal aunt. She was tall and dark-haired, a keen student with a good mind and an unbridled desire for learning. At the time of her sister Clara's birth she was a teacher in North Oxford. Like her mother, Dolly had a magnificent temper and an excitable nature, though she possessed enough patience to do intricate embroidery and to write poetry in a flowing, ornate script. She seems to have been especially interested in Clara, and much of the baby's daily attention came from this quarter. Sensitive and scholarly, Dolly longed to obtain a higher education than that offered in the village school and wept when made to attend classes with a less bookish brother, who she felt disgraced the family. In later years Clara was to remember her eldest sister's tender care and "ever watchful hand," and to give Dolly credit for much of her own interest in intellectual pursuits. "Under suitable conditions . . . ," maintained Clara, "she should have been the flower of the flock."[28]

But Dolly Barton's nervous and sensitive nature led to tragedy when Clara was six years old. In 1827 Dolly had a mental breakdown from which she never recovered. In an era in which mental illness was regarded as shameful and virtually no treatment was available, the best the Barton family could do was to keep Dolly away from society and try to control her flaring temper. In time Dolly became actually dangerous. She cut her beautiful embroidery into shreds, and the rockers on her favorite chair had to be halted with a restraining strip of wood to keep her from rocking too furiously. As her condition worsened she was kept in a locked room with barred windows to control her rages. She would often beat on the door and scream to be let out. Once she escaped and spent the night in the deep woods outside of the village. Another time she tried to violently attack the wife of her brother David with an axe; the young woman was saved only when her husband ran from a nearby field and restrained Dolly.[29]

The Bartons never knew what caused Dolly's insanity, but the tragedy of this sister, "so bright, so scholarly, so promising, and so early blighted," haunted Clara throughout her life.[30] In the late 1870s Clara confided to a doctor that she believed it was due to "some menstrual obstruction which was not understood or treated"—a common medical misunderstanding of the time.[31] Later, however, Clara told a niece that she believed Dolly would not have lost her mind if she had been able to obtain proper schooling and fulfill her ambitions in the world of letters. Her constant brooding and inward reflection only increased her unhappiness and finally drove her to despair. Significantly, Barton never referred to her sister's insanity publicly and only rarely did so in private. In her autobiography, *The Story of My Childhood*, she notes only that her eldest sister was "an invalid."[32]

Of Barton's siblings, the most dominant personality seems to have been Stephen junior. He was fifteen when his youngest sister was born and had already gone through his own maturing trials. He was physically strong and athletically inclined but, like his mother, was excitable and nervous. As a child he found it difficult to settle down to studying—at twelve he was still unable to read.[33] He resisted his parents' admonitions, then suddenly decided for himself that he would like an education. By studying at night after a day of farm chores, Stephen surpassed the rest of the town's pupils within a year, being especially noted for his "power and quick wits in mathematics."[34] While Clara was still a child he became a teacher. After a few years, however, his father deeded the Barton mills to his sons and they became two of the town's noted industrialists. He had a keen business sense, and during the years Clara was growing up Stephen was gaining a reputation as a sharp trader, his mathematical ability apparently sometimes overriding the strict morality of his Universalist upbringing.[35]

If rumors of slightly shady dealings at the S & D Barton Mills were circulating, so was a growing feeling that Captain Barton's eldest son was destined to be a town leader. Like his father, he sympathized with the area's poor and took several underprivileged boys to live with him when he established his own household. Between 1825 and 1840 he used his influence to evaluate the school system, design a well-graded and straight road from the village of North Oxford to the depot of the Norwich Railroad, and plan and maintain a new town cemetery. He was elected town assessor in 1834 and 1837, and simultaneously served on two school committees.[36] Stephen's business and civic duties kept him too busy to spend a great deal of time with his sister Clara, but she later recalled his patience in teaching her arithmetic. "Multiplication, division, subtraction, halfs, quarters and wholes, soon ceased to be a mystery," she recalled, "and no toy equalled my little slate."[37] Although he spent less time with Clara than the other Barton children did, Stephen's example was constant in the Barton household, where pride in his success as a town leader was coupled with a nagging doubt about the nature of his business transactions.

Stephen's partner in the mills was David Barton, his junior by two years. David also possessed the manly build and athletic interests of the Barton men. He never became involved in the family's more intellectual pursuits, though some faded sheets of verse, carefully saved by Clara, show an attempt at composing poetry.[38] Instead he was a dashing daredevil, a handsome neighborhood strongman, "the Buffalo Bill of the surrounding countryside."[39] He was fond of horses, and to Clara he became something of a hero, a gentle giant who talked to her about the ways of animals and initiated her into the joys of riding. She saw herself as his "little protege" and constant companion.[40] While Clara was still a girl he began seriously working at the mills, seeing them prosper but also gaining with his brother a slightly dishonest reputation. "Has David had an opportunity to toll any more grain for Capt. DeWitt so as to make right the mistake in tolling?" a family friend anxiously asked Clara a few years after David began running the mill. "He took I believe the toll of 4 quarts too much."[41] In Clara's mind, however, his reputation was never tarnished. She loyally upheld him throughout her life, later remembering that "he had been my ideal from earliest memory."[42]

Sally Barton was the sister closest to Clara in age, yet very little of her influence is seen in Clara's childhood. It is possible that she was absent from home a good deal, for a receipt from the Nicholas Academy shows that Stephen Barton paid for his daughter to attend boarding school for at least one year.[43] Sally was, by all accounts, a fair-haired, graceful, and intelligent girl, who grew into a gracious and kind woman; she was "lovely as a summer morning and never so lovely as she was good and womanly," Clara recalled.[44] Like her older sister and her brother Stephen, Sally taught school for a short time, indulging her literary taste in the study of poetry. Clara Barton later believed that her own taste in literature stemmed from this sister's influence. Together Sally and Clara read the works of Sir Walter Scott, then "all the train of English poetry that a child could take in." After Dolly's mental collapse, Sally watched anxiously over Clara, vigilantly protecting her small sister's interest and welfare in the unsettled atmosphere of the Barton home.[45]

9

Throughout her life, Clara Barton showed a great deal of ambivalence about the experience of growing up in this household of matured and unusual personalities. Though she often recalled individual incidents with pleasure and wrote sunny descriptions in her autobiography of horseback riding and playing with cousins in the beautiful countryside, the overall impression of her childhood is one of sadness and a struggle for acceptance. As she sat down in 1907 to begin *The Story of My Childhood*, she questioned "whether to tell the truth about the little girl," and once wrote in her diary that she had not "had the happy home life of a little girl that most children have, I knew I had hard days then."[46] Even to the world at large she admitted that "in the earlier years of my life I remember nothing but fear."[47]

Fear she felt from the natural terrors of childhood—snakes and thunderstorms and runaway horses—but also from the imposing conflicts that surrounded her. Barton's ambivalence is also reflective of the sporadic and inconsistent attention she received at home. She wrote that her mother, thinking there were plenty of others to care for her small daughter, "attempted very little," and that family attitudes toward her wavered between a kind of intense individual instruction and total disregard for her needs and desires.[48] At times Clara felt that her very identity was submerged in the priorities of the rest of the grown-up family, that she was little more than a slate to mark with her teachers' personalities. Her childhood became a series of repeated attempts to express her own needs and proclivities, to shake off dependence, and to overcome the neglect and ridicule she felt were so often her lot.

There was a sense, too, that the others, with their larger experience, had an edge in family discussions that she could not hope to match. Her earnest attempts to be helpful or add to a conversation seemed childish and amusing to even the youngest of the other Barton children. Clara came to feel that the merriment made at her expense went beyond family teasing, and she grew to be self-conscious about her efforts and resentful that she was the brunt of so many jokes. The family watched as Clara dutifully shared candy given to her, carefully counting the number of recipients but forgetting to include herself. The look of bewilderment on her face when she discovered that everyone had a piece but her caused, in Clara's words, "an amusing bit of sport for the family at my expense as was their wont." The Bartons similarly joked at her misconceptions of various political figures, setting her up in front of them to give her naive impressions. "To the amusement of the family," Clara allowed that she believed the president to be the size of the meetinghouse and the vice-president the size of a barn—and green. Their laughter hardly encouraged the young girl to express herself. As she grew older they joked about Clara's rapid work in her brother's mill, intimating that a fire there had been caused by friction from her clattering loom—"that joke on me lasted many years." So bitter did Clara become that she came to mistrust even the family's motives for sending her to school at an early age, feeling that it probably stemmed from "a touch of mischievous curiosity . . . to see what my performance at school might be."[49]

Clara's earliest reaction to the dominant personalities at home was to retreat into an acute and painful timidity. Immersed in a situation in which responses to her would be unpredictable at best, she shrank away from contact with strangers and withdrew from scenes in which she would be noticed and possibly made the focus of a joke or argument. The reticence that resulted from her home life was exacerbated by an almost total lack of the physical charms usually meted out to young girls. Short, plump, and homely, she had yet to gain the character that would render her face so interesting. Clara's mother also neglected the child's thick and lustrous dark brown hair—her one good feature—by having it close-cropped, which only served to emphasize her broad forehead and sallow complexion.[50] In addition, a mild speech impediment caused her to lisp, increasing her bashfulness. Clara long remembered the humiliation at school of mispronouncing and lisping words. In one instance, having studied diligently to learn the names of the ancient Egyptians, she mangled the name Ptolomy, pronouncing it "Potlomy." Although the teacher checked the laughter of the older children, Clara was "overcome by mortification" and left the room in tears.[51]

Barton's excessive timidity also caused her actively to avoid a feeling that she was "giving trouble." Aware of the contrast between herself and the rest of the family, she felt keenly her dependence. She was continually afraid to mention the clothing and comforts she needed. Her memories of Sundays in the old Oxford Universalist Church more frequently mention the cold and her need for gloves than exhortations from the pulpit.[52] On one occasion she was given a dress at a child's Christmas party and, instead of expressing polite thanks, burst into tears and ran from the room. Evidently the dress had been sorely needed for some time. But, as she recalled, "I was too sensitive to represent my wants, even to my father, kind and generous as he was."[53] Yet Clara's timidity cannot have been the only problem. Perhaps too absorbed in their own temperamental relationship or overly casual in the upbringing of their youngest daughter, the Bartons seem to have neglected to notice the child's everyday necessities. Far from taking special notice of the bashful child, Clara's mother seems generally to have regarded her shy, self-effacing daughter as troublesome and "difficult to manage," an attitude that only reinforced Clara's own sense of being a burden.[54]

Clara's timidity was at once heightened and tempered by her experiences at school. She soon found she could gain much-needed attention by her unusual intellectual abilities, but she had difficulties fitting in with the shouting, rambunctious children.

Clara began her formal education at the age of three—a practice not uncommon in New England at that time. Even at this age she was no novice, having already the rudiments of a basic education. Indeed she could not recall a time that she could not read and startled her teacher on the first day by spelling words as advanced as *artichoke*.[55] One of her earliest schools was conducted by Richard Stone, a converted Universalist like her father, whose belief in bringing out the best in each child helped him to attract pupils from all over New England. This school, like so many she would attend, crowded up to a hundred scholars in one or two rooms and stressed reading, writing, and arithmetic, learned largely through rote. Stone, however, was unusual in his commitment to challenging his better pupils, and Clara was among those who enjoyed the benefits of individual attention.[56] She especially recalled the pleasure of discovering the field of geography at his school, becoming so intrigued that she "persisted in waking my poor drowsy sister in the cold winter mornings to sit up in bed and by the light of a tallow candle, help to find mountains, rivers, counties, oceans, lakes."[57] Barton's earliest school papers also show that Stone inculcated her with the patriotic, moral, and religious precepts thought appropriate to the proper formation of character. "Death is the only thing certain in the world," a nine-year-old Clara carefully copied into her penmanship book. She followed it with "Govern your passions" and "Knowledge is gained Only by Constant Study."[58]

The strong personal relationship between Clara and Richard Stone seems to have been repeated with all of her teachers. They found in the serious young girl an eagerness to learn that was both touching and challenging. Another teacher, Lucien Burleigh, treated her "with consideration and kindness," and developed a series of advanced studies—including astronomy, ancient history, and poetry—for her questing mind. Long after she left his school, Burleigh continued to show an affectionate interest in her affairs and concern for her spiritual and intellectual development.[59] Clara next attended an Oxford school taught by Jonathan Dana, and once more the pupil-teacher relationship proved to be a close one. Barton wrote of this friendship that she had "no words to describe the value of his instruction, nor the pains he took with his eager pupil." There again she was permitted to dabble in the higher branches of learning and was given special instruction outside of school hours. Thankful for any individual attention, Clara remembered her experiences at Jonathan Dana's school with affection: "My grateful Homage for my inestimable teacher and his interest in his early pupil, became memories of a lifetime."[60]

Clara's family was proud of her scholarship, and she basked in their approbation. Her sisters helped her to expand her literary tastes, sharing poetry and their favorite books, while Stephen, she recalled, "inducted me into the mystery of figures."[61] The Bartons' encouragement of Clara's intellectual talents speaks of their liberalism, for many girls of her day were dissuaded from intellectual pursuits or actively barred from the more advanced fields of study. It also strongly shaped her perception of the skills needed to gain recognition and acceptance at home and in the world at large. While other girls were honing the traditional traits of womanhood—humility and nurturing—Clara found that achievement and "hard-thinking" won her the respect she so anxiously sought.[62]

Clara's school experiences gave her scope for intellectual growth and lessened somewhat her family tensions, but they made only minimal inroads into her chronic social malaise. On her first day of school, finding herself away from the familiar scenes of home, she "was seized with an intense fear . . . at finding no member of the family near."[63] She gradually adjusted to this, of course, but continued to feel alienated from the other pupils and fearful of new faces. An attempt to reduce her bashfulness by sending her to Richard Stone's new boarding school turned into a disaster as Clara, "in constant dread of doing something wrong," could not adjust and would not talk or eat. Despite the kind attentions of teachers, she finally had to be sent home. Clara bitterly resented the whole episode, characterizing it as a decision "to throw me among strangers."[64] As an older pupil, Clara found the majority of her peers to be less earnest than she about their studies, and they consequently seemed to her frivolous and immature. Though at least one fellow pupil admired her ("she was very studious and had a remarkable memory"), she also sensed that most of her schoolmates found her "unaccountable and prudish." Her memories of school days are filled with remembrances of teachers and curriculum, not carefree frolics and school fellowship.[65]

Recognition for Clara's scholarship reinforced in her a taste for masculine accomplishments and pursuits that caused her to identify strongly with men both during her childhood and in her adult life. "Your father always said you are more boy than girl," Clara reminded herself in 1907.[66] She idolized her father, and her favorite memory as a very small child was of sitting and listening "breathlessly" to his stories of war and wilderness living until she could recite the names of his heroes with a "parrot-like readiness."[67] The tales were transformed into playtime mock battles, complete with drums, banners, and stick bayonets— unusual games for a young girl. "The army played havock with each other, had fearful encounters, and . . . suffered disastrous results," Clara recalled.[68] The men in her family led her in pastimes that tested her strength and courage: David had her riding bareback before she was five, and her father's present of a spirited horse, "Billy," increased her ability until, galloping out in all kinds of weather, she would leave her companions far behind.[69] Eschewing dolls, she followed instead the pleasures and work of Stephen and David; they, in turn, taught her well, allowing few excuses for performance that was not up to their standard. "I must throw a ball or a stone with an underswing like a boy and not a girl, and must make it go where I sent it, and not fall at my feet and foolishly laugh at it," Clara proudly stated. "If I would drive a nail, strike it fairly on the head every time and not split the board. If I would draw a screw, turn it right the first time. I must tie a square knot that would hold."[70]

At the age of seven or eight, Clara found herself in a situation that allowed her to exercise and hone her tastes for boys' play and boys' company. About that time her father moved the family to the nearby Learned farmstead. Jeremiah Learned, a dashing but indiscriminate nephew of Captain Stephen Barton, had died, leaving a wife and four children and a farm that had suffered badly during his long illness. There were large debts, children to be clothed, and only the scantiest crops in the ground. To retain the land—nearly three hundred acres—

13

for the family, Captain Barton, together with another relative, purchased the farm. The Learneds were allowed to stay on, but Clara's family also moved into the house. The Learned boys, Jerry and Otis, and their friend Lovett Simpson, became her firm friends. "Wild" Jerry and mischievous Otis set the tone for the activities of the little band of cousins, and the next four years were filled with adventurous and daring escapades. In describing the happy events of this time Clara rarely mentions her girl cousins.[71]

The old Learned homestead, built in the early eighteenth century, was a much larger and more commodious house than the one in which Clara was born. Two stories high, of strong clapboarding, and with a pitched roof, it was surrounded by orchards, gardens, and intriguing outbuildings. The new place presented an array of interesting nooks and crannies to explore. Thus the little troop of cousins and friends roamed the farm's territory, running through "broad beautiful meadows" and up the rocky and wooded hills. They hunted chestnuts, explored caves, and dogged snakes near the French River. Clara recalled with obvious pleasure the lure of "three temptingly great barns. . . . Was there ever a better opportunity for hide-and-seek, for jumping and climbing?"[72] The saw and grain mills also held a special fascination. The children rode the long saw carriage out over the raceway, jumping off quickly after the sawn log was drawn back. They dared each other to balance on a pole thrown across the mill stream, and they gasped and whooped as it "swayed and teetered from the moment the foot touched it till it left it." Oblivious to the danger, the children merrily tempted the odds, and, miraculously, none was ever hurt.[73]

It was a time of revelations and a burst of freedom for Clara. She was away from the watchful eyes of six surrogate parents and removed from the scenes of Dolly's rages. She idolized Otis and Jerry, and they admired her extravagantly, for she "could run as fast and ride better" than they.[74] She enjoyed the varied wildlife of the place and had special care of ducks, chickens, cats, and kittens, as well as her own little dog, "Button." Even the hired hands adored her, teasing and pampering her in a way her own family was not wont to do. Indeed, she remembered this as the happiest time of her life. "Oh, what a houseful that was up there on that grand old hill," Clara would exclaim. "I would not say what I would give for one day of that just as it was then, and we be just the same."[75]

It was perhaps inevitable that Clara's long tether would eventually be pulled in, especially when the benign neglect afforded her by her parents had had some unfortunate repercussions. Once, accustomed to roaming the outbuildings and meadows at will, Clara wandered into a barn during butchering time. The sensitive child was startled to see a large ox struck on the head with an axe, and she fell as if she herself had been struck. Her father was furious with his hired men, though Clara came staunchly to their rescue: "I was altogether too friendly with the farm hands to hear them blamed."[76] Worse, her parents began to question the appropriateness of the little girl's tomboy ways. Her father forbade her to learn to skate, something her male companions enjoyed tremendously. Undaunted, she slipped out at night, tempted by the smooth glare ice and bright stars. The boys tied a woolen comforter around her waist, and while one pulled her along, the other two skated on either side to help keep her steady. "Swifter and swifter we went," reminisced Clara, "until at length we reached a spot where the ice had been cracked and was full of sharp edges. These threw me and the speed with which we were progressing . . . gave terrific opportunity for cuts and wounded knees." Seriously hurt, her disobedience was discovered. For several weeks she endured the isolation and disappointed looks that were her punishment.[77] Despite her mother's reassurance that other little girls had probably done as badly, Clara wrote that she "despised herself and failed to sleep or eat."

Her parents' ambivalence about her escapades continued, and, as the mistrust of Clara's wild sports increased, her mother began encouraging the female arts and girlish play. An enormous fuss was made over a little girls' party: a poem learned, a new apron made, and a rare kiss bestowed for successful conduct.[78] Mother provided the accoutrements for playhouses on the farm's hills and taught Clara to build fires and cook little dinners or make "real butter in a teacup."[79] Friendships with cousin Elvira Stone and a neighbor, Nancy Fitts, were actively promoted. This was obviously a contradictory signal, as was her earlier punishment for her proficiency in masculine ways that had so often led to acceptance or praise. It confused Clara, who was invigorated by adventure, leadership, and daring, and who by now realized that her abilities equaled those of her male companions. Struggling to draw from the world the same esteem, freedom, and power that she sensed they possessed, she was occasionally applauded but increasingly chastised.

The alternation of pride in belonging to the world of men—of their acceptance and camaraderie, and her strong identification with them—and the distress over the frowns of family and society for forsaking her proper role as a woman, was to become a constant theme in Barton's life. From childhood she straddled the fence, a visitor to both worlds, a member of neither. As an adult this access gave her an ability to move freely through all elements of society in a way that few others—male or female—could. As a child it served mostly to increase her sense of isolation and drive her to continue her search for a niche.

One way Clara hoped to establish a stronger role in her family's life was through work. To some extent this was an accepted and necessary part of her childhood, for like farm children of all times, her work and play were inextricably tied together. As a tiny child she learned to call the hired men to dinner, then giggled with pleasure as the chief hand tossed her up on his shoulder to give her a ride back to the house. Clara's fondness for animals led her to adopt several milch cows, which she learned to care for. "I went faithfully every evening to the yards to receive and look after them," she recalled. "My little milk pail went as well, and I became proficient in an art never forgotten." In the springtime she watched the soap making and learned to stir the bubbling mass. Tending ducks, turkeys, and lambs was also her duty. She viewed the creatures as pets, but like her cherished "Button," they were also obligations. The care of farm animals taught a pattern of responsibility that was the backbone of the New England farm.[80]

Clara Barton's reminiscences of her childhood thus show that she was exposed at an early age to a strong belief in the value of hard work. It is doubtful that anyone consciously stressed this idea, although the Bartons were a quintessentially industrious family, striving for achievement from both personal amibition and nervous energy. Rather it was an influence that pervaded a New Englander's existence and was accepted as an unquestionable truth. Lucy Larcom, who much to Barton's admiration recorded her own memories of a New England girlhood, reflected that she "learned no theories about 'the dignity of labor,' but we were taught to work almost as if it were a religion; to keep at work expecting nothing else."[81] Though the way of life of the Bartons in the 1820s seems mild in comparison with the rugged conditions of their early ancestors, a rigorous schedule was still needed to maintain their comfort. Molasses and cloth might be bought from local merchants, but soap and medicine were made at home. In the rush of harvest, in the continual need to produce food and clothing, and in the relentless effort to look after stock, an affirmation was made of the ritual of work and of its rewards.[82]

From an early age, therefore, Clara Barton found diligence and usefulness to be methods by which she could gain favor, and she began to define her worth through her service to others. She looked for opportunities beyond the usual farm and school chores, and found one when a painter came to refresh the walls of the Learned place. Fascinated by the tools and scents of his trade, she begged to help and was allowed to do so. "I was taught how to hold my brushes, to take care of them, allowed to help grind my paints, shown how to mix and blend them, how to make putty and use it, to prepare oils and drying . . . was taught to trim paper neatly, to match and help to hang it, to make the most approved paste, and even varnished the kitchen chairs," was her exuberant recollection. At the month's end Clara could only "look on sadly" as the painter packed up his brushes and left. The gift of a locket, inscribed "To a faithful worker," was scanty compensation for the loneliness she felt.[83]

Perhaps the most dramatic example of her pressing need to be useful—and the one that has traditionally been accredited with foreshadowing her future vocation—revolved around a long and painful stint Clara spent nursing her brother David. Renowned for his agility and physical courage, David had been chosen to affix the rafters to the ridgepole of a newly raised barn. When a timber broke under his weight, he fell on his feet, apparently unharmed, but a persistent headache and slight fever caused the family physician to be called. The doctor prescribed cupping and leeching—the standard remedies available to the early-nineteenth-century medical expert—confident that these would clear the blood and break the fever. Instead the system weakened David and prolonged his infirmity, greatly alarming his family, especially his eleven-year-old sister Clara. She begged to help to nurse him. Her hands "became schooled to handling the great loathsome crawling leeches which were at first so many snakes"; she learned to painlessly dress the angry blisters. As her family "carefully and apprehensively watched the little nurse," she gained confidence and surprised herself at her own competence and indispensability. At the same time she merged her needs with David's, refusing to leave his side for nearly two years and acquiescing to his demands that she alone administer his medicine. Finally, after nearly two years of the treatments, when doctors from twenty miles around had thrown up their hands, a young practitioner suggested a "steam cure." Though the steam worked few miracles on David, this change did in fact effect a cure, largely through its secondary prescriptions of rest, healthful foods, and banishment of the leeches.[84]

Despite her relief, however, Clara sensed a loss of her own purpose: "I was again free; my occupation gone. Life seemed very strange and idle to me." Feeling that her own place and position had been removed, she withdrew into herself, afraid that she was "giving trouble" or not contributing to the family. She felt a uselessness, a void, which she sought for the rest of her life to fill. "Instead of feeling that my freedom gave me time for recreation or play," she remarked in The Story of My Childhood, "it seemed to me like time wasted, and I looked anxiously about for some useful occupation."[85]

Clara found it in caring for her sister Sally's children and helping with the unremitting household chores. For a short time she enthusiastically worked in her brothers' satinet mill, enjoying the newness of the clattering machinery and mastering the intricacies of warp and woof with alacrity, despite the laughing derision of her family. But after only two weeks the mills burned, and, Clara remembered, "no heart was heavier than mine." Once again she was without the work that gave scope and value to her life.[86]

To fill the void she began to look for ways to be of service outside of her family. Consequently she befriended many of North Oxford's poorer families, tutoring children, helping poor mothers cope with their uncertain lot, and advising her father about which families were most in need of financial assistance. During a smallpox epidemic that occurred in her early teens, she and a neighbor girl nursed several families until she herself came down with the disease. They held the hands of the sick, cooled foreheads with damp cloths, and brought food to families too ill to prepare their own. In one instance Clara "carried a lantern and led the way out in the midnight darkness while [a] Mr. Clemence carried the casket of one of his children and buried it."[87] Her services were so timely, her style so appropriate, that the memory of this early charitable work was treasured throughout life by its recipients. "Clara, don't you remember coming to our house once when my brother James died?" queried Thomas Lamb in 1876. "You went home with me & staid all night he died when you . . . was giving him some tea in your arms . . . do you suppose I forget that—we wer[e] Poor, very poor."[88] As she grew into adolescence, Clara increasingly derived most of her satisfaction from directly alleviating sickness or trouble. She liked situations in which her personal ministrations improved the conditions of others, liked emulating her father's charitable ways, and enjoyed the role of benefactress.

17

Clara Barton's parents encouraged her in these charitable activities. Her father's own strong interest in helping the poor was reflected here of course, but also they believed it brought her out of herself, at least temporarily. (Perhaps also they felt nursing to be a more appropriate activity for a maturing young woman than the ball throwing and horse racing encouraged by her brothers.[89]) Yet the Barton family still worried about their introspective daughter, who was so timid in her demands and spent so much time in her room reading *Paradise Lost* or copying poetry. The years nursing David had retarded her social progress, and, if anything, she had grown more aloof. As she grew older she was still physically immature; in height she had grown only one inch since her ninth year and at thirteen or fourteen "was still a 'little girl'" in appearance. She had a troublesome tendency to obesity; to control it she "made long fasts," which caused a dyspeptic stomach and insomnia. At an uneasy age of self-consciousness about physical development, the already shy girl withdrew even more.[90]

Trapped once more at home, Clara associated mainly with relatives and childhood chums. Her grandmother, Dorothy Moore Barton, came to live with her son for the last few years of her life. This exposed Clara to the whims and stories of this spunky woman, who had raised twelve children, had lived through the Revolution and two other wars, and had chosen to lead an independent life in North Oxford rather than acquiesce to her husband's desire to move to the Maine wilderness. Dorothy Barton had precise and demanding ways, and by the time she moved to Stephen Barton's household she was blind. She needed too much close attention for either Clara or her mother to give, and so another granddaughter, Julia Ann Porter, came to North Oxford from Maine to help care for the old lady.[91]

Julia, the daughter of Stephen Barton's sister Pamela, did a good deal to help Clara shed her introspective ways. She was a tall, attractive girl, the youngest of twelve children, with an outgoing personality and headstrong manner. She was a few years older than Clara, and this younger cousin held her somewhat in awe. They became friends, if not close confidantes. Julia shared Clara's love of horseback riding and indulged in it with her, Elvira Stone, and a neighbor girl. Taking their cue from their grandmother, they galloped happily around the countryside, despite the fact that they were now young ladies. Once they were caught in a storm, which frightened the horses and sent them dashing uncontrollably home. "We must have presented a striking miniature portrait of the veritable 'Three Furies' on a rampage," recalled Clara, "[Elvira] and myself each rushing directly past our own homes unobserved in the storm until at length we rounded the curve that brought the flying horse in sight of his own stable."[92] The merry rides bound the girls together, leaving them with pleasant memories of girlhood laughter and narrow escapes. "I don't believe any two girls . . . in that town got as much *actual fun,* out of riding and driving about as we have," wrote Clara to Julia years later.[93]

Exposure to cousins, some recreational associations with girls her own age, and even her brief period of work at the mill eventually helped to make Clara more relaxed socially. Moreover, she was exposed to the society of strangers and the stimulation of new ideas, since her father's reputation for hospitality and a liberal mind made his house a favorite stopping place for lecturers and other travelers. But Clara's overall termperament remained shy and self-effacing. Her tendency to run to her room weeping when disappointed, rather than tell her family of her needs, continued to concern her parents. Her mother especially became increasingly perplexed about this "difficult" daughter, finally viewing her as "incomprehensible."[94] After one incident involving a teary scene over a pair of worn-out gloves, Sarah Barton poured out her frustration to a sympathetic visiting lecturer.

This confidential conversation was to have a considerable impact on Clara Barton's life. The visitor was L. N. Fowler, who was gaining a large following from his lectures on phrenology. He and his brother had done much to popularize this pseudoscience, which offered the theory that the different aspects of human behavior were controlled by discrete portions of the brain. The relative power or sensitivity of these areas—the categories included such traits as intellect, amativeness, and courage—could be determined by cranial bumps and the profile of one's head. Although phrenology was based on a number of wrong assumptions, it fell short of quackery. Indeed in many of its conclusions it was the forerunner of modern psychology, especially in the belief that no two humans, or human reactions, are alike. Phrenology attempted to find the distinctive traits of each person and to guide each individual toward those pursuits which most suited his or her temperament.[95]

Fowler proved to be insightful about Clara's personality. He told her mother that Clara herself suffered more from her bashfulness than anyone else and that although she might appear to outgrow the traits "the sensitive nature will always remain." He also acknowledged her need to work and to feel appreciated by recommending that she be given some responsibility, preferably in the form of teaching. "She has all the qualities of a teacher," Fowler observed. Clara could not have agreed less. She was home with the mumps and had overheard with dismay her least desirable traits aired before the stranger. Yet she had had to agree with the pronouncements and frustrations described by her mother and had hoped for advice that would help. But this suggestion was a shock. To stand before a schoolroom of children, to be alone each day among strangers, without the guiding hand of her brothers, seemed unthinkable. Barton's memoirs do not reveal how she was persuaded to quell her fears and try teaching, but persuaded she was, for the next spring it was arranged that she begin teaching in the old schoolhouse in district no. 9.[96]

two

Clara stood by the large stone fireplace in her family's house and trained frightened and questioning eyes on the assembled Barton family. "But what am I to do with only two little old waifish dresses?" she asked. Her cousin Julia recognized at once that Clara was right—with her new occupation as teacher she needed an image that would inspire confidence and respect, especially since her appearance was so small and childlike. Convinced that clothes would indeed make the woman, the women of the house began lengthening skirts and putting up hair— a bustle of activity aimed at making the insecure schoolmarm look older and larger.[1] At least one new dress was forthcoming. It was a fashionable green outfit that Clara wore on her first day of teaching and sentimentally saved for the rest of her life.[2]

Barton was probably about eighteen when she first began teaching. In later years she often stated that she was fifteen at the start of this, her earliest career. A letter from a close friend, dated in the spring of 1838, however, indicates that if she taught before this date he knew nothing about it. Moreover, her mill work, which she admitted was finished before she began to teach school, took place in 1839 when she was seventeen. Elsewhere Clara mentions that she was sixteen when she undertook her first summer session, yet her earliest extant teaching certificate (won after "an examination of the learned committee of one clergyman, one lawyer and one justice of the peace") is dated 1839.[3] Whatever her age, she felt the handicap of being but slightly older than her pupils. She had been treated as a child at home and had had little experience with the responsibilities of the working world, save two weeks at the looms of her brother's mill. "We had all been children together," Barton wrote of her first pupils.[4]

Barton taught her first classes in a barren stone building, "neither large nor new," she recalled. An ungraded school, it was filled with rows of shabby desks into which were crammed forty curious pupils, ranging in age from toddlers to

20

four young men in their late teens. In summer schools such as these, the pupils were apt to be girls and little boys who were not needed at home to help with the farm work. (School boards thought the sessions easier for that reason and paid the young women who taught them a salary substantially below the going rate for winter schools.) Facing her pupils from the teacher's platform the first day, Clara felt no optimism about the ease of her task. She found the pupils distracted by the sweet smell of meadow grass and the warm breezes, and knew the boys stood ready to test her. With a rush of panic, she realized she had no idea how to open a school. Lighting on the first object at hand, she opened a Bible. Too shy to address the pupils, she directed them to read from the text of the Sermon on the Mount. She was pleased to find them responsive and amusing, and to discover that the four larger boys could be checked with a stinging glance.[5]

Elvira Stone recalled that her cousin Clara "took to teaching as natural as could be."[6] Clara was, in fact, a gifted pedagogue who formed an immediate and strong rapport with her pupils. Her own interest in learning was infectious, and her agile mind kept the pupils continually challenged. Moreover, she knew instinctively that if she made her expectations known her pupils would rise to the mark and that this would be an effective disciplinary tool. She coupled this with an unerring ability to earn their respect. When Miss Barton found that the boys played too roughly at the noon recess she joined the game, winning them over with her admirable talent for throwing a ball. "My four lads soon perceived that I was no stranger to their sports or their tricks. . . . When they found . . . that if they won a game it was because I permitted it, their respect knew no bounds." Their admiration was carried over into the schoolhouse, and she found little need for the harsh punishments that characterized many common schools.[7] A girl who sat in Barton's school attested to this when she wrote to her former teacher with fond memories. "I remember you walking about with your ruler in your hand. . . . I don't remember that you ever punished anyone, you used your ruler for other purposes."[8] At the end of the term Barton's school received the highest standing in North Oxford for discipline. The young teacher remonstrated, stating that there had been no disciplinary actions during the whole term. "Child that I was," Barton later wrote, "I did not know that the surest test of discipline is its absence."[9]

This ability to gain her pupils' affections and discipline them gave her an unequaled reputation in the town, and she was soon in demand as a teacher. Initially Barton herself was uncertain about continuing to teach because she still felt that her own education was lacking. Her family, however, was far too pleased with her progress to allow her to decline. At the end of the next term, therefore, she reluctantly accepted a position with a school in Charlton, a village adjoining North Oxford. It was, again, a summer school, but one with a reputation for boisterous children and a need for discipline.[10]

Charlton was just far enough away that Barton could not continue to live at home during the school term. Outwardly she faced the move from her family with more serenity than she had felt on former separations. Yet when her father drove her to the school at the commencement of her term, she admitted that her "cheery good-bye" was only "typical of most of the things said and done in practical life, altogether unlike the thing felt or meant." She believed that she had reached a turning point in her life, a branch of the road along which she would have to find her way alone. This thought sobered her and reinforced her already pensive turn of mind, but the confidence she had gained from her teaching success helped to allay the sting of terror she had felt before on such occasions. Fortunately, too, the ache of separation from home was eased by the cozy and genial residence in which she boarded.[11]

The school in Charlton, like so many others Barton would see, had "a rather time worn edifice." She taught fifty pupils, for which she received around two dollars a week. No advanced teaching was required. The schoolroom resounded only with the monotonous drone of ABCs, multiplication tables, and recitation of state capitals. Despite the easy curriculum, however, Barton worked hard for her salary, since the school was not only large but lived up to its rough reputation. She soon discovered that it was dominated by a group of unruly boys, whose leader was "contrary, sullen and half-insolent," and that the members of this gang were not as easily managed as their counterparts in North Oxford. Attempts to win them over with smiles and respect brought only jeers and the exchange of knowing glances among the rowdies, who were certain that this schoolmarm would be broken as quickly as the rest.[12]

When they began to seriously disrupt the classes and an attempt to contact the ringleader's mother gave no satisfaction, Barton was left with little choice but to save her school by drastic means. One morning, when the most troublesome boy swaggered tardily into the classroom, annoying the pupils and mocking Barton by refusing to make even a pretext of correctly reciting his lessons, she took action. She requested him to come forward, and as he walked saucily up the aisle, she pulled a long riding whip from her desk, lashing out and tripping him while the other pupils watched with horror. Barton continued to wield the whip, jerking him to his knees until he apologized to the school for his actions. She then dismissed the shaken students for the day and suggested that they have a picnic in the meadow near the school. Barton herself was shocked by this episode, which was her only experience with corporal punishment. It made an impression so lasting that in 1908 she would write that "all these years have not been able to efface [it]." Needless to say, it put an end to trouble in the school for that term. "I had learnt what discipline meant, and it was for all time as far as that school was concerned; none ever needed more than a kindly smile."[13]

The control Barton exercised over this school further enhanced her reputation. She was asked to teach it again the next year, and for nearly ten years her services were actively sought in both Oxford and the surrounding area. Rarely did she teach the same school twice. Though she allowed her older students a certain leeway in the subjects they studied, she was not an innovator in matters of curriculum; rather, she was challenged by the organization and discipline of the school. It intrigued her to ferret out the unique problems of each schoolhouse and to channel her pupils' energies into study instead of mischief. But once the problems were conquered and the school settled down to a contented routine, Clara's active mind became distracted. For this reason she refused to teach again in Charlton, and after a short, unchallenging term at another neighboring town called West Millbury, she again sought a more demanding position. She was pleased, therefore, when the school board in Oxford requested that she teach the winter term of a particularly difficult school. When they offered her the salary usually paid women for the shorter and easier summer session, however, she declined. "I may sometimes be willing to teach for nothing," she told the board, "but if paid at all, I shall never do a man's work for less than a man's pay." It was a measure of Barton's growing confidence that she felt emboldened to make such a demand, and of her value as a teacher that the school board withdrew the original offer and paid what she requested.[14]

Clara's monetary rewards were matched by increasing satisfaction in her work during these early years. She viewed herself as a serious, professional teacher, and unlike many young men and women, who saw teaching as a temporary station between the end of their own schooling and the beginning of a profession or marriage, she seems to have embraced her work as a long-term career. Accordingly, she invested many hours expanding her own expertise with self-study. In addition, she actively sought advice on method and curriculum from Sally and Stephen, both of whom had been accomplished teachers, and from her father and brother David, who had seen the trials and successes of many schools from the vantage point of school board members.[15] She further reinforced and rounded out her own fine instincts in a lengthy correspondence with her former tutor, Lucien Burleigh. He challenged her to treat both individual pupils and even the most routine aspects of the work with respect. "It is a responsible station, and one that demands much thought and meditation," he cautioned her. To her query about personal bonds formed in the classroom, he replied unequivocally: "If the instructor succeeds in securing the affection of his pupils, he will be able by being judicious to forward them rapidly in their studies."[16]

Whether directly heeding this advice or acting on her own strong impulses, Barton excelled in capturing not only the respect but the love of her pupils. She had a ready wit, and an absence of condescension which pleased them, and her sense of fairness destroyed the jealousies of favoritism. "She had such a happy way with her that she won everybody over to her side," recalled one admirer.[17] Poor children received the same care as the others, with a personalized attention that sometimes changed their lives. (One such boy was rescued from the drudgery of factory work to develop his exceptional mathematical skills, a favor he never forgot.[18]) She was, moreover, unabashedly loyal, even possessive of her pupils. "They were all mine," she recalled in an autobiographical sketch, "second only to the claims and interests of the real mother. . . . And so they have remained." [19]

Her pupils returned the favor. They fulfilled beyond Clara's wildest expectations her self-expressed need for "approval, encouragement, trust, confidence," without which she felt her soul might "go awreck." [20] In the shining faces of her students, the boys filled with regard for her fairness and sportsmanship, she felt the acceptance and admiration that had so long eluded her. One pupil liked to think of "the days we spent together at the old no 9 school at Oxford and how proud I was if I could take hold of your dress as you had but too [sic] hands, and walk a little ways with you, how we all loved you then." For the rest of her life Barton received letters such as this, and the loyalty of her pupils was a continual source of pleasure. "Their life-long loyal allegiance to me is beyond my comprehension," she wrote at the age of eighty. "Little as many of them were, trifling as the days must have seemed among a whole life of scholarship, which so many of them followed, it is a most remarkable thing that all have remembered those few months and cherished them with a loyalty that the most ambitious teacher could but prize." [21]

Self-respect and a sense of place in the community increased Barton's social confidence. As L. N. Fowler had predicted, the experience diminished her chronic introspection; through successful interaction with people she lost some of her shyness, or at least learned to effectively hide it. The social growth was also at least partly due to a conscious effort on her part to face the world with poise, and to please her brother David.

Soon after Clara began teaching, David had become engaged to Julia Ann Porter, the same cousin who had lived with the Bartons during their mutual grandmother's illness. One day David gave his younger sister an invitation that, she later wrote, "took my breath away": he wished her to join the wedding party by accompanying him to Maine to serve as bridesmaid. Fearful that she would appear awkward or embarrass her brother, she at first demurred but at his insistence was finally persuaded to go. The thought of standing beside the lovely Julia, whose charms could only serve as a contrast to her plain, dumpy figure, and of being called on to graciously introduce cousins and friends, filled her with dread. Yet once it was decided that she would go, she silently determined to act in the most obliging manner possible. Clara cared less what the citizens of Winsor, Maine, thought of her than that she might disappoint her brother and lose his love and support. "I was not distressed about what might be thought of me . . . ," she reminisced, "but how it might reflect upon my brother, and the mortification that my awkwardness could not fail to inflict on him." Thus Clara's "tearful resolution" conquered her debilitating shyness. It was yet another turning point during the important years of her teaching career, and she was keenly aware of it at the time. The desire to take responsibility for her actions and to prevail over personal qualities that she herself found unacceptable, she noted, "seemed to throw the whole wide world open to me."[22]

For Clara, David Barton's wedding proved to be a memorable experience, not only because of the personal growth she experienced during the time but because it was her earliest adventure away from home. The party traveled up the New England coast by boat, and she felt the thrill of seeing the ocean in its vastness and mystery.[23] With wide eyes she encountered "a whole townful of uncles and cousins," and came to know a place and part of her family that had heretofore been merely characters in stories or names penned on envelopes.[24] On the eve of her departure Vester Vassall, her brother-in-law, gave her a Morocco-covered autograph album. At socials and teas she asked her new friends to write a few lines, and they filled the book with their good wishes. Evidently she had conquered not only her own social malaise but the hearts of her relations in Maine. The little green album was carefully preserved with her treasures as a tangible piece of the pride she felt in overcoming her fears.[25]

As the boundaries of her known world had expanded on the trip, so had her emotional horizons broadened. Barton continued to feel the disadvantage of her homely face and round figure. Yet her quick wit and adventurous and sporting manner were appealing, and several young men in the vicinity of Oxford came to call on her. One swain let her know that whenever he saw her he "made up my face for a really good time," and another praised both her intelligence and her capacity for laughter.[26] Clara's romances remain elusive, however, for they were, to her, intensely private, and she rarely spoke or wrote about them. The few people in whom she confided were rewarded with conflicting or cryptic allusions to gentlemen who were impossible to identify.

According to family tradition Barton formed an early and strong attachment to Jerry Learned, the cousin with whom she had grown up. She was fond of his high spirits and merry ways and felt comfortable in his familiar company. The boyhood recklessness of the Learned cousins, however, was still in evidence in their maturity. Some dubious ventures, and their financial dealings seemed always to have a shadowy edge to them. Jerry in particular appeared wedded to the life of a speculator. A nephew close to Clara believed she realized with sad reluctance that Jerry Learned lacked the strength of character she thought necessary for a close relationship. A girlhood chum, however, had a different explanation. "Jerry Learned was real good-looking," confided Fanny Childs Vassall, "and Clara once said to me that she shouldn't want the man to have all the good looks in the family."[27]

While Clara was still in her teens she enjoyed the company of another young man, L. T. Bacon (his first name has unfortunately escaped record). He evidently did not live in Oxford, but he and Clara still managed to meet, ride horseback, crack hickory nuts, or roam the hills in search of blackberries. Mr. Bacon evidently took the romance seriously, since he noted that it pleased him to hear that she had been learning some household arts, "for it is not entirely impossible that such *accomplishments* may be some *practical* use."[28] Close-mouthed

Clara does not tell us what became of this relationship, but the tenor of their light-hearted romance has not been entirely lost. It shines through the semi-poetic ramblings Bacon sent to Clara soon after one of their meetings, in which he praises her as "much more a sister so dear as you are to me," and remembers "a fine walk home which place we reached soon enough (being favored with a moon and thoug[h] near noon) for a nap which we enjoyed first rate and no mistake."[29]

Still another suitor during her teaching days was Oliver Williams. Barton had boarded with his family during one school term. After the session ended they corresponded, and diary entries for 1849 show that she spent considerable time in his company. During one week she visited every day with him, save one, and on that day she noted in her journal that it was "a lonesome day."[30] It is difficult to tell, however, whether Barton's interest in Williams was based on simple friendship or bespoke a deeper affection. Williams was the illegitimate son of a woman with whom Barton was familiar, and she had befriended and helped to educate him. He had responded to her teaching with a steadfast love that lasted over many years. But, although she enjoyed his company, Barton saw little chance of their friendship ripening into a permanent attachment. Fanny Childs again held the view that Williams was not a very interesting man and that Barton failed to see in him "the possibility of a husband such as she would have chosen."[31] Before Clara was thirty, Williams had left North Oxford to bury his sore heart in the gold fields of California.

It was indeed a time when most girls of her age and social status were considering marriage, both as romantic fulfillment and as their highest calling in life. There is every indication that Clara Barton also assumed that marriage would come to her in due course. She liked the company of men; as a girl she had preferred the companionship of her brothers, father, and male cousins. She was no political feminist—she admitted that in her youth she never heard of the work of Susan B. Anthony or Elizabeth Cady Stanton—but her entire background had encouraged her to view herself as the compatriot and match of any man. The men in her family had treated her—indeed trained her—as an equal, and her personality grew as strong and dominant as theirs.[32] By comparison her beaus seem to be always in her shadow. A friend wrote that "more men were interested in her than she was ever interested in," then added that Clara was so pronounced in her opinions that most men, used to more submissive women, "stood somewhat in awe of her."[33] They admired her extravagantly, and Clara enjoyed their adulation, but she could not take any of them seriously as a life partner. Moreover, she came to disdain many men who she thought treated women in a patronizing way. The case of Sam Healy, a young man who for a time paid attentions to Elvira Stone, is indicative of Clara Barton's strong sense of the respect she felt was due women. Healy escorted her cousin for a time, but his intention was more to gain social acceptance than to have the pleasure of Elvira's company. Barton was outraged when she heard that Healy had stopped seeing Elvira after securing his social toehold and had spoken poorly of her in company.

"Ah Sam Healy," Barton wrote, "that was the day ye died in my estimation and there was no Resurrection for Ye."[34] Incidents such as these convinced her that it would be a rare man who could live up to her standards of intelligence and at the same time respect her for her own abilities and aspirations. Fanny Childs Vassall, who knew Clara intimately during her twenties, acknowledged this. "I do not think she ever had a love affair that stirred the depths of her being," she wrote. "Clara Barton was herself so much stronger a character than any of the men who made love to her that I do not think she was ever seriously tempted to marry any of them."[35]

Yet a mystery hangs around the emotions involved in many of Barton's romantic relationships. In later life she often alluded to serious affairs, including one that was terminated not by her desire but by the gentleman's death in the Mexican War. She never mentioned the man's name, but she gave at least one person the impression that the two had been engaged.[36] Clara's diaries also show that she was capable of a strong emotional response to men.[37] Her disinclination to marry, at least during these early years, stemmed more from the unavailability of a suitable mate than from a strong prejudice against the subordinate role of women in marriage or a dislike of men.

Clara's social life during the years of teaching was not dominated by amorous adventures. Captain Barton, recognizing the emotional burden that teaching often placed on her, bought her a spirited saddle horse.[38] She often rode alone, leaving her cares behind as she flew through the wooded country lanes, but she also occasionally shared her rides with the more adventurous of her acquaintances.[39] She played whist, apparently with some indifference, and tried her hand at making artificial flowers and painting.[40] Between school terms, when she had an unusual amount of spare time, she wrote copious letters—a habit of correspondence she was to keep all her life—and went chestnuting with her favorite nephew.[41] Literary pursuits, too, occupied her time, and she wrote verses (generally more doggerel than poetry) for her friends and copied works by others in a scrapbook pasted together from her old school copybooks.[42] Her days were filled with social calls, as a diary entry for February 24, 1849, shows: "Received a call from Mrs. Cummings, visited David in the afternoon. Went to Webster [a neighboring town] in the evening. E P. called and left in the evening."[43]

Clara could hardly be accused of being asocial now, yet she still preferred to spend her time in some productive occupation. Restless and impatient, she searched for ways to be useful. She often found an outlet in keeping the books for her brothers' mills, and when the mills burned in 1839, she helped to straighten the financial records so that a new complex could be built. She was anxious, too, to be of help at home. During the final illness of her grandmother, Dorothy Barton, who died in 1838, she aided her mother as best she could, and when her sister Dolly finally succumbed in 1842 to the sad collapse of her mental powers, Clara was by her side.[44] In addition, she participated actively in the work of the

Universalist church. When a new church was to be erected, around 1844, she pitched in to help raise money for the building. As always, it gratified her to work toward a goal. She noted with pride that "no body of church people ever worked harder than we. We held fairs, public and home, begged, and gave all but the clothes we wore, we cleaned windows, scrubbed [up] paint after workmen, bought and nailed down carpets." Barton also helped to furnish the parsonage and was pleased when she was chosen to stay in the house to welcome the new minister and his young bride.[45]

Yet her church work, dedicated as it was, was not an indication of deep religious feelings. Though aware of her father's devotion to Universalist principles, Clara did not share his strong religious convictions. From childhood on she remembered the town church as an austere place of "tall box pews and high narrow seats" in which there was ever an "incongruous winter atmosphere" that pinched her fingers and toes, and where faith was not easy but was "hammered out."[46] Despite the efforts of friends such as Lucien Burleigh, who advised her to search her soul and give more attention to religious beliefs, Barton remained aloof from the doctrines of the church. She had trouble meshing the Universalist notion of ultimate joy with the poverty and unhappiness she saw around her, and if anything she became increasingly pessimistic during this period. After confiding to a friend about this trend in her personal feelings in 1843, he replied with a note of sadness: "You announce to me a change in your religious view from a hope in the final infinite happiness of all mankind you have become a believer in the endless misery of a part, that is truly a change."[47] Barton never completely relinquished her faith but remained, as she pronounced it, a "well-disposed pagan."[48] Still she enjoyed the tie to the church's organization, which provided a welcome outlet for her enormous energy and capability.

Barton's most ambitious project during the 1840s, however, was worked in tandem with her brother Stephen. For several years Clara had been aware of the need to redistrict the schools in the town of Oxford. Owing to the success of the various mills, the town had grown rapidly, and the centers of population had shifted so that the locations of the old schools were no longer suitable. Oxford had no large central schools. Instead it relied on several small, dilapidated buildings that were empty half of the year and served only a few pupils. Clara had seen similar problems in other areas. In the early 1840s, during the time she had taught in Millbury, she had persuaded the local school board to endorse a report that deplored the poor attendance, lack of uniform textbooks, inadequate facilities, and superficial community attention to school problems.[49] In 1844 she began in earnest to try to remedy similar problems in Oxford, and she found in Stephen, who was then a member of the town school board, a willing and able compatriot.

After several sessions, during which they consumed "more or less midnight oil," Clara and Stephen set out to convince the town of the need for a new system of school organization. They met with strong opposition. Many Oxford citizens believed that such an effort would cost the town dearly and that sufficient funds were already spent on education. Others saw a problem in requiring their children to walk across town to school; they liked the system of neighborhood schools, which kept the boys and girls close to home where they could be called quickly if they were needed to help with farm or shop. Moreover, the Bartons' original plan had grown to encompass a scheme for educating the millworkers and their children. As a mill owner, Stephen was well aware that low wages and long hours conspired to keep these people from obtaining an education, and that, furthermore, no district school existed in the area in which the millworkers lived. Although this situation outraged Clara, few of the citizens of Oxford were convinced that the town was obligated to educate those from the lower social ranks. Their objections were reinforced by similar opposition from two of the town's most powerful men, Deacon Peter Butler and Clara's own father, Captain Stephen Barton. So influential were they that it took Clara and Stephen junior over a year even to bring the matter before a town meeting.[50]

In the spring of 1845 the issue was finally presented to the town. Clara had labored arduously over the major speech in favor of redistricting. The argument was read by a popular mill owner, "of course as his own," for as a woman she had no voice in the meeting. Despite her long and respected years of teaching, in matters such as these she sadly recognized that "I was nobody." The scene was tense as speakers from each side aired their views and emotions rose. Those in favor of redistricting watched anxiously to see if the moderator—Captain Barton—would show any favoritism. But Clara and her brother had canvassed well, and just as the vote was to be taken, eighty-two workers from the local factories marched in and packed the ballot box with a solid block of votes in favor of redistricting.[51]

That night Clara celebrated at a special dinner cooked by her mother. The whole family assembled to share their triumph and to reconcile the split family views. Captain Barton showed no animosity over defeat at the hands of his children. Wrote Clara, "my father's first hearty toast was to the 'new fangled folly.'"[52]

It had been a rewarding effort, the first of many crusades Clara was to fight for the distressed or underprivileged, and she found the habit of altruism addictive. Thus she continued the good work by advising and aiding the redistricting board and undertaking the design of one of the new enlarged district schools. "I had ample opportunity for original design for I had never seen a schoolhouse that in its construction was not nearly as well-adapted to any other ordinary use than a school," she dryly noted. (Her design called for maps, blackboards, and a clock for teaching purposes, as well as a sloping center aisle to compensate for the uniformly sized desks, which overwhelmed six-year-olds and cramped the older pupils. A few years later Clara proudly described the classroom to a former student as "chang'd indeed . . . within, without and around.") This project completed, she embraced yet another social cause—the still-controversial establishment and teaching of the mill school.[53]

The school was established initially in one of the largest local mills. It was a small, dark pocket whose only light came from a large doorway facing a public street. To provide enough light for reading, the door had to be kept open, and the noise from the road was as constant distraction. Every passing dog and cat skipped in, as well as "goats that searched the neighborhood for dainties." In addition, there was the problem of the diversity in age and nationality of the students. Clara taught a total of seventy pupils, who ranged from four to twenty-four years of age. There were American-born scholars in the school, but also English, Irish, and French, which resulted in conflicts of language and culture. To keep order under such circumstances, Clara appointed monitors—to be one was deemed a high honor among the students—and arranged classes with an eye to preserving each pupil's self-esteem. By using a combination of "gentle restraint, calm reasoning, confidence and encouragement," she guided her school to success.[54]

Those who had doubted the effectiveness of such a school were surprised to find the makeshift classroom abuzz with productive activity. "There was not a minute of the day for me to lose," Barton acknowledged, noting that her classes studied not only "the 3 R's," but algebra, bookkeeping, philosophy, chemistry, and ancient and natural history. In one area the school so excelled that it gained a regional reputation. Convinced that reading aloud would improve the language skills of her foreign pupils, Barton encouraged recreational reading and rewarded those who skillfully dramatized their favorite pieces. To her surprise crowds began to gather outside the open doorway on the days when the readings took place. What had originated as a spontaneous and pragmatic exercise charmed the public into recognizing the school's potential, and the mill school became widely known for its distinguished "concert readings."[55]

Once she had met the challenge of the mill school successfully, however, Barton became increasingly dissatisfied with the cycle of teaching, which left her with sporadic months of aimless leisure. She was now in her late twenties and had mastered every situation that had been presented to her. She had tamed the unruly boys in countless towns and country schools, fostered the hopes of the area's illiterate mill hands, and helped to bring about educational reforms, which had seemed to her such obvious necessities. In her mind the years of dull routine stretched endlessly before her. With no jobs open to women save teaching or factory work, she could not imagine from what direction she would find new and stimulating work. Instead Barton began to think seriously of leaving the teacher's podium for a pupil's desk, to find, in her words, "a school, the object of which was to teach *me* something."[56]

It was not the first time Clara had considered advanced schooling. She was, however, uncertain about the possibilities open to women and the methods of gaining admission to the few institutions that had opened their doors to gifted females. As early as 1838 she had asked Lucien Burleigh for advice on the subject, questioning him also about her potential for earning money while a student. Burleigh recommended a school in Uxbridge, Massachusetts, and one nearby in Charlestown, "where young ladies have an opportunity of paying their board by their labor." [57] Money problems and indecision stalled her, and nothing came of the idea at this time. Ten years later, with her capital enlarged by scrupulous savings, Barton again began to actively look at colleges and academies. Only two colleges accepted women at this time: Mount Holyoke and Oberlin. Barton seems not to have been at all interested in Mount Holyoke, possibly because the school was close to her home. She was determined to go far enough away that a run of bad luck at an Oxford school would not lure her back. She gave Oberlin, a coeducational school in Ohio, serious consideration, but after talking with a trusted neighbor on the subject, she dropped her plan of going there for reasons which are not altogether clear. [58]

Barton deliberated her future quietly, telling few people of her plans and continuing to trudge through the day-to-day activities in her school. While she worried over inadequate fuel for heating the classroom and the necessity of expelling two unruly students, her mind wandered to her own educational needs. [59] She watched with interest as her brothers enlarged their mill complex until it was "quite a village" of two factories, five dwelling houses, barns, shops, and offices, but she could not really feel a part of it as she had in the past. Her health was good but her mind was dissatisfied, and her spirit tired of "working oneself to death to get a living." [60] Finally, late in 1850, she determined to go to the Clinton Liberal Institute, a well-respected coeducational academy run by the Universalist church in Clinton, New York. For Barton this would be much more than an academic opportunity. Almost two hundred miles from home, the school would broaden her experience beyond the familiar hills of central Massachusetts and entwine her life with friendships that would have a major impact on her growth and aspirations. [61]

three

On a blustery day at the end of December 1850, Clara Barton tucked herself under the lap robes in her brother Stephen's sleigh and set off for the Worcester train depot. Her heart felt as cold as the frozen ground, for she at last realized that if she was leaving scenes that worried and oppressed her, she was also leaving her family and all that had been familiar and comforting.[1] It was, moreover, a bad time to leave Oxford. Her mother had been sick, indeed "quite feeble," for much of the year and did not sustain much hope of recovering.[2] That autumn tragedy had struck her brothers, too. The mill complex had burned again, this time leaving only one wall standing, and the loss was much heavier than the insurance would cover. The distress Clara felt over this incident was heightened by the belief that the fire had been intentionally set, possibly as a result of the Barton brothers' slightly shady dealings. It was thus with sadness at leaving her distraught family, mingled with relief, that she boarded the train for New York.[3]

The trip was long and frustrating, delayed by closely missed connections and frozen rivers. Barton met no one along the way, and even late in life she could remember the slow, unsettling journey, which was "passed in silence."[4] The trip to New York City took twenty-five hours, and as she was too late for a morning boat up the Hudson River, she stayed at the Irving House until evening, when she boarded the *Isaac Newton*. The game little boat tried dutifully to help pull another vessel out of the ice; it finally succeeded, only to find itself stuck more firmly than the other boat had been. "She was thumped and heaved since," Barton noted in her journal, "and Heaven only knows which way she will stray if she ever starts."[5] After much ado, and to the passengers' great relief, the boat loosed itself and kept on its way toward Albany. From there Barton took the train for Utica and thence on to Clinton.

In Clinton she made her way to the Clinton House, "a typical old time tavern," where Mr. and Mrs. Samuel Bertram rented rooms to students. She was disappointed to find school would not start on the first Monday in January as advertised.[6] Although the institute had been established twenty years previously, in the year that Barton arrived it was undergoing vast structural and academic changes. A new building called the "White Seminary," an imposing structure with a broad portico supported by Ionic columns, was being built to house the female portion of the school, and classes could not be resumed until it was finished.[7] Meanwhile, the faculty was working to institute a program of studies that they believed would give the students an academic foundation "as good as can be obtained in most colleges of the country."[8] While these changes were taking place, the opening of school was delayed several weeks.

Clara spent the time exploring the town. The home of Hamilton College as well as the Clinton Liberal Institute, Clinton wore the traditional college air of youthful frivolousness and scholarly gravity. Over half of the population in 1850 were students, hailing chiefly from New England but occasionally coming from as far away as Canada or Alabama. They slept in plainly furnished rooms in the several lodging houses around town, living on a shoestring and socializing in the debating and Philomien societies, which were then popular.[9] Yet Clara could not rejoice in the abundance of young people; she felt only the frigid atmosphere of the dark January days. Even the appealing buildings looked cold and hostile to her, and the "two plank walk with a two feet space between, leading up from the town was not suggestive of the warmest degree of sociability to say the least of it."[10] Wondering whether her decision to leave Oxford had been wise, she wandered alone through the town every day. At night she wrote cheerful letters home, crafted to reveal little of her anxiety.

Clara was much relieved when school began and life once more had a purpose. The newly finished schoolrooms still seemed cold and forbidding to her, but she found to her delight that the girls' principal, Louise Barker, was a rare leader, with qualities that could truly inspire her pupils. "I found an unlooked-for activity, a cordiality, and an irresistible charm of manner that none could have foreseen—a winning indescribable grace which I have met in only a few persons in a whole lifetime," recalled Barton. Louise Barker not only made the timid young woman feel at ease, she encouraged her to lead a balanced life at the institute. Barton, eager to gain the widest education possible in her year in Clinton, often tried to forego the pleasures and sociability of student life. It was Barker who unfailingly steered her toward a more active existence and instilled in her the importance of developing her confidence as well as her intellect.[11]

Clara was probably in the third class at the institute, although the scanty documents related to her year at Clinton never state this precisely. The studies of this course were well beyond those of secondary school and included analytic geometry, French and German, ancient history, philosophy, calculus, astronomy, and religious studies. The male and female students were physically separated, but girls were encouraged to "pursue the Languages, the Mathematics, and the

Natural Sciences, to any extent they may wish."[12] This policy, rare for the time, had enormous appeal for Barton. Unfortunately, however, the institute limited the number of studies allowed each term. Barton, convinced of the necessity of utilizing every moment, begged and cajoled the faculty until they had stretched the limit to the utmost. "I recall with some amusement, the last evening I entered with my request," wrote Barton. "The teachers were assembled in the parlor and, divining my errand, as I never had any other, Miss Barker broke into a merry laugh—with 'Miss Barton, we have a few studies left; you had better take what there are, and we will say nothing about it.'" Thereafter Clara took what courses she liked, studying with "a burning anxiety to make the most of lost time."[13]

For this privilege she paid, as did the other female students, a flat rate of thirty-five dollars per term, which included tuition, room and board, and laundry. She had moved from the old Clinton House into the dormitory rooms of the White Seminary. The accommodations were bare but adequate, and the building included, besides the sleeping compartments and classrooms, a parlor, sitting room, and library. But while Clara was comfortable in her living situation, socially she decidedly was not.[14]

Barton had purposely refrained from revealing her past teaching experiences, which she believed might cause discomfort to either the teachers or other students. She hoped instead to blend in without noticeable difference among the other pupils, and to glean what she could from the instructors without prejudice. "There was no reason why I should volunteer my history or step in among that crowd of eager pupils as a 'school marm', expected to know everything."[15] But the maturity of her experiences, as well as her years, kept her distinct from her fellow students. Most of Barton's classmates were ten or more years her junior, and she had trouble assimilating herself with the 'frolicsome girls.'"[16] While they found her "a perfect mystery," unassuming yet with a forbidding aloofness, she saw them as narrow in their prejudices and immature.[17] One roommate noted "some peculiarities," such as her habit of eating only two meals a day, but charitably announced that none of her oddities were "bad ones."[18] Barton was also self-conscious about her clothes. With characteristic thrift she had had two dresses cut from one length of material in her favorite shade of green. Though the garments had different trimmings, the other girls thought it odd that she should wear such similar clothes day after day and attached a mysterious significance to the color. Fortunately, among the 150 pupils at the institute she did find several kindred spirits. Barton long remembered "Gentle Clara Hurd" affectionately, but Abby Barker, from Connecticut, and Mary Norton, a Quaker from Hightstown, New Jersey, became her closest chums. These girls, whose jokes and secrets she shared, were to remain lifelong friends and supporters.[19]

"When at school, her photograph, would have shown you a rather thick-set girl, with head bent a little forward, looking up with small black eyes, through heavy, low eyebrows," wrote a classmate. Despite this unflattering description, Barton seems to have attracted the attention of a number of men while at Clinton. Indeed, the same writer went on to admit that she "was much admired."[20] One of her most ardent beaus was Charles Norton, her friend Mary's brother, who also attended the institute. He was a genial and intelligent fellow who appreciated Barton's sense of humor, but he was ten years younger than Clara, and she found it difficult to take him seriously. "While she esteemed him as friend," wrote an acquaintance, "I don't think she regarded him as a lover."[21] Another person who was intrigued by this dark, serious girl was Samuel Ramsey, a professor of mathematics at Hamilton College. He admired her fine horsemanship, and their long afternoons riding together aroused much speculation among the young women of the institute. Here, too, Clara seems to have drawn the line at friendship. Nonetheless, Ramsey, like Charles Norton, remained a devoted and lifelong friend to Clara Barton, and rumors about a possible romance between the two were whispered until well after the Civil War.[22]

Other references to men crop up in Barton's writings at this time, but they are generally cryptic, identifying these friends only by their initials. Years later she was to share with Abby Barker happy memories of exchanging secrets about gentlemen friends. The two of them, she recalled, would stand giggling and talking at the top of the stairs before the gas was turned out at ten o'clock. "I have a letter in the pocket of this *green* dress," Barton wrote, conjuring up the scene,

> you may take it to your room, and tell me tomorrow night, as we stand here gain, *what you think of it*. . . . And while Louise Clap is fandangling around, and Sarah Stoddard is putting up the stray locks that *won't* stay in place . . . Abby Barker and the strange girl in the green gown will *exchange views* over the letter and say how it *seems to us*, and you can give it back to me, & tell me how *you* would answer it if you were in my place, & *must* do it.[23]

These good friends helped to break the intensity with which Clara pursued her work. Driven by her "habit of study," she put in long hours at her desk and left an impressive record of scholarship at Clinton. Yet the discipline to study did not always come easily. "It is hard work to sit and study all day," she commiserated with a nephew who was complaining of school. But she rationalized the effort on the grounds of "future benefit," not "present happiness," and so admonished him: "let us bear it cheerfully." So dogged was she that even her vacations were spent in study. Concerned that Barton would overtax herself and thus lose all she had worked so hard to gain, Louise Barker encouraged her to ride in the countryside and even resorted to employing Samuel Ramsey to lure her out of the library.[24]

It was an effective technique. Barton still relished outdoor exercise and enjoyed displaying her considerable equestrian skills. When a gentleman alighted from his horse she could, to the amazement of the other girls, "spring upon his horse and ride, to the astonishment of all, without change of saddle."[25] She liked to explore the countryside, so very different from that of Massachusetts. Dashing across the broad, level acres, Barton wondered at the immensity of these western farms and sensed her own provinciality when she realized how narrow her expectations of even the physical world had been. Everything in New York, she told a favorite nephew, was on a larger scale than she had come to expect in Massachusetts. "What we are accustomed to call rivers become brooks and creeks in New York and what we call ponds they don't think worth calling at all, but what they call lakes we cannot call for we have nothing like them." She was intrigued, too, by the Erie Canal, with its long, flat boats, the chant of the boatmen, and its strings of mules.[26] As much as her studies broadened her intellectual world, so did this close examination of a different landscape broaden her outlook. She never again faced a journey to unknown parts with trepidation. Rather, she welcomed travel with its new vistas, its risk, and its element of surprise.

The kindness of Louise Barker, the close friendship of a few girls, and admiring glances of several young men eased Barton's stay in Clinton, but overall the year was a difficult one for her. She felt divorced from her family, on whom she had always relied for support, and longed, as she told a cousin, to "be situated near each other again so as to enable us to *speak* our thoughts and feelings to each other."[27] She never completely relinquished the feeling that she did not quite belong with the younger students, but she masked it by a show of aloofness. Rather than attempt to be a part of the student community, she simply withdrew and followed her own inclinations in study, dress, and recreation. When a classmate fell sick she volunteered to nurse her and responsibly accompanied the girl home, much to the admiration of the younger girls.[28] But her classmates felt more awe than fellowship with her. As one recalled, "she was treated with . . . deference by her associates who always seemed to concede to her the right of doing just as she pleased."[29]

Barton also faced financial difficulties during the year. It was with a start that she realized that her carefully saved earnings were barely going to keep her through the three terms of school. Barton therefore eschewed many of the frivolities of the more affluent students, spending increasing amounts of her leisure time in study. Monetary considerations also prevented her from leaving Clinton during the school holidays in spring and summer, and she spent this time alone in a hotel in town.[30] Despite her economies, however, her worst fears materialized: before the final term had ended she was out of funds. Barton did not write to her immediate family—perhaps for reasons of pride—but instead called upon her old childhood playmate, Jerry Learned. He bailed her out, saw to it that she was comfortably situated for the remainder of the year, and paid her expenses home.[31]

Clara's reluctance to mingle too much with other students may also have been heightened by shocking news she received in May 1851. Her brother Stephen, whom she had always revered and even emulated, was indicted on charges of bank robbery in Otsego County, New York. The Learneds, who had been under surveillance for some time for less than honest business practices, were also implicated. An article in the *Boston Courier* stated that "the people of Oxford did not believe Barton had any connection" with the robbery, but a credit agent found that this was not really the case. Many Oxford citizens had long been suspicious of the ways in which the Barton brothers had found the funds to acquire such extensive real estate. Stephen Barton's immediate problem became the loss of faith by his creditors, who began calling in his debts. "His C^r has received a shock difficult to get over," wrote an agent of R. G. Dun and Company, "his large R[eal] E[state] is under allocat[ion], & will not be enough in all prob. to pay his C^{r}s." Not only was his financial position in peril, but his reputation of town leader, cherished for so long, was now irrevocably tarnished. As one observer wrote, "it will be extremely difficult for him to remove the unfavorable impression."[32]

Stephen Barton was not convicted of the robbery, though many circumstances connected him with it. Clara has left no impression of the event or of the grief it must have caused her to learn of it. Otsego County was a jurisdiction bordering on the county in which she was attending school, and her brother may have been in the vicinity in connection with a visit to her. Clara appears never to have chastised her brother; instead she showed her strong sense of loyalty by upholding him in her mind and continuing to rely on him as her principal advisor. During the long years of her fame, when biographers were anxious for any detail of her family life, she effectively shielded this and other questionable activities from the public view. The extent to which this outward loyalty was inwardly felt is difficult to tell. Surely her brother's indictment and trial shook the very roots of her admiration for the energy and honor of her family. It probably contributed to her shy and aloof manner, for in attracting attention to herself, she might possibly attract attention to her brother's troubles.

Clara had barely recovered from this tragedy when she received more news of family sorrows. In early July she opened a letter from her brother that began: "Our excelent [sic] mother is no more. She died this afternoon at a quarter after five o'clock her last end was without a struggle and apparently easy."[33] Clara knew that Sarah Barton had been ill for several months and that she had not expected to live much longer, but like the indictment of her brother, this death flung her away from the anchors of the past, pressing her to rely more on herself. Helplessness overwhelmed her. She could not even attend the funeral, for her mother had already been buried in the new cemetery in Oxford by the time the news reached her. She locked herself in for nearly a week in order to be alone with her grief, telling no one of her sorrow.[34] Her brother, sensing her isolation, tried to comfort her as best he could. "Dear Clara how much I think of you and what your feelings must be when this sad news reaches you," he wrote. "I think of you as far away from connections and acquaintances in a strange country and among strangers and none to comfort and sympathize with you in this stroke of affliction. Yet I trust and hope that you will bear it meekly and with fortitude."[35] At last Louise Barker, hearing of the loss, sent for her; by pulling her out of her deep introspection she helped Clara to make the first small steps toward over-coming her loss.[36]

At the end of her term at the Clinton Liberal Institute, Barton had accom-plished her goal of increasing her academic expertise, yet she had no idea how to shape a career or what direction her life should now take. Teaching, factory work, and domestic service were the only respectable choices widely available to women. Of these, teaching was by far the most prestigious. But to return to Ox-ford, to the same round of one-room schools and unruly boys, to the thorough familiarity of countryside and citizens, seemed a backward step, lacking in either challenge or productivity. Determined that she should not dry up in the static atmosphere of Oxford schools, Barton elected to avoid her old home town alto-gether while she debated her future. She boarded a train for New England Vil-lage, a neighboring community and the home of her adventurous cousin Jerry Learned.[37]

four

Clara's visit to the Learneds lasted only a few months. In the hazy days of late summer 1851 she returned to her family at North Oxford, still without plans and in a depressed state of mind. Despite her fine scholarship in Clinton, she had been forced to leave before completing the entire course, and for the remainder of her life she considered her education lacking. Though others would view her as learned and erudite, Barton felt that her formal instruction had been rather haphazardly won. She would fill every little gap between jobs or while ill with study. When well into her eighties she embarked on the study of Thucydides and Xenophon because she felt "ignorant" without the benefit of their insight.

Barton's arrival at her home was unceremonious, and she experienced a distressing feeling of never having left. The hills and wooded streams surrounding North Oxford looked pleasantly familiar, but nothing compelled her to stay in the town. She had left because she saw that her talents were under-used and her time wasted there. If she stayed now, her bold escape to Clinton would be meaningless, and she could look forward to little beyond simple teaching and family association.[1]

Back once more in the scenes of her childhood and the ten years of teaching, which she later wrote "always haunted me as lost," Barton felt again the old agonies of uselessness and dependence.[2] Her brothers were busily rebuilding their mills; the school she founded for the laborers was thriving without her assistance; sister Sally was thoroughly preoccupied with raising her two sons. Her mother's recent death had broken up the household, and Clara wrote sadly that she felt she was returning to a "home that was still a home, and yet not all a home."[3] Barton wished her father would remarry and keep the old farm going.[4] Realizing, however, that he was over seventy, "still hale" but comfortably established at brother David's house, she knew there was little she could do to further influence or help him.[5] Gradually she reached the uncomfortable conclusion that everything was thriving without her and that to remain in North Oxford would be to eat again the bread of dependence. "I know too well how bitter it is," Barton lamented.[6] Forty years later she could still recall the discomfort of that time and summed up her reasons for leaving in a single forceful phrase: "I was not needed."[7]

Throughout August and the lingering brightness of Indian summer she pondered her future. Distracted and more self-contained than ever, she spent the time riding horseback. One fellow townsman later recalled how "stately and noble" she appeared to him at this time. Preoccupation with her immediate plans probably kept Barton from noticing that it shocked several people when she chose not to dress in mourning for her mother. (It startled them further to hear her declare that she did not grieve and that it would thus be insincere for her to wear the traditional black.[8]) She made some effort to socialize by enjoying the opportunity to renew acquaintances with Elvira Stone, Annie and Frances Childs, and her nephew Bernard Vassall. But behind her ready humor and easy conversation was a nagging doubt about the future. "I could feel no other way at home," Barton wrote a few months later, admitting that she was preoccupied with plans to get away. She knew that she must leave; deciding how to go was the only rub. "I had no where to go no one to go [to] nothing to go with and no way of earning my living if I did go anywhere, at least I had no employment or situation in view."[9]

In this frame of mind Barton was eager to seize an opportunity that presented itself in the early fall. Charles and Mary Norton had remained favorites among her acquaintances at the Clinton Liberal Institute. Anxious to retain the friendship, they wrote to Clara, asking her to visit them in Hightstown, New Jersey. Mary was a mature and deeply religious girl of sixteen; in Clinton she had looked to her friend Clara for guidance and viewed her with a young girl's idolizing eyes. Both Clara and Mary had enjoyed the relationship and had used the mentor and protégé roles to help bridge their fourteen-year age gap. And of course there was Charlie, now a handsome and ebullient twenty-one-year-old, with whom she felt a strong intellectual tie. When her friends' parents wrote to underscore the invitation, Barton accepted readily. In mid-October she set off, with no knowledge of the future but grateful to escape the stifling atmosphere of home.[10]

Traveling by train and steamer, Barton arrived in Hightstown, where she was met by "the familiar contours of my old friend Charlie Norton."[11] He drove her through the village—a simple community consisting of a railroad depot, general store, and post office, and Universalist and Baptist churches—to the Nortons' farm three miles away. It was a prosperous place, containing 178 acres of level, fertile land on which the Nortons grew wheat, corn, and fruits, and raised sheep, cattle, and dairy cows. The mixed farming, aiming as it did at self-sufficiency, must have pleased Clara, reminding her of the similar farms on which she had grown up.[12] The house too was inviting. She would remember it as "a commodious country house," with a sitting room geared to family activities. Books and papers covered a center table, a piano stood in the corner, and a settee and potted plants gave a cozy and comfortable air to the room.[13]

She soon found that the Nortons were "the XYZ in Hightstown," dominating local activities and commanding unparalleled respect.[14] Richard Norton, the family patriarch, had been raised a Quaker but converted to Universalism as a young man, much as Barton's own father had. Once convinced of the truth of Universalist doctrines, Richard Norton enthusiastically espoused them to his neighbors and relatives. His own position in the community had been consolidated by locally prestigious family connections. His wife, who was affectionately known as "Mistress Nelly," let her husband dominate her as he did the rest of the family. Charged with running the household, she appeared to Clara to be "slight, active, orderly, busy" and to possess "nervous hands and, clear blue eyes full of capacity and care." The family further consisted of the Nortons' six children, four of whom still lived at home. Besides Mary—the youngest and the only girl— and Charlie, there were James and Joshua, who were in their late twenties when Barton arrived. A housekeeper, Margaret Haskins, completed the household.[15]

The Nortons embraced Clara wholeheartedly, and her early days in New Jersey were filled with pleasure in the company of this merry group. "A sterling family it is," she told her nephew, "good as gold and true as the sun, every one of them."[16] They included her in church activities and weddings, barn raisings and nut-gathering expeditions. She especially enjoyed Charlie's company. Together they explored neighboring towns or sat in the Nortons' drawing room writing letters on a shared lap desk.[17] The evenings of teasing and piano music, of the boys' antics as they "telegraphed" secret messages to her through the wall, gave her a strong sense of fellowship, which the Nortons shared.[18] "I have learned a Quaker welcome and a warm hearty one it is too," she reported.[19] When, after two weeks, she talked of returning to Massachusetts, the family refused to listen.

The Nortons sensed, however, that Barton could not long remain comfortable without an occupation. Soon after her arrival, Richard Norton asked her if she thought she would be able to teach school. She had chosen not to reveal her past history in Clinton and had kept the policy—"it is *my* way you know"—in Hightstown.[20] Thus it was with skepticism that Norton approached her, and with hesitancy that she replied. The position that was offered was at the nearby Cedarville School, renowned for its rough gang of boys, who were especially fearsome during the winter term. The troubles outlined to her at the school must have seemed an old familiar story by now, but she told the Nortons only that she would try, if they would send Mary along to help her.[21]

"Commenced school," Clara noted in her diary on October 23, 1851. Her practiced eye must have noticed, with mingled pleasure and frustration, the similarities between this country school and those over which she had presided for the past ten years. The building itself was woefully like the ramshackle structures she had fought to improve in North Oxford, and the expressions that showed on

41

the faces of her pupils were also familiar. She read expectation and timidity on the countenances of the younger children, but among the older boys the looks were challenging and defiant.[22]

Clara Barton was in her element in these simple surroundings. She let Mary introduce the children to her one by one, and when she came to one large boy, Hart Bodine, she startled him by stating that she knew him to have "the reputation of a great rogue in school" but expected him to behave now. She further abashed the boy by asking him to help her remove the switches that had been used by the previous teacher. "When she had him carry them all outdoors and break them into small bits," the boy's mother recalled, "and tenderly took him by the hand, assuring him she would never need them, for he was one of her big boys and she could depend on him to help keep order in the school, he was simply overwhelmed." Barton saw that the students had come to expect chastisement and received it almost as recreation. When she told them there would be no punishment, the game was over.[23]

She also won over her pupils by her "entire want of all formality" and her habit of "taking the pupils into her confidence."[24] One student noted that she rarely sat at her desk, preferring to walk among the children or to stand at the stove "with one foot crossed in somewhat masculine fashion and resting on the hearth."[25] At recess she played ball with the boys or talked with them of philosophy. "Button" was the favorite game on nasty days, and she sometimes joined in the fun. "Then they are so overwhelmed they can find no means of expressing this gratitude but by giving me the button every time they go 'round," she told Bernard.[26] By setting herself with the pupils instead of against them, and by establishing clear standards at the outset, she kept discipline by simply expecting them to conform to her behavioral norms. By the end of November, her reputation was so well established that she had eight or ten pupils from other districts in the school and at one time crowded sixty pupils under the leaky roof.[27] "To all who remember Clara Barton as a teacher at Cedarville," wrote one Hightstown resident, "her success is still a tale of wonder."[28]

At the time Barton wrote that it was "the most pleasant school thus far that I ever had."[29] Nevertheless, there were elements of the job that disturbed her. The children had been poorly trained academically; they had been exposed only to spelling and simple arithmetic, a shocking state of affairs for pupils in their teens. The students were anxious to learn, however, and Barton instituted classes in geography, American history, and natural philosophy. More bothersome to Barton was her discovery that the school was not free. Each student paid two dollars per term for basic studies and an additional dollar for higher branches of learning. The proceeds went to the teacher and constituted her pay. Imbued with the long and sacred traditions of free public education in Massachusetts, Barton found it a difficult situation to accept. She acknowledged that teaching here was more profitable than in New England, but it dismayed her to bill the students at term's end, and she relieved herself of this burden by soliciting the aid of Mary and Charles during the accounting process. "I had kept time for grown men,"

Clara remarked, "but never for little children."[30] Although she quietly sought aid from the state, she received only $19.10 for the term, barely enough to keep the schoolhouse repaired.[31] After considering starting a campaign to rid the area of subscription schools, Clara decided against it. "I was in a different social atmosphere, and realizing in a way the value of discretion, I kept my reflections to myself."[32]

Barton's school was going well, but troubles appeared in other areas of her life. Chief among these was the lack of privacy she felt in the Norton household. What had begun as a pleasant feeling of inclusion in the family's activities had become a social burden. By January 1852 she had grown tired of the entertainments, which consisted "chiefly in the attempt to have as many kinds of cake as possible on one's table."[33] Used to interspersing companionship with solitude, Clara found tedious the expectation that even letter writing would take place in the family drawing room amidst the distractions of piano playing and conversation. Worse yet, her presence was required on every family outing. The situation became absurd one Sunday morning when Barton decided not to accompany the Nortons to church. "I . . . thought that need make no difference with the rest of them," she wrote in exasperation to Bernard Vassall, "but not an inch would one of them go. . . . I offered to go when I see [sic] the effect I was producing but they would not allow it on any consideration."[34] To avoid the confusion, she resorted to writing her diary and correspondence in the schoolroom while her pupils studied, and privately sought a way to remedy the problem. Spring found Barton still complaining to her diary of her inability to determine her own activities, however. She had just begun writing a letter to her brother when "a wild set of company came from church and everything must be laid aside—pass a foolish and unsatisfactory day with which I am morally sure no one could have been much pleased."[35]

At this time, too, a set of romantic entanglements left her confused and alternately exhilarated or depressed. It was a period when Clara indulged in flirtation and several young men seriously courted her. Charlie Norton was still among the suitors, and she was as attracted to his fine intellect, genial nature, and good looks as ever. Together they visited Trenton and Philadelphia, went sleigh riding, and roamed the woods. When he returned to Clinton she missed him and anxiously awaited his arrival home. But Charlie was her junior by nearly a decade. Whether he knew of the age difference or not—for, as she wrote, the good citizens of Hightstown had no idea of her past, and she might "have been taken for any age from 15 to 25"—there was a difference in experience that gave a certain adulation to his view of her. Barton found this flattering, but, as with Oliver Williams and others she would relate to in this way, it fostered on her part a sense of superiority that precluded a response to Charlie's affectionate gestures. The situation was further complicated by the flirtation of Charlie's brothers, James and Joshua. They liked to tease her by "bearding" her, their term for drawing their rough beards across her face in mock kisses. Her protests were generally ignored; indeed, as James reported, they "only set Joshua on all the more." [36]

Another Hightstown swain, Edgar Ely, put in his appearance soon after Clara's arrival in the town. A lawyer and self-taught scholar, Ely impressed her as "one of the most unpretending men I ever met." [37] He patiently accompanied her as she walked to and from school in her tall rubber boots, took her sleigh riding, and invited her to use his extensive library. [38] The Nortons liked to rib Barton about his habit of meeting her in the road and abruptly turning around to walk the other way with her. [39] Clara showed some initial enthusiasm for this admirer, but after a short time his attentions barely rated a mention in her diary.

Clara was, in fact, preoccupied with an interest of her own. Noted generally in her diary as "JLE," he was Joshua Ely, a farmer who lived near Philadelphia. How and when Barton met this young man is unclear, but by the time of her removal to Hightstown they were regular correspondents. The frequency of their letters increased during Barton's stay there, as did the anticipation with which she awaited the mail. She became "rather melancholy" when she received no letters; then her feelings soared when the familiar envelopes arrived. "Alone, quite happy," she wrote in her diary on March 19, 1852; "J's letter was longer than usual and of course pleased me in proportion to its length." [40] This was, however, to be the last such jubilant notation. By March 31 Clara was expressing surprise that she had not heard "from JLE think must be sick or worse but fear to imagine." [41] When a few days later she still had received no letter, she was so agitated that she could not concentrate on work or conversation. Acutely sensitive to the fact that at thirty she had had no serious love affair, she concluded that "there is no such thing as true friendship, at least not for me." She evidently determined to find the root of Ely's silence, for a fortnight later, having still received no letter, she visited her friend. The details of their meeting are omitted from Barton's diary, but that it dashed her romantic hopes is evident from her entry of April 20: "Have kept no journal for a month or more had nothing to note as I had done nothing but some things have transpired in the time which are registered where they will never be effaced in my lifetime." [42] No further communication with Joshua Ely is recorded after this date.

During this period of turmoil—exacerbated by news of yet another burning at the Barton Mills in North Oxford and squabbles with the parents of a few of her pupils—Barton's mood was characterized by a heightened depression. Amidst the laughing (and ever-present) Nortons she felt alone and under pressure to maintain a cheery countenance. "I have seldom felt more friendless," she lamented. "True I laugh and joke but could weep that very moment and be the happier for it." [43] The depth of her despair caused her to lose confidence in herself and the world. Even as she struggled to stop her "useless complaints," she seriously considered suicide. [44] "There is not a living thing but would be just as well off without me," she wrote on March 11; "I contribute to the happiness of not a single object and often to the unhappiness of many and always my own, for I am never happy." [45] The whole world seemed false and brought her to her "old inquiry again, what is the use of living in it." "I have grown weary of life," she concluded, "at an age when other people are enjoying it most."[46]

It is tempting to view these musings as Barton's earliest struggle with what was to become a lifelong battle against chronic depression. Her words suggest, however, that this low period in the spring of 1852 was simply part of a continuum; Barton's diary entries are the first daily recording of her depression, not evidence of the first instance of it. It was an "old inquiry," this questioning of life's purpose. She alluded to a long history of such despair when she confidentially told her nephew that she had "lived over years wishing myself dead. . . . I could feel no other way at home."[47] Moreover, the problems that faced Barton in Hightstown were much the same as those she encountered in the years before she broke "away from the long shackles" and went to Clinton—they were simply heightened by her unfortunate love affair. She had left her home town, with its unhappy associations of dependence and unrewarding work, only to find herself again a member of a domineering family and submerged in the minutiae of a job that held no challenge. Bound by a society that required far less of an educated spinster than she had to give, Barton was haunted by the horrible spectre of an unchanging and unfulfilled life. Thus, as she again contemplated her future in the thin warmth of the March days, Barton saw little reason to be optimistic. "I know how it will be at length," she surmised. "I shall take a strange sudden start and be off somewhere and all will wonder at and judge and condemn, but like the past I shall survive it all and go on working at some trifling unsatisfactory thing, and half paid at that."[48]

The final term at Barton's school ended on April 20. It had been a most pleasant group of children: "I have never been able to find a blemish in them," she told her nephew.[49] With Charlie's help she completed the repugnant task of billing the students, swept the room, and closed the door for the last time. Barton's feelings at term's end were mixed, for she recognized that the school had filled a distinct need in her. "Would scarce know how to pass my time without it," she admitted. "Should be very lonely I am sure."[50] Yet she was glad that this obligation was fulfilled and that she was now free to leave Hightstown. A few pleasant excursions with the Nortons, a few days of dressmaking, and she suddenly announced, just as she had foretold, her intention of leaving. She had formulated her plans by herself and preferred to reveal as little as possible to the Nortons. As they accompanied her to the Hightstown depot on May 25, her hosts talked excitedly of activities they would share when she came back. "They thought it a visit, and that I would soon return," Barton remembered. "I knew that I never would."[51]

The train on which she embarked carried her only a short ten miles to the town of Bordentown, New Jersey. Barton herself seems not to have known what drew her to this community. Fifty years later she believed it might have been "historical associations." The town was, in fact, well endowed in this regard, having served as a home for Francis Hopkinson, a signer of the Declaration of Independence, and political theorist Thomas Paine. The town's most famous resident, however, was Joseph Bonaparte, the exiled king of Spain and brother of Napoleon I. The stately villa that had served as his residence had burned to the ground years before Clara Barton arrived, but the stories of his life in Bordentown gave the place a prestige and intrigue that she found seductive. The town had first taken her fancy on a trip she made there in January 1852. She had thought the lack of paint on some buildings gave it a shabby aspect, but its spectacular situation on the Delaware River had filled her with wonder. As headquarters for the Camden-Amboy railroad and the Delaware and Raritan Canal, Bordentown was something of a crossroads of transportation in the 1850s, a thriving community of granite buildings and tobacco factories. Bordentown also had a drawing card in the form of Charlie Norton, who had arrived in late April to teach school. On yet another journey with an uncertain future, it comforted Clara to see a familiar face.[52]

She did not have an exact goal in mind, and her initial efforts at finding a job in Bordentown proved fruitless. After a few days, Barton traveled the short distance to Trenton, where she spoke with the local school trustee about establishing a public school. Their conversation was lengthy and cordial but inconclusive. She jotted a brief and discouraging memo in her diary—"am just where I was this morning as far as employment is concerned"—but she was forming a challenging idea. The lack of free public schools in New Jersey had disturbed Barton, and she had wondered at the antiquated public opinion that forestalled efforts to alleviate the situation. Why not start a free school, which would serve as a model for other communities in the state? With a renewed sense of purpose she contacted several prominent men in Trenton, who addressed her questions sympathetically but showed no signs of acting on her ideas. One gentleman, a Mr. Cunningham, found Miss Barton herself more appealing than her philanthropic notions, and he spent several days escorting her around the city, holding her attention with promises of influence with the state school board. One afternoon while he was driving her to the local orphan asylum, she caught wind of his less honorable intentions. The next day, angered and depressed over having lost valuable time and opportunities, she journeyed back to Bordentown.[53]

It was easy for Barton to picture a system of public schools, which would mirror those she had known in Massachusetts. But in New Jersey there were few models that would activate the imaginations of school boards or public officials. Laws providing for the creation of free schools had been passed in the state as early as 1817, though there was no comprehensive legislation until 1846. Public opinion, however, which was concerned with inequities in the distribution of public school funds and the social stigma attached to those attending "pauper" schools, did not keep pace with the legislation. A free school had been established in

Nottingham in 1844, and by 1850 there were public classrooms in Trenton and several smaller towns, but these were isolated and often temporary, and the movement failed to catch the public fancy. Not until 1866 did a statewide effort at providing public education find real support in New Jersey.[54]

It was thus necessary for Barton to marshal every conceivable argument to persuade officials in Bordentown to accept the idea of public education. She talked first to Peter Suydam, the editor of the *Bordentown Register* and a member of the school board. A genial man and something of a jack-of-all-trades, Suydam was to become one of Clara's favorite companions. At this meeting, however, he seemed to her only a tense and official obstacle to overcome. She told him she had observed that the local subscription schools were taught by persons who were well-meaning and often "elegant," but whose educational qualifications were strictly limited. When the children's knowledge grew beyond that of the matrons, they became an embarrassment and were barred from the classroom. Worse yet, Barton believed that the brightest children were the first to be "graduated into the street," for they most blatantly challenged the teacher and pointed up her weaknesses. As a final, if not tactful, argument, she maintained that New England had proved the worth of universal education with its superior productivity and ingenuity. It was time the citizens of Bordentown recognized the "force of ignorance, blind prejudice, and the tyranny of an obsolete public opinion," and joined the ranks of the more civilized states.[55]

Suydam listened with interest to the articulate young woman, but he came back with arguments of his own. There had actually been a free school a few years earlier, he explained, but an unsuitable teacher and inadequate class space had caused the experiment to fail. Housing for a school was indeed a problem in the town, as one official school report explained: "Bordentown district . . . does not possess a single school building which it can claim as its own." Consequently, should the town wish to revoke a teacher's license or establish a school, it was hampered by being solely dependent on using the private teachers' quarters for holding classes. These private teachers, Suydam explained, were greatly opposed to free schools, and their dissatisfaction would carry considerable influence among the townspeople. He believed Barton would be ostracized socially, if not subjected to outright ridicule. Finally, Suydam told her, the children themselves would not come because of their fear of the disgrace of being a public charge. Used to roaming the streets aimlessly, the boys would threaten and bully her and keep smaller children from coming to learn.[56]

Suydam's arguments failed to discourage Barton. She cared little for the approbation of the town and thought the previous failures had been due to the teacher's personality, not the inappropriateness of the free school idea. As for the boys—well, she had already talked with them. Walking through Bordentown's narrow streets, she had encountered "little knots of them" on every corner. When she asked them why they were not in school they dispensed with the expected bravado and replied plaintively, "Lady, there is no school for us." Barton found nothing derelict in the boys' behavior; she believed they were mischievous simply because they were idle and bored. "I had studied the character of these boys," she told Suydam, "and had interest and pity for, but no fear of them."[57]

Her poise and determined manner clearly impressed Peter Suydam, and Barton now underscored her persuasiveness with a trump card. She was, she told him, not an inexperienced and naive young woman but a veteran teacher of nearly fifteen years who had handled rougher boys than these, in rougher towns. Neither an adventuress nor a crusading idealist, she simply saw a chronic situation that needed remedying, and the idea of fulfilling that need challenged her.

Suydam was inspired by her words. He agreed to call a meeting of the school board to discuss the issue and invited Barton to attend. At the meeting she reiterated her arguments and effectively convinced the board that they should value her estimation of the situation, for as an experienced educator she had insight into the nature of the children. By the end of the evening she had won the confidence of the officials, who agreed to endorse a free school in the town. Moreover, she had won the school on her own terms, terms which would do much to establish the credibility of the experiment. Barton informed the board that she was willing to teach without salary, that they need provide only classroom space, but that the school must be supported and publicized by the school board. Without their approval she knew it would be considered merely another private school. "In fact," she wrote adamantly, "it must stand by their order, leaving the work and results to me."[58]

With some difficulty the board found an old brick schoolhouse—reportedly first erected in 1798—on Crosswicks Street, several blocks from the center of town. Its dilapidated condition delayed the school's opening, and Barton waited impatiently for the repairs to be completed. "You see I am making a stir among them don't you?" she boasted to the ever-faithful Bernard; "Well it will never hurt them, it is time they stired [sic] themselves to fit up school houses in Jersey—of all old sheds you never saw the like."[59] Not content with merely airing the house (whose smell she claimed rivaled that of Cologne, Germany, said to be the worst-smelling city in Europe) and building new seats and benches, she instructed Peter Suydam to provide her with maps and blackboards. Blackboards were apparently something of an innovation in the town, but when Barton insisted that she would install them if he did not, Suydam laughingly acquiesced. "Yes, yes," he replied, "*you shall have them* although no such mention is made in the contract."[60]

The contract, in fact, stated little beyond licensing "Clara H. Barton to teach or keep school in said district for the space of one year." Under the auspices of the school board, the opening of the school was announced in the local paper and on signs posted throughout the community. Finally in early July, after more delays and with much anticipation, Barton set out for her first day of class.[61]

She was greeted by a schoolhouse and yard devoid of children, save a few curious boys perched on the rail fence that surrounded the grounds. Bidding them a cheerful good morning, she strolled around the yard, pointing out birds' nests and butterflies and speaking all the while of pleasantries, not of books or studies. The six boys followed her into the schoolhouse, where she still refrained from playing the rigid schoolmarm. Instead she asked them about themselves and slowly eased into the role of teacher. Using the most striking objects in the room—the large, colorful maps of the United States, world, and Europe—as focal points, she began to answer their questions about the great oceans and foreign lands. She wooed them into the fascination of learning, with the mysteries of continents and customs, with every dramatic tale she could remember. With a certain smugness she noted that they "seemed to find my stories and my conversation generally quite entertaining." She feared they would not return after the noon recess. To her relief, however, their numbers grew. The afternoon wore on in the same vein, as she used friendship and adventure to convert her audience. "In that three hours until four o'clock we had travelled the world over," she recalled. Clara left at the end of the day, still without speaking of books or slates, commenting only that she would be back the next day.[62]

Twenty boys stood outside the schoolhouse the next morning; by week's end she had nearly forty young faces to greet her. Barton had been confident of the school's success, but this ready response far surpassed her expectations or even her hopes. She believed the school would hold only fifty students, but in another week, teacher and pupils alike shoved and rearranged to squeeze in fifty-five. Barton gave up her own chair to an eager youngster, and when the news of this reached the school board, Peter Suydam sent a chair to her from his own parlor. She still attempted only a minimum of traditional instruction. "We were studying each other, more than books, and the chapters opened pleasantly." Like her pupils in Hightstown, she found Bordentown students lacking in sound educational background but exceptionally well behaved.[63]

The students, bored with their previous enforced idleness and anxious to make up for lost time, were such eager learners that they surprised even their teacher. "I have two hours intermission . . . it yet lacks twenty minutes of that time and here they have all set studying as if their lives depended on it," Barton wrote to Mary Norton soon after the school opened, "for the last 3/4 of an hour, I have invited them to play instead but they don't want to, I think they *are* so queer, don't you?"[64] She set them to work learning to do sums, teaching arithmetic as a game—much as her brother Stephen had taught it to her—until they begged her to let them do more. While the fundamental branches of knowledge were honored, she let the advanced students experiment with the studies that interested them most. When she herself read the newly published *Uncle Tom's Cabin* and found it to be "excellent," she gave it to the older boys. "My school boys . . . are reading and crying over it and wishing all sorts of good luck to Uncle Tom and the contrary to his oppressors," she told a friend.[65] As her reputation for academic excellence and discipline grew she found some girls anxious to join the classes. Although she had vowed to take no more pupils into the overcrowded room and each morning found boys crying to get in, she could not turn these girls away. "The large boys met the emergency by smuggling in a little boy beside ea·h," she noted proudly, "and my timid gentle girls found place."[66]

So ʹnʺ ʹ pupils, and such crowded quarters taxed even Barton's considerable disciplinary talent. She discoverʹ ; that it took "the best powers of thought and invention" to control the schoʋ. Her solution was to relate the rules of self-government, which her classes in United States history were studying, to the school situation. Consulting the class in the matter, she asked their opinion— and approval—of a code of laws under which each pupil would be responsible for his or her own behavior. Although the students responded favorably to these proposals, the school board became alarmed when the news inevitably reached them. Their confidence in Barton's ability, which had risen so rapidly as the school flourished, sank, and they feared the experiment would end in defeat and mortification. Summoning the entire force of her personality and once again es-chewing bombast for the art of persuasion, Barton secured a trial period for her disciplinary system. Promising that she would inform the board if the children became uncontrollable, she returned to the school and laid the case before the pupils themselves. "Now boys," she said, "you see by this the reputation you bear among the best people of the town—how you are regarded by them. . . . You must either remain as you are or redeem yourselves." As she had hoped, her stu-dents succeeded in proving the school board wrong.[67]

Like their counterparts in Charlton, Oxford, and Hightstown, the Borden-town pupils became Barton's devoted admirers. George Ferguson, a member of the group that Barton had encountered on the first day, treasured the memory of this teacher who had recognized and made the boys feel important both inside and outside of the classroom. Writing to Barton more than twenty years later, he gratefully recalled that "you was never ashamed to speak to one of your scholars in school or out it mattered not how our toilets were, ragged or dirty, we always received a kind word and smile of recognition."[68] Another observer also com-mented on the children's devotion: "I was often with her on little walks about town; and the girls and boys seemed to vie with each other in forestalling any wish of hers. Their affection and chivalry was received so graciously and natu-rally that it was a pleasure to witness."[69]

Before the end of the term the number of children clamoring to get into the school had reached such proportions that Barton wrote to her brother for advice about alleviating the situation. Stephen recommended opening a second school, a project that was endorsed by the school board. In the fall of 1852, an addi-tional classroom, located above a tailor's shop, was outfitted. On Barton's recom-mendation, the board hired Frances Childs to teach the younger grades. Clara must have carried great weight with the school committee by this time, for she persuaded them to retain Childs—her old friend from North Oxford—over any of the local candidates. The two schools coexisted amicably, but even doubling the size failed to provide enough room for the children who wished to attend. When the citizens finally realized that nearly four hundred children still needed accommodation, they began talking seriously of erecting a larger building.[70]

It was an unusually rewarding and happy time for Barton. The unqualified success of her school provided her with the dignity and confidence she had felt so lacking in Hightstown. Remembrances of the tangled and pained romances of the previous spring were ebbing slowly away, and she relished outings with Charlie Norton and a visit from Oliver Williams with a renewed detachment.[71] If she missed the thrill of passion her letters do not show it. Fanny Childs also brought an enjoyable companionship to her life. Together they shared rooms in a boarding house run by Peter Jacques and his wife. The Jacques were amiable, Maria Jacques was an excellent cook, and the other boarders, who included Peter Suydam, were equally congenial. Indeed Fanny Childs remembered it chiefly as a time of laughter. Suydam, she noted, "frequently commented on the fact that when Clara and I were in our room together, we were always talking and laughing. It was a constant wonder to him. He could not understand how we found so much to laugh at."[72] By now Barton was something of a heroine in the town and, far from being socially ostracized, found herself a coveted guest. Underscoring Clara's pleasure was the great accomplishment she felt in having escaped the untenable situation in Hightstown by fearlessly moving on without friends or certain job to act as a safety net. She had come to trust her self-reliance, and this had renewed her faith in the world. Boldly she told a friend, "I have learned to think I have as good a right to live as any body and I will in spite of them."[73]

Throughout the winter term of 1853, Barton and Childs taught while admiration of their work grew. They were pressed to accept salaries of $250 per year and were greatly encouraged by the now almost universal support for free public education in the city.[74] With pride the Bordentown school board informed the state superintendent that "during the past year great advances have been made in . . . the cause of education. . . . We have an advance in the character of our teachers, an advance in the attendance of children, an advance in system and order within school, and an advance in the public interest felt in schools."[75] Once convinced of the advantages of public schools, the town had no desire to keep the children not accommodated in the two schools on the streets. As a result, at a public meeting the townspeople enthusiastically approved a plan to raise four thousand dollars to build a new public schoolhouse, large enough to house all six hundred school-age children.[76]

In March 1853, at the height of this triumph, Barton returned home for a visit. Ever mindful of her students, she required them to write to her as an exercise in letter writing; one pupil remembered with a certain amount of awe that she answered all with a personal note. She was not, however, completely preoccupied by her students. It had been eighteen months since she had been home, and she relished the thought of meeting the "kind friends waiting there." Now, independent and successful, she could come home without apology to anyone. The pleasures of a triumphal visit were cut short, however, by a serious groin infection, which she recalled years later as one of the most uncomfortable illnesses of her life. Recovery was slow, but by late spring she was again in Bordentown supervising the erection of the enlarged school.[77]

The handsome new school building of plastered brick was a teacher's dream, with new desks, maps, and equipment of every sort. Two stories high, it contained eight classrooms, with the distinct advantages of graded classes. The rooms gave a great deal of privacy, yet enough proximity to promote healthy competition between teachers. The town looked with pride on the rapid completion of Schoolhouse Number 1, and the opening of the school in the fall of 1853 was the "event of the season."[78]

Beneath the freshly plastered facade, however, were cracks of discontent and disappointment, especially for Barton. She was distressed to find several religious groups clamoring for state funds for their sectarian schools. Under New Jersey law, they were entitled to a share of the funds that were distributed locally, but the monies would have to come from those already earmarked for the large public school. Another minor flurry arose over the dissatisfaction of those who had previously taught the private schools. As the free schools gained in reputation, the old subscription schools gradually closed. This was the only form of livelihood open to many of the teachers. Although the school board tried to help place the teachers, some accusations worried Barton and marred her pleasure.[79]

The gravest blow of all, however, was the discovery that the school was to be headed by an outsider named J. Kirby Burnham. It was Barton's sex, not her skills, to which the town objected. Having been raised in an atmosphere that encouraged her intellectual skills, having conquered rough winter schools that had shaken many a schoolmaster, and having demanded and received pay equal to a man's, she had not expected to meet such prejudice in Bordentown. It shocked her to be classed as a "female assistant" in this school, thereby ranking no higher than the other seven women who taught in the building. Not knowing what to do, she stayed on, helping with examination and classification of the six hundred pupils. But her heart was no longer in the work. She believed Burnham to be ungrateful and highhanded and resented deeply the necessity of taking orders from him. He created strict rules for governing the children, of which Barton did not approve. Burnham may indeed have possessed dictatorial qualities, or perhaps he was merely trying to establish himself in what must have been an extremely uncomfortable working relationship. In any case, Barton grew increasingly resentful of his presence, complaining vehemently that she needed "no one to give *me directions* and tell me what I shall and shall not do."[80] She may also have resented the lower salary she received, for Burnham was making $600 to her $250. Her brother tried to console her: "Those that do the hardest work generally get the least pay."[81]

Barton was not the only teacher who was put off by Burnham. The teachers were split in their loyalties, and the resulting disunity hampered the school's progress during the first year. Fanny Childs followed Barton's lead in deploring the unfortunate Burnham, as did another teacher, Ellen Bartine. Together these three nicknamed him "the Critter" and spent much time poking fun at his mannerisms and occupations. But another teacher, a Miss Stinton, had formed a romantic attachment to Burnham, and she rallied the other teachers to his defense.[82] Hostility among the staff rubbed off on the children. "I don't see why Miss Barton could not have taught in *our* room," one student complained when assigned to another teacher's class.[83] A scathing editorial in the *Bordentown Register* condemned the teachers for their squabblings and unprofessional attitude. The school, it noted, had "stringent rules and regulations made to govern innocent and unoffending children, but none for those who needed them the most viz: the teachers." The common knowledge of their quarrels was dividing the town, the paper continued, and had "completely disunited our school, destroyed its usefulness and intrinsic worth, bred war and contention in our midst, and instead of yielding the long sought blessing, is crushing us with the iron power of a despotism and covering us with the mantle of confusion and shame."[84]

Under the pressure of rivalry, unhappiness, and the bitter collapse of her hopes, Clara's health broke down. She became weak and faint, and her spirited voice first hushed to a whisper, then gave out altogether. Although she blamed it on the damp new building, lime dust, and the strain of constant speaking during the five days of pupil examinations, she would experience these symptoms again and again during her lifetime in situations in which there was no lime dust or plaster, only tension, or disappointment and overwork. She tried to remain at her post, "but it was a vain effort." Finally, seeing that there would be no change in her status in the new school and needing desperately to escape the stressful situation, she and Fanny Childs resigned. The town protested, hoping she would stay and appear occasionally at the school to lend it her prestige and a sense of continuity, but "the strain was too great." In February 1854 she left Bordentown, her heart broken, her future again uncertain.[85]

The town, misunderstanding her motives and seeing no reason for self-blame, condemned the act. The *Bordentown Register* called it a "wrong" against the community and criticized Barton and Childs for "forsaking their posts without leave or warning."[86] But they could hardly blame Clara for the school's troubles, which remained acute after she left. In May 1854, the strife culminated with Burnham's dismissal and an entire revamping of the school's structure.

Barton's family had only an inkling of the trial through which she was passing. The clues in her letters were too scanty to give a full picture of the problem, but Stephen "thought there was something in the wind" and begged her to come home, to relax from business and spend time with their aging father.[87] The family would be glad of her presence, he wrote, for they had troubles of their own. Otis Learned, the mischievous playmate of Clara's youth, was accused of robbing a safe in the company in which he worked. "I can hardly tell why," complained Stephen, "only that his name is Larned [*sic*]."[88] After she finally wrote "a long history" of her "trials and perplexities," her brothers made a special effort to encourage her. "I suppose that you have done much to establish the system of free schools in the city and in so doing have done an infinite amount of good to the rising generations," wrote Stephen.[89] And later: "I am sorry that things have taken such a turn in the public schools, and think it must be unpleasant to you after you have done so much to help to establish them to feel that you cannot with propriety and respect to yourself continue to assist them."[90]

Despite this show of support, Clara could scarcely imagine returning home. Whereas, less than a year earlier, her plans and prospects had been on the verge of fulfillment, they now lay wasted and scattered. Her own health was, to her, a sign of her failure to meet her ambitious goals and to accept with grace the blow to her pride. To return home again at thirty-two, with no future plans, was, in her mind, to cast herself once more into subservience. Moreover, there was, in the Learned robbery, yet another family scandal to be faced. After years of small-town gossip centering on robberies, Dolly's tragic insanity, and the storms and rages of her mother, Barton felt she could not bear another such disgrace.

Clara left Bordentown in February, but it was not until mid-March that her brother received word from her. Picking up the envelope with the familiar copperplate handwriting, he was surprised to see that the postmark read "Washington, D.C."

five

In her hasty departure from the rivalries in Bordentown, Clara Barton herself seems hardly to have known why she headed south. "I wanted the mild air for my throat," she later claimed, stating that she believed Washington to be the furthest point south an unescorted woman could go with propriety. At other times she maintained that the decision was influenced by her interest in politics or the presence of the Library of Congress in the capital. Since the library offered her access to a greater variety of materials than she had ever before encountered, Barton hoped to spend her time in therapeutic study.[1]

Certainly her decision had little to do with any lure of city lights, for Washington in the early 1850s was hardly a stimulating metropolis. The capital had been plopped down into the wilderness a half century earlier, and unfinished public buildings still stood like splendidly incongruous islands in a sea of seedy and temporary structures. These lent an air of hesitancy to the city, as did the transient population that flocked to it, anxious to receive the favors of the men who governed there, and then, with unabashed fickleness, left town when better prospects were seen elsewhere. The existence of slavery in the capital, the sleepy tempo, and a lack of adequate public water or sewage facilities often startled those visiting from Europe or the northern United States. Social and political life ebbed and flowed with the sessions of Congress. Those seeking entertainment could look chiefly to the galleries of the Senate or House of Representatives, a stroll on the Capitol grounds, or to private levees, to which everyone, from lowly government clerks to foreign diplomats, was invited. Both the government and the social arena were dominated by those from below the Mason-Dixon line; the city spoke with a decidedly southern drawl.[2]

Barton welcomed the slow pace and balmy spring air, for she was battered by the overwork and disappointment she had met in Bordentown. She and Fanny Childs took rooms near the Capitol in one of the city's innumerable boarding houses. While her friend looked for a new school in which to teach, Barton settled in to the "dim quiet of the alcoves" and arranged an ambitious course of reading for herself. Still eager to make up for her "lost 10 years" of teaching, she sped through books until, even as her throat grew better, her eyes suffered from the strain. "I enjoyed my quiet, almost friendless and unknown life," Barton wrote.[3] Her belief that she had done the right thing in escaping the situation in Bordentown was reinforced when the news reached her from New Jersey that the town had lost faith in the schools and had dismissed the principal and several teachers. "We have . . . all come to the conclusion that you took a prudent course with the Bordentown school and left it at just the right time," wrote Stephen in May 1854. "I think it will be a long time before they can have a peaceable publick school and they had better have none than to have any other."[4]

Barton's life was "almost friendless," but not completely so. Among her first acquaintances in Washington was Alexander DeWitt, congressman from her home district. A tall, congenial man and a distant cousin, he made it his business to offer Clara hospitality and to act as an influential "sympathizer and benefactor."[5] Through DeWitt, Barton met another early friend and patron: Charles Mason, the commissioner of patents. Calm, self-effacing, and with an imposing intellectual curiosity, Mason proved to be a stimulating companion. Moreover, he shared many of Barton's views about public-spirited philanthropy and impressed her with his earnest efforts to conduct Patent Office business in an atmosphere of scrupulous fairness. For his part, Mason found Barton to be an excellent conversationalist and an astute political observer.[6]

Impressed with Barton's motivation and credentials, Mason asked her to become governess to his twelve-year-old daughter, Mary.[7] Before the arrangements could be settled, however, DeWitt used his influence to persuade Mason that she would be much more suited to work as a clerk in the Patent Office. To her surprise she was requested to attend a formal interview, and the commissioner went so far as to send his private carriage to pick her up.[8] At the interview Mason offered her a job as a clerk, copying patent applications, caveats, and regulations at the very respectable salary of fourteen hundred dollars a year. By July 1854, she had put her reading aside and had taken on the new role of office worker.[9]

Barton had a naturally inquisitive mind, and the Patent Office must have seemed an especially stimulating atmosphere. Her working life had been dominated before by children, among whom she had neither peers nor competition. Now she was challenged and amused by a whole office of fellow workers. Moreover, the work of the office encompassed an enticing range of pursuits—not only the regulation and granting of patents but many types of scientific research and acquisition. Although the office was under the auspices of the Department of the Interior, it carried out many of the functions of the later Department of Agriculture, Smithsonian Institution, and Weather Bureau. It sponsored scientific expeditions around the world and had amassed a large collection of specimens, many relating to the natural history of North America and the background and inventiveness of its people. Charles Mason believed these articles were too valuable and too interesting to sit in the cellar in which he had discovered them. After he cajoled Congress into appropriating money to construct a large addition to the already imposing Greek Revival building, the Patent Office took on some aspects of a museum. A march up the high steps and along its arched and marbelized corridors became a necessary stop for visitors to the capital. "It contains many of the rarest curiosities in the United States," Clara wrote enthusiastically to a former pupil, including "Jackson's dress worn at the battle of New Orleans, and scores of relics too numerous to mention." Like other branches of the government, the Patent Office had its spindles of red tape, petty spoils, and wasteful paper shuffle, but with its emphasis on innovation, it kept its reputation as one of the more dynamic places to work in Washington.[10]

The office employed lawyers, patent examiners, and clerks, whose number was strictly regulated by law. The commissioner had the option of hiring temporary clerks when the rush of business required it, however. Mason had chosen to use a very liberal interpretation of the patent laws, for he believed that promotion of technological progress was the most effective way of developing the country. The results of his policy showed themselves in simpler procedures and more open competition for the securing of patents—and a consequent flood of applications. The commissioner was therefore forced to be equally liberal in the number of temporary clerks he hired. It was as one of these impermanent workers that Barton was first employed.[11]

Barton's position, though insecure, was nonetheless an unusual one for a woman. The government had very few women in its employ in 1854, and those who were hired were chiefly the widows or daughters of former employees, who kept the job in the deceased man's name. Few officials felt comfortable with the presence of women in the offices, but no firm policy had been established. Barton knew of only four other female clerks in Washington at the time of her appointment, though a year later there were at least that number working in the Patent Office alone. Her position was all the more unusual in that she was receiving a salary equal to that of the office's male clerks. Even in this favor-oriented metropolis, her job was precarious, and Mason took care to keep the situation unadvertised. During the six years she was in government service, not once was she included in the official roll sent annually to Congress.[12]

From nine o'clock in the morning until three in the afternoon, Barton labored with the other clerks. Her exquisitely formed and highly legible handwriting made her valuable to the office, as did her trustworthiness in confidential matters. In these first months of her employment she relished the novelty and responsibility of her position. "My situation is delightfully pleasant," she wrote in October 1854. "There is nothing in the world connected with it to trouble me and not a single disagreeable thing to do, and no one to complain of me."[13] Her status and pay were far beyond any she had known as a schoolteacher. Following on the heels of her inequitable treatment by the Bordentown school board, the compensations of this job must have been especially gratifying.

She was easing, too, into Washington society, enjoying its personalities and eccentric social life. After walking in the golden autumn weather she wrote to her friends of the quiet confidence she felt.[14] She took every opportunity to visit the Senate debates, where, from the gallery of the new red and gold Senate chamber, she came to know the faces and style of the era's great politicians: Sam Houston, Henry Clay, Daniel Webster, and Charles Sumner were among those who particularly impressed her. She was surprised, like other young clerks, to find herself invited to numerous parties, and her early friendless condition rapidly changed. "I should be happy to see your nice collection of choise [sic] friends," her brother told her, adding, "I think I can conceive the value you set on them for you and I value friends about alike."[15]

Barton was boarding now with Joseph Fales, a fellow Patent Office worker, and his thin, jolly wife, Almira. Their companionship was light-hearted and added laughter to the satisfaction of hard work. Almira, whose exuberance especially impressed Clara, was a tall, plainly dressed woman with, as one friend noted, "few of the fashionable and stereotyped graces of manner." She was a storyteller, a devotee of the jovial manner, gangly, abrupt, and disconcerting. Almira Fales believed strongly in the necessities of charity and pursued her private projects with a drive that matched Barton's own. Her enthusiasm and passionate devotion to her northern background would cause her to wholeheartedly embrace relief work during the Civil War—work that was to have a direct effect on Barton's own role in that conflict. But in 1854 Almira was for the most part simply an amusing personality in Barton's gallery of friends and acquaintances, providing a nice contrast to the more sophisticated and serious society of Alexander DeWitt and the Masons.[16]

Clara worked in this contented and ambitious spirit for nearly a year. Then, to her dismay, her "valuable ally," Commissioner Mason, decided to resign his position and return to his home in Iowa. A difference of opinion with the secretary of the interior over internal administrative affairs was the immediate cause, but Mason was also anxious to oversee the affairs on his farm and remove his family from the heat of the Washington summer. His decision resulted in a good deal of confusion in the Patent Office and had some unfortunate consequences for Clara Barton.[17]

Mason left in mid-July 1855, and Samuel T. Shugert, his chief clerk, was appointed acting commissioner. Shugert was eager to please Secretary McClelland, and one of his first steps—despite his personal friendship with Clara Barton—was to consider removing the four female clerks from the office. Their presence had long annoyed McClelland, an old-line politician who considered that the women were taking jobs from deserving men who, even if not more competent,

were at least voters. The sight of teapots and hoopskirts in the office irrita___
him; he could not see that they were only the female equivalent of the omnipre-
sent cigars and spittoons. Barton's appointment as recording clerk was immediately dropped, and in August 1855 she was placed on the rolls as a copyist, to
be paid according to the amount of work she completed each month.[18] Ten cents
per hundred words was the standard rate for both men and women. Even the
most industrious copyist rarely made over nine hundred dollars a year. Worse yet,
Shugert, though retaining their names as employees, gave the women no work to
do; Barton drew no salary at all for the months of July, August, and September
1855.[19] She and her colleagues were further discouraged when Shugert announced
that by the end of August they must vacate the basement room in which they
worked.[20] Back in Iowa, Mason heard the news and was greatly saddened. "I
have some grave objections if I understand the matter rightly," he remarked.
"They were some of my best clerks and besides charity dictated their appointment and retention."[21]

Barton began to mobilize her partisans almost as soon as she heard of Shugert's
scheme. She wrote to her cousin, Judge Ira Barton, asking for his support, and she
hoped that her father's membership in the Masonic order might also aid her. After
reading her lengthy explanation of the situation, her brother Stephen expressed
his sympathy and assured her that she had the support of her cousin, as well as
Isaac Davis, a prominent politician.[22] More importantly, Barton solicited the aid
of Alexander DeWitt. He too wrote to McClelland and used all the influence at
his command to have her retained. "Having understood the Department had
decided to remove the ladies in the Patent Office on the first of October," DeWitt
wrote to McClelland, "I have taken the liberty to address a line on behalf of Miss
Clara Barton, a native of my town and district, who has been employed in the past
year in the Patent Office, and I trust to the entire satisfaction of the Commissioner."[23] But McClelland was seemingly unswayable. On September 27, 1855, he
replied sharply, telling DeWitt that though he wished to help Barton, he would
stop short of retaining "her, or any of the other females at work in the rooms of the
Patent Office." He allowed that they might do piecework in their own homes but
balked at the "obvious impropriety in the mixing of the two sexes within the walls
of a public office." He was, he concluded, "determined to arrest the practice."[24]

It was not uncommon to send work out to be done in the home, and it is
probably in this capacity that Barton worked in October 1855. She collected
$73.56 that month, a rate well over that of most clerks. Why she was not dis-
missed on October 1, as McClelland had ordered, is not altogether clear, but
perhaps, if his real complaint was the proximity of the women to other office
workers, he did not object to her copying outside the building. Like the other
women she would walk every morning along Seventh Street, past the bustling
city market, and up the stairs of the Patent Office to pick up her work and hand
in completed projects. She was not allowed to stay in the offices or linger with
the other clerks.[25]

What Barton thought of this drastic cut in pay and stature, whether she believed it preferable to dismissal or accepted it only on temporary terms while she looked for work elsewhere, has gone unrecorded, but it surely reinforced her growing objection to the unequal chances women had for earning a livelihood. She did not have long to debate the case, however, for in late October she received news that Charles Mason was returning from Iowa. The demand for his reinstatement had risen from the scientific grassroots of the nation. Inventors from all over the country sent petitions to him and to the government bemoaning the loss of his services. Bored after only a few months of the staid rural life he had previously coveted, Mason yielded. He arrived back in Washington on November 1, and with his return Barton's fortunes again rose.[26]

In November 1855 Barton received pay of $135, nearly double that of the previous month and again consistent with her old salary of $1,400 per year. She was, however, kept on the rolls as a temporary copyist at the standard rate. Mason, anxious to retain Barton's good services but reluctant to make any move that might goad McClelland into dismissing the female clerks entirely, probably developed the system of classifying Barton as one type of employee and rewarding her as another. As Barton was to declare, it was all a little "subrosa."[27] It may also have served Mason's purposes to keep Barton's real status a secret, for he again needed her help in straightening out intraoffice problems.

"I have been this day in my old place in the Patent Office," noted Mason in his diary on November 3. "I do not know how well I shall be pleased with it after all. I shall have some very unpleasant duties to discharge in general of the clerks and examiners. . . . I fear I shall be obliged to discharge some of them."[28] Intemperance was a problem among the employees, a sticky situation since several prominent political appointees were among the offenders. Worse, however, was a network of frauds he believed was threatening the impartiality of the office. Several clerks were evidently selling patent privileges illegally, an old temptation about which he had complained to Congress as early as 1853.[29] Moreover, there were apparently a number of in-house rivalries and jealousies cropping up, which were difficult to control and damaging to morale. "I have been so disgusted with the office seeking manoeuvering all around me," a Patent Officer worker declared.[30] Calling on Barton's tight-lipped assistance, Mason set about untangling the personnel knots.

Clara viewed Mason's efforts as a righteous crusade and something of a witch hunt. It appealed to her strong moral outlook and allowed her to indulge herself in a short period of sanctimoniousness. "I found the frauds," she told a female reporter proudly. "It made a great commotion among the clerks; they knew what it meant and they tried to make the place too hard for me."[31] The only woman regularly in the office now, she took the brunt of any animosity that the men felt against women workers. She wore victory with smugness, and this exacerbated the bitterness that she felt the men had secretly harbored because of her ability to equal or surpass them in their duties. That she made no attempt to hide her close social ties with Mason may also have increased the resentment against her. Lining the halls as she came in to work, the men made catcalls, spit tobacco juice at her, and blew smoke in her face.[32] "It wasn't a pleasant experience," Barton conceded, "in fact, it was very trying, but I thought perhaps there was some question of principle involved and I lived it through."[33] Indeed, she rose above them, though it did little to dissipate her reputation for haughtiness. In a tone of marked superiority she told a friend that "there is not a spot upon my system that is not perfectly invulnerable to any touch of theirs, all the world who know as I know the relation they have sustained toward me, and know what to expect from them. Any blow that they could slanderously aim at me in *these* days, would make about as much impression upon me a[s] a sling shot would upon the hide of a Shark—I have got above them."[34] The job that had once been "delightfully pleasant" was now possible to endure only to win her point. By September 1857, the daily trip to the office had become a "weary pilgrimage."[35]

It is difficult today to imagine the degree to which Barton's aggressiveness and capability appeared unusual—and in many ways unacceptable—in the 1850s. Such traits as ambition, bureaucratic competence, and leadership were the opposite of those preferred in the Victorian woman. However "accomplished" she might be, a lady was expected to be demure, self-effacing, easily controlled, and interested primarily in children and the home. Within this sphere a woman was exalted and idolized by society, which saw her as the protector of moral values and family sanctity. Outside of it there was little or no place for her. A woman who was not married—who chose not to be married—was already suspect; a woman who enjoyed men's company and forged brazenly into their fields of occupation was due for reproach. When Barton encountered the rows of men who spat upon her each morning, she was, in a sense, facing the judgment of contemporary society, which could not quite believe that it was "nice" for a woman to earn her living or strive for occupational fulfillment. It was for these reasons more than personal habits or proclivities that women who were pioneers in government service often gained a tainted reputation, despite the fact that most of them came from respectable middle-class backgrounds and conducted themselves with self-conscious decorum. There was a rumor that the early clerks "painted" themselves and used indelicate language, but few specific examples could be given.

Similarly, Barton's own reputation for lax sexual conduct during this period was probably based more on the boldness of her employment than any real promiscuity. Reports that she arrived in Washington in the company of Samuel Ramsey, her friend from Clinton, and that her talk of free love and unwillingness to live apart from the professor caused her sister to shun her company are thus suspect, as are later stories of a similar nature about Barton and Senator Henry Wilson. Although Clara may well have been an advocate of free love, neither Sally Barton Vassall nor Ramsey lived in Washington at the time of her early Patent Office employment; the latter story, which featured the birth of two illegitimate children with Negroid features, seems equally unlikely. It is doubtful that men of the stature of Alexander DeWitt or Charles Mason would continue to keep company with a woman who this blatantly breached society's rules. Because she enjoyed and sought the company of men and was adept at their amusements and repartee, Barton was always open to criticism of her feminine conduct. (In later life she would diminish it by modest dress, a low, soft voice, and by actively avoiding confrontation.) Given in addition her persistent drive to work and her air of superiority, there was a rich field for those who wished to gossip or who felt threatened by her unwillingness to abide by a smug society's standards. For the rest of her life Barton would be prey to those who could not or would not understand her motives . There were those who would point to her even at the age of seventy-eight with accusations of lax morality or loose living.[36]

Employee relations at the Patent Office were strained enough, but the work of the office had also reached a fever pitch. An examiner complained that he had to get to the office at 5:00 A.M. to make any headway in his workload. Barton was copying over a thousand pages a month of "dry lawyer writing" into a ledger too heavy for her to lift. "My arm is tired," she told her sister-in-law, Julia Barton, "and my poor thumb is all calloused holding my pen."[37] She began to feel that the efforts were not worth the rewards of the job. "We are tired as a dog and almost sick," she complained in half jest to Bernard, "and it wouldn't much matter if we were turned out to grass." Whatever pressures emanated from the office were multiplied by Barton's own compulsion to drive herself, inability to relax, and tendency to set unattainable standards. After taking a few days off to visit Jamestown with a friend, she copied at a frightful pace to make up her work.[38] Despite intermittent bouts of malaria, she continued on the job, frequently working until late at night. She took a guilty view of her own foibles and rarely indulged herself either materially or mentally. Once when she misplaced a parasol, she would not buy another of good quality, forcing herself instead to carry a cheap one. In a strangely proud confession of this self-denial, she told Julia that "it was the best I have had all summer, and I walked to church under it today, so much to pay for carelessness."[39]

She was tired, her fingers were sore, yet she managed to maintain the intense correspondence with friends, former pupils, and relatives that was so important to her. Barton rarely spoke of her troubles in these letters; even brother Stephen had to plead with her not to bottle up her feelings.[40] Her sense of humor was particularly keen at this point in her life, and she joked about many of the rougher aspects of Washington life. Complaining in a light vein of the beastly summer weather, she wrote, "I have no idea where the thermometer stands, if indeed it *stands* at all, it does better than most people can."[41] And she told Julia, with regard to a current scandal that involved the shooting of a Pension Department worker by a jealous fellow employee, "We are at our same old tricks yet here in the capitol [sic], i.e. killing off everybody who doesn't just happen to suit us or our peculiar humor at the moment."[42] Barton wrote of politics and her view of the South, which, like that of many New Englanders, tended to be one of both fascination and disdain. Southerners peppered their food—and their arguments—too much for her taste. She had a gift for letter writing, an ability to make the most mundane actions seem fresh and interesting. The enthusiasm she had in the small pleasures of her life was infectious, and the demands her correspondents made for letters almost smothered her in an embarrassment of popularity.

Barton was pleased, too, in these days, with the strength of her finances, which allowed her to buy presents for her father and Bernard, save extensively, and even purchase some valuable prairie land in Iowa, perhaps at the instigation of Charles Mason.[43] "We are in fact in a state of prosperity," she told a friend, obviously tickled.[44] Free from monetary worries, she could enjoy the company of a fellow boarder, Mr. Harbour, a bricklayer from Iowa whose sense of humor matched her own: "We have laughed since he has been here until we are sore."[45] Even merrier was the first of a number of extended visits of sister Sally and her younger son Irving Vassall to Washington. Clara escorted them to the city's important sites, talking enthusiastically of the local politics and gossip. With the unjaded eye of a sixteen-year-old, Irving surveyed the self-conscious Washington scene and found it wanting. Far from adulating the heroic statesmen of the age, he found their peccadillos a source of amusement. James Buchanan, the newly elected president, had hair "combed so as to stick up exactly straight something in the fashion of an Indian. He tips his head to one side and squints with one eye horribly." Old General Cass, long a respected member of the Senate, was ridiculed because he did little except frequently move for an adjournment. "He has a funny way of smacking his lips every few moments," Irving told his grandfather, "so loud that it can be heard distinctly all over the Senate chamber."[46]

Irving's Aunt Clara laughed at his irreverence but overall viewed the Washington circus a bit more seriously. She took advantage of every opportunity to watch the proceedings of the Senate and House, whose debates now centered upon the fiery question of slavery. One evening in 1856 she sat spellbound in the Senate gallery while Massachusetts senator Charles Sumner delivered an impassioned speech against expanding slavery into the territories. So vehement were his arguments in this speech, entitled "The Crimes Against Kansas," that the next day he was struck down and beaten by Congressman Pierce Butler from South Carolina. Dour Charles Sumner with his staid speech and imperious ways was not a man to inspire adulation, but the assault on him caused a flurry of emotion both North and South. This scene, more than anything else she had witnessed in Washington, sobered Barton to the terrible divisions within the country. "I have often said that *that night war began!*" she told a friend years later. "It began not at Sumter, but at Sumner."[47]

She was beginning to realize, too, that her own political star was descending. The men who had sponsored her were, one by one, leaving Washington. Much to her regret, Colonel Alexander DeWitt was not reelected in Clara's home district, and he returned to Massachusetts in March 1857. "I would attempt to tell you something of how sorry I am that the Colonel is going home to return to us no more," Barton confided to Julia, "but if I wrote all night I should not have half expressed it."[48] Barton herself was out of step with the new Buchanan administration, which advocated unconditional political allegiance as a prerequisite to government jobs. Buchanan, like all presidents, sought to reward his own followers, but he also hoped to avoid the strife and delay caused by factions within the government. Though she could not vote, Barton's liberal views had made her sympathetic to the supporters of Buchanan's rival, the antislavery candidate John C. Fremont, and she realized her position was in jeopardy. When she joked about it at a political levee, a fellow office worker tried to smooth over the incident, saying that she was not responsible for anything she "might say on the present occasion, as the *coffee* was exceedingly strong."[49] Charles Mason was also worried. On June 27, 1857, he noted in his diary that the secretary of the interior had that day "asked me what I thought of the policy of removals in the patent office for political differences of opinion. Being thus asked I stated to him briefly my notions, that it would not be wise . . . to remove good officers . . . merely because they differed from us in political views."[50] Barton was agitated, yet she tried to make light of it to her family and friends: "there is great talk about cutting off official heads," she told a nephew, "but no specimens of decapitation yet."[51]

That summer the Patent Office was in a frenzy of activity. June 1857 was the busiest month in its history, and Barton put in long hours to keep up with the workload.[52] In six days she did two weeks' work, all in an oppressive heat wave that overwhelmed the city that month. As the summer wore on she tried to keep up with the work, though a severe case of malaria sapped her strength. She took "Bitter bitters" to rid herself of the disease, but her skin turned yellow and her spirits flagged.[53, 54] Any hopes she had for keeping her job were finally dashed when Commissioner Mason resigned on August 4, 1857. Without DeWitt or Mason, her two staunch advocates, she had little chance of retaining her already controversial appointment.[55] "I begin to feel that my Washington life is drawing to a close," she wrote home early in September. She had prized the work and welcomed the experience, but her uncomfortable position vis-à-vis the other clerks and the infighting between the secretary and commissioner allowed her to leave in a state of mind more philosophic and relieved than regretful. It "had not been *all* sunshine," she concluded, but "a steady battle, hard-fought, and I trust well won."[56] A month later, after being told that her place was wanted, she packed her bags and headed north.[57]

Barton was free and had a substantial savings account, but she had formulated few ideas about her future, immediate or otherwise. Washington seemed a less attractive place to remain, even temporarily, now that her friends were gone, and a hostile administration virtually foreclosed any possibility of employment. But, as always, she was loath to return home permanently. Giving herself time to think and a much needed rest, Barton boarded a train for Auburn, New York. There she visited the Bertram family, with whom she had stayed years before while a student at the Clinton Liberal Institute.[58]

Barton was a good house guest, cheerful, helpful, and unobtrusive, and the Bertrams pampered her and urged her to stay for an extended visit. They tried to interest her in settling in the area, possibly to start an academy for young ladies. Barton, however, was in no mood to set up a school or to overstay her welcome. Perhaps remembering her uncomfortable subservience at the Nortons', she determined not to settle in New York. After a stay of nearly two months, she made a long-promised Christmas visit to her family.

She found that North Oxford was still little changed from her childhood and youth. The same families wielded the same influence. A few new mills had sprung up, but population, enterprise, and interest generally remained stagnant. Her father was growing deaf and saw with difficulty, but he still insisted on setting out his beloved garden and walking miles over the rocky hills to chat with his old comrades. Clara was living in the little house in which she was born, a guest of David and Julie, and that situation, too, was reminiscent of old times. The same climbing rose grew over the door, the same underlying tensions puzzled and disturbed her. Julie's acerbic tongue made her at once witty and disquieting to be around. David she found as charming and erratic as ever, personifying the family trait of overworking himself to the point of nervous exhaustion. Their active, bustling household reflected the varied life of an extended family, but to Clara it seemed to encompass everyone except her, and she felt again that she was the fifth wheel, the sore thumb, the one who did not quite fit.

Only Stephen was missing, his absence keenly felt by Clara. Early in 1856 he had moved to North Carolina to establish a new milling complex. His reputation had never completely recovered from the association with the Learned bank robbery in New York, and this, coupled with a conviction that labor and land were cheaper in the South, and chronic medical problems that made him uncomfortable during the cold New England winters, convinced him to make a move. He sold his share of the S & D Barton Mills to David, recruited twenty excellent workers, uprooted his wife, son Sam, and Bernard Vassall, and settled on the Chowan River in Hertford County. The first year was a lonely and anxious struggle to establish himself as a farmer and businessman. Still, he kept a tight cork on his liberal attitudes, availed himself of the local black labor supply, and determined to succeed. Two years later his business was thriving, but his wise counsel was sorely missed by his youngest sister.[59]

Clara's visit to North Oxford was meant to be only a short one, but it lengthened to a stay of over two years. During this time she was suspended in a semipermanent limbo. She refused all offers to teach that would commit her to staying in the vicinity. Yet she had no dreams that would precipitate a move. Long a pragmatic dweller in the present, Barton was not given to making elaborate plans. Decisions about the future—a hazy and alien place to her—came with difficulty. She seems to have decided that if she would have to teach she would undertake a position in an academy or as a governess. With a partial eye to this, and with her ever-present zeal for further education egging her on, she embarked on a series of French classes, painting lessons, and other art courses. Languages and art were considered necessary attainments for a well-taught lady and indispensable to the private teacher. In 1858, Clara moved to Worcester, boarded with the family of Judge Barton, and commenced taking classes at a local academy.[60]

Barton did well in her French courses and earned a little pocket money here and there, chiefly as a companion to an elderly woman friend.[61] In addition, she lived off her savings, thus making herself financially independent. Nevertheless, she did not flourish in this, her own most-hated role of subservience and uselessness, and she felt obliged to explain herself and her actions or to conform to the family's standards when in their presence. For all of 1858, she continued her studies, half hoping that something more enticing would come along. Undecided about the future and unhappy with the present, she seemed incapable of acting decisively to relieve her depression.

Determined to make at least a small change, Barton switched from languages to drawing courses in September 1858. Throughout that fall she sketched from nature or models, then graduated to painting and work with ceramics. The few pieces of her artistic work remaining show a detailed and technically competent style, but one that lacks originality or freedom of movement. Though she found her efforts mildly interesting, she did not regard them as work and could not embrace them seriously. Rather, they encouraged her fears that she was not developing but only idly filling time.[62]

What Barton sorely needed was a sense of purpose. She found a focus in two young relatives, both of whom looked to her for help at this time. She was distracted by their troubles and, more importantly, could bolster her own feelings of self-worth by working out their problems. But ultimately she undertook too much responsibility for these children, and they proved a costly emotional and financial drain. Their success or failure became entangled with her own sense of achievement; their progress dictated her own elation or sorrow.

It was concern for her nephew, Irving Vassall, that most seriously affected Barton's mood. She was closer as a peer to Irving and his brother Bernard than perhaps any other members of the family. To these two she confided her own darkest self-doubts, and with them she was at her most playful. For years she had exchanged poems with Bubby, as she nicknamed Irving, and enjoyed his witty and inquiring mind. In his late teens, he had "grown to be a young man, full of promise, noble and intellectual beyond all reasonable expectations."[63] Now she watched with alarm as his health declined and his vitality sputtered and died. He was, at sixteen, consumptive, and he was beginning to experience the full effects of this debilitating disease. By the time his Aunt Clara moved to North Oxford, his spirits and constitution were precariously low. He and his mother had moved to Washington: they hoped the mild climate would improve his health. In fact it had deteriorated seriously during their first months there. To make matters worse, Vester Vassall, his father, had proven to be an inadequate provider. The Barton family was constantly called on to help, for Irving's own family could afford neither expensive medical care nor a permanent move to a less rigorous climate. Worried that the boy would be allowed to waste away, Barton began to confer with Bernard about the best possible course for his recovery.

Neither Bernard nor his father was working at that time, and thus they could contribute little. But Clara and Bernard together devised a plan to collect funds to send Irving to Minnesota. The "prairie cure," which relied on the clear dry air of the Midwest to allay the disease, was popular at the time, and Barton hoped the change in climate would help her nephew. Sure that if she explained the case each of Irving's many friends would contribute a little toward the journey, Clara hoped to collect over one thousand dollars. She was, however, disappointed. Stephen Barton gave a good deal of money, and several Oxford families contributed five or ten dollars to the fund, but the net collection was something under two hundred dollars.[64]

The family believed the proposed cure was unlikely to aid Irving's health and would be a waste of money on a boy who, though charming and talented, they considered thoroughly spoiled. This attitude annoyed and hurt Clara, and coupled with legitimate worries over Irving's condition and her own sense of futility, it created an intense period of anxiety for her. To her diary she complained that her nerves were "ticklish" and her sleep fitful. In early February 1859, she became so distraught that she could accomplish nothing and spent her time wandering aimlessly.[65] A month later, after receiving a letter from Irving that spoke of a greatly worsened condition, her old insomnia returned, and with it the painful physical symptoms that accompanied her periods of mental stress. "I became satisfied then," she told Elvira Stone, "of what I had mistrusted before, i.e., where the difficulty in my back originates."[66] Her low spirits increased throughout the year until she began again to think life not worth living and meditated forlornly on "the strange duplicity of mankind."[67]

It was not only Irving Vassall's case that depressed her but other family obligations as well. Her Aunt Hannah died in February 1859, leaving her "sad and desolate" and saddled with most of the responsibility for the funeral arrangements. Moreover, she worried about her father's increasingly feeble state. When David fell ill that spring, she felt obliged to care for him as of old. She returned to North Oxford to "nurse up" her brother, who was slow to mend, and her own affairs were left in disarray for nearly two months.[68] At the same time she took up the cause of Mattie Poor, another young relative. Mattie, then studying music in Boston with high hopes of becoming a concert pianist, had more ambition than talent. Naive and profligate, she ran through the $125 Barton sent her in March 1859 in less than three weeks. Horrified, but unwilling to see the girl's education go unfinished, Barton burdened herself with this additional responsibility.[69]

She tried to raise her spirits by attending the lectures of fashionable speakers such as poet Oliver Wendell Holmes and travel author Bayard Taylor. She pieced together a quilt, kept up her voluminous correspondence, and took pleasure in a few outings with old friends.[70] As the summer wore on, however, her thoughts were increasingly black, her mood ensnared in some terrible, dark cavern of depression. Irving's situation was worsening gradually, and it seemed apparent that her sister and other family members would do little or nothing to aid him. Worse yet, Irving himself had apparently begun to lose courage and seemed reluctant to try the prairie cure or anything else that might help his condition. Finally, convinced that she must shoulder this burden alone if she could not find others to help, Barton sent Irving a bank draft for three hundred dollars. Then, after a thorough check of her finances, she penned him a forceful letter. *"You are going to Minnesota as soon as you are able to start, and your mother is going with you,"* she wrote, adding that the expense was little to her in comparison with the prospect of his recovery. More money would be forthcoming, she promised, concluding: "So My Boy dont puzzle over it, but get ready, get off and get well, as fast as you can."[71]

She felt better with the decision made, despite the worrisome drain on her finances. (The last check to Irving, she confided to a friend, had "exceeded my limit."[72]) But, her guilt erased and optimism restored, she could now wax philosophic about her prospects. "I have taken the 'rough and tumble' of life and outlived aspirations enough to know something of it," she told Bernard. "I have helped do just such things as I desire done for Irving and it was a pleasure then, and surely is now to remember it."[73] Feeling more useful and self-satisfied than she had in a year, Barton decided to escalate her role in the matter. Sometime in August she announced that she would accompany Sally and Irving on their trip west and stay to see them settled.

It was a long and difficult journey. Irving's illness was more pronounced than she had been led to hope. His thin, shaky frame was wracked by hemorrhages, during which he lay coughing up blood for hours. Barton met the Vassalls in Washington, where they took the dirty and rattling cars for Chicago. They sat stiff and tired for the three day trip, arriving in Chicago's raw wooden railway terminal on September 18. Irving was sick and worn; he had to lie prone and quiet for a week before they continued on. Though it was her first trip west of New York, Barton was too preoccupied with Irving to experience much beyond a grim determination to settle him in a healthful atmosphere; she recorded no impression of Chicago's rough streets or the wide stretches of waving prairie grass, so different from the rocks and rills of Massachusetts. Before her opinion could be formed, they traveled on from Chicago to Duluth, where they stopped for several days.[74]

Barton stayed with her sister and Irving until late November. They tried a number of towns in their search for a place to settle permanently but could not find one that suited them exactly. Irving, in despair over his ebbing strength, became pettish and was rarely satisfied with food, lodging, or location. Sally Vassall was also tired and exasperated, and it fell to Clara to keep them in good cheer. A woman who met them at this time remembered her as "a small person with a very bright face and at times very serious. Often she was gay, too." Clara talked with Irving of slavery and politics, took him on excursions to see the Mississippi River, and tried to make herself useful to the families who generously put them up.[75] One family was surprised to find her building a cupboard from rough boards when she saw that they had need for one. Another man remembered the gracious and cheerful way in which Clara "refused to deprive the 'little sisters' of their bed, and slept on the floor," and how she loaned her "dancing slippers" to a disappointed girl whose own had been forgotten. Later in life the girl would brag that "she stood in Clara Barton's shoes a whole evening."[76]

Finally, short of money and recognizing her own need to find a job, Barton returned home. Once there, however, her depression only worsened. To her discomfort she found her finances even less secure than she had supposed. Her old nervous condition was back and within a few weeks was so bad that she could scarcely leave her bed. She was also distressed to hear that both Bernard and his father were still essentially unemployed and unable to contribute to Irving's support. Worse yet, she either sensed or imagined a lack of hospitality on the part of David and Julie. Convinced that they wished her to leave, she felt more beholden than ever. In despair, she told Bernard that she had sent Irving thirty dollars more, but that he "must meet the next demand. I have *very little money,* no credit, no business, no prospect of any, and sick in bed, and unlike either of you, *no home.*"[77]

Two weeks later Irving sent a request for additional funds, which Barton felt unable to raise. He also wrote that he disliked Minnesota, found it unbearably cold, and wanted to return to Washington for the winter. To underscore his point he allowed that his health had worsened in the Midwest. Alarmed that the boy might leave Minnesota before the cure had a chance to work and completely exasperated at his demanding and ungrateful attitude, Barton's patience gave way. "Can it be that he is so trifling and selfish?" she asked Bernard. "Would he subject us to all he has . . . and then after we are all beggared, rob us of all the little chance of gratification we could possibly have, viz to see him *try* to improve a little under our exertions." If so, she concluded, "if there's not more than this *to* him, he is not worth *trying to save.*"[78]

Her reserves of cheer and strength were giving out now, eaten away by worries real and imagined. Mattie Poor, who had also overrun her funds, refused to leave her studies, though she was now more than qualified to teach music. She demanded Clara's continued aid but rejected any advice along with the check; "she is only a counterpart of Bub on my hands," Clara sadly noted.[79] At the same time, Clara was worried about her father's health. When he was again sick in February, she became so distraught that she exhausted herself, as she had so many times before, nursing him.[80] When she at length looked up from his sickbed she found the winter nearly over. Another season had passed without profit or serenity.

At home, Barton received no support, comfort, or even understanding for her misery. Friends and kinfolk thought her foolish for pampering Irving and Mattie and believed she had brought her troubles on herself. They could not understand why Clara did not take a teaching job, settle down, and rid herself of her nervous affliction. Julie Barton seemed concerned that her sister-in-law would become a permanent charge, for Clara had not been able to pay for her board for several months. Furthermore, Clara was—or felt she was—socially shunned. She had no idea what was expected of her, did not know how to fit in, felt every move was the wrong one.[81] "I work all day to keep things as straight as possible and cry half the night . . . ," she wrote, adding sarcastically, "now you will naturally see that things look 'bright to me.'"[82]

Well aware that she needed to get away, find work, and recapture her self-esteem, Barton wrote, "I must not rust much longer . . . [but] push out and do *something somewhere*, or *anything, anywhere*."[83] Just what she would do was another question. She would consider the subservient and poorly paid life of teaching only as a last resort. "I gave outgrown that, or that me," she recognized. "I have no desire to do it now."[84] Having ruled out the most easily obtainable position, she wearied of mulling over the other limited possibilities. Clerking, starting a school, and escaping to South America were all considered. Frustration mounted as she used her influence to gain lucrative positions for Bernard, Elvira Stone, and other friends, and saw herself still empty-handed. After two jobs—a clerkship and an administrative job with a school—failed to materialize, Clara's emotional state became so desperate that she was immobilized by panic. She had, she acknowledged, "added more than ten years right into my life in the last two months."[85]

Her frustrations were heightened by the difficulty she was experiencing because of her sex. The very clerkships that Barton's influence gained for Bernard were not open to her. It was a fact of which she was acutely conscious and which increasingly rankled her. The outright discrimination she had suffered in Bordentown and the prejudice of the official policy during her years in Washington had done a good deal to politicize her feminism. Like many other early women's leaders, personal experience gave bite to the shadowy liberal notions with which she had been raised. Knowledge of her own capabilities and the way in which these were bound by society began to give her reason to believe a radical change in the social structure must be accomplished. She was angry that she could not win the same political favors her untried nephew could, simply because she "couldn't wear broadcloth." Barton acknowledged that her political friends had always encouraged her to call on them for aid. There was a difference, however, between such hearty reassurances and the actual initiation of some help. Still shy when asking favors, Clara did not see how she could approach her friends and was thus reluctant to ask them "until some change should open the way."[86]

Perhaps, she surmised, a permanent government appointment was too much to expect. Then, in a burst of fury, she recognized her own tendency to limit her expectations to the level of the men around her. She vented her anger to Bernard, in one of the most succinct statements she was to make about the oppression she felt surrounded her and others of her sex:

> When you have pictured my past life and habits and training for the past number of years, you will . . . forgive such an aspiration in me. Were you in my place you would feel it too, and wish and pine and fret in your cage as I do, and if the very gentlemen who *have* the *power* could only know for one twenty-four hours all that oppresses and gnaws at my peace, they could offer me something to do in accordance with my old habits and capabilities before I am a day older, but they will never know and I shall always be oppressed no doubt. I am naturally businesslike and habit has made me just as much so as a man (and *were* I a man I would never do a four penny business). . . . I should be 'perfectly happy' today if someone would tell me that my desk and salary were waiting for me—that once more I had something to do that *was* something.[87]

But the prejudice continued to haunt her. On yet another job search in official quarters she found to her dismay that "the registrar says he has no room for ladies . . . and fears to have papers taken out of the office to be copied."[88]

Word from Irving was as discouraging as her search for a job. He was dissatisfied, in need of money, and weaker than ever. Clara, her patience strained to the limit, could not see how he and Sally could run through so much money. Clara was not a natural altruist, and much of her pleasure in helping was bound up in the gratitude, love, and dependence that were shifted back to her. She resented those who did not give her this recognition, and the news from the Vassalls was thus doubly exasperating. Irving complained so much of Minnesota and its negative effect on his condition that his aunt dryly allowed that "the child's disease must have removed from his lungs to his head."[89] Feeling that for all her good intentions she was to blame for Irving's plight, Barton's nerves gave way. Once again suicidal thoughts crept upon her. "I wished we were all at rest . . . ," she remarked upon receiving yet another sad epistle from the West. "I am not quite myself and don't know when I shall be again. . . . I am weak and nervous ever since, and I am good for nothing at all."[90]

Barton now had virtually no money to send Irving and Sally. Her long-term finances had taken a turn for the better in February when Captain Barton sold her twenty acres of valuable timberland at a bargain-rate price. He took a note for the property, though she felt obliged to pay him for it later in the year.[91] But this transaction did nothing to help her immediate need for cash. To make ends meet she returned to Boston in late April for another brief tour as a companion to an older woman. This was little better than doing nothing; its only advantage was to remove her from the critical eyes of Julie and David.[92] She endured it for a month, then, deciding that she *must* take control of her life and earn some money, she suddenly packed her bags and left for New York.

Barton was sick and nervous when she left North Oxford, "in a better condition," she admitted to a friend, "to go to bed than New York City."[93] She had hoped to look for a job in the business community, but she arrived barely able to make it to the offices of her old friend, phrenologist L. N. Fowler. He took her in hand, charted her personality traits (giving her high marks for friendship, low for self-esteem), and sent her to a hotel run by a son of the Bertrams, bidding her rest and get well before trying to find work.[94]

After a week the hotel proprietor decided to send her home to his parents. Determined to go "where I could be sick and feel that I was not committing an unpardonable sin thereby," she retreated to the Bertrams, where she was received with open arms.[95] The contrast between her treatment there and that afforded her by her own family could not have been sharper. "I was almost cheated in belief that I *had* come home and had a home to come to," she told Bernard sadly.[96] For two months they harbored her, pampering her, encouraging her to stay with them indefinitely. They again tried to talk her into starting an academy or teaching in their area "It is really a temptation, Ber," she told her nephew, "if it were anything but teaching I would."[97] She was more relaxed with the Bertrams, yet she knew it was only one more temporary stopping place. And with no immediate prospect of work, home, or any sense of permanence, she could not quite shake her morbid thoughts. In late July she was still feeling that there was "nothing . . . *so welcome as perfect rest*." She was happy when she slept and, she noted, had felt "for long years . . . that when the command should come, Lay down thy burden and rest, it must be the sweetest hour of my whole existence . . . sometimes my stubborn heart rebels and I murmur to myself, how long Oh Lord how long."[98]

six

In rooms that were the "cosiest and prettiest that one could ask," Clara pondered and recovered, let the Bertrams wait on her, worried about Irving, weighed her options. Still "weak and bilious" in August but gaining strength, she was determined to go back to New York City, trade her accounting skills to the business world, and rely on friends, not family, for support.[1] Outside events, however, influenced her to follow a different course. Through circumstances that are not altogether clear, for her correspondence was minimal during these uncertain months, Barton was recalled to her post in the Patent Office. After the election of Abraham Lincoln in November 1860, her politics did not seem so offensive.

It was the government's lame duck period between the election and the March 4 inauguration, when work was slack, and appointments were up for grabs. Some unnamed "personal friends" engineered Barton's appointment as a temporary copyist, charged with "recording specifications and making office copies."[2] This did not equal the status of her earlier job with the Patent Office, and the salary too was lowered, for women could now earn only eight cents per hundred words copied, or a maximum of nine hundred dollars per year.[3] But she was hardly in a position to complain, and she accepted the appointment with relief and even delight.

By December she had bid her final adieus to the Bertrams and, with a lighter heart than she had known in months, arrived back in Washington. The scenes and faces seemed so familiar. Samuel Shugert and Joseph Fales were still in the Patent Office; Charles Mason resided in the city, earning his living as a patent lawyer. Clara's old room in Almira Fales's boarding house was available. The two impressive fountains in the courtyards of the Patent Office building still made "cool the air in the sultry days of summer." Picking her way through the muddy streets and up the long stairs to the office door, newfangled hoopskirts in hand, she felt as though her absence had been nothing but a pause in a long continuum.[4]

73

Washington itself was much the same. "As in 1800 and 1850, so in 1860," Henry Adams wrote, "the same rude colony was camped in the same forest, with the same unfinished Greek Temples for workrooms, and sloughs for roads."[5] Yet the political air had a different quality in the days following the election of Abraham Lincoln. The southern states had long agitated over the policies of this man and his party, whose platform against the expansion of slavery seemed at odds with everything they valued. About the time Barton was patiently enduring the twelve-hour railroad journey from New York to Washington, the state of South Carolina declared the end of its own patience with the Union's policies toward slavery and tariffs, and the nation's capital became a whirligig of excitement. Those with Southern leanings predominated in the town; they guffawed at the pretenses of that awkward lawyer from Illinois and slapped each other on the back in congratulation of the South's audacity and spirit. Just what the action of South Carolina and the states that followed it would lead to was anyone's guess, and everybody did guess. A spirit of debate and the airing of long pent-up opinions filled the atmosphere, and the speculation about the country's future was the favorite topic in drawing rooms and alleys.[6]

Miss Barton, sitting at her desk in the ladies' section of the Patent Office, held close to her conviction that a moderate course would prevail. No rabid abolitionist, she had opposed the mass meetings and fiery oratory that the North had offered a year earlier in support of John Brown's raid on the federal arsenal at Harpers Ferry. The South, she believed, had a right to feel fearful in the face of such misplaced zealotry. But she had scarcely expected them to dissolve the Union, and now, in January 1861, she did not think their hotheaded move would be permanent. "Would it be of the least interest if I should talk to you of political excitement and 'secession'?" she asked cousin Elvira Stone. "I believe the latter to be wearing out in its infancy and if wisely left alone will die a natural death, long before maturity."[7] Like Robert E. Lee, who expected that "the wisdom and patriotism of the country will devise some way of saving it,"[8] like countless others with hope or naiveté in their hearts, Barton chose to view the Union as undividable. What rankled her was the bravado shown by Southern sympathizers, who saw triumph for the culture of the slave states and boasted of it in the streets of the nation's capital. "Nothing is or has been more common than to see little spruce clerks and even boys strutting about the streets and asserting that 'we had no government—it merely amounted to a *compact* but had no strength,'" she wrote furiously a few months later. "I have listened to harangues of this nature in the few past months until my very brain whirled—and now from the bottom of my heart—I pray that the thing may be tested."[9]

The political fever in Washington reached its highest degree with Abraham Lincoln's arrival in the city. Threats on his life and rumors of rioting had been so numerous that the lean westerner had quietly entered the town the day before he had planned to, disguised in an old slouch hat and baggy coat. Many thought he would not live to become president, but Barton reported to her friend Annie Childs that the "4th of March has come and gone, and we have a *live Republican* President, and, what is perhaps singular, during the whole day we saw no one who appeared to manifest the least dislike to his living." She had attended the inauguration, thought the speech acceptable and the delivery good, but had turned down an invitation to the inaugural ball because of a bad cold. Sensing few of the ominous rumblings that foretold the coming conflict, she retained a haughty indifference to the earnest Southern leaders, viewing them as something akin to naughty children, who, if ignored, would come sheepishly back to the bosom of the family. Her letter to Childs ended, not on a note of foreboding about the national crisis, but in raptures over the spring weather and concern for the tawdry state of her wardrobe.[10]

Perhaps it was that she was less concerned with the Union's safety than with her own vulnerability in the Patent Office at that time. Recognizing that the political friends who had obtained her position would soon be out of power and that she had no guarantee of support from the new administration, she devised a plan to win some political influence. When last in Washington, as Clara told a friend, "I never formed any acquaintance with the Republican members of our Delegation as it would have been worse than nothing and now that it has come to be worth everything I have none of it."[11] She spent some time observing those who represented Massachusetts and decided that Henry Wilson, one of the state's two senators, could best support her. She initially tried to spark an acquaintance by persuading Cousin Elvira, who knew Wilson, to write a letter of introduction interesting enough that he would go to the trouble of calling on her.[12] But six weeks later the inauguration had come and gone, her job was in jeopardy, and she had as yet found no guardian angel. On a chilly March afternoon she therefore put on her bonnet and set off for the Capitol. Rather than ask for personal favors, she planned to speak to the senator about the generally crowded and overworked conditions of the Patent Office, in which she knew he had an interest.

This time her scheme succeeded. Scarcely had Clara called Wilson out of the Senate chambers than "he set away his hat, arranged his coat sleeves, and settled himself into a conversable posture which seemed to say 'let us talk, I am ready', and we did talk."[13] Their understanding had been immediate; it was the beginning of a long and important friendship. They talked that afternoon, walked home together through the fashionable Capitol grounds, and then met again, only a few hours later. "Oh yes he is married," Barton joked to Elvira.[14]

Barton made a savvy choice in picking Wilson to be her patron. Ambitious and effective in his work (one observer called him "the most skilful political organizer in the country"[15]), Wilson exuded a calculated geniality that made him almost a caricature of the successful politician. His big florid face shifted easily to delight or anger. He had had a poverty-stricken childhood in Massachusetts and

pprenticeship as a cobbler; the memories of these early years were not
and he strove to overcome them with each decisive political maneu-
he time he met Clara, Wilson was completing his first Senate term and
had already become an impressive force in that body. His influence would grow
rapidly with the coming of war, when, as chairman of the Military Affairs Committee, and with the complete confidence of Mr. Lincoln, he wielded enormous
power. In March 1861 Barton had little concept of what Wilson's influence would
mean for her in the next four years. She thought only that her clerkship might
not be lost under the Lincoln administration, that her future in the Patent Office
was more secure.

She was in fact pleased with her prospects under Lincoln. The new commissioner of patents, D. P. Holloway, seemed to have no objection to women in his
office. On the contrary, rumors had it that he enjoyed their presence.[16] Wilson,
who had once told some prejudiced office seekers that he "supposed that it was
the design of the Almighty that women should *exist*, or he never would have
created them, although it is a scanty chance we give them,"[17] was inclined to
promote her interests simply because she was a woman. Instead of losing her precarious hold on a temporary clerkship, which was netting her only $35 to $61
per month, Barton had hopes that she would be given a permanent position and
that her success would open the doors for other talented women. If this should
happen, she told Elvira, "I had just as lief they made an experiment of me as not,
you know it does not hurt me to pioneer."[18] Though the situation was far from
settled, she sensed that she had beat the narrow prejudice of the government
officials at last—indeed had beat them at their own game of spoils and patronage. With "all the influence of my State—personal at that" behind her, she
wrote giddily that she "should like to see that little click reprove me in this
matter—just let them try it will be fun—nuts, for me, I like it."[19]

Her own future secured, Barton began concentrating on helping friends who
were coping with similar problems with the government or the uncertainties of
the times. There were many who were impressed with the tireless energy she had
at this time for the problems and sorrows of friends, acquaintances, and relatives. One admirer recalled that he

> rarely saw her without some pet scheme of benevolence on her hands which she pur-
> sued with an enthusiasm that was quite heroic and sometimes amusing. The roll of
> those she has helped, or tried to help, with her purse, her personal influence or her
> counsels, would be a long one; orphan children, deserted wives, destitute women, sick
> or unsuccessful relatives, men who had failed in business—all who were in want, or in
> trouble, and could claim the slightest acquaintance came to her for aid and were never
> repulsed. Strange it was to see this generous girl, whose own hands ministered to all
> her wants, always giving to those around her, instead of receiving, strengthening the
> hands and directing the steps of so many who would have seemed better calculated to
> help her.[20]

She had not lost sight of her concerns for Mattie Poor and Irving Vassall, but their situations seemed in abeyance for the time being. More pressing now was a crisis for Elvira Stone, which brought to the fore all of Barton's anger at injustices to her sex. Since 1857 Stone had been postmistress of North Oxford, a political appointment that became vulnerable when the new administration took office. More than one gentleman in the town had his eye on Elvira's sinecure, which involved little work but brought in a significant revenue. When Elvira wrote of her worries, Barton acted quickly to inform Senators Wilson and Sumner that the pretext for which Stone might be removed had little to do with politics and everything to do with sex. Tempted to draw up a petition that began "*Mankind being naturally prone to selfishness we hereby . . .* ," Clara settled for reporting to Sumner and Wilson that she had been able to find no complaint against Stone's performance "except that she is guilty of being a woman."[21] With the aid of the two senators and some timely petitions from North Oxford's citizens, Stone's appointment was eventually secured. Triumphant against the "forces of blind prejudice and ignorance" that so annoyed her, Barton felt a modicum of satisfaction with her own abilities to overcome society's narrow standards. But the incident reinforced her awareness, too, of the disadvantage that even talented and willing women faced in male-dominated society; it glued one more rung in the ladder that would lead her to an active role as a feminist leader, bent on sweeping reform in government policies.[22]

Success in these matters, an outlet for her work-hungry mind, and cheerful diversion at plays and levees made her confidence again unshakable. A handsome new companion in the Patent Office, R. O. Sidney, amused her with his stories of the South and an obvious admiration. Once there was an end to the dependence, the boredom, and the uncertainty of the previous six months, the despondency vanished. She felt ready to face anything. In all too short a time she would be surrounded by an emergency that would require all of her powers.[23]

Fort Sumter was fired upon and captured by Southern rebels on a Friday. It was April 12, a memorable day when vague dreams, which pictured two peaceful nations existing side by side or the ultimate peaceful submission of the South, were shattered. The president was alarmed at the defenselessness of the capital and called for a force of seventy-five thousand volunteers to protect it from the rebels across the Potomac. Militiamen, and companies based on neighborhood groups and local associations, quickly heeded the call. Clara, as quick to rally as any volunteer, felt sure the Union would win. "She was confident, even enthusiastic," marveled a friend. If Sumter truly meant war, she would embrace the fray with all of her resources. "For herself, she had saved a little in time of peace, and she intended to devote it and herself to the service of her country, and of humanity. If war must be she neither expected nor desired to come out of it with a dollar."[24]

Barton was pleased that men from Worcester County mirrored her own enthusiasm. Among the earliest troops to muster in and board a train, amid cheers and tears and fluttering handkerchiefs, was the Sixth Massachusetts Regiment. Many of them were fresh-faced farm boys who had never before left their native New England, and nearly forty had once been Barton's pupils. Only four days after the firing on Fort Sumter, the Sixth Massachusetts left Worcester. On April 19 they arrived in Baltimore.

Baltimore's citizens were overwhelmingly secessionist in spirit. It was they who had threatened the safety of the president-elect, and they saw both insult and opportunity in the parade of Union soldiers about to pass through their city. The trains from the North would not merely stop at the station or chug slowly by the brick row houses with distinctive marble stoops. The configuration of railroad tracks and stations was such that passengers were forced to alight, find transportation to another platform some half mile distant, and wait for the arrival of the cars, which were being drawn by mules along a precarious piece of track. The soldiers would have to leave the protection of the cars and march through the streets of the city in full view of the hostile Baltimoreans.[25]

On April 19 exaggerated gossip proved true and worst fears were realized. The officers in charge of the Massachusetts men had ordered them to endure whatever the Baltimore mobs hurled at them—insults, profanities, or bricks—unless they were actually fired on. With raw troops and an angry crowd, however, there was little hope for restraint. Three men were killed and thirty wounded from the regiment that day—the war's first casualties. In Baltimore the rebellious mood was heightened, as defiance or determination grew stronger in every breast.[26]

In Washington, news of the attack flashed across the telegraph wires, and crowds began to form in the street. Barton, hearing the noise, joined the throng and was "thrilled and bewildered" to hear of the atrocities in Baltimore.[27] Her sister (who had returned to Washington with Irving) was with her; together they were swept up in the current that flowed toward the depot of the Baltimore and Ohio Railroad. Southern partisans predominated in the tumultuous crowd, jeering and shouting congratulatory slogans. By the time she and Sally reached the station, Clara was so "indignant, excited, alarmed" that she determined to render any aid possible to the weary and wounded men.[28]

The city was unprepared for the arrival of so many soldiers, let alone wounded and frightened raw recruits. Hasty quarters had been arranged in, among other inappropriate places, the Senate chamber. There were no hospitals or even barracks, and Barton filled this immediate need by bringing the most severely wounded to Sally Vassall's house. From the patients there she learned that the men's luggage had been seized in Baltimore and that many had "*nothing* but their heavy woolen clothes—not a cotton shirt and many of them not even a pocket handkerchief."[29] Hearing also that no rations had been issued them, Barton hastily set to work to alleviate the problems as best she could. The next morning, ignoring the fact that it was Sunday, she rose early to persuade neighboring grocers to sell her as many provisions as they would, hired a train of Negro servants, and proceeded to march down Pennsylvania Avenue, laden with parcels in wicker baskets. Besides food Barton packed every useful article she could dream of; she had emptied her pockets and drawers of combs, "sewing utensils, thread, needles, thimbles, scissors, pens, buttons, strings, salves, tallow, etc." Old sheets were torn up for towels and handkerchiefs. With such a cargo she had no trouble passing the guards at the Capitol. Once inside, her former pupils crowded around her, anxious for news. She had only one copy of the *Worcester Spy*, so she sat in the chair reserved for the president of the Senate and read aloud to the men, joking later that it was "better attention than I have been accustomed to see there in the old time." The troops were homesick and misunderstood the country's expectations, she noted, and pledged: "So far as our poor efforts can reach, they shall never lack a kindly hand or a sister's sympathy if they come."[30]

It was a crucial moment for Barton: this place and time united her self-confidence and strength of purpose with a glaring need. She had once told a friend that it would be a "strange pass when the *Bartons* get fanatical,"[31] but she became so, both in her devotion to the Union and her attachment to "her boys." Inside the woman remained the little girl who shunned Mother Goose's melodies, asking instead for "more stories about the war" as she sat on her soldier-father's knee. She had always looked first to her father for pride and inspiration, and she saw now a chance to emulate his philanthropic nature, to fulfill his teaching that "next to Heaven our highest duty was to . . . serve our country and . . . support its laws."[32] Remembering the spirit of mission that she felt in these early weeks of the war, Barton would later acknowledge: "The patriot blood of my fathers was warm in my veins."[33]

The troops from Massachusetts were soon followed by trains from New Jersey and Herkimer County, New York, all bearing old friends and former pupils. With the arrival of each new company, Barton's exhilaration rose, as did her determination to be a part of this great drama. She was amazed at the change in sleepy, rustic Washington, now a bustling place "grown up so strangely like a gourd all in a night."[34] Over seventy-five thousand troops were camped in and around the city. Their white tents were everywhere, they marched and drilled and loafed in the streets, and at night the stars were blotted out by the haze and glare from their campfires. Many Washington women feared the strange men; one acquaintance of Barton's recalled that although she had had no unpleasant experiences, she spent the war years avoiding the throngs of soldiers. Clara felt no such intimidation. The presence of the troops brought a feeling of intimacy to her that had been missing in the city, and their numbers thrilled and cheered her. In an early war letter she informed her father, "I don't know how long it has been since my ear has been free from the roll of a drum, it is the music I sleep by, and I love it."[35]

Clara and Sally visited the troops often. The DeWitt Guards, in which Bernard was now a fourth lieutenant, was a favorite company, as were the Fourth and Eighth New Jersey regiments, home for the familiar faces from Bordentown and

Hightstown. The two women played whist with the officers in their tents, joked with correspondents from eastern newspapers, and shook hands all around. They also discovered the small miseries to which the soldiers were exposed. Disease and vermin were prevalent in the unsanitary camps. Clothing was shabby, meals inadequate, shelter sometimes completely lacking. Clara felt some envy but no sympathy for the "few privileged, elegantly dressed ladies who ride over and sit in their carriages to witness 'splendid services' and 'inspect the Army of the Potomac' and come away 'delighted'."[36] Increasingly, she brought delicacies from home for the men: homemade jellies, cloth-lined sewing kits called "housewives," even whole pies and cakes. The soldiers wrote to their families with a myriad gripes in the early months of the war; at the top of the list were complaints over the inadequate food and the poor preparations the army had made for them. Energetic mothers and wives baked, preserved, and mended in answer to these grumblings, then sought a way to ensure delivery of their precious wares. Through a chance mention of Clara in a soldier's letter, someone's remembrance that she lived and worked in the Union's capital, or through Elvira Stone, who tirelessly began to solicit goods, individual women and relief societies started to connect Barton with philanthropic work with the troops. They began to send their boxes to Barton, certain that they could not go astray in her care.[37]

By early June she was so inundated with supplies that she moved her quarters to a larger room in a business block. Though less homelike, it had enough space for both Barton and her stores. Behind a wooden partition she kept the boxes and barrels; her own belongings were crowded into the remaining space. "It was a kind of tent life," noted Fanny Childs, "but she was happy in it."[38] The importance she had assigned her work in the Patent Office now seemed misplaced. She had not meant to start the rush of boxes from Massachusetts, but when she realized the distribution of the provisions would serve a significant need, she committed herself to the work totally. She determined also to remain in the capital, despite the fact that, like most other citizens, she thought it would come under attack shortly. "I will remain here while anyone remains and do whatever comes to my hand," she declared stoutly. "I may be compelled to face danger, but never *fear it,* and while our soldiers can stand and *fight,* I can stand and feed and nurse them."[39]

Barton was proud of the army in that late spring and summer of 1861, and as she sat calmly on the Treasury building steps watching campfires and Roman candles on Independence Day, she longed for their gleaming sabers to be called into service.[40] Even so she was unprepared for the outbreak of fighting only two weeks later. After Confederate troops, massed near Manassas, Virginia, held back the Union army's first advance with a decided rout on July 21, she watched the "sad, painful, and mortifying" scene of their return.[41] Hundreds of wounded began to pour into Washington, filling makeshift hospitals in Armory Square, Judiciary Square, and even the exhibit hall of the Patent Office. Then a new phase of her work began. She unpacked the cartons so carefully piled near her bed and distributed combs and compresses, dainty cordials and embroidered neckerchiefs to the patients. The personal contact with the soldiers in the wards pleased her, and she enthusiastically wrote letters, smoothed brows, and fed disabled men, but it sobered her, too. The bright banners and flashing hooves that had been her chief inspiration faded. It was the grim reality of war, the overwhelming, numbing misery, that activated her now.[42]

With something of a shock Barton realized how necessary her stores were. The hospitals were devoid of even the smallest niceties, and often the bare necessities as well. In its haste to establish an army, the government had sadly overlooked its medical needs, and now surgeons, nurses, and supplies were at a premium. She was further distressed by the neglect the wounded suffered. Some had gone days without food in the hot July sun; others had painful, festering wounds, which were left untreated until their arrival at a Washington hospital. One man, finally brought to Sally's home, had been left to rot until "all parts of the body which had rested hard upon whatever was under him had decayed . . . his toes were matted and grown together and . . . now *dropping off at the joints.*"[43]

Henceforth Barton would not simply receive supplies but would actively solicit them. An advertisement in the *Worcester Spy* called for the women to keep busy—"The cause is holy; do not neglect an opportunity to aid it."[44] She wrote personally to her old friends in Massachusetts and New Jersey, asking them to send what they could. "It is *said,* upon proper authority, that 'our army is supplied,'" she told the Worcester Ladies' Relief Committee. "How this can be so I fail to see." Begging them to continue to supply her, though no immediate danger was evident, she queried anxiously, "in the event of battle who can tell what their necessities might grow to in a single day? They would want *then* faster than you could make."[45]

In the next year Barton was overwhelmed with supplies. The women sent raspberry vinegar, pickled grapes, honey, soap, and lemons. What they did not send she bought from her own purse, spending up to fifteen dollars a day for bread alone. She became something of an expert on the vagaries of shipping, and she took time to instruct the women on the proper way of packing a box (small packages were preferable, and clothes were not to be packed with stewed fruits, which might easily spill and ruin the garments).[46] When the boxes overflowed her room, she rented space in a warehouse; six months later she had completely filled three.[47] Not content with accepting just what came to hand, Clara asked an officer what the troops needed most. To her surprise he answered "tobacco." Far from flinching at this, she took the part of the men against the reproving frowns of her own sex. "It is needless to say that I trust soon to be a good judge of the product as it has become an article of commerce with me," she told Vira Stone in some amusement.

> You would smile at the sight of the half yard slabs of plug lying this moment on my table waiting for Dr. Sidney's Basket of Whiskey to arrive to accompany it to Kalorama. *Dainty gifts,* you will say, but all necessary my dear Coz—this I conceive to be no time to prate of moral influences. Our men's nerves require their accustomed nar-

cotics and a glass of whiskey is a powerful friend in a sunstroke and these poor fellows fall senseless on their heavy drills.[48]

Barton's love for "her boys" and fierce patriotism were further stimulated and reinforced by her former landlady, the plain-spoken Almira Fales. Fales was surely the first woman to engage in army relief work. She had not waited for a declaration of war to begin her ministrations but had commenced garnering supplies the moment South Carolina seceded. Others might mistrust the outcome of this action, but Fales had had no doubt it would lead to fratricidal war, and she simply ignored the laughter of acquaintances who gazed at her work and "thought it was a 'freak.'" She continued to hoard delicacies and distribute them at her pleasure after the firing on Fort Sumter. Her snappy blue eyes and brash way of telling stories from a memorable fund of anecdotes made her a favorite in the hospital. Although her patriotism did not lack zeal—she once erected a tent in her front yard to minister to any suffering soldier who might happen by—she was extremely modest about the contributions she made. Before, during, and after the war she declined to discuss them, simply forging ahead in her blundering way, without fanfare or praise.[49]

Fales was also one of the first to sense the terrors endured by the wounded on hospital transports and as they waited for help on the battlefield. The injured men needed a middleman between the bullet and the surgeon. As early as the battles of Corinth and Pittsburg Landing, she made her way directly to the line of battle, and she continued working in that capacity—tending wounds, encouraging, and nourishing—until the end of the war. She plied the Potomac River in hospital transports during the tedious Peninsular campaign and, when not actually with the army, met the wounded as they arrived at the wharves near Washington. After one of her own sons was killed at the Battle of Fredericksburg, she redoubled her efforts.[50]

Fales's activities further galvanized Barton, who was beginning to acknowledge that the Washington hospitals were becoming pretty well supplied with luxuries and willing ladies to hand them out.[51] Soon after the battle at Manassas, therefore, she began to take her supplies to meet the ships and train loads of disabled and sick men and, like Fales, found the effort more rewarding than mere hospital service. It reinforced her belief that many men perished for lack of simple attention. She once told a reporter that she was, at this time, "deeply impressed with the importance of early attention to the wounded, and was made to see how much more efficient her service would be if it could be promptly rendered on the field of battle."[52] As she recognized the need, Barton felt a growing urgency and pursued her course with uncamouflaged intensity. Oblivious to the opinions of the more dignified townspeople, she transported her wares in any conveyance, and at any time, that seemed handy. More than one person could recall her small figure perched atop a ludicrously large wagonload of goods, clutching the seat and sides as best she could, while crowds of well-dressed people walked sedately to church.[53]

Throughout the fall of 1861 and the winter of 1862, Barton pursued this self-appointed task. It was above, and in addition to, her duties at the Patent Office, where she continued her chores on the "ladies side" at the same low salary. Clara later claimed that in her zeal for the Union she refused to accept any payment from the overtaxed United States Treasury, but government records show that she drew her salary throughout the war. She was, however, given additional responsibilities in December 1861. "I have been a great deal *more* than busy for the past three weeks," she lamented to Fanny Childs, soon after the New Year, "owing to some new arrangements in the office, mostly, by which I lead the Record, and hurry up the others who lag."[54]

The tenor of the Patent Office was notoriously pro-South, which aggravated Barton no end. There and elsewhere she began a new crusade—routing out those disloyal to the Union. In the office she offered to take over the work of two blatantly Confederate clerks, at no extra salary, if they were dismissed. The proposal was politely refused and served only to make her unpopular.[55] Her familiarity with the parcel section of the post office caused her also to lead a campaign there, when she found that unclaimed parcels were being auctioned off to gentlemen who sent them on to the Confederate army. Barton had the pleasure of seeing that the rebels were arrested, though a hoped-for bonus in the form of an appointment to the army's sanitary committee never materialized. Still, she was content as long as her "precious freights" arrived directly.[56]

The vagaries of the Patent Office and the treacherous dealings of local Southern sympathizers seemed of slight significance compared to a personal blow that befell Barton in February 1862. For months, cousins, nephews, and neighbors had kept her informed about her father's health. He had lost his robustness years before, and there had been a serious alarm in December 1860, but the old man's "oak and iron constitution" had forestalled the family's worst fears.[57] Clara had often thought of visiting her father, yet the image of North Oxford and the unhappiness she had felt there kept her from returning home, even when Sam, Stephen's boy, told her that the Captain "spoke in high terms of Julie and of the excellent care she had taken of him, but said after all there was no one like you."[58] Now the end was truly near. Barton turned over her work to another Patent Office clerk and went home to do her "last and highest" duties.[59]

Clara and her father talked much of the war in the last few weeks they had together. Captain Barton believed the Union would triumph but knew he would not live to see it; he therefore "committed himself and his country into the hands of a good and just God."[60] Clara sat patiently at his bedside, listening to the old soldier and telling him of her own war work. She worried aloud about the sick and wounded soldiers, soliciting her father's advice about how and where to give the most expedient aid. She had hoped to go to the battlefield, she told him, but was struggling with her sense of propriety, for women in the camps were often considered—and treated as—prostitutes. He brushed aside her fears, maintaining that a respectable woman would meet with respect from even the roughest soldiers. He then gave Clara a command that she would always recall:

"As a patriot he bade me serve my country with all I had, even my life if need be; as the daughter of an accepted Mason, he bade me seek and comfort the afflicted everywhere, and as a Christian he charged me to honor God and love mankind."[61] As a symbol of his faith in her decision he handed her his gold Masonic badge to wear for luck and protection.

Near mid-March Stephen Barton's condition worsened, his imminent death evident in the wasting away of his desire to live. He wrote his will and put his other business affairs in order but took no food or water for some days. Late in the evening on March 21, in Clara's words he "straightened himself in bed, closed his mouth firmly, gave one hand to Julia and the other to me, and left us."[62] The local papers heralded Captain Barton as a "brave and true man," and the house and grounds were crowded for the funeral, held in David's home.[63] Clara watched as they lowered him into the grave, next to her mother—gone over a decade now—and recognized that she was alone in a way she had never been before. Her "last earthly guide" was gone, her mentor, the most inspired and inspiring of her kin.[64]

The long hours of vigil at her father's deathbed had given Clara an opportunity to mull over her urge to join the army in the field and to determine the best method of preparing to do so. She had Henry Wilson's backing, but she needed someone with direct influence in the army who would supply her with passes and protection if she moved toward the lines. Most officials were not anxious to see Barton, or any woman, in the field, asserting that the women caused serious morale problems and at the first sight of a gun would "skeedaddle and create a panic." Their wealth of supplies was viewed as a slap in the face of the quartermaster's department, and their presence in hospitals was an embarrassment to the obviously needy medical corps.[65] General Ethan Allen Hitchcock, an aging leader of the volunteer forces, given to nosebleeds and esoteric philosophic quotations, refused Barton permission on the grounds that she would be an "unreasonable, meddlesome body, requiring more waiting upon" than she would give to others.[66] Barton had already begun to badger friends in official Washington for permission to go to the front. While in Massachusetts she decided to petition John Andrew, the governor and commander-in-chief of the Massachusetts forces, for a recommendation. Accordingly, the day before her father's death she wrote him a stilted, calculating letter, full of self-justification, references to venerable Bartonian service to the country, and allusions to her rebel-hunting activities in Washington. Assuring him that she had "none but right motives," she waited anxiously for a reply.[67] Governor Andrew answered her letter quickly with the promise of a "letter of introduction, with hearty approval of your visit [to the troops] and my testimony to the value of the service to our sick and wounded." As she was soon to find, however, it would take far more than this to get her official permission to follow troops to the field.[68]

Barton did not leave North Oxford immediately but remained to help clear away her father's effects and settle his estate, of which she was virtually the sole legatee. Captain Barton had believed in disposing of his property where it could be of the greatest benefit. David and Stephen Barton had been given land and milling equipment as young men; Sally received a generous settlement at her marriage, not to mention continual handouts during the financial ups and downs of her life with Vester Vassall. Only Clara had gone uncared for. Now she was the recipient of a modest acreage, a house, two horses, and some antiquated farming equipment. It was not a large legacy, but she was determined to administer it properly and as her father would have wished. One of her first acts was to make provision for the perpetual care of the family graves in the old North Oxford cemetery.[69]

Frustration grew upon Clara, along with boredom and a feeling of uselessness. "You must feel lonely there and anxious to get away," Irving sympathized, proceeding to give detailed war news, which only heightened her desire to get into the fray.[70] A few weeks later she wrote plainly of her envy to a young cousin, stationed in the muggy swamps of North Carolina. No account of his hardships could diminish her ardor for the soldier's life. "Why can't *I* come and have a tent there and take care of your poor sick fellows?" she asked with some resentment. "I should go in five minutes if I could be told that I might." She hinted that Dr. S. L. Bigelon, a brigade surgeon and distant relative, could request her services if he wanted to, but she feared that he disliked women.[71] Finally, feeling she had done all she could for her family and herself in Massachusetts, she returned to the martial spirit and frantic activity of Washington.

Surrounded again by scenes of war that had seemed far removed in her home town, Barton felt a heightened urge to follow the cannon. Almira Fales had gone down the peninsula between the York and James rivers that spring; she was hardly talkative about her experiences, but her strength of purpose reinforced Clara's own. She was "full to aching" when she viewed the teeming hospitals, and touched beyond words by the frequent visits of hometown boys and former pupils who often left some personal items with her to be sent home if their names should appear on the black list.[72] Yet she thought these urban hospitals abundantly supplied, and her aid seemed hollow and effortless. "I cannot rest satisfied," she complained to Captain Denney, "it is little that one woman can do, still I crave the privilege of doing that."[73] She was certain there were numerous ways she could be useful at the field, and though General Hitchcock might think otherwise, she was convinced that she was "stronger, better acclimated, had firmer health, better able to forego comforts than ladies in general. I had almost said *men*." She raged mostly at the injustice of the accusation that she would hike up her crinoline and flee at the very first threat of danger. Time and again she assured herself that she would not "either run or complain if I were left under fire."[7]

Completely frustrated, she tried to forget the war, at least temporarily. But the heroic scenes and simple life of the soldiers continued to challenge, exhilarate, and haunt her as nothing had before. She was sensible of the discordant serenity of commonplace events when acted out against the backdrop of the terrible conflict. She read avidly the poets' prolific works in every penny journal and ladies' magazine, musing, "What did our poets do for subjects before the war?" She might as well have asked what she herself had done for conversation, for dreams, for paragraphs in her cherished correspondence. "I'm as bad as England," she finally concluded after a last attempt to purge herself of the martial spirit, "the fight is in me, and I will find a pretext." [75]

seven

Colonel Daniel H. Rucker scanned the crowded waiting room of his office somewhat impatiently. It was a hot July day and the quartermaster's office was, as usual, filled with petitioning citizens and irate soldiers, who had come to leave baskets for favorite sons or brothers, collect their back pay, or angrily demand remuneration for property confiscated or damaged by the Union army. The sea of faces had paraded by Rucker for so many days now that he had stopped seeing them individually, and although he was a kindly man, with a genial face and comfortable stomach, he could no longer view these cases as particular tragedies. Checks went out, answers and small comfort were dispensed, but the actions had become automatic, the responses given by rote.[1]

He was surprised therefore to find his eye caught by a small, plainly dressed woman sitting in the corner. She was not beautiful; at best her face was full of interest and the character of middle age. Yet there was an arresting quality to this woman, something that commanded attention and respect.[2] Rucker called her over to his desk; to his surprise she burst into tears when he asked what she wanted. "I want to go to the front," she choked out. Attempting to keep his patience, Rucker explained that the front was no place for a lady, there was to be a battle soon, and it would be next to impossible to find any relatives she might have in the army. But with a studied meekness she told him she wanted only to distribute some stores she had collected for the soldiers. She needed a pass and some wagons. Then she played her final card, telling him this was no basket of made-by-loving-hands delicacies she was describing, but three warehouses full of hospital stores and food—everything, in fact, that the soldiers needed.[3]

In an instant Barton's world changed. With a haste that seemed absurd in light of the months of tedious waiting, Rucker wrote out an order for six wagons, teamsters and men to load them, and requests to the surgeon general, secretary of war, military governor of Washington, D.C., and other crucial officers to allow

87

Miss Clara Barton to pass through the lines "with such stores as she may wish to take for the comfort of the sick and wounded."[4] Where logical and patient petitioning had failed, influential friends and loyal relatives had been unsuccessful, and demonstration of sincerity and need had been ineffectual, tears had worked. If Barton's incipient feminist views were at odds with this, she never admitted it. It was a trick she would use with success on many occasions, and she always recounted the episodes dramatically, without a hint of apology.

The Army of the Potomac was camped near Fredericksburg, Virginia, and this is where she intended to deliver her supplies. But she did not leave at once, preferring first to visit her family in Massachusetts, supply a few more Washington hospitals, and get her stores in order. She began to feel an interest around this time in the plight of runaway and freed slaves—"contraband" as they were called—who were crowding the Union lines, and she shared some of her supplies with them. Feeling that she would need some protection on the ninety-mile journey through rebel country, Barton also spent time arranging for additional passes for two gentlemen and a lady companion.[5]

On August 2 they set off, reaching the Union camps the next day. Barton and her comrades distributed their stores and were cordially received by both officers and men. She breakfasted at the Lacy House—a gracious eighteenth-century structure where elegant entertainments had been held for Fitzhughs, Washingtons, and Lees—with the officers of the Twenty-first New York Regiment, not knowing that in four months the house would be the site of some of the most grisly scenes she would see in the war. The next day, she found her beloved Twenty-first Massachusetts, greeted privates and officers, took special pains to cultivate the friendship of Dr. Clarence Cutter, the old regimental surgeon, and enjoyed the cheers and adulation of her boys. The cheers could not, however, hide the deprivation in the army, which more than fulfilled her expectations. She returned to Washington on August 5 to gather more supplies to send along to her co-workers who had stayed on in the camps.[6]

Scarcely had she arrived back than news of a clash between the two armies near Culpeper, Virginia sent dots of panic along the telegraph lines. The battle, variously referred to as Cedar Mountain, Cedar Run, and Culpeper, took place on August 9. General Lee's Southern army and the Union army under John Pope had met in a vast cornfield on a sweltering day. Despite a valiant and somewhat desperate charge by Union forces under General Nathaniel Banks, the North was soundly beaten, and their casualties numbered almost two thousand. On a Monday morning Barton learned these details; imagining the groans and suffering, she determined to go to the front.

It was here, as she later recalled, that she "broke the shackles and went to the field."[7] She did not ask for new passes, for they would most likely be denied. Instead she used the old ones meant only for safe transportation to an unengaged army in camp. On this sultry August day she gave up her last concerns over the propriety of her army work, letting the immediate need forestall her fears of insults or abuse. The "groans of suffering men dying like dogs, for the life of every institution" she valued drowned the doubts in the back of her mind, the chief one being "the appalling fact that I was only a woman."[8]

Once decided, Clara was impatient to go and promised herself she would leave the first moment access could be obtained.[9] She went to the Massachusetts state supply agent to get additional supplies and arranged to have them sent by rail to the scene of the battle. She then rounded up Cornelius Welles and a Mrs. Carner, who had helped her in Fredericksburg. Carner, a middle-aged woman with plump, capable hands and a ready smile, was able to work tirelessly in the soldiers' hospitals but was skittish near the battlefield. Welles complemented her skills. He had been sent by a missionary society from his home church in Hartford, Connecticut, to work in freedman's schools in Washington, but as the war commenced he began to work chiefly with the wounded. He had a tendency to talk to pain-wracked soldiers of the "Physician of the Soul," a habit which annoyed Barton. But they worked well together because he subordinated himself, instinctively following Clara's commands in the heat and confusion of battle. She later described him in terms that revealed her ideal of a fellow worker: he was "a meek, patient, faithful" follower.[10]

On August 13, Barton and the other workers clambered aboard the creaking cars to Culpeper, arriving about five o'clock. Though the battle had been over for four days, Barton immediately saw the suffering she had imagined for eighteen months, suffering that made her shudder and despair. "I cannot describe it," she jotted in her diary.[11] Almost at once she began transferring her stores from the freight car to wagons. Dr. James Dunn, a Pennsylvania surgeon who would become one of Barton's special admirers, told his wife of her midnight visits to his hospital. The poorly equipped surgeons were out of dressings of every kind and gratefully received her bandages, salves, and stimulants. "I thought that night," Dunn wrote, "if heaven ever sent out a homely angel, she must be one her assistance was so timely."[12] It was the commencement of "such a course of labor," Barton later told a group of women, "as I hope you may be spared from ever participating in, unless you have sinews of steel and nerves of iron."[13]

Barton found that the doctors and wounded needed all she had brought and more. The next day, at the Main Street hospital and at countless private houses that had been converted to shelter for the wounded, she saw that the anguished men covered the bare floors, lying in their own blood and filth, some without arms and legs, others with jaws or hands blown away. Many of the wounded had lain on the field in the blistering sun until a flag of truce allowed them to be cleared off. Sunstroke, dehydration, and shock increased their suffering. When thanking the women who had sent boxes of cooling cordials and soft linen shirts, she could write: "You will believe they were welcome when I tell you that we put shirts on men who had been stripped on the field and lain with naked breast in the scorching sun two days."[14]

Barton labored with "the strength of desperation" for two days and nights, without food or sleep, hardly knowing how to face the enormity of the suffering and able only to relieve small pockets of it. She, Welles, and Carner cooked food, made bandages, held hands, and helped the surgeons whenever they could. They drafted every available bystander for the work of cleaning the "hospitals" and the men, both of which were filthy.[15] When her supplies had given out "with a rapidity truly appalling," Barton was relieved to see the stringy form of Almira Fales jump with tight-lipped determination from the side of a freight car of reinforcements. She also saw that no matter what desperate scenes her mind had formerly conjured up, she had not anticipated this overwhelming carnage. Barton had believed herself bold and realistic. To her dismay she found that her ministrations were not completely effective because the horrors of the battlefield had been beyond the reach of her imagination. Her naiveté had left her unprepared.[16]

At Culpeper she was away from the battle, removed from the powder and noise she would come to know only too well, but she was initiated into the chaos and want that so characterized the Union's medical activities. No trained ambulance corps brought in the wounded. Supplies reached the surgeon days after the conflict, or not at all. At one station there was nothing but rooms of wounded and one broad table that served as stretcher, operating theater, and occasional bed. Simple necessities such as fresh water or clean bandages were luxuries in some hospitals, and she saw that most of the shelters were furnished "without a single convenience of life, without one cheering thought or view."[17]

Barton visited every makeshift ward she could, staying until her last shirt had been handed out. Before leaving Culpeper she visited a hospital of wounded Confederate prisoners, who had been badly neglected in the furious rush to supply the Union casualties. Believing her to be a local resident, they begged her to bring them sheets and clothing—anything that would lighten their suffering. When she told them she was from Massachusetts, their faces fell, but an observer recalled that tears came into some eyes as she brought in every article she could for their comfort. Impartiality became a watchword of her war work. Pain and anguish, she believed, were scarcely held in monopoly by the Union men, and she could not bear to see unmitigated distress. Moreover, she had always liked helping the lowliest underdogs, for they heaped on her the greatest praise and gratitude. The feelings of the boys in blue came close to adulation, but, after all, she was a staunch Unionist, and these were her friends, her defenders. To the Confederate soldier who was surprised by her aid, who believed he would find neglect and brutality within the Union lines, her spot of comfort was an unexpected gift, for which he was generous in praise and gratitude. If there were tears in the rebels' eyes, if they hailed her as an exception to the hated "damn Yankee," Barton relished it and solicited their worship.[18]

Barton later told lecture audiences—in theatrical tones, which both heightened the image of her work and distorted it—that she had worked for five days and nights at Cedar Mountain. Her diary shows, however, that after two days she left Culpeper, went home, and slept for twenty-four hours.[19] This would not

be the only time she exaggerated. Believing in the power of strongly stated publicity, she also wrote a series of letters that, though theoretically penned to
friends during the press of work, were in reality written afterward with the
knowledge that their calculated drama would lend them to publication. Clara
had long combined a swift, sure, and witty style of writing with a heightened
sense of the tragedy and tension in human life. The conflict that surrounded her
now accentuated these skills. The extent of her own naiveté led her to realize
the total ignorance of the North about the real conditions of the war. In bold
phrases, well planned to horrify and inspire, she described the patience of the
men, their wants, and their noble cause. After Culpeper, she wrote the first of
these letters, describing the "golden ringlets of the fair-cheeked boy, the weeping, waiting, mother's idol," and "the blood-matted and tangled locks of the
sterner, braver man, who has faced death on many a field. . . . The bright
stream that trickles . . . to the floor—is it wine? Ah, who shall count the value
of the wine of life?"[20] In a frenzy of patriotic fervor she rallied her reader to uphold the Union cause for which these men were so valiantly fighting. "At no
moment of my life has our country seemed worth so much or her institutions so
sacred as now," she stated, "in the fearful trial of fire and blood, she shows us that
she can produce, and nurture, and educate, and sacrifice such sons."[21]

Barton hardly knew how to return to normal life after this experience. She
could not react to commonplace sights and sounds but spent her time mending
socks for the soldiers and pleading with her contacts in New Jersey and Massachusetts to send her more supplies. In one battle she had emptied her three warehouses, and now to meet the army's "terrible necessities" she had only her empty
hands.[22] She was no longer working at the Patent Office, though her name remained on the registers, presumably keeping her place open for the day that hostilities would cease. "Miss C. H. Barton" also collected her pay throughout the
war, but half of the salary went for the use of a substitute, who did her work and
collected the pay under Barton's name.[23] Such a practice was common in D. P.
Holloway's Patent Office. The commissioner's unqualified support for the North
led him to make exceptions and allowances for anyone helping the army—not
always to the satisfaction of the other department clerks who were required to
take up the slack. One, who became so annoyed that he petitioned Congress
with his complaints, noted that by thus paying salaries to absent clerks the commissioner was "taxing the office *twice* for *one* service."[24] But for Barton, the fact
that her place was held was a measure of security in what was an otherwise disturbing and chaotic, if exciting, period of her life.

On August 30 Barton made one of her routine trips to the hospital on Armory
Square. She was taking some small toilet articles to one of her boys of the
Twenty-first Massachusetts when she chanced to hear the news of a battle that
had taken place on the old Bull Run battlefield near Manassas, Virginia. Crowds
of people were flocking to the Sixth Street wharf for news of the encounter, and

Clara went along, anxious to verify the rumors.[25] What she heard was more disastrous news for the Union. General John Pope's troops had retreated from their defeat at Cedar Mountain along the Rappahannock River, hoping to meet General George McClellan and the Army of the Potomac. But Robert E. Lee's Army of Northern Virginia had cut them off and forced a battle on the site of the first Battle of Bull Run. The troops were exhausted and leaders hesitant or entirely absent. Union casualties were, as usual, heavy; Clara heard reports that over eight thousand were wounded, though this later proved an exaggeration. Union medical care was, as ever, inadequate.

Barton rushed home suffused with excitement and energy. From Colonel Rucker and the burgeoning Sanitary Commission (a relief agency started by northerners concerned about the Union army's lack of supplies) she requisitioned stores. Before daybreak the next morning, she donned her battlefield uniform—a plain, dark print skirt and blouse, which for pragmatic reasons eschewed the fashionable hoopskirts and furbelows of the era—and alerted Cornelius Welles, Almira Fales, and two friends from New Jersey, Lydia Haskell and Ada Morrell. Pausing only long enough to pen a hasty letter to her brother David, she prepared to depart.[26] "I leave immediately for the Battlefield," she wrote, "don't know when I can return. If anything happens [to] me you David must come and take all my effects home with you and Julie will know how to dispose of them." She dashed off a similar note to Vira and was on her way.[27]

Rucker had supplied her with men to load a boxcar that night, and the next morning in a drenching rain she joined the train as it "steamed and rattled out of Washington."[28] She managed to squeeze herself into a spot atop the boxes and barrels and spent the trip wondering whether she would be thrown out of the open side door. It took two hours to make the eight-mile trip to Fairfax Station, where the federal wounded were being taken. This was excellent time compared with the experiences of many trains that day. The medical officials had thrown up their hands in the face of the slaughter at Second Bull Run and reluctantly advertised in newspapers for "surgeons and nurses (male) to attend to the wounded." The thought of adventure and easy pay attracted a whole range of unsuitable men, who held up the trains or celebrated their delays by breaking open the casks of wine and brandy meant to revive the wounded. One train took eleven hours to travel from Alexandria to Fairfax Station, and when it arrived the bands of workers more resembled brigands than conveyors of mercy.[29]

At ten o'clock the train rolled to a stop and Barton stepped gingerly from her precarious perch. She had believed herself a little inured to the agonized visages of the wounded, but the scene at Fairfax Station shocked and frightened her. The station was surrounded by thinly wooded hills, their grass burnt yellow and dry from the scorching Virginia sun. Stretched out on these hills were thousands of wounded men, covering the landscape in every direction.[30] "The eye wearied, the heart grew faint in seeing them," wrote a chaplain who was there that Sunday morning.[31] A threadbare procession of stretchers came in from the field to the temporary operating theaters. Frantic surgeons worked there, horrible with "their knives and uprolled sleeves and blood-smeared aprons, and by their sides ghastly heaps of cut off legs and arms." Surrounded by the shrieks and wailings of the wounded, Clara, for a moment, panicked.[32] They were the earliest relief workers to arrive, and with a start she realized that they were but "a little band of almost empty handed workers, literally by ourselves in the wild woods of Virginia with 3000 suffering men crowded upon the few acres within our reach."[33] But it was not like her to give up or complain, and she quickly plucked up her courage.

This was not a hospital with tents or beds but a way station for those wounded who were to be taken on to Washington. The most fortunate lay on rough straw that had been hastily laid on the hillside. Many had been transported over twenty-five miles of rough roads in ill-designed and crowded ambulances; most had not had food or water for two days. These were the simple needs Barton hoped to meet. Her place, she later acknowledged, was "anywhere between the bullet and the hospital." Her work was to keep as many men alive as she could before they could reach expert assistance.[34]

With a box of motley tinware and some cornmeal, she began to cook. When the meal gave out she made a concoction of crushed army biscuits, wine, water, and brown sugar to feed the languishing men. "Not very inviting you will think, but I assure you always acceptable." She lacked receptacles in which to hand it round, relying on empty jelly jars and wine bottles for the purpose.[35] In moments away from the kettle, she ministered to whatever need she found among the men. For many she bound wounds, to others she gave last rites or a clean shirt, or simply closed their glazed eyes. Many needed encouragement and a friendly voice as much as they needed water. One young boy, who haunted Barton for the remainder of her life, mistook her for his sister, and she sat with him through a fever-raged night, then pleaded with surgeons to include him on the hospital train, though his case was hopeless. If in her own estimation her resources were inadequate, her assistance again seemed a godsend to those about her. Dr. Dunn who had seen her as a "homely angel" at Culpeper, remembered the despair of the surgeons at Fairfax Station, where he said, "we had nothing but our instruments, not even a bottle of wine." To his amazement and joy he saw that "when the cars whistled up to the station, the first person on the platform was Miss Barton to again supply us with bandages, brandy, wine, prepared soup, jellies, meals, and every article that could be thought of."[36]

The inadequate medical services of the Union army made Barton's work at this battlefield station among the most difficult—and important—that she would perform. No system of hospital care or emergency relief had yet been established, though Dr. Jonathan Letterman, an earnest and creative surgeon, had been brought on a month earlier to tackle the problem. Care for those who were shot or ill was left to the individual regiments, and this generally collapsed in the pandemonium that followed a battle. Among the worst problems was the lack of trained ambulance workers, not to mention the disastrous design of the ambulances themselves, which were ungainly, two-wheeled ox carts that swayed and tipped on the rough roads so that a man had not even the consolation of a level bed. If he survived the trip he could look forward to medical care that included ignorance of bacterial infection. "We operated in old blood-stained and often pus-stained coats . . . with undisinfected hands," wrote a Union surgeon. "We used undisinfected instruments . . . and marine sponges which had been used in prior pus cases and only washed in tap water." Quinine and morphia were practically the only drugs available for whatever ailed the men, and the mortality rate among the wounded during this early part of the war was truly dismaying. Nearly 90 percent of those suffering abdominal wounds died despite hospital ministrations, as did 62 percent of those with other wounds. The statistics were even higher at the field of Second Bull Run. On the long retreat down the Rappahannock the valuable medical supplies, considered cumbersome and expendable, were left by the roadside as the men wearied. In all only two wagons of medical supplies reached hospital personnel at this battle.[37]

Though Barton would rail against the "heartless officers" whom she thought responsible for these statistics, it was impossible for her to view her wounded boys in aggregate numbers, for she was caught up with the private suffering of each individual soldier. Her accounts of this most personal of wars, which touched Americans as no other conflict, appear not as a continuum but a collection of stories and scenes, strung together like beads on string by a memory so jumbled with weariness, blood, and a thousand small crises, that it could not possibly sort them into consecutive facts. She was too busy to note each day's events in the small pocket diaries she always carried with her, but they are filled with the names of dying men and last messages, each one too precious at that instant to be overshadowed by the larger reality of war. With more grief than surprise she recognized some powder-stained faces. It was not "a light thing . . . to pick up a shattered arm to bind and sling it and find the other suddenly thrown across your neck in recognition. Oh what a place," she lamented, "to meet an old-time friend."[38]

Thus she worked on through that night and the next day, overwhelmed by the numbers yet never losing sight of new ambulance trains leaving more men to take the place of those already transferred to Washington. At night the horrors were increased, for the wounded men lay so close to each other that the workers could not step for fear of injuring them. The candles they carried made fire an ever-present risk on the windy, hay-covered hillside, and Clara lived "in terror lest some ones candle fall into the hay and consume them all."[39] Their supplies gave out with woeful rapidity. "I never realized until that day how little a human being could be grateful for—and that day's experience also taught me the utter worthlessness of that which could not be made to contribute directly to our necessities," Barton acknowledged. "Of what real value was that which could not save life? the bit of bread which would rest on the surface of a gold [coin] was worth more than the coin itself."[40] She feared, and rightly so, that whatever measure of aid she gave, it was not enough.

All day Monday she labored as she had on Sunday, unable to think of anything beyond the crisis of immediate need. She was working by rote now, squeezing out her own last drops of strength, for she had had no sleep for two days and had eaten nothing. As food became scarce she and the other workers took the meat from their own sandwiches and gave it to the stricken men. Clara and the others were demoralized, overwhelmed by the ceaseless parade of ambulances, the seeming indifference among army officials, and the confirmed reports of disastrous defeat at the hands of the Southerners. "It is no light thing to travel days and nights among acres of wounded and dying men, to feel that your last mouthful is gone and still they famish at your feet."[41]

Barton and the other relief workers could hear the shots of rebel skirmishers in the nearby hills, reminding them of Confederate dominance of the area and warning them that they must hurry.[42] Ebbing strength and fear of the guerrillas caused two women of the party to scurry home to Washington, leaving only Reverend Welles to labor beside Clara.[43] And beyond every impersonal sorrow was the dreadful start of recognition Clara felt when she saw the faces of friends and former pupils among the sufferers. "*Seven times!* in one train of ambulances, I passed this ordeal," she mourned, "you will not wonder that my heart is sore."[44]

Late that afternoon a thunderstorm blew up, and so did the sounds of another battle. Pope's ragged and angry men were retreating along country roads to the west when they encountered Stonewall Jackson's forces. Jackson's men challenged the Unionists to make a stand near the tiny hamlet of Chantilly. It was a brief battle, fought furiously in the rain, and two popular Union generals, Isaac Stevens and Philip Kearny, were lost here. Though it was a small victory for the South, it heightened the already serious demoralization of the United States troops.

This "cavalry charge in a cornfield," as a curious bystander described it, inevitably meant yet more ambulances, more stunned and bleeding men, more need and fewer supplies to relieve it.[45] Barton had caught a catnap by huddling in a waterlogged tent among baskets and boxes, unable to completely lie down. After sleeping for two hours, she sprang again to action after removing the matted grass and leaves from her hair and wringing the muddy water from her skirts. She spent the next day climbing from the wheel hub to the brake of every ambulance, determined to see that no man faced the long trip to the hospital without some water or a small portion of food.[46]

Rebel scouts appeared more frequently now among the rain-glistening trees. An officer rode up to Clara and asked her if she could ride a horse bareback. "Then you can risk another hour," he shouted to her affirmative reply. Should the Confederates close in, Barton knew, she would have to ride an unfamiliar horse cross-country through enemy lines to reach Washington. Fortunately this emergency did not arise. At breakneck speed Barton and Welles loaded the last man on the train about five o'clock Tuesday afternoon, then jumped aboard themselves, escaping just as a band of rebel cavalrymen galloped up to the station. Barton peered out from the boxcar as the engine puffed away and saw them setting fire to the little station, which had sheltered the helpless. "Two hours later," she told Vira, "and Fairfax Station is no more."[47]

In the days that followed, the carnage she had witnessed seemed almost too much for Clara to comprehend. The well-known scenes of Washington life, the fashion-conscious patina and nonchalance—even gaiety—appeared brutal and yet steeped in a familiarity that made the desperate days with the wounded only a horrible fantasy. She slept and wrote letters, including some for public consumption, and though she described events, she could not bring herself to retell the grisly details. "My heart is too sore today to recount to you the scenes of suffering I have witnessed," she told her friends. "Some future day, when their wounds and mine are less fresh, I will find strength to tell you."[48]

If Barton felt any small pleasure or pride in her recent experience it was in the knowledge that she had labored to her capacity and that her courage and energy had been tried and not found wanting. Four months earlier she had thought she "would not . . . run if left under fire." She had faced sniper fire and the threat of capture at Fairfax Station, and an eyewitness later asserted that her willingness to stay until the last man was aboard the train was "one of the most courageous acts of the war."[49] She had proved her value to the army, to the surgeons, and most importantly, to herself. Now she would tackle her work with a new energy, conditioned by an understanding of the tremendous need for her services and the confidence that she had the strength, as well as the desire, to meet it.

Barton had come to believe in "the folly or wickedness of remaining quietly at home" while the army was in the field, and she regretted to the end of her life that social mores had kept her from the field for over a year. "I said that I struggled with my sense of propriety," she told friends nearly twenty years afterward, "and I say it with humiliation and shame. I am ashamed that I thought of such a thing."[50] She rushed off again almost immediately, therefore, following the army to Hammond Hospital in Point Lookout, Maryland. Her young cousin Leander Poor was amazed to find her "just as usual," fired with enthusiasm, even after the experience she had undergone during the previous fortnight. "It has been more than a common soldier could endure," he noted proudly, "yet I find her with head, heart and hands full of business: calm, methodical, and cheerful."[51]

Thin fingers of light were creeping over the eastern sky a few mornings later when an army messenger slipped a paper into her hand. "Harper's [sic] Ferry—not a moment to be lost" it ran. She read it, then burned it in front of the courier, who told her when her wagons and supplies would be ready. The army that had been so reluctant to accept her services now offered her supplies and the best mules and teamsters, as well as privileged information about anticipated battles.[52] Robert E. Lee's self-assured men had headed toward Maryland in the belief that an invasion of the North would both inflict psychological damage on the already shaken Union and provide new fields to plunder. The Union army followed lamely, unable to prevent wily Stonewall Jackson from capturing the strategic mountain town of Harpers Ferry and taking thirteen thousand prisoners on September 12, and two days later handing them defeat at South Mountain some miles distant.

Only the faithful "Cornie" accompanied Barton, for she no longer felt the need of a female companion to protect her against the barbs of society's judgment. Although she would later laud the role of women in the Civil War and claim their bravery and competence for a victory over the doubts and superstitions of men, in actuality she scorned the women who surrounded her. She could feel nothing but contempt for the well-meaning ladies who

> When the charge is rammed home
> and the fire belches hot . . .
> never will wait for the answering shot.[53]

Even Almira Fales had hurried off at the first sign of danger, and though she only "went for stores," Barton could not forgive her: "*I* know I should *never leave a wounded* man there if I knew it, though I were taken prisoner forty times."[54] Women helpers caused Clara more hindrance than help when they were shaken or tired; moreover, they vied with her for recognition and the honor of equaling the men in nobility and courage. She came to agree with Colonel Rucker and the other officers who had tried to keep her from the front for these very reasons. Never again was she accompanied at the battlefield by a woman.[55]

Barton would test her strength again at the fields of South Mountain. At first her wagons passed the straggling blue-clad soldiers, and she revived them as best she could by passing out chunks of bread from a supply she replenished at each town. Then debris and grotesque forms began to appear along the road. The fighting was barely over when she finally arrived at the battlefield. Almost more dreadful than she could contemplate, the sight merited the only description she would write of a field of war. It was "all blood and carnage," she wrote with revulsion, "our wagon wheels within six feet of yet unburied dead. A mingled mass of stiffened, blackened men, horses, muskets, bayonets, knapsacks, haversacks, blankets, coats, canteens, broken wheels, and cannon balls which had done this deadly work—the very earth plowed with shot. . . . It was a fearful way to learn of a battle, a hard page to read."[56] She and Welles, "shocked and sick at heart," climbed over the hills and ledges to find the last wounded man and see that he got medical attention, then trod through the field to answer screams and whimpers. The last she saw of "that field of death" was the lingering haze of smoke and a "hideous pile of mangled and dismembered bodies."[57]

She joined the army then. Her four wagons became part of the ten-mile train, which crawled through Maryland's western valleys. The golden, peaceful country was beautiful, but Barton knew, as did the dispirited ranks surrounding her, that the incidents at Harpers Ferry and South Mountain amounted to little more than a dress rehearsal for an imminent and terrible clash. Barton was more frus-trated than demoralized at this point, however. Her carts and stores, which she believed should be ready the instant there was need, stood at the back of the creeping train, hours, even days, away from the troops destined for battle. The officers and drivers ahead of her refused to let her pass. They would "no more change position than one of the planets," she remarked.[58] Feeling a "terrible sense of oppression" as the armies approached the little community of Sharpsburg, Maryland, she devised a plan to travel all night through the caravan of wagons, which had pulled off the road for a few hours of fitful sleep. By daybreak, as the fetid air of men and beasts began to fill the muggy, somnolent valley, Clara was where she wanted to be: just behind the cannon.[59]

With the first roar of the artillery, Barton, feeling sorrowful for the men but as exhilarated as any general in anticipating the battle, urged her teams to a gallop, taking them eight miles across the fields to what appeared to be a dressing station on the right. Wading through a field of ripe corn so high that it hid everything from view, she came upon the farm of Joseph Poffenberger, a German immigrant who had fled with his family at the first sign of the armies. To Barton the whole wretched scene in the house already overloaded with the wounded was too famil-iar. Even the surgeons were those with whom she had previously worked. The first face she saw on reaching the house was that of Dr. James Dunn.[60]

His round face brightened at the sight of Barton, and his lips formed the praise that made her efforts worthwhile: "The Lord has remembered us; you are here again."[61] Their necessities were terrible, he told her. The house was so close to the field that shells burst among the workers, lighting up the sky in a brilliant display. The worst cases were brought here, those that could neither stay on the field nor endure the long passage to the distant field hospital. Those with entire thighs gone, with faces blown away or abdomens penetrated, were tenderly transported by comrades who believed there was still hope in the surgeon's small knife and rolls of cotton bandaging. Until Barton's arrival, however, there was little comfort for the agonized. Doctors Dunn and Chaddock had rolled up their sleeves to begin work with nothing but their instruments and a little chloroform they had hastily crammed into their pockets. Not only were the wagon trains as slow as molasses, but a railroad shipment of stores had failed to reach them. Men were bleeding to death from shell wounds, with only green corn leaves to cover, but not stop, the flow. Four tables with patients ready for surgery stood on the porch of the bullet-ridden house. With relief the surgeons accepted Barton's armfuls of bandages and stimulants and began their awful labor. Barton sized up the situation, drafted twelve loitering soldiers (who, to her delight, were from the Twenty-first Massachusetts) to help locate the wounded, and together with Reverend Welles began to answer the screams which echoed on all sides.[62]

On this, the "bloodiest day in American history," nearly forty thousand lives were lost. There were few survivors at the Poffenberger farm, where one of the relief workers estimated fifteen hundred men were crammed into barns, corn cribs, and mangers. Welles told his flock in New York that their work centered largely on "a grateful privilege to bathe their faces and close their eyes for the sake of loved ones at home."[63] Oliver Wendell Holmes, who went to the field at Antietam Creek to find his wounded son, wrote that it was "a pitiable sight, truly pitiable; yet so vast, so far beyond the possibility of relief, that many single sorrows of small dimensions have wrought upon my feelings more than this great caravan of maimed pilgrims."[64] This was how Barton too remembered the battle of Antietam—not as a sea of faces but as the bright image of one or two which appeared through the smoke that blinded and choked and sickened them. She extracted her first bullet at this battle from the face of a youngster who begged her to relieve his pain and let more seriously wounded men be attended to by the surgeons. With her pocketknife she severed for the first time "the nerves and fibers of human flesh," while a veteran, wounded in the thigh, held the boy's head. "I do not think a surgeon would have pronounced it a scientific operation," she said with a quiet pride, "but that it was successful I dared to hope from the gratitude of the patient." She held another face, offering the man a drink of cool well water, only to hear a soft whir and see his body quiver and lie still: "a bullet sped its full and easy way between us, tearing a hole in my sleeve and found its way into his body." Still another face that peered anxiously through that sooty haze looked to Clara too soft to be a soldier; the boy was suspiciously hesitant to have his wounded breast dressed. After gentle probing, Barton ascertained that the soldier's name was Mary Galloway. Barton could sympathize with this girl's spirited defiance of custom and her determination to join her menfolk at the front. She shepherded and shielded the girl, and subsequently located her lover in a Washington hospital. In later years Barton liked to recall that the two had named their eldest daughter for her.[65]

She cut an eccentric figure, standing over a kettle of gruel, with the hem of her skirt pinned up about her waist, her hair astray, her face covered with gunpowder.[66] But no surgeon would have thought to laugh at the sight. She had the habit of command and comfort, and the soldier aides turned naturally to her for instructions, which she always gave in a calm and sometimes infuriatingly unhurried manner. When, exhausted from the unrelieved misery, the medical men denounced the indifferent government that left them to cope in the dark without a single candle, she gently told them of the candles and lanterns she had brought. She would not flinch as she held a leg that was to be hacked off without chloroform, did not cry at the ghastly death of some former pupil. "Now what do you think of Miss Barton?" Surgeon Dunn asked his wife, after describing to her some of these feats. "In my feeble estimation, General McClellan, with all his laurels, sinks into insignificance beside the true heroine of the age, *the angel of the battlefield.*[67]

At the Poffenberger farm Barton saw the worst of the day's fighting and the worst excesses of medical disorder, despite the fact that medical services overall improved markedly at the battle of Antietam. Dr. Letterman had rounded up a team of competent and well-rehearsed ambulance workers, who could proudly claim at day's end that no man was left on the field more than twenty-four hours. Letterman had also begun to slyly supplant the ineffective regimental hospital system, proposing instead field hospitals on the division level with supplies distributed only to the surgeons in charge. It was a radical change for the slow-moving medical department, and one that did not evolve completely until the campaigns of 1864. The conservative career doctors of the army medical bureaucracy frowned on these humane innovations, believing they would cost the army money or slow its ability to move. They had reluctantly supported the newfangled ambulances, only to see the army order large numbers of the ridiculous two-wheeled carts, which caused more misery than relief. But Letterman had the support of Dr. William Alexander Hammond, the aggressive and self-confident surgeon general whose "immense energy and capability" made his promotion of new ideas a valuable asset. Together Letterman and Hammond fought to eliminate "the total want of organization, the drunkenness and incompetency" they had seen at Second Bull Run.[68]

The Sanitary Commission was also a crucial source of relief supplies during this battle. The organization had been started early in the war when disease and demoralization from filthy camps and inadequate food threatened to undermine the hastily assembled Union army. The prominent New Yorkers who headed the organization rightly predicted that disease and malnutrition would decimate the men more quickly than bullets, and they formed their own army of civilians to inspect camps and distribute everything from onions (to prevent scurvy) to cotton drawers. They fought favoritism to particular regiments with equitable distribution of supplies, administered from a network of regional and local auxiliaries. Not surprisingly, the medical department refused at first to acknowledge them. The Sanitary Commission went blithely on, however, cleverly harnessing the energetic spirits of volunteers from Maine to Kansas. Women from Chicago and Philadelphia organized huge "Sanitary Fairs" to raise money to outfit hospital ships and purchase supplies, and women at home knitted, preserved, and stitched, packing every kind of ware under the label of "sanitary stores." The goods they collected resembled those solicited by Barton, and they established warehouses similar to hers for collection and distribution. Eventually effective publicity and obvious impact on several battlefields won the commission both recognition with the army medical staff and nationwide fame.[69]

Alongside the Sanitary Commission labored the Christian Commission and a bevy of female nurses under the superintendence of Miss Dorothea Dix. The Christian Commission, whose purported goal was to "give relief and sympathy and then the gospel," was a branch of the YMCA.[70] It did seek to convert the soldier and warn him against the campfire sins of gambling and drinking, but especially in the latter part of the war, it also provided many of the same comforts as other civilian groups. Dix's nurses, on the other hand, were a breed apart. Experienced medical men might be unused to women in the sanctity of their wards, but the work of Florence Nightingale in the Crimea in 1859 had pointed up the terrible need for that routine care and cleaning for which surgeons had little time or inclination. Able-bodied men were needed in the army, and the use of women, however controversial, seemed a pragmatic solution for the under-staffed hospitals. Dorothea Lynn Dix, who had gained national prominence for her exposure of the scandalous treatment afforded inmates of prisons and insane asylums, was appointed to head the Department of Female Nurses. She was a small, birdlike woman, flighty and energetic, with a prim, pointed face. At sixty she was determined that no scandal should taint her nurses. She required that the volunteers be over thirty, plain of dress, and strong enough to singlehandedly turn a man in bed. Pretty girls with hoopskirts and wasp waists, or bold person-alities who craved adventure, were turned away. For the most part these nurses staffed Washington hospitals and, later, the divisional field hospitals established by Letterman. But Dix lacked executive ability, and this, coupled with her rigidity and nervous temperament, confirmed many a medical man's worst fears about female nurses. At war's end Dix left the organization with personal regrets: "This is not the work I would have my life judged by." [71]

In addition to Dix's workers there were countless unaffiliated women who la-bored as Barton did, with individual initiative and hand-to-mouth resources. Heavyset Mary "Mother" Bickerdyke worked with the western armies, alter-nately bullying and soothing the men until she gained the respect of surgeons and generals. Upon receiving complaints about her high-handed tactics, Gen-eral William T. Sherman stated to an aide that he could not correct her for "she ranks me." [72] Frances D. Gage fought in South Carolina for the rights of black soldiers, bucking prejudice in every rank as she struggled for impartiality of treatment. Mary A. Livermore directed the Western Sanitary Commission. Katherine Wormely took hospital ships as her special jurisdiction. In a tribute to these women, written in the 1880s, Barton acknowledged their contribution, and lauded the "hinderance and pain, and effort and cost" of their individual sacrifices. [73]

But it was only after the war that Barton came to identify with these fellow heroines. She wrote that her labor and the work of the Sanitary Commission were "in perfect accord, mutual respect and friendliness," and she frequently called on them for stores or transportation. [74] She did not, however, align herself too closely with any of these groups. She could not admire Henry Bellows, presi-dent of the Sanitary Commission, when on the eve of the Peninsular campaign he told her hard-working Worcester ladies that they needed to do nothing for a while because the army had "hospital stores enough . . . to supply all de-mands." [75] This was evidence to Barton of the inexperience and impracticality of the commissions: "a fudge," she called the Sanitary Commission in her journal. [76] On the battlefield Barton was often exasperated by clergymen who "erected a tent or two," then stood about "evidently considering what to do next." And she despaired of commission officers who refused to give a pair of socks to a barefoot soldier because they were saving them to put on the dead.[77] She was not the only field worker who complained of these organizations. Walt Whitman, strolling through the wards of the hospitals to cheer and sustain the soldiers, remarked on the unsuitability of handing out religious literature and the "way the men as they lie helpless in beds turn away their faces from the sight of these Agents, Chaplains, etc. . . . (they seem to me always a set of foxes and wolves.)"[78] As for the dour band led by Dorothea Dix, Clara wanted nothing to do with them. Hospital wards were the very arena she hoped to avoid, and she found the strong personality of Dix equally unappealing. Sensing that two women who had always prided themselves on working alone were unlikely to work well together, she avoided any work that would fall into Dix's jurisdiction.

Indeed, Barton was deadly serious when she referred to the Army of the Potomac as "my own army."[79] She was proud that she had cut the army's red tape and pioneered on her own long before the commissions became at all successful at field work. She was tireless and personally fearless, but she did not work well with others, for she disliked interference or competition. Feeling "cramped and unhappy" alongside other workers, she went to great lengths to avoid being "compromised by them in the least."[80] Furthermore, Clara Barton liked the praise that greeted her efforts and was disinclined to see it bestowed on an impersonal organization. "I do not believe in missions," she concluded.[81]

Welles and Barton stayed at the little farmhouse hospital for over twenty-four hours, getting only scanty bits of sleep, despite the relief nurses who took over after dark. "We could not think of rest, although we had had none for two or three days," recalled Welles, "for all around us were dying men, calling for water, for friends, for God to deliver them from their miseries."[82] When most of those who could convalesce had been removed, Welles and Barton began the journey home, distributing the few supplies that remained to hospitals en route. Clara had worked virtually nonstop for six weeks, and now, with her supplies and strength gone, she began to feel the nervous effects of too much work and too much sorrow. Her drivers, she wrote, "made up a bed for me of an old coverlid on the floor of a wagon; and I lay down on it, and was jogged back to Washington, eighty miles."[83] She arrived in the city dazed and with a violent fever, collapsing gratefully into Sally's arms. "When I . . . looked in a mirror," Barton stated, "my face was still the color of gunpowder, a deep blue."[84]

While the nation, impatient for the Union troops to pursue Lee's forces in western Virginia, watched McClellan's army keep camp in Maryland, Clara lay exhausted and ill of typhoid fever in the boarding house on Seventh Street. She wrote few letters during the fine fall days and only rarely received callers. Finally, after nearly a month, she gained strength, even as McClellan's army roused itself from its exhaustion in Maryland. On October 25, the quartermaster's office put a horse at her disposal in hopes that she would join the army, which had at last crossed the Potomac and was camped near Winchester, Virginia. Lee had placed his men at Culpeper Court House, between the Union troops and Richmond. President Lincoln, infuriated at the string of lost opportunities that McClellan had allowed, had brought in Ambrose E. Burnside to carry on the fall campaign. Burnside was pleasant and confident but not conspicuously gifted as a soldier. Nevertheless he devised an elaborate plan to outflank Lee and reach Richmond by way of Fredericksburg. Some action on this march seemed inevitable, and the army hoped both to improve morale and to anticipate any medical catastrophe by including Barton as part of the entourage.[85]

She caught up with the army at Harpers Ferry, taking with her a string of loaded wagons and the ever-faithful Welles, who she now referred to as an assistant, despite the fact that their labor had been planned and carried out in tandem. She took her own supplies and, following the Ninth Corps, ministered to the sick and those wounded by snipers.[86] A member of her beloved Twenty-first Massachusetts recalled that she brought along her knitting and "went among the officers and men chatting in the pleasantest way." One night a dress parade was held in her honor, and amidst fanfare and the flashing swords and trooping colors she so loved, Barton was made a daughter of the Twenty-first Massachusetts Regiment. "She made a little speech," wrote an onlooker, "and there was cemented a friendship begun under fire which was destined to last to the end of the lives of all participants."[87]

Barton reveled in these military trappings and never failed to look back on the "grand old marches down beside the Virginia mountains" with nostalgia.[88] The march was, in actuality, an ill-planned and arduous one, with skirmishes taking place both front and rear nearly every day. Food was in short supply, and one unit became so disgruntled that the men spent a day bellowing a chorus of "Bread, bread, bread" as they tramped wearily on.[89] Dysentery and scurvy spread quickly through the lines. Having seen the hideousness of war, its ugly purposes, and small cruelties, Barton would often speak as a pacifist in the remaining fifty years of her life. "Deck it as you will," she would proclaim, paraphrasing General Sherman, "war is hell."[90] Yet she could not hide her enthusiasm for army life, with its valor, camaraderie, selflessness, and color: "I am a U.S. soldier you know and therefore not supposed to be susceptible to fear."[91] On this march she was truly part of the army as she was never to be again. It was here that she could proudly claim that she had "always refused a tent unless the Army had them also and . . . never eaten a mouthful of . . . soft bread or fresh meat until the sick of the army were abundantly supplied."[92] Her memories of these days reflected few of the hardships and many of the most romantic elements of camp life. "Those bright autumnal days!" she exclaimed. "And at night the blaze of a thousand camp fires lighting up the forest tops, while from 10,000 voices rang out the never ending chorus of the Union army [singing] John Brown's Body."[93] She had shared all of their experiences now, battle and camp. There was "something sublime" about these young men. Identifying strongly with the common soldier who idolized her, she spent her time with the privates, eschewing the privileges of officers who glanced at her skeptically or hindered her work.[94] This was her badge of honor: that she was deprived when they were in want, sick when they fell ill, exhausted when the lines faltered and fell back.

She could barely admit to herself her need for soldiering. Instead, she and her champions explained her actions in terms that would gain approval despite the narrowest Victorian prejudice. "Clara Barton gave expression to the sympathy and tenderness of all the hearts of all the women in the world," wrote one enthusiast. Her womanly sympathy was lauded, not her executive ability or nursing skill. She was mothering her boys, nurturing them, smoothing brows as a sister and wife. Even the term "my boys" bespoke a womanly care and possessiveness. Beneath this crown of acceptable female virtues, however, Barton wore a boastful satisfaction at having bested the skeptics, proved them wrong, and outsuffered them to boot. During a terrific artillery charge at Antietam she saw every male surgical assistant run; she stayed, held the rolling table so that the operation could be finished, and did not fail to mention it afterward. Barton knew that her own bravery shamed many men into working under fire, and she deliberately took risks to prove her superior courage.[95] She raised protests of indignation among teamsters assigned to her, who were suspicious of her motives and resentful of her womanhood. One such rough group challenged her authority by working only a half day and thereby delaying the train. When she ordered them on they perversely drove until late at night. Her reply to this was a little speech crafted to acquaint them with both her magnanimity and ability to suffer. As "long as I *had* any food, I should share it with them, that when *they* were hungry and supperless, I should be, that if *harm* befell them I should care for them, if *sick*, I should nurse them." The men shuffled their feet, looked embarrassed and apologetic, and realized that they were up against someone who would use both her personal strength and the social considerations they were expected to accord a woman in order to dominate them. As for her being a woman, "they would get used to that." It was, she wrote with satisfaction, "one of the best moments of my life."[96]

After a few weeks Barton reluctantly left the army to accompany sick soldiers to Washington. Although her spirits were exhilarated, she suffered from hands chapped by "water and cold and burns and bruises and frosts." In addition, one hand had been disabled by a felon, which had had to be lanced in the field before her departure.[97] Once in Washington, for a short time Barton collapsed gratefully into the less arduous tasks of soliciting supplies, visiting hospitals, and writing letters. Her nephew Sam was worried about her, thought she looked shabby and tired, and hinted to friends that she did not have enough clothes to cut a decent figure away from the less fashion-conscious circles of the army. When, early in December, she set off again for the army, he begged her to "dispose of her stores if there was to be no battle and return to the city."[98]

The Army of the Potomac was now camped at Falmouth, a village across the Rappahannock River from Fredericksburg. It was an awful field, a stinking "wallow-hole" crammed full of unpaid, unfed, disenchanted troops. Barton and Welles took the "largest stores ever" to these men in army wagons requisitioned for them by General Charles Sturgis.[99] At Falmouth Barton established a hospital in the Lacy House, whose broad veranda faced the river that separated the two armies. She distributed stores as well as she could among the other hospitals but, sensing how near to battle she was, could not respect Sam's wishes about returning home. Instead, she stood by forlornly as the generals strode about, awaiting the engineers who were to make the pontoon bridges so crucial to crossing the river. Her spirits were lightened a little by the fuss with which she was received. "General Sturgis had his [ambulance] taken down for me and had supper arranged and a splendid serenade," she told a friend in North Oxford. "I don't know how we could have had a warmer '*welcome home*' as the officers termed it."[100]

The pontoon bridges that would have made the Federal army's entrance into Fredericksburg both timely and untroubled were not built until it was too late. Lee's men had a chance to catch up, establishing posts throughout the city until it resembled a ghostly garrison, for the citizens had long since fled. The rebels hid themselves in attics, cellars, and abandoned stables. Barton watched with anxiety as Burnside went recklessly ahead with his plan; a man of little imagination, he could not adapt to the changed circumstances. In the frosty moonlight on December 12 she waited for the morrow's battle and, unable to sleep, wrote of it to Vira. Though the letter was calculatedly poetic to make it suitable for publication, it was no less stirring or sad for its self-consciousness:

> The camp fires blaze with unwanted brightness, the sentry's tread is still but quick— the acres of little shelter tents are dark and still as death, no wonder for as I gazed sorrowfully upon them, I thought I could almost hear the slow flap of the grim messenger's wings as, one by one, he sought and selected his victims for the morning sacrifice—sleep weary ones, sleep and rest for tomorrow's toil. Oh! sleep and visit in dreams once more, the loved ones nestling at home. They may yet live to dream of you, cold, lifeless and bloody, but this dream, soldier, is the last, paint it bright, dream it well. Oh northern mothers, wives and sisters, all unconscious of the hour, would to Heaven that I could bear for you, the concentrated woe which is so soon to follow. . . .
>
> Mine are not the only waking hours, the light yet burns brightly in our kind-hearted general's tent, where he pens, what may be a last farewell to his wife and children, and thinks sadly of his fated men.
>
> Already the roll of the moving artillery is sounding in my ears, the battle draws near, and I must catch one hour's sleep for tomorrow's labor.[101]

Barton's dire expectations were only too well fulfilled. From every window and every sheltered ledge Confederate gunmen fired on the men crossing the river by the frail bridges and hastily constructed boats: "ere ten paces of the bridge were gained, they fell like grass before the scythe." She did what she could at

Falmouth, then received a note from a surgeon stationed in the beleaguered city. "Come to me—your place is here," read the note. A dying Confederate officer, appreciative of her ministrations, tried to dissuade her from going. Every house was the refuge of some eagle-eyed rebel. She would not stand a chance, he warned. With marked defiance she ignored his pleas, crossing the swaying bridge under heavy fire. As an officer helped her over the debris at the end of the bridge, a piece of exploding shell tore away a portion of her skirt and his coattail. A few minutes later a shell burst only thirty feet away, killing a cavalryman. "Leaving the kind-hearted officer," Barton wrote, "I passed on alone to the hospital. In less than half an hour he was brought to me—dead."[102]

She was working in the division hospital run by Clarence Cutter, the old regimental surgeon of the Twenty-first Massachusetts. The divisional hospitals were working well at this battle; Letterman's system had had the benefit of the experience at Antietam as well as time to train orderlies and ambulance teams. The supply system was also greatly improved, though Walt Whitman wrote after seeing this battle that there was "an unaccountable and almost total deficiency of everything for the wounded. . . . No thorough preparation, no system, no foresight, no genius. Always plenty of stores no doubt, but always miles away."[103] Barton and Welles established a soup kitchen large enough to feed several hundred wounded for many days, and Welles could tell his parishioners that "everything we took was needed; our noble brothers were actually suffering for these very articles."[104] While the men fought on desperately at Marye's Heights and hand-to-hand in the streets, Barton worked quietly among the tortured forms on the floors about her. Once again she smoothed brows, stopped the flow of blood, and gave what nourishment she could. Once more the faces were tragically familiar. Hart Bodine, the wayward boy that she had so effectively tamed in Hightstown, appeared as if in a dream, though he was one of the lucky ones who would recover. A man, smothering under a mask of dried blood, was revealed a bit at a time by her patient hands to be the sexton of the North Oxford church. His face, which she had known from childhood, was now hardly recognizable.[105]

The battle had been a staggering defeat for the Union troops, with over twelve thousand men lost. As the North clucked and cried over the news of "Burnside's Blunder" and the South gloated over a victory that Jeb Stuart called "one of the neatest and cheapest of the war," the relief workers gazed once more with shock at the carnage surrounding them. At Marye's Heights General Lee had refused a truce, and the wounded lay for three days in the December cold, adding frostbite and skin frozen fast to the ground to their woes.[106] Near the stone wall that had hidden their enemy lay eleven hundred dead men in a hideous heap. One Confederate officer could never forget the sight of these wretches lying "in every conceivable posture . . . here one without a head, there one without legs, yonder a head and legs without a trunk, everywhere horrible expressions, fear, rage, agony, madness, torture, lying in pools of blood, lying with heads half-buried in mud, with fragments of shell sticking in oozing brain."[107] The pile of dead weighed heavily on the minds of humanitarian workers, already numbed by the spectral streets filled with smashed crockery and the carcasses of horses, silent but for the occasional muffled hoofbeat. This time there was no victory in the slaughter, and it seemed that the men's bravery had been used in charges that were senseless and cruel.

Barton was everywhere in that pinched and unhappy town, saw every wretched collection of wounded men, knew every ugly corner. What stayed in her memory, though, was the dreadful confusion of the Lacy House. Clara did not flinch, as did fellow worker Walt Whitman, at the pile of amputated arms, legs, and feet that graced the door of the mansion—she had seen them piled to the shoulders of operating surgeons during the heat of battle.[108] But even a soul as inured as hers gasped at the spectacle of hundreds of sufferers crammed onto floors slippery with blood, balanced on the shelves of china cupboards, and wedged under the legs of tables. The agony there, within the physical remnant of a gracious way of life, seemed so immense that she later estimated that twelve hundred men were at the Lacy House, though official reports claimed something under three hundred. "All that was elegant is wretched," wrote a surgeon stationed there; "all that was noble is shabby; all that once told of civilized elegance now speaks of ruthless barbarism."[109] Individual names and faces from the house came back to Barton over the years:—a man saved by a tourniquet repeatedly saying as he clutched at her skirt, "You saved my life"; an officer, fatally shot, believing in his delirium that she was his wife. Recalling to a friend the terrors of this place, Barton remarked that when she rose from the side of one soldier, "I wrung the blood from the bottom of my clothing, before I could step, for the weight about my feet." For her the Lacy House became synonymous with inefficiency, needless suffering, and all the collected misery of the war.[110]

Until the last week in December she worked on, living in a tent beside her wagon. When her supplies ran out and the majority of the wounded had died or been sent on to Washington, she too made her way back to that overtaxed metropolis. She had no spirit left to toast the New Year. Instead she waded through the mud from the Sixth Street wharf, climbed the long flight of stairs to her room, "cheerless, in confusion, and alone," and sank down upon the floor and wept.[111]

eight

During the winter of 1863 Barton followed the example of the Union army by settling into sluggish semiactivity. She shared with the soldiers a bone-weariness, and like them she spent the dreary months living on memories of the past and expectation for the spring campaigns. She had neglected herself, her clothes, and her surroundings, but those seemed of small consequence after the privation she had witnessed. Indeed, she wore her shabby dress with pride, feeling it was one more link between her and the tattered foot soldiers. "I am glad too that I have not time always to make me a comfortable clothing," she told Mary Norton, "for I think I discern the shivers running under a soldier's thin shirt all the sooner." [1]

Her resources were very low now. She relied on the army for rations and her friends for discreet donations. After Cousin Leander sent home a description of Barton's scanty wardrobe, seamstress Annie Childs and other admiring Worcester County women posted her a box of elegant tailor-made clothes that left her weeping with gratitude. [2] Henry Wilson dropped by and pressed her for information about her finances. When he heard that she was denying herself so that the men in hospitals might have a few luxuries, he said in a choked voice, "*Our cause ought not to fail.*" Wilson hastily set down two five-dollar notes on the table, which Barton accepted without the least humiliation. "I prize it," she noted soon after, "from the source and the circumstances." [3]

Though her finances were weak and the soles of her shoes thin and patched, Barton's courage and self-assurance had soared under the seasoning of the guns. Her enormous capacity for work and commitment to the ideals of her patriotic father had festered within her before the war offered her an outlet. Much of her energy had been turned into useless self-pity or aimed uncertainly toward vague and everchanging targets. She had sensed that the undercurrents of her personality were strong, but as she admitted, "I did not know their strength—or where they would lead, or where come out to the surface and I was a little afraid of them myself and tried to cover them."[4] With the war even the most troublesome personal traits seemed to have suddenly turned to assets. The crisis had cemented the vari-hued bits of her discontent—the yearning to be useful, the need to exercise her courage, the constant desire for male companionship, and the love of adventure—to complete a perfect mosaic. In addition, the surge of confidence had helped Barton to shed some of her morbid introspection. "You no longer have an identity at such times . . . ," she would later acknowledge, "you are merely a channel through which flows hardest work . . . [and] you would never have to worry about your feelings, if you were as busy as the women who went to the front."[5] As she began to enjoy her new self-esteem, all the cares and memories of restless years seemed to vanish. "I was not as certain of my ground as I am now," Clara confided to a friend; "you would find me much more accessible, and easy now. . . . I am more open and 'don't care' and all in all I am better and happier."[6]

Much of her confidence came from the unabashed adoration in which she was held by the common soldiers. If she missed the attentions of a husband or the fulfillment of her romantic dreams, she now claimed a thousand ardent lovers who exalted her name or shyly brought her gifts of nosegays and apples. Officers saluted her, and a steady stream of young fellows in blue made their way toward her door on Seventh Street. They came to thank her, to show her their improvement in health, or to chat about the battles they had been through together. The man from the doorway of the Lacy House, whose leg Clara had bound in a life-saving tourniquet, called one afternoon. To her surprise he dispensed with traditional greetings, blurting out instead, "You saved my life." Neither thought that any other explanation for his arrival was necessary.[7] Sometimes there was more dramatic evidence of the army's appreciation. Soon after she arrived back in Washington she received an invitation to visit the men in Ward 17 of Lincoln Hospital. Each man had been wounded at Fredericksburg and treated at the Lacy House before being brought to the capital city. As she entered the room they shouted and applauded, some poor fellows falling back in their beds from the effort. She would not exchange the memory of their three great cheers, Barton later admitted, "for the wildest hurrahs that ever greeted the ear of conqueror or king."[8]

During the slow months when there was no pressing army work to be done, Barton used her influence to fight for pensions and favors. Among those she championed was Thomas Plunkett, whose arms had been shot away while carrying his company's standard and who had remained on the field keeping the flag erect with his feet. She also promoted a bill to institute Jonathan Letterman's far-reaching reforms in the ambulance and hospital corps. The remainder of her time was spent preparing herself and her stores for the bloodshed that was sure to come. The long string of battles from Culpeper to Fredericksburg had convinced her that even the most generous ladies' auxiliary could not hope to supply the army. She had had to draw stores from the Sanitary Commission, an uncomfortable procedure that both diminished her sense of autonomy and made its justification difficult. Early in January 1863, therefore, she petitioned Henry Wilson for permission to draw directly on the medical supplies of the government. Flannel underclothing and blankets were needed, she contended, as well as wine, condensed milk, tableware, and meat. "You have, I hope sufficient assurance of their being prudently and properly applied," she added somewhat defensively.[9] Though Wilson conscientiously tried to help her in every possible way, this was one request he could not grant.

Ironically, much of her lobbying worked against her. The very improvements in medical service that Barton had promoted were finally being implemented, and the medical department, in its grudging way, hoped the new ambulance corps and hospital system would satisfy the public outrage and coax the civilians from the field. Moreover, they had finally, and with great reluctance, recognized the Sanitary Commission as the official civilian relief agency late in 1862. That body had won its recognition at least partly on the understanding that it would channel the diverse charitable work of the war toward one really effective relief system. The Sanitary Commission and the army sought to eliminate the individual efforts that Clara Barton came to personify. The self-styled humanitarians who straggled after the army were, for the most part, a sorry lot who created more problems than they solved. Barton was a shining exception to the well-meaning but bumbling amateurs, but inevitably her name was linked with them. Nurses, packages, tents, and bandages were thus being bureaucratized. As Wilson said, in the climate of early 1863 it was impossible to give one lone worker, no matter how reputable, access to army stores. Such permission would mean official sanction for her efforts—efforts which already raised eyebrows since they were outside the jurisdiction of Dorothea Dix, the Sanitary Commission, or the medical department. Barton could not recognize, in this time of high personal confidence, that partially through her own effective propaganda the army had come to believe it alone must care for its wounded. The improvements she so fiercely advocated nearly made her obsolete. In January 1862, when over two years of the war's bloodiest fighting was still to come, she had already given her greatest service and seen her most direct action. Never again would she serve under fire as she had at Antietam and Fredericksburg. Increasingly she would find her work blocked by medical directors, nursing superintendents, commission officials, and generals.

What Wilson did do was to submit David Barton's name to the Senate for appointment as a quartermaster. Neither Clara nor her brother had sought the commission, and he received it with mixed emotions. David, now in his late fifties, was well past the age at which he would have expected to join the army. His prospering mills and family ties complicated his leaving Massachusetts, and his total want of experience and interest in military matters made him hesitant to accept the post. Both he and his wife thought that Clara, in her patriotic zealotry, had instigated the matter, and this, despite her protests to the contrary, caused a certain amount of friction between them. In fact, Wilson appears to have conceived the idea alone, as a roundabout method of gaining protection for Clara as well as giving her access to the quartermaster's stores. Clara viewed the plan—which she took as a compliment to herself—with delight. It was "completely what I needed," she wrote, thanking Wilson, "would so facilitate my movements, increase my usefulness and relieve me at once of all that I have ever found unpleasant in my field labors—viz the necessary contact with strangers upon business matters." She convinced David that it was his patriotic duty to accept the assignment, and he reluctantly conceded.[10]

Her program was now linked to his, and she waited impatiently in the next six weeks to hear where he would be posted. She marked time with her usual correspondence, excursions to the Senate gallery, and a hurried trip to Massachusetts, during which she badgered David to let his fifteen-year-old son, Stephen Emory, join the army. Julia Barton, already annoyed with Clara for whisking her husband away to a war that had heretofore seemed remote, was incensed. But Aunt Clara won the day, personally marching the boy into Worcester to see him outfitted. "Never was I so proud in my life as when I walked out of James store with my Aunt Clara, in my new blue uniform," he would later recall.[11] While in Worcester she took time to pay a visit to the women whose busy fingers had kept her own hands filled in so many crises. Yet Clara continued to find these trips to her old home unsettling and somehow vaguely compromising, and she returned to her makeshift Washington quarters after only a few days.

Toward the end of March David received orders to report to Hilton Head, South Carolina, where the Eighteenth Army Corps was preparing to bombard Charleston, that most sanctimonious of rebel cities. Clara easily received permission from the War Department to accompany him, and on April 2 she set sail from New York on the *Argo*, a trim boat that carried several other women as well as the inevitable swarms of military men. She experienced seasickness (from which she would suffer all her life), and was relieved to arrive on April 7. To Barton's surprise and secret delight she found that the bombardment of Fort Sumter, a key point in Charleston harbor, was to begin that very afternoon. "When I left Washington everyone said it boded no peace, it was a bad omen for *me* to start," she wrote gleefully in her journal. "I had never missed of finding the trouble I went to find, and was never late."[12] If she hoped for a major assault that day, however, she was disappointed. The guns began a pounding that would continue, to little purpose, for eight long months.

The Sea Islands to which the Bartons had come were a chain of irregular pieces of land, cut through by salt marshes and sluggish creeks to make a composite of islands and inlets. Many were little more than sand bars, with coarse, scruffy grass on one side and a wide expanse of sea on the other. The islands were famed for their excellent cotton, and there had been highly successful plantations on them before 1861, though the steamy climate caused many of the estates to be run as absentee holdings. The large population of blacks therefore had little contact with whites, and they retained their African customs and language to an unusual degree. The absence of white protectors made the islands easily accessible to the Union army, whose early sea blockade had given them control of the local waters. The large number of blacks posed something of a puzzle to the army, which could not possibly support them but was reluctant to see them starve. In an experiment that was to have a far-reaching effect on the nation's reconstruction policies, the army kept the blacks working on their home plantations while offering them some education and a chance to keep a measure of their earnings. A small band of workers had volunteered to run the experimental program, and they alternately relieved and irritated the settled monotony of garrison life on the Sea Islands.[13]

The first movements of the expedition to Charleston failed, though Barton dryly remarked that she had "seen worse retreats if this be one."[14] She was disappointed in being excluded from what little action did take place and was surprised to find that she had time to settle in and become accustomed to the pace of life at Hilton Head. She and David were given two rooms next to the chief quartermaster, furnished with a colleciton of makeshift furniture and castoffs from the local plantations: a large mahogany table "evidently once very costly," a rocking chair, an Egyptian marble-topped bureau, mosquito netting for curtains, and Clara's army trunk that unfolded into a bed.[15] They were assigned to the officers' mess—a situation which Clara relished but which made David feel awkward and bashful. To her further delight, several of the officers were old friends, including Captain Samuel T. Lamb, whose father had been the Barton family physician. His two sons also joined the party; both were bright young men in their early twenties, with hearty appetites and jolly laughs. Equally notable among the company was Colonel John J. Elwell of Cleveland, Ohio, the chief quartermaster for the Department of the South. He "possessed the rare combination of intellect, scholarship, business talent, spirit and gentleness, firm like a man and tender like a girl," Barton was to write of him; he was a kindred spirit with a broken leg, and she could pour on him her solicitude and companionship. Frances Dana Gage, a worker among the freedmen, and her daughter, Mary, were also much in evidence. Their challenging minds and easy natures were a welcomed addition to the already merry group. The table was resplendent with coastal delicacies—oranges, terrapin, shrimp, and fresh vegetables—and Clara told a friend, "You would smile to see *us soldiers* eating our dinner from the whitest of linen table covers with *silver knives and forks* but so it is." It was a different army altogether from that in which she had shared salt beef and weevily crackers with muddy men. She reveled in the glitter of gold braid and the starched linens, but she also had an uncomfortable sense that the real war was far removed from these civilized quarters and witty companions.[16]

Almost immediately Clara was engulfed in a social life, the equal of which she had rarely enjoyed. The gallant Captain Lamb and elegant Colonel Elwell vied for her company, sending bouquets of local blooms and baskets of fruit to her room and inviting her to ride with them along the beaches and old plantation roads. Taking a girlish pleasure in playing them off against each other, she flirted and teased and waited until the last minute to decide whose invitation to accept.[17] She liked to think of herself as among peers, a valued and accepted part of the army, and even had a riding habit made of blue officer's cloth with brass buttons.[18] Defending their pleasures, she wrote, "It is not the days of active service, marching and fighting that spoil an army but, lying *idle* in camp, the mind getting sour and rusty."[19]

Yet, in spite of the neat rationalization, Barton could not quite justify this "decidedly *fashionable* and splendidly *gay*" society.[20] Unable to forget that it was wartime, she found little comfort in dancing flirtatiously while the spectres of hunger and death haunted many of her boys. Less than a fortnight after her arrival she began feeling the pangs of guilt. "I cannot feel settled to remain here without some object . . . ," she confided to her diary; "I feel out of place."[21] Worrying that the army would find her a nuisance or brand her as a glorified camp follower, Clara defended her position to herself—"the Lord knows best"— then decided to leave, only to reiterate the old justifications for staying. She balanced thus between her desire to stay and her need for more active involvement, without being entirely happy about pursuing either possibility, for eight months.[22] In the end she stayed, partly because it was easier than a flight back to Washington, and partly because David, already disgruntled and lonely, would be abandoned. (His much-heralded appointment to the quartermaster's department was proving to be a travesty; it was a burden to the army and an embarrassment to her.) As time passed she felt increasingly sorry for her lost opportunities. "I am sick at heart . . . ," she told Mary Norton; "I only wish I could work to some *purpose*. I have no right to these easy comfortable days and our poor men suffering and dying, thirsting in this hot sun, and I so quiet here in want of nothing. It is not rightfully distributed, my lot is too easy—and I am sorry for it."[23]

But she could not make the decision to leave. In her uncertainty she wanted decisive counsel; this her acquaintances freely gave, but they were strongly against her leaving. "Still unsettled, my inclination says go, but others do not," she jotted in her diary.[24]

Of those encouraging her to stay, Colonel Elwell was the most ardent. From the first moment they met, he and Clara had rejoiced in an instinctive understanding of one another. "Words could scarcely describe all his kindness," she wrote on the day of her arrival. Within a week they were exchanging poetry and visiting each other two or three times a day.

Colonel Elwell's apartment was hardly commodious. Indeed it was a "dull, dingy room, with bare floor, . . . half a dozen shaky chairs," and a great fireplace, which served both to heat and light the room.[25] But Elwell's brilliant conversation, his "wit and humor, and scholarship lit up the dingy room." For him,

Clara was a welcome diversion from illness and trouble. "[You] who when I was disabled and strapped down . . . in a hot room—dark and dismal—," he told her a dozen years later, "came to me one evening and helped me more than medicine, surgeons, generals and all."[26] They spent their time with books and laughter, read Wilkie Collins's No Name together, and talked of Barton's heightened feelings about the war. "Called on the Col. had intellectual feast," she happily recorded.[27] It had been a long time since she had had an admirer who could at once charm her and appreciate her fine mind.

To add to their pleasure, they shared a love of horseback riding and were caught in a beautiful spot in which to indulge the passion. Like Clara, Elwell was a fine equestrian, and as quartermaster he had access to the best horses in the army's stable. In the early hours of the morning they galloped together along the beaches by water "as blue as romance could paint it, and virtually filled and glowing with phosphorescent light." They picked blackberries from the saddle and chased after sea turtles, then arrived late for dinner, mumbling excuses and trying to hide their blushes and exultation. Clara liked to test her riding ability against the men, and her success at both this sport and the game of repartee gave her a glowing confidence. She ordered another new riding habit and saddle, declaring that if affairs kept up in this fashion she should consider abandoning her foot-sore soldiers and join the cavalry.[28]

Dozens of notes passed between Barton and Elwell, and as their feelings grew, the friendly messages developed into love letters. Elwell's notes had at first been addressed to "My dear sister," but as the weeks passed they more often saluted "My pet" or "Birdie," his nickname for the flighty Clara. He begged her to come often to his rooms and ignored gossips who frowned on his own frequent visits to his "Birdie's Nest." Social engagements and propriety were forgotten in their absorption in each other. "I cannot forget the expression of your face while we were talking," Elwell wrote after an especially intimate evening. "It was the expression of happiness, the deepest happiness, not the evanescent flash of joy, but the deep realization of what only comes to us now and then. Was I mistaken? Was it but a reflection of what I feel in my own heart? I think not."[29] And Clara, bursting with pleasure at the romance, told him tenderly that "some of those hours and words were to be in after life *golden threads* woven into the web of life; there to shine forever and ever."[30]

The intimacy of their letters strongly suggests a relationship of the closest kind. Barton had always been liberal in her sexual views, and her passage through menopause a few months earlier would have dispelled any fear of pregnancy.[31] Elwell admitted that he "loved her all the law allowed and a little more perhaps,"[32] and Clara spoke rapturously of leaving his rooms at dawn in a glow of love.[33] The only jarring note was that Elwell was married to a tender and patient wife who waited in Ohio. Of the many men with whom Barton associated, Elwell was the only one who ever came near her exacting standards for a husband. Yet she made no play for him to leave his wife. Elwell wrote blissfully of their future: "Ah! the *future!* the *great* future! Ooo the last night. How it opened to us!"[34] Yet both were apparently content to "be let into the paths of duty," and seemed to accept the boundaries of their love.[35] After leaving Elwell one early morning, Barton walked thoughtfully home along the shore and noted that the waves seemed to whisper "thus far shall thou go and no farther."[36] Though it filled her heart as no other love affair would, Barton wisely recognized that her passion was best appreciated and treasured in the strange wartime context in which it had been formed. Rather than bemoan their constraints, they made the most of the moments they had. "Our time is precious," Colonel Elwell sighed. "I do not know how to forego your companionship for even two or three hours."[37]

In strong middle life a genuine love affair had come to Clara and so caught up was she that even the war seemed distant and unaffecting. Only occasionally did she hear the news from David or pick up gleanings from officers of her acquaintance. The continual bombardment of Charleston had sent the rebel defenders scurrying and had struck a small note of alarm among the Southern ladies, who nonetheless remained steadfastly in the delicately tinted houses. The Union was no closer to occupying that proud city than it had been in 1861. The many steamers that stopped in the tiny port of Beaufort brought word of the great battles farther north, of Chancellorsville and the Confederacy's crushing loss of Stonewall Jackson, and Gettysburg, where three days of terrible fighting had horrified both the North and South. Despite the reassurance of John Elwell, this news made Barton ever more unsure of the value of being in South Carolina. She was somewhat relieved, therefore, to hear rumors that the general in charge, Quincy A. Gillmore, was planning to escalate the attack on Charleston by an attempt to take Fort Wagner. The fort was a relatively unimportant garrison on a slim sand bar named Morris Island, but Gillmore, a taciturn and unimaginative career officer whose experience had been chiefly with the Corps of Engineers, saw it as the first hurdle in his plan to systematically topple the defenses of Charleston harbor. He began to rouse the indolent troops, lazy after so much loafing in the tropical climate, and cajole them into an aggressive confrontation with the enemy. On July 10, Gillmore led his men across narrow Lighthouse Inlet and up the long beach toward the fort.[38]

Barton was informed of these maneuvers two days before the battle. It stunned her out of her dream world, and she swiftly began preparing to work. On the whole Gillmore had shown a cordial indifference to her presence. Nevertheless, he now allowed her and Elwell to accompany him aboard the flagship *Fulton* as it plied its way some seventy-five miles toward the fort. It was probably due more to Elwell's influence as quartermaster than any good will on Gillmore's part, however, that Barton was so excellently equipped for the attack. Thirty-five years later Elwell would recall how he had stolen wares from the commissary department for Barton's use. In addition to her own stores, she thus benefited from numerous items slipped off the quartermaster's shelves and was fitted up with a saddle horse and ambulance. The ambulance had been equipped with a bed and other small necessities and would double as her house.[39]

With these supplies, Barton boarded the *Fulton*, which arrived in time for her to see the first moments of the siege. She watched the guns blare away at the walls of Fort Wagner, the hot charges sending up geysers of sand, apparently to little effect. The bombardment lasted a week. For most of that time the defenders simply stayed inside the bomb shelters of the fort, suffering dreadfully from water that had become fouled and lack of food, but guarding the secret of their strength from those so anxious to overwhelm them. Finally, believing that Wagner was deserted, the Federal troops made a night assault. Struggling through the sand in strict regimental formation, they made a perfect target for the rebels, who opened a blistering fire on them. "I shudder as I think of that awful charge," wrote a man who was treated by Barton. "I could hear the sickening thud of case and canister shot slushing through the bodies of men."[40] Barton watched the scene with fascinated horror and penned an excited note to Vira, describing the action as it unfolded. "Lo! Our troops were leaping from the boats like wild cats, and scarce waiting to form, on they went, in one wild charge, across the marsh and up the banks, and into the entrenchments."[41] She gasped as she saw her beloved Elwell gallop madly toward the fort to rally the men and then fall from his horse, badly wounded by an Enfield cartridge. He was one of fifteen hundred—nearly a third of the charging forces—who would be wounded or killed in this battle.

Somehow she got ashore in the midst of this fury. There was still some danger from shot, and it was a struggle to wade through the pitted and blowing sand, but she reached Elwell and bathed his face until he regained consciousness. His ordeal was similar to many of the wounded there, for he had to crawl on his hands and knees down the beach "in a most unmartial manner . . . like a turtle," his wound filling with sand and the shifting earth affecting his balance and vision. The surgeons were, as ever, too hurried to spend time with anyone not critically wounded, and many of those whom Clara reached remembered her best for the hope she gave them in the face of the impersonal medical system. A man who suffered terribly, yet was passed over by three doctors because they could not agree whether his wound was fatal or slight, appreciated the kind words and cool drink she offered. More than one fellow claimed that the little she could offer gave him the strength to recover. Left to die because he was too weak to undergo surgery, a colonel in the Tenth Connecticut Volunteers awoke to find her bathing his temples and murmuring "poor sufferer." As he felt the pulse surging again through his body he thought a miracle had happened and, like many another crippled soldier, envisioned her as an angel, a miraculous embodiment of mercy in the midst of death and destruction.[42]

Barton later claimed that she was the only woman at Morris Island, but in fact she was actively assisted by Mary Gage, a plain, hard-working woman about her own age. Barton set up camp on the island in an army tent and worked once again at a breakneck pace trying to obtain needed personnel and supplies. She covered the men with rubber blankets to protect them from the rain, helped the regimental surgeon establish a field hospital and tried to find supplies and utensils enough to feed the wounded. For men in shock, with gaping abdominal wounds or newly amputated limbs, the army provided such delicacies as dried salted beef, moldy hardtack, and an occasional spoonful of rice. Barton begged and borrowed what she could, emptied the crates consigned to her by loving hands, then badgered the medical officials until they grew weary of seeing her. Her diary record and correspondence fell by the way during this frustrating period, and she had time only to jot: "Cannot give details as I have neglected to keep up my journal in my haste to do, and all the inconveniences I have to suffer in the way of being able to get anything ready for the men to eat." Even Elwell, who assisted Barton after his wounds healed, could not obtain supplies from his abundantly stocked larder seventy-five miles away. She had seen immediate want many times, but she had never before encountered such sustained inadequacy of food and comforts.[43]

The siege wore steadily on. The Union men finally took Fort Wagner and hauled the mammoth guns, destined to hammer away at proud Charleston, into place. The pride of the artillery was an eight-inch cannon nicknamed the "Swamp Angel." General Gillmore gallantly warned the citizens of Charleston to evacuate their city, but they refused to budge, staying more out of snobbery than courage and stoutly declaring that they disbelieved that any Yankee general could force them out. They proved to be right. The Swamp Angel belched fire and smoke for thirty-six impressive rounds, then blew itself up. Aided by gunboats in the harbor, the Angel had managed to reduce defiant Fort Sumter to a pile of rubble. It was, however, an empty prize, for the now worthless fortification could not help the Union gain closer access to the city. Charleston would not fall, as one historian would later put it, until the Confederacy had run its course.[44]

Barton watched part of the bombardment from the steamer *Philadelphia,* but during most of the siege she was living in her tent, advancing with the army, and sharing the bleak accommodations on deserted Morris Island. There was no terrapin soup to dine on now; she felt fortunate to have wormy crackers. Often even the water was not fresh; frequently she took her share from that which had leached through sand filled with the decaying bodies. The elements were as relentless as the guns. She and her workers, she wrote, were "scorched by the sun, chilled by the waves, rocked by the tempest, buried in the shifting sand, toiling day after day in the trenches."[45]

In addition to the physical deprivation, Barton felt emotionally vulnerable at this time. Army officials, believing Barton's methods haphazard and her presence threatening to their own strict regimen, did not actively support her work at Morris Island. In their view, her bold demands for supplies and food, for "decent care" of the soldiers, amounted to little more than criticism of their methods. Barton was used to higher officials than these listening to her, but she had no sponsor here, and no official sanction. Tired of her presence and her high-handed ways, the medical officers tried to force her out by reclaiming her tent and demanding that she use only her own stores. Clara maintained that the tent was hers, and a long "piece of petty spite and unmanly persecution" followed.[46] Lamb and Elwell took her part, of course, but the situation eventually became unbearable, rendering her work ineffectual. Unable to stand the strain and disinclined to argue her case to a deaf jury, she gave way instead to a physical collapse. As she had at Bordentown, she let her emotions and bodily fatigue prey on each other, creating a situation in which the mental anguish could scarcely be detached from the physical. As always, it affected her eyes, her nerves, and her voice. "I—no longer able to see, was lying weak and helpless as a child," she wrote some months later, "little knowing and less minding, towards what goal my way was wending."[47] The commanding officer sent for a boat, and with her work at Morris Island unfinished, she was taken back to Hilton Head.

Cousin Leander Poor, who had again been posted near his aunt's hospital operations, thought she was less sick than after the battle of Antietam, yet believed she was close to death. But her infirmities healed rapidly. She received solicitous attention from Poor, Elwell, and the Lambs, as well as care from poor, bewildered David. John Elwell sat by her side for hours at a time, and all brought every delicacy they could. "Luxuries are rarities here, but comforts she has not wanted for," reported Poor. Dysentery seemed to be Barton's physical trouble, but the emotional turmoil caused by Gillmore's dissatisfaction was her most serious complaint. Two weeks of attention soothed it away. While she lay helpless her partisans worked feverishly to have her reinstated with the medical department. She was cheered back to health when Elwell secured a reluctant order requesting her presence on Morris Island.[48]

Barton was optimistic when she returned to the island again on September 7, believing that her friends had settled her scores and that the supply and housing problem had been cleared up. But barely had she arrived when she suffered a severe setback. On September 15 she received a command from General Gillmore stating that her "services will be no longer required in connection with the hospital in the field" and advising her to return to Beaufort. The terse note contained a gratuitous postscript stating that while the general appreciated her little efforts, she really was not needed.[49] The letter caused her such a shock that she sunk into despondency for three days, a period she termed "the severest ordeal of my life."[50] When she finally roused herself she wrote a lengthy and melodramatic reply to the general, informing him of her past virtues, the extent to which she was misunderstood, and her willingness to leave his department.

Barton then lapsed into a defensive and bitter mood, manifested by a childish

118

mixture of self-pity and sanctimony. Echoing the tone of her sentiments, a friend wrote that Clara simply could not work unless "some proper location be made where she could feel that she was not encroaching upon the right of anyone, where she could be apart from those who think her services are of so little value, or rather who have no thought or care for others."[51] Barton had labored with tireless and honest devotion for the Union, and if she needed recognition and a certain amount of privilege, she felt it was but little to ask. She had certainly never expected to meet with active criticism or hostile stares and uncomfortable silence when she requested food or supplies. Heretofore Barton had showed pride when she spoke of her work, but her comments were tempered by a becoming humility. Now her words became defensive. She gave little speeches on her achievements, delivered in a self-congratulatory tone that was indicative less of pride than justification. She would never again drop this dark cloak of self-righteous apology. For the remaining fifty years of her career, Barton would feel the need to anticipate dissatisfaction, even to falsify information, to avoid unfavorable comment.

But Gillmore was fed up with Barton and her entourage of relatives, who one by one had been thrust upon him: a fifteen-year-old boy who ran skittishly from the telegraph office at the first rumor of attack; a portly middle-aged man who knew nothing about his duties as quartermaster and languished and grew sick in the southern climate; two cousins who were to be kept at all costs well out of rifle range. He was already exasperated by the continual demands of the civilians in the area; this was trouble enough for a man trying to wage a prolonged siege. Under such pressures Gillmore declined to reconsider Barton's position at Morris Island, declined, in fact, even to respond to her letter. When Barton failed to receive a reply she had no choice but to return on the next boat to Beaufort.[52]

She landed once more in Hilton Head, heartsick and uncertain, with time and supplies on her hands. Riding and socializing seemed more trivial than ever now. She choked on the fine dinners and longed for an honest army cracker. Her romance with Elwell was but a tiny glow in the general despondency, for she knew that inevitably she must leave and that he would return to his wife. Even the hospitals near Hilton Head were closed to her. The Sanitary Commission and nurses under Dorothea Dix had established a strong foothold here, and they were constrained by rules and a ripe distrust of Barton's growing reputation for temperamental, authoritarian ways. Barton wished to help, for she had heard rumors that the hospitals were poorly supplied and gave inadequate care, but her services would scarcely be utilized where there were so many suspicious workers. In her frustration she burst into a torrent of words in her diary:

What can I do? First it is not *my* province; I should be out of place there; next Miss Dix is supreme, and her appointed nurse is matron; next the surgeons will not brook any interference, and will in my opinion, resent and resist the smallest effort to break over their own arrangements. What *others* may be able to do I am unable to conjecture, but I feel that my guns are effectually silenced. . . . Should I prepare my food and thrust it against the outer wall, in the hope it might strengthen the patients inside? Should I tie up my bundle of clothing and creep in and deposit it on the doorstep and slink away like a guilty mother . . .? [53]

Thus Barton was left idle, and, but for the stimulating company of Frances D. Gage, it would have been an autumn of regrets and self-debasement. Gage, an Ohioan thirteen years Barton's senior, had arrived in Port Royal to take charge of one of the contraband plantations. Thin and of stately bearing, with a sharp eye that rarely failed to judge the character of a person or situation accurately, she had long been an advocate of a number of liberal issues. As a young girl her father had once admonished her for being a tomboy. "Then and there sprang my hatred to the limitations of sex . . . ," Gage admitted. "I was outspoken forever after." She had as her forum *The Ohio Cultivator*, in which she wrote articles, advice, stories, and poems under the pseudonym of Aunt Fanny. To her strong feminist leanings she added two other campaigns to form what she termed her "triune cause": temperance and the abolition of slavery. In 1862 she had recognized the plight of the abandoned slave and, leaving her husband and seven of her eight children, had journeyed to South Carolina, where she labored without official status or pay. Parris Island was her domain. She taught, supervised, sewed, and punished, and meanwhile made the plantation bloom with a garden that was famous throughout that country. [54]

It is impossible to overestimate the influence this woman had on Clara Barton. Both had been raised in the Universalist church, both loved to read poetry and indulge in a little versifying of their own. And both had a burning sense of fairness, of the moral right of democratic justice. "Justice is inborn if not perverted," Barton had written, and Gage gave shape and a scope of action to her sentiments. [55] Clara's experiences in Bordentown, the Patent Office, and even among her own family had made her a loosely dedicated feminist, taking action and feeling injustice when it affected her personally. Rarely, however, had her feelings been expanded to include a larger community. Gage sharpened her personal discomfort into a realization that all women needed more rights and that all women needed to work for them. "She has such excellent judgement and such correct and large views," Barton wrote of her first encounter with Gage. [56] The older woman wasted little time in educating the unhappy Barton. "For whom are you going to vote?" Gage would taunt her in letters before the election of 1864, and she encouraged her to speak out on the work women performed on the battlefield. [57] Under Gage's tutelage Barton's perceptions begin to change significantly. Her letters and comments show an increasingly feminist slant, and for the first time she began to view herself as an active proponent of woman suffrage. She did not mind being taxed, she told Mary Norton, in November 1863. Indeed, she rejoiced in helping her country during this time of crisis. But, wrote

Barton, "I think 'taxation and representation are and of right ought to be insepa-rable.' I most devoutly wish that intellect, education and moral worth decided a voter's privileges and not sex, or money or land or any other unintelligent principle."[58]

Gage's influence also caused Barton to widen her conception of equal rights to include rights for Negroes. For all of her broad-minded ways, Clara had never had a particular interest in this cause. Her mother had signed several early aboli-tionist petitions, and brother Stephen had worked as well as he could in North Carolina to help the blacks. But Clara had rather scrupulously avoided any such action. She had, on the contrary, considered living in the slave society of the South, denounced John Brown's attempt at insurrection, and taken more than a few pains to deny that slavery was the primary cause of the war. Now her eyes were opened to the difficult position of the newly emancipated blacks. They were free but had no property, no education, no way to earn a living beyond serving their former masters in a capacity that differed little from their former bondage. The cause for which Gage was laboring so hard suddenly gained new meaning for Barton, and soon after her arrival in Hilton Head, she began teach-ing a number of blacks to read, though it was a sporadic effort. She gave gifts of clothing and food to the poorer freedmen around her and helped Gage nurse those on Parris and St. Helen's islands who were ill with smallpox.[59] Her experi-ence among the black soldiers at the siege of Morris Island heightened her admi-ration for those strong people, for she found them especially uncomplaining and dedicated. Her meant-for-publication letters now frequently contained para-graphs devoted to praise of the freedmen, particularly those fighting for the Union: "Whiter blood than their's has often failed to exhibit traits as high and noble."[60] She also began to believe, as did Gage, that the tragic and costly war was being fought for the sins of the South: it was God's terrible retribution on the American people. Six months after leaving Hilton Head, she wrote: "God has made it so that for every African enslaved, an Anglo-Saxon must suffer."[61]

Gage and Barton were more than political allies. Their temperaments and personalities suited each other; they laughed and commiserated, talked of their similar girlhoods, and shared their love of literature and a deep appreciation for nature. They cheered each other by exchanging informal verses, ridiculing themselves and their predicaments:

> Two old grey-headed women lived all by themselves
> Kept salt in the cupboard & tea on the shelves
> Ate when they were hungary & cooked their own oats
> Laughed or *cryed* as it suited and gargled their throats
> So these grey-headed women first time, at their ease
> Shake their fists at the M.D. & do as they please.[62]

Gage admired Clara's work tremendously but thought her overanxious and morbidly introspective. Aunt Fanny chided her gently, always attempting to make her take the larger view of problems. "Think of a heroine, who to fields of battle could march unflinchingly," Gage wrote in a teasing verse,

Staining her soft white fingers with the flowing of some heroe's blood.
Catch up the last word of the spirit going from battlefield to God.
Think of the noble generous self-poised woman.
So nobly true & free
That it seems sacriledge to call her human
Fretting about a flea.[63]

Barton came to greatly cherish Aunt Fanny's wisdom and kindness. She seemed to personify all of the intellectual attributes and humanitarian spirit Clara herself was striving to achieve. She would never consciously admit Gage's influence on her, but its spark was consistently present during Clara's lifetime. Long after her death, Gage continued to inspire Clara, and even forty years later she would be among the ranks of Barton's "Most honored spirits."

The company of Frances Gage helped Barton enormously during the difficult autumn of 1863, but frustration and anxiety mounted as the weeks of inactivity wore on. She wanted to see if the intrigue surrounding hospital matters would subside but was unable to infiltrate the rigid system of the commissions and Dix. In December she was extremely annoyed by a visit from a flighty woman who relayed the news that the hospitals needed a bit more care in the way of food preparation and wondered what Barton thought of sending in volunteers. The woman evidently thought this an original idea and was surprised to find Barton barely able to control an angry retort. "I listened attentively, gave it as my opinion that there would be no difficulty in obtaining supplies . . . but of the manner and feasibility of delivering and distributing them among the patients I said nothing. *I had nothing to say.* . . . What I have *thought* is quite another thing."[64] News from the North further depressed her. Her old comrade, Cornelius Welles, had died suddenly while on a visit to California, and the loss of this friend, with whom she had experienced so much, shook her deeply.[65] The cheerful tidings of the marriage of Fanny Childs and her favorite nephew, Bernard Vassall, seemed to point up the unhappy difference between her and everyone else.[66] David also caused worry. His health and spirits had become so low that he was finally forced to leave the army; his entire tour had been a failure and an embarrassment. Even Clara's romance with Colonel Elwell had calmed to the point that, as in all once-ardent relationships, they now felt only a lingering fondness and mild embarrassment when they were together. Elwell's invitations to ride or dine went unanswered. Around the beginning of December, Barton predicted that "Mrs. E. would come in two or three weeks. I should go home soon after that."[67] A cordial society with her former lover's wife was an experience she would choose to forego.

And yet one more strain took its toll. Barton's arrangement with the Patent Office, by which her position was retained and half of her salary collected, had come under question. What hurt her most was that it was the female office workers who had filed a complaint, the very women in whose behalf she had pioneered. They maintained that she was being paid for her field work by the army or Sanitary Commission, and they wanted the position vacated for another woman. Barton knew that her relationship with the Patent Office was an extraordinary one, but she felt that it was fully justified under the circumstances. Immediately she wrote to Commissioner Holloway in her most vehement tone of martyrdom. Although she justifiably denied that she retained any supplemental salary and maintained that all monies she received from the Patent Office went only to help the soldiers, her letter degenerated into self-pity. "It is not for those accustomed to face death twenty times a day, in nearly all possible shapes, to become appalled by a little *future want*, and sue for mercy," ran one line. The women's accusation, she concluded, was "niggardly in its nature and derogatory to every feeling of humanity and patriotism and as such I reject and scorn it."[68] Holloway, clearly abashed, responded a few weeks later, assuring her that he had misunderstood the situation and that her position was secure as long as he was in office. The matter was dropped there, and she had no further battles in that arena for the rest of the war.[69]

Heartsick, resentful, and convinced that she had been "sadly abused," Clara determined to leave South Carolina. She concluded bitterly that her great mistake had been to underestimate the "amount of maneuvering space needed by field officers."[70] With much ado she boarded the boat for home on the last day of December, in a mood so low that even Aunt Fanny was at a loss to give advice or render comfort. She saw the very irony of Barton's nature: that of embracing the world with so great and trusting a heart that she left herself vulnerable. As Clara boarded the ship, sympathetic Frances Gage pressed a little poem into her hand.

Thy heart so rich my Clara dear
Is tender almost spoiling
What shall I do to save its love
And stop its endless boiling?
Hearts should be warm we all know that
And free to overflowing
But too much heart may make them blot
And barely worth bestowing
So tell me darling what to do
With your dear heart; I pray you do.[71]

Barton had thought that her wounded spirit would rally once she was among her friends and sponsors in Washington. But she found little work to do during the winter season of encampments. The Sanitary Commission and Dix were as strong—perhaps stronger—in Washington as they had been in Hilton Head. In any case, she would decline to work with them, for she doubted that they would prove "as faithful and efficient as they have grown powerful and wealthy." So she began again the seemingly endless search to find a niche, and her mind started to harp on the old spectres of inactivity and dejection. Fearless as she was on the battlefield, she had little courage to face personal disappointments. On a trip to Brooklyn in February 1864, she went to hear the famed minister Henry Ward Beecher speak on the daily heroism he witnessed in devoted mothers, scrimping, saving, servant girls, and a thousand other consistantly courageous individuals. To her diary she acknowledged the truth of his sermon: "how forcibly I felt that my bravery if ever I had any had not been exhibited on the field—I had nothing to dare or endure in those days." [72] When a scheme to establish a private ware-house for her supplies did not work out, she sank into deep depression, vowing to "have done . . . with my efforts on behalf of others. I must take the little rem-nant of life, that may remain to me, as my own special property, and appropriate it accordingly." [73] Barton considered devoting her life to literature and letters, or lecturing about her experiences as Frances Gage had done. But she could barely face those possibilities and instead shuffled blindly through the dark days. [74]

Nerves taut, she was many mornings unable to get up for sheer depression. [75] Friends tried to distract her, but by March she was ready to snap. To Henry Wilson, the one man whose support had been unshakable, she wrote a petty, whining, accusatory letter, stating that she had only the purest motives for help-ing soldiers and that he had done nothing to aid her. "Alone, in constant danger from rank and buffoonery and selfishness, I cannot accomplish it." "Please do not misunderstand me, this is not a complaining letter. . . .," she finished loft-ily; "destroy this letter, forgive me for writing it and forget it." [76] When Wilson kindly came to her the next day and asked her what it was she wanted, Barton admitted that "like a spoiled child I looked down, winked fast, bit my nails, drummed with my foot on the floor and wouldn't answer." [77] A week later the world still looked treacherous and hostile. She was, in fact, considering suicide. "Have been sad all day," she confided to her diary. "I cannot raise my spirits, the old temptation to go from all the world. I think it will come to that some day, it is a struggle to keep in society at all. I want to leave all." [78]

Her dejection was lifted finally by her only true remedy—a need for her ser-vices. The Union army's spring campaign had started early. General Ulysses S. Grant had been brought to Washington from the west to take command of the Army of the Potomac. His effective if ruthless strategy was to use the Union's numerical superiority to drive the Confederates into submission. He began by fighting relentlessly in a wilderness area of Spotsylvania County, Virginia, where men were slaughtered by the thousands, and the army pushed on, never stopping to recover, always driving at the enemy. No one had anticipated such carnage as occurred at the Bloody Angle and Spotsylvania Courthouse, and the public was outraged. Even those as pro-war as Barton found this type of fighting shocking. "I am holding my breath in awe at the vastness of the shadow that floats like a pall over our head," she exclaimed to Gage; "it has come that man has no longer an individual existence but is counted in thousands and measured in miles."[79] With the opening of the spring campaigns, supplies and volunteers were needed, much as they had been during the early days of the war. The Sanitary and Christian Commissions, on whom the army now relied, had drastically underestimated what would be required. "They all said that enough and even a surplus of stores had gone forward," wrote Dr. Hitchcock. "In this respect they were all mistaken."[80] Whereas two months earlier the secretary of war had ignored Barton's requests for passes and transportation, he now embraced her services enthusiastically. At last she again had a place, a purpose, and a need to fulfill.

On receipt of her pass, Barton stayed in Washington for a week, finishing her plans and collecting supplies while the battles raged one hundred miles to the south. Finally she was granted transportation on a boat from Aquia Creek to Fredericksburg, where many of the wounded were being brought. She found conditions so appalling that even her later descriptions of this time reveal a choked inability to express the depth of her emotion. "I believe it would be impossible to *comprehend* the magnitude of the necessity without witnessing it," she jotted down at the time.[81] In 1862 a lack of ambulances and skilled rescue workers had caused untold misery. Now there were ambulance trains in abundance, but a conspiracy of weather and geography made the removal of the wounded as impossible as it had been at Fairfax Station. Rain streamed down onto a flat plain (inappropriately named "Belle') of notorious Virginia red clay. Wagons were stuck for days in the quagmire or jolted and heaved until the soldiers died of exposure and shock. Barton stepped from the boat to see nearly two hundred such conveyances buried to the hubs of their wheels, with no way to move and no supplies. The best she could do was to round up some terrified Christian Commission workers and wade through the sticky red mud to deliver a few crackers and some coffee to the men in the wagons.[82] She made her way to Fredericksburg and found conditions equally bad there. "Went to the Old National Hotel found some hundreds (perhaps 400) western men—sadly wounded," she reported in a brief pause from the work, "all on the floors—had nothing to eat. I carried a basket of crackers—and gave two apiece as far as they went and some pails of coffee, they had no food that day and there was none for them. I saw them again at ten o'clock at night, they had had nothing to eat—a great number of them were to undergo amputation sometime, but no surgeons yet."[83] Barton also noted that beyond the obvious want, there was unquestionably something wrong in Fredericksburg. There were plenty of houses but no space for the wounded, cellars filled with meal but no gruel to feed starving men. She believed that the Union officers were responsible for this state of affairs, for they were too proud (or, as she thought, too disloyal) to ask the rebel civilians to open their houses to the maimed and dying Union army. For Barton, who had seen men lying helpless upon "bare, wet, bloody floors, hold up their cold bloodless dingy hands, as I passed, and beg me in Heaven's name for a cracker to keep them from starving," this was an outrage verging on treason. She gave out the supplies she had and hurried back to Washington, determined to change the situation.[84]

Once in the capital she sent immediately for Henry Wilson. The officers in charge were faithless, she maintained, "overcome by the blandishments of the wily inhabitants." Wilson, stirred by a profound grief over the army's suffering and confident of Barton's ability to judge a situation, took immediate action. He stepped briskly around to the War Department, found them ignorant of the dire state of affairs in Fredericksburg, and gave them an ultimatum: either they would dispatch an official to relieve the situation, or Wilson, as chairman of the powerful Military Affairs Committee, would send his own representative. By two o'clock the next morning, noted Barton with sarcastic satisfaction, the city's elegant houses "were opened to the '*dirty, lousy soldiers*' of the Union Army."[85]

Barton paused in Washington long enough to scavenge all the bandages, food, and clothing that she could and to send out emergency pleas for help to newspapers and relief organizations. "For the first time in the history of the war, the magnitude and intensity of suffering and want are so appalling as to wring from me a public call for aid," she explained. Taking care not to criticize the army directly, she nonetheless made a dramatic plea for articles of every description. "There is time for all to labor," it concluded, "and grow weary in well doing."[86]

This line described well her work in the next few weeks. She returned to the crowded Fredericksburg hospitals, returned to shrieking men and never-ending death. A fellow worker saw her as a cheerful spirit, breezing through the wards in a blue dress and white apron, rousing the men by singing "Rally Round the Flag, Boys" in a none-too-melodious voice.[87] Barton's inner thoughts were sober, however. "I have had but one night's sleep since last Thursday," she wrote on a Tuesday late in May. "I had so many personal friends that were mortally wounded, and just reached our city to die—we are waiting at the cotside and closing their eyes one by one as they pass away."[88] On June 3 soldiers dazed from the battle of Cold Harbor, during which seven thousand men had been killed or wounded in a few minutes, arrived in Fredericksburg. It seemed impossible now, she told friends, to hold the body and soul of the wounded together—even more impossible to contemplate the sheer numbers being slain. "I cannot but think that we shall win at last," she declared, "but *Oh the cost*—a regiment reduced to a score and a corporal commanding."[89] With one ear cocked for the favorable news from the front and the other attuned to the pitiable cries around her, she carried on for three more weeks.

The army was holed up near Petersburg now; Grant proposed to fight it out "if it takes all summer." Barton wanted desperately to go with the Union troops, and to this end she badgered Wilson until he promised to do what he could. His June 20 letter of introduction to General Benjamin Butler, then commanding the Army of the James, resulted in an interview a few days later, at which the two New Englanders evidently exchanged a good deal of mutual admiration.[90]

On June 23, 1864, Barton wrote in her diary: "Need not note the interview for I shall never forget it. I am satisfied with my success with Genl Butler."[91] Butler was an assertive man, imperious and without a shred of military skill. Round of body, bald of head, he had a twisted squinty eye that made his pompous attitude seem ridiculous. Southerners hated him as they did no other general because of an order dispatched during the occupation of New Orleans that decreed that women who insulted Union men were to be considered ladies of the town and treated accordingly; "Beast" Butler the rebels called him.[92] Barton liked him because he was from Massachusetts and because, in notable contrast to General Gillmore, he flattered her by listening to her suggestions. On this day he offered her a job at a corps hospital near Point of Rocks, Virginia; she would be in charge of diet and nursing but directly beneath the surgeon who supervised the hospital. Barton later claimed that he had appointed her superintendent of nursing for the Army of the James. Whatever Butler may have told her unofficially, no such position was ever created, recorded, or officially approved by the War Department. Her duties, though supervisory within the hospital, were by no means so broad; many other nurses of equal rank labored with that army. Nonetheless, Barton had found a place under a sympathetic general and a niche that would hold her for the duration of the war.[93]

The field hospital, a receiving and convalescent center located on the James River, consisted of a collection of twenty large and yellowing tents set up on an abandoned plantation. From time to time a few men suffering from gunshot wounds were brought in, but they usually died within a few hours or were removed by boat to the better-equipped hospitals in Washington. Barton generally cared for between forty and one hundred men, sufferers from typhoid fever, pneumonia, or, in the majority of cases, dysentery induced by an inadequate diet and unhealthy water. Lifesaving emergency measures were rarely needed; the care was of a slower and gentler sort. The hospital folded its tents and camp cots and moved with the army, for no agreement protected the wounded men from being mistreated by the enemy. Thus called a "flying hospital," it was much less a permanent facility than a part of the baggage of the corps.[94]

Barton arrived at the hospital in an uncomfortable heat wave. "It has not rained for a month and the poor wounded fellows lie all about me, suffering intensely from heat and flies," wrote a surgeon in the hospital. "The atmosphere is almost intolerable from the immense quantity of decomposing animal and vegetable matter upon the ground."[95] Surgeons and nurses also suffered from the thick and oppressive air, and Barton found in her first days with the hospital that she had to fight constantly to keep up with the work required. Her routine was varied, but she quickly recognized that the most pressing need was for a strong hand in the kitchen. Armed with a scanty supply of tinware and a castoff wood-burning stove, she took on the role of cook. On a day soon after she arrived, with the temperature over one hundred degrees, Barton reported that she had made a barrel of applesauce "and have given out every spoonful with my own hands. I have cooked ten dozen eggs, made cracker toast, corn starch blanc mange, milk punch, arrow-root pudding." What little time she had left was spent in the wards. On the same day she had "washed faces and hands, put ice on hot heads, mustard on cold feet, written six soldier's letters home, stood beside three death beds."[96]

Supplies were abundant because City Point, one of the army's chief warehouse centers, was directly across the river. These were comparative riches, and Barton, a firm believer that food was good for the soul as well as body, set about fixing the little specialties that she could for her boys. On July 4, there was a gala dinner that included roast beef begged from a jealous quartermaster and a musical presentation by some local players of dubious talent. She somehow found salt cod and shaped it into "one hundred and fifty gallons of nice home codfish," so reminiscent of more peaceful days that the taste of it made several Yankees burst into tears. Apple pies and gingerbread were not too much trouble, and she even attempted to make doughnuts. For the soldiers, many of whom could be moved at the sight of a fresh egg, the good home cooking worked wonders. There were very few deaths among the patients, and most were able to leave the hospital within a month.[97]

Barton's days were now filled less with death than with improvement and relief, and the work was correspondingly satisfying. To take a feverish man, filthy from the trenches near Petersburg, bathe and feed him, and then lay him on a cool sheet was a daily pleasure. "You will fail to comprehend the magnitude of the change," Clara told one group of women, "because it will be impossible for you to realize the depths of the misery they were taken from."[98] Nonetheless she was tiring. The generous heart that wished to be everywhere, to cook one meal after another on the stove, to hand it round with strong, steady hands, then to be sister or mother to the emotionally spent, had an overly optimistic view of what one person could do. The surgeons—Doctors Kitlinger and Craven—liked her and left her alone, but they unwittingly created more work for her by spontaneously changing diets, moving patients, and forgetting to keep her informed. Then, without telling her, they accepted four other nurses into the hospital, to be under her care and to help her.

Alone Barton would "keep cheerful and toil on," tirelessly trying to fill every gap.[99] With the new nurses, however, she felt uncomfortable. All five were forced to share one stove, and she felt awkward planning a division of duties. Furthermore, she felt unhappy and resentful at the thought of relinquishing any of her prerogatives. She had never learned to supervise without dictating or accept suggestion without condemning it as criticism. Yet the difficulties were not all Barton's fault. Many of the women who became nurses were unskilled or inexperienced, or had temperaments ill-suited to the hard work and unpleasant sights of the hospital. As one fellow matron working across the river put it, "hospital nurses were of all sorts and came from various sources of supply."[100] Barton never dignified her nurses with a description of their characters. It was enough that they were aliens in her little world, and that they competed with her for the attentions of doctors and soldiers.

Disgruntled and testy, Clara dashed to Washington at the end of July after hearing rumors of Jubel Early's raid on that city. She was concerned about her belongings and spent about a week securing them. Returning to Point of Rocks, she found that one of Dorothea Dix's nurses, Adelaide Smith, had been sent to take over the hospital. The girl had, apparently by mistake, been given Barton's room to stay in, and the older woman felt her authority violated and her future threatened. "All that I had feared so long had transpired and I was not near and could have done nothing if I had been. Things change a little and I do not feel at home, things combine to grieve me," she sadly confided to her diary. Smith would leave, but not before she cast a critical eye around the premises, noted her annoyance at Barton's careful, methodical ways, and made Barton feel thoroughly unwanted and out of place. For her part, Barton retaliated by being just as uncooperative as she could. Once when Smith had run to her for some bandages needed in an emergency, Smith remembered, she deliberately kept the girl waiting. "She asked about my health, urged me to take a seat, and very slowly rumaged about for the necessary supplies."[101]

Tension remained high until the latter part of August when the hospital was moved closer to the field armies at Petersburg. Action at this location was always imminent, and of the women only Barton accompanied the long train of surgeons, equipment, ambulances, and tents. They were moving before the enemy, trying to stay as close to the lines as possible without endangering the sick soldiers in their care. "I cannot tell you how many times I have moved with my whole family of a thousand or fifteen hundred," Barton told Vira Stone, "and with a half hours notice in the night."[102] The already grueling work of the hospital was increased by this constant "flying"; at each stop boxes had to be packed and unpacked, quarters found, wards cleaned and straightened. Barton, who now had virtually no leisure time at all, lamented "still I leave *so much* undone, night comes and I chide me that I have done so little, and morning returns and I feel that I should not have spent so many hours in sleep when so many about me perhaps could not sleep at all." She heard little news of the battles and no longer knew whether or not the Union was making progress. "I do not bother my poor head about the end," Barton wrote, "but plod on day by day, trying to perform my round of duty faithfully."[103]

She encountered in the hospitals a number of soldiers of whom she would grow especially fond, and groups of men for which she would form a tremendous admiration. Clara was particularly attracted to the young foreign nationals, who were drawn to the Union cause by adventure or ideology. Jules Golay and Emile Clare, two Swiss boys among the wounded, amused her with their continental charm.[104] She renewed her respect also for the black soldiers who passed through the hospital. Following the precepts of Frances Gage, she treated them with courtesy and continued to write "public" letters on their behalf. "They are ever the objects of my deep commiseration and care," ran one such epistle, "so patient and cheerful, so uniformly polite and soldierly. They are brave men and make no complaints. . . . They have wants as . . . soldier's [sic] now, as well as 'freedmen', and I sincerely hope this fact may not be overlooked by their northern friends."[105] She found to her delight that the former slaves made excellent nurses, and consequently drafted them whenever possible for hospital duty. She continued to fight the stereotype that they were not brave or aggressive soldiers. "I am well satisfied," she informed her Northern correspondents, "that they are not a class of men that an enemy would desire to meet on a charge."[106] She felt haunted, too, as did so many Northerners staying for the first time in the South, by the strange and beautiful singing of the black troops that rose with the evening mist across the countryside. Here was a rich culture, she informed her friends, worthy both of admiration and protection.

On October 14, Barton had barely settled into the latest encampment of the Tenth Army Corps (this time only six miles from Richmond) when she received a letter that she had long both anticipated and dreaded. It was from her nephew Sam, and it contained disturbing news about brother Stephen. All during the war years, Clara and her family had anxiously tried to keep in touch with him. Now he had been captured by Union troops, Sam wrote, and was being held a prisoner of war in Norfolk. Sam begged Clara to use her influence with General Butler to secure his release. Outraged and nearly overcome with worry, she obtained the earliest possible interview with Butler, dramatically telling her brother's story. To her great joy, Butler, who felt the army owed Clara a great deal, ordered that Stephen be brought to his command to be held under his sister's care, and that all papers relating to the case be forwarded directly to him.[107]

Stephen arrived at the hospital a few days later, and the story of his long ordeal in North Carolina began to unfold. After years of working to establish himself in the state, he feared that the war would ruin his business. He had stayed at "Bartonsville" to protect his property and for three years had walked a fine line between his Union sympathies and his need to win the confidence of his Southern neighbors. The Chowan River, on which he had established mills and farms, had changed hands several times, making his already tenuous situation even more precarious. In mid-1863 the rebels again controlled the river, and a Confederate colonel, Joel R. Griffin, learned of Barton, paid him a visit, and questioned him at length about his loyalties and intentions. Griffin was impressed with Stephen, whom he considered a "candid and consistent man," and decided to place him under the personal protection of his troops. He warned Barton, however, against holding further communication with the Federal gunboats that prowled along the Chowan. It "served to raise prejudice and render his property and himself liable to molestation, and . . . I knew of threats by the Confederates to burn him out," Griffin later told Clara.[108]

Stephen Barton was given permission about this time to trade a little cotton to the Northern troops across the Chowan River for badly needed foodstuffs. The arrangement was under the personal protection of several officers but was not strictly legal. In his later statements, Barton maintained that the wheat and corn he had obtained in trade had been given away to the poor in the area.[109] Whatever truth there was in this statement, it reflected only part of Barton's trading activities. He had also been selling cotton to factories in the North, in turn obtaining drugs and medicines that were badly needed in the South. For these he received substantial sums.[110] This was strictly in violation of the Federal blockade, and could have been interpreted by some as treason. Stephen's motives were undoubtedly less those of a traitor than a shrewd Yankee businessman. "I guess between you and I that he has been making a good thing out of the war, both for himself and federals or Rebes," Sam wrote to his mother in a letter marked "confidential." "For my part I am glad if some of us can make something out of the war."[111] On September 25, while driving toward Elizabeth City, North Carolina, to continue his trading, Stephen was arrested by Union soldiers. They found that he was carrying a thousand dollars in cash—an enormous sum for that time and place—which Stephen claimed was to purchase bagging. His money and papers were confiscated, and he was ordered to a prison in Norfolk.[112]

Stephen was treated harshly in Norfolk. The Federal authorities threw him into a cell without furnishings or adequate food and refused to give him medicines or hospital treatment for the chronic diarrhea that was rapidly wasting his body. Stephen finally smuggled out a note to Sam through a Negro guard, which of course led to Clara's intervention with General Butler. By the time he stepped from the wagon at the flying hospital he was so ill that his sister, who had not seen him for years, was shocked by his appearance. "Six years before I had seen Stephen, strong, muscular, erect, two hundred pounds. . . . He walked into my presence now, pale, tottering, a hundred and thirty, his thin white locks resting upon his shoulders, bent and walking feebly with a cane." She brought him to her quarters—a rude hut that had once been a slave cabin—and nursed him while he awaited a hearing on the charges against him.[113]

Late in November an impromptu (and probably illegal) court-martial was held in Butler's tent. Stephen's worn condition and his sister's dramatic testimony did much to sway the general in favor of the Bartons. His captors were roundly castigated for the rough and unorthodox manner of seizing him, and a demand was made for the return of his property. Little was said of the trading in cotton or drugs. Loyal Clara, never able to believe anything but the best about her brothers, aptly viewed the incident as an enjoyable round of besting a few petty officers. Stephen, of course, was also pleased at the outcome. It was "most interesting, happy and amusing," he wrote in glee to his brother David's children, "to all present, exept the officers who commanded the raid that arrested me and took my property."[114] Clara took him back to the hospital in the hope that she could help him regain his strength, and the family set about hushing up the story. Said his son: "I don't care to have it sounded all over town that he is a prisoner of war."[115]

When he was strong enough, Clara sent Stephen to Washington, where he would be better able to petition for the protection of his Carolina property while still under the watchful eye of Sally Vassall. Clara followed her brother home early in January 1865. Things were not going well in the Tenth Army Corps. Butler was relieved of his command on January 7 for alleged incompetence; because of this the troops' movements were constantly changed and rearranged. Moreover, Barton had had several quarrels with officers' wives who were anxious to work in the hospital but disinclined to take orders. Without Butler's willing ear to receive her appeals, Barton thought it best to quietly retreat. She had, however, every intention of returning again to the army.[116]

Butler's dismissal and Clara's worry over Stephen's worsening health made it difficult to return to Virginia right away, however. Her future, with or without the army, seemed uncertain. It was clear that the war was drawing to a close and that her humanitarian work would end with it. She could not go backward, could not retreat to Massachusetts or to the Patent Office. She wished to remain with the army, yet she realized that she had never really been accepted by the military; they had tolerated her temporarily only because of immense need. As she contemplated her long-term problems, she socialized, nursed Stephen, and was distracted by several of the receptions given by President and Mrs. Lincoln. She even worked up a little enthusiasm for the inaugural ball, borrowing a green silk skirt to wear with her white lace bodice and enjoying the attentions of her escorts, Admiral Farragut and Senator Wilson.[117] Jules Golay was in town, and he and other friends, elated over the anticipated peace, called frequently. She fussed with her clothes and fussed over Irving Vassall, whose health was as precarious as ever. He kept up his cheerful spirits, but it was clear that his tuberculosis was reaching the last, exhaustive stages.

Despite his poor health, Irving had worked tirelessly during the war. Now it was he who gave Clara an idea for prolonging her service to the soldiers. At the express office where he worked, Irving had heard that prisoners were coming in from the South in pitiable condition. The starved and ragged men needed food and clothing, and the government needed help taking statements and corresponding with their relatives. Barton was excited by the idea of expanding her work in this direction, and she approached Wilson for help. Wilson gave his hearty approval to her plan and promised he would arrange a meeting with the president to discuss it. Barton fretted nervously about her hair, borrowed furs and a hat for the occasion, only to be disappointed: the president was out when they called. Several more attempts to call on Mr. Lincoln, this time with the additional support of Dr. Hitchcock and Senator Elihu B. Washburne, proved equally disappointing.[118] Struck by the contrast between her high hopes and her inability to cut through the labyrinthian bureaucracy, she began again to slip into despondency. Her diary notes were a refrain of the previous year's frustrations: "I feel that some hand above mine rules and is staying my progress. I cannot understand but try to be patient—still it is hard. I was never more tempted to break down with disappointment."[119]

Worst of all, she could no longer ignore the fact that both Stephen and Irving were dying. Since late January her brother had been too weak to stand alone. Clara tried to help him both physically and spiritually by applying "injudicious remedies" and by making a trip to Fortress Monroe to see about his affairs. None of his property had been returned, and the thought of its loss vexed him. Early in March she knew he could not recover, and on the tenth of that month his end came quietly. It was left to Clara to make all the funeral arrangements, for Sally was ill-equipped to handle such responsibilities. She traveled with the body and saw him put to rest in the shady North Oxford cemetery he had helped to found.[120] Only two weeks later she sat at another lonely deathbed, as poor, long-suffering Irving hemorrhaged his way out of her life. She was so torn that she had no heart to express her anguish to her journal and noted only the fact of her nephew's death and the time. The loss of Irving overshadowed even the glad news of Lee's surrender at Appomattox Court House on April 9. He had lived to the age of twenty-six, yet Clara could think only of the lost promise, the wasted talent.[121]

It was nearly a year before Barton could comment on the loss of these two family members, and even then the pain was sharp. "I have parted with the two who perhaps in the old time has [sic] twined most deeply about my heart," she wrote, "who h[a]d traits of character more in common with myself than any others, whose love for me was a mine of wealth, and around whose dear memories the tenderest fibers of my heart still cling, and crushed & torn, and buried still ache & bleed."[122] Few except Henry Wilson seemed to know the depths of her misery at this time. He appeared at her door soon after Stephen's death and humbly asked her to accept him as a brother to replace the one she had lost. He assured her that he was continuing to try to obtain official sanction for her to work with the returning prisoners. In mid-March Wilson won Lincoln's approval for the plan but kindly advised Clara to "bury her dead" and recover before continuing in her good service. Tight-lipped and sore of heart, Clara wandered through Washington as it jubilantly proclaimed victory, then joined her fellow citizens in shocked disbelief at the death of Abraham Lincoln.[123]

nine

In her sorrow Barton once again instinctively turned to work for comfort and escape. She had won Lincoln's approval for her plan to work with released prisoners of war, and his word was, if anything, more revered now than before his death. His legacy to her had been a scrap of paper that read:

To the Friends of Missing Persons:

Miss Clara Barton has kindly offered to search for the missing prisoners of war. Please address her at Annapolis, giving her name, regiment, and company of any missing prisoner.

Signed
A. Lincoln[1]

Armed with this letter and a vague notion that there were men arriving at Annapolis who needed attention, Clara confidently set off for the port town. She found there a confusing mix of cacophany and pathos; the noisy bustle of departing soldiers and the strange silence of the skeletal men arriving from the South. The neatly laid-out streets of Annapolis, its elegant circles, and the grounds of the Maryland state capitol were lined with little tent cities, whose inhabitants destroyed the green lawns and tall, graceful trees. The arrival of the prisoners had brought doctors, hopeful women with poke bonnets shading their careworn faces, and government officials to the already crowded town. Annapolis was so filled with people that Barton could not find lodgings. She was forced to camp for a few days at a time as a "scarce welcome guest" in private homes, while the trunks and other baggage she brought with her stood out in the snow.[2]

Her hosts were poorly equipped to cater to a stranger, and she found that in this hectic time the army was equally ill-prepared for her. After several days of discouraged wandering through this confusion, Barton discovered that, despite her note from Lincoln, generals in the War Department in Annapolis had no idea where to place her or what she ought to do. The public had been told to inquire for sons and lovers through the Annapolis bureau of the army. From every corner they came to Maryland to ask advice, beg favors, or chastize those responsible for death or demotion. The tiny section of the War Department handling the exchange of prisoners was overwhelmed, as the ghostlike figures began arriving from Belle Isle and Andersonville. It could barely keep up with recording their deaths—for most of the men died within a few days of their arrival—let alone cope with the demands of the public. Though Barton was offering the very help they needed, her petition was lost in the sea of inquiring and anxious faces. Repeatedly she was turned away or told to report to another bureau.

Attempts to keep organized reports on the incoming prisoners, or to register their deaths accurately, were continually frustrated by the fraudulent, incomplete, or incorrect records of exchange. When Barton inquired for the official rolls of prisoners she was informed that in many cases prisoners had been exchanged without any record at all. She knew from firsthand experience the inconsistent records kept at hospitals. Men who had been lost enroute to Annapolis appeared on few lists, existing only in the memories of comrades, who might chance to tell an official of the death. With the army thus harried and public records so poor, it appeared for nearly eight weeks that her scheme of working with the government to identify those who had been prisoners would fail. But finally, late in the spring, a busy general loaned her a tent and gave her permission to begin.[3]

Thousands of letters, anxiously requesting word of a beloved soldier, some of whom had been missing since the early months of the war, lay unopened in piles on tent floors. As she walked through the dirty streets, thronged with soldiers' relations who hoped to recognize one of the haggard faces coming off the boats, it struck Barton that the identification of those men listed as missing constituted an even more significant problem for the nation than she had at first realized. Over half of the Union men known to have been killed were unidentified. Some 190,000 graves were unmarked.[4] Barton could never view these as mere statistics; they were "her boys," the men she had seen fighting with so much determination on so many hard-won fields. Yet she understood now that she could not identify the prisoners through the maze of army and government offices. The only people who seemed to have the ability to distinguish the dead from the living were the returning soldiers, who had seen their friends fall or watched them recover. Determined to carry on in spite of bureaucratic obstacles, Clara decided to make use of the soldiers themselves.

She drew up a rather convoluted plan, which relied heavily on chance and the initiative of the Union veterans. As she received each inquiry, Barton placed the missing soldier's name on a master list which was subdivided by state. She decided that she would periodically publish the lists in newspapers, display them in post offices, and circulate them through organizations such as the Masons.

She would then ask the veterans to check the lists for any name about which they had knowledge and to send that information to her. She in turn would send the intelligence to the original inquirer. It was an optimistic scheme, but with so little in the way of official information, and with the army evidently too preoccupied to spend time on correspondence with distraught families, she saw no other way to alleviate the problem.[5]

"In view of the great anxiety felt throughout the country for the welfare of our prisoners now being exchanged and arriving in Annapolis, Maryland," read an article inserted in the newspaper,

> Miss Clara Barton, by permission of Genl. Hitchcock, Commissioner of Exchange, with the sanction of the President, has kindly undertaken to furnish information by correspondence in regard to the condition of the returned soldiers, especially those in the hospitals in Annapolis, and also as far as possible to learn the facts in reference to those who have died in prison or elsewhere. All letters addressed to Miss Clara Barton, Annapolis, will meet with prompt attention.[6]

Almost immediately Barton was inundated with letters from all over the country, adding to the bushels of mail already requiring answers. Those who wrote had only a vague idea of her methods, often believing she would personally undertake a detailed search for every soldier. "People tell me the color of hair & eyes of the friends they have lost, as if I were expected to go about the country and search them," Clara wrote. "They ask me to send them full lists of all the lost men of the army, they tell me that they have looked all through my list of missing men, and the name [of] their son or husband or somebodies [sic] elses is not on it and desire to be informed why it is made an exception."[7] The naiveté and sincerity of the letters touched her deeply. Only rarely was there a jarring note. Soldiers who wished to start a new life, those who had deserted or were attached to a Southern sweetheart, often preferred to remain missing. One young man, who saw his name on a list in the newspaper, angrily asked Barton what he had done to have his name "blazoned all over the country." Barton had little time for such antics. "What you have done . . . I certainly *do not* know," she told the soldier. "It seems to have been the misfortune of your family to think more of you than you did of them, and probably more than you deserve from the manner in which you treat them. . . . I shall inform them of your existence lest you should not 'see fit' to do so yourself."[8]

By mid-June Barton had published a list of twenty thousand names and was already compiling a second roll. "I am oh so busy," she wrote enthusiastically to Elvira. "My plan is a perfect success and is growing popular I think—at least no one condemns it that I know of."[9] The army, the Sanitary Commission, and several private organizations all referred requests to her.[10] She was delighted to find that information about the missing came pouring in and later claimed that almost half of the first list were identified, though statistics about her search show that this was quite an exaggeration.[11] The "Office of Correspondence with Friends of the Missing Men of the United States Army" came to have the aspect of a regular office, with letterhead stationery, several clerks, desks, ledgers, and messengers.

All of this cost money, and funding was a continuing problem. A number of those who wrote so imploringly to Miss Barton believed she charged a fee and asked her "price as if I hunted men at so much a head."[12] Most believed that she was well paid, either by the government or some other organization. In fact, she received no salary at all and was compelled to run the operation on a shoestring. In her initial letter to President Lincoln she had promised that she would do her work at little cost to the government.[13] As the project progressed, however, she found that she had to rely heavily on the War Department to meet expenses. The tent and camp table from which she worked in the pleasant mornings of early summer were not enough to carry on an operation that involved hundreds of letters daily. She was forced therefore to petition the government for free transportation between Annapolis and Washington, for stationery and supplies, for a postage allowance, and late in May, for the actual printing of the lists of missing men by the Government Printing Office.[14] Though Barton continued to retain her Patent Office clerkship, she had virtually no money of her own to use, and her efforts to solicit private contributions failed. Hers was only one of a multitude of requests pouring onto the desk of every government official from widows, disabled veterans, former slaves, and those who had lost property at the hands of the Union army. Barton's small office, though noble in sentiment, was lost among the more pressing needs of the war-torn Republic. The need for money, and Barton's poor ability to raise any, would keep it from ever becoming large and really effective.[15]

Barton's greatest help came one day, late in June, in the form of a letter, written in a rather shaky hand. "Can you send one of your lists of missing men to me?" read the letter. "I can inform you of a good many of them." It was from a young man named Dorence Atwater, a fellow New Englander who had endured twenty-two months at Andersonville Prison. A few days after she received his letter, Atwater arrived in person to tell his tale. His gaunt appearance and prematurely wrinkled brow could hide neither his extreme youth nor the innate dash and gentility of his manner. At eighteen he had joined the army in New York, though his native state was Connecticut. He was taken prisoner shortly thereafter while carrying a dispatch between the lines. At Andersonville he had been put into the hospital, then assigned to the task of recording the name, rank, and cause of death of each prisoner who expired. It was a grisly job for such a sensitive man, and one which grew more sorrowful by the day. When the numbers of dead topped seven hundred per week, Atwater began to suspect that Confederate officials might try to hide evidence of the brutal treatment they meted out by falsifying the records. He therefore began to copy the official registers secretly. Each night he hid his own copy in the lining of his jacket, and at the war's end he was able to smuggle it safely to the North.[16]

Atwater realized that his record was of great value to the War Department, and in late April he traveled to Washington to place it at the disposal of the authorities. The army offered to pay him three hundred dollars for the list, but he held out until he was offered a clerkship in the department in addition to the money. Atwater believed he had sold to the army only the right to copy the death rolls. He was adamant that the original be returned to him when the department clerks finished copying it, for he feared that the army would not communicate with the families of the dead men, and he knew from firsthand experience how anxious the prisoners had been for their relatives to know their fate. A rift developed between Atwater and the army over the matter when, after several months, the roll had not yet been returned to him, and it appeared that the army had stopped the copying process. By the time Atwater appeared at Barton's tent in early July, he still did not have his death list.[17]

In addition to the name, unit, and cause of death of each prisoner, Atwater told Barton, his list carried a number that marked the soldier's position in the long rows of trench graves. No names had been placed on the graves, but each place had been marked by a small numbered stick. This fact came to the attention of the secretary of war, Edward Stanton, early in the summer of 1865. Believing that those who had endured the horrors at Andersonville should be officially acknowledged by the nation and their graves marked in a proper manner, he ordered an expedition to the site of the old prison. The party was to be led by Captain James B. Moore, an army regular in charge of battlefield cemeteries. Atwater was invited to accompany the group so that he could give firsthand information about the burials.

A few days after Stanton's decision, Barton was summoned to an interview with the secretary. He flattered and praised her, then consulted her about embellishing the cemetery at Andersonville. To her delight, he told her that he had decided to invite her "to accompany Capt. Moore, with Atwater and his register to Andersonville, and see [her] suggestions carried out to [her] entire satisfaction." (Barton later claimed that she had originated the idea of an expedition, but Stanton's correspondence and her own papers indicate that she was invited along, almost as an afterthought.)[18]

The group, consisting of Captain Moore, Atwater, and a crew of forty laborers and craftsmen, boarded the U.S.S. *Virginia* on July 8. A slight mix-up in transportation arrangements caused Clara to arrive hours after the scheduled departure, irritating James Moore to the point that he reportedly shouted "God damn it to hell! Some people don't deserve to go anywhere. And what in hell does she want to go for?"[19] The mishap foreshadowed a spirit of animosity between Moore and Barton that flourished during the trip. As soon as she stepped on board,

138

Barton sensed the strain and bemoaned this extra burden on an already tension-filled journey. Moore ignored her, choosing to show her only superficial courtesies. "I cannot understand Capt. Moore, he does not seem friendly, is silent; and abstract as if I were an intruder," Clara recorded in the early days of the expedition. She chose to try to make amends, but as the days went on she realized that Moore's hostility was not to be tempered. She had lived among large numbers of men before, of course, but there had always been a loyal friend of the Twenty-first Massachusetts or a gallant surgeon or officer to look after her. Barton was more a product of her times than she cared to admit, and when Moore pointedly refused to accompany her to dinner or drive with her through Savannah upon their arrival, she stayed in her cabin rather than appear before the world without an escort.[20] "How alone I am and on such a trip," she wrote sorrowfully in her diary; "how little people at home can realize my situation and what it will cost me."[21]

The snub rankled her out of proportion, and she began to lose perspective on Moore and the expedition. When poor roads and nonexistent railroad and river transportation made Moore consider rerouting or postponing the journey to the interior of Georgia, Barton believed it was a conscious plot to undermine her efforts. They set off for Andersonville on a roundabout route that led them hundreds of miles out of their way and required traveling by slow boat up the Savannah River, transferring halfway to an antiquated railroad car, and completing the journey by mule train.[22] They traveled through Atlanta, "*torn in fragments*, a shocking place," and made the many changes, each of which required unloading and loading headboards, lumber, and equipment with agonizing slowness in the unrelenting July heat. Emotionally drained and bone weary, Clara's only comfort during the trip was an occasional snort of "Mr. Tuffts Blackberry Brandy."[23]

They arrived at Andersonville on July 25 feeling some trepidation, for they were the first official group to enter the prison since it had ceased functioning. The horrendous reports of the few surviving prisoners left them wondering what to expect from this place of misery and death. The prison had been placed in this remote part of Georgia because of either the abundance of food or the unhealthy climate (depending on whether the account was from the South or the North). It consisted of an open stockade enclosing twenty-five acres of treeless ground, through which ran a sluggish stream. The prisoners, up to twenty-five thousand at one time, were herded into this enclosure and kept, without benefit of shelter, fresh water, or sufficient clothing, through the merciless drizzle of winter and endless days of summer heat. The stream dried to a trickle in July and August and became so mired with grease and filth from latrines and cooking tents that the residue still clung to the banks at the time of Barton's visit. Inside the stockade the ground was pockmarked with burrows and wells, the pitiful attempts of the soldiers to live decently under inhuman conditions. Food had been worse than inadequate (often the entire day's ration was half a cup of rice), with no firewood over which to cook it. Men died by the hundreds of pneumonia, ty-phoid fever, starvation, and most frequently, scurvy. Fear was added to this pri-vation, for the stockade was surrounded by a well-patrolled line of demarcation, the "dead line," over which no one was allowed to venture. Men were shot for accidentally stepping on it, for putting their hand on it, or, occasionally, for merely coming too near it. Perhaps the greatest tragedy of Andersonville was that conditions need not have been so bad. There was abundant timber nearby from which barracks could have been made, and a wide stream, named Sweet Water Creek, flowed briskly a mile away. The country produced food abundantly throughout the war. As for escape, the area was so remote that the prisoners would have easily been recaptured.[24]

Rumors of half-buried bodies and lingering pestilence had reached the band of workers, and they were relieved that, in this respect, the sight of Andersonville was better than they had expected. A local farmer had taken the trouble to re-bury those bodies that were exposed and to maintain the cemetery in a cursory fashion. But, though she had been forewarned with stories of maltreatment, Bar-ton gazed upon the stockade and rude semblance of a hospital with shock. She had maintained a certain objectivity during the war; her beloved Massachusetts boys had had no monopoly on suffering, and she had been quick to see the needs of the fallen on both sides. Now, as she walked the pitted and filthy prison ground, she questioned for the first time that spirit of impartiality. Bitterness, which had not before tinged her patriotism, flowed quickly through her veins.[25] She would never again give the South the benefit of the doubt, and henceforth would actively give her support to the radical Republicans. The most dramatic and poignant writings of her life would be addressed to the subject of this prison and its ghosts. "I have looked upon its terrible face," she would tell lecture audi-ences scarcely a year later, "but friends, not in the same breath in which I would speak of anything else in the Heavens above, or the earth beneath, would I speak of this. . . . My heart sickened and stood still, my brain whirled, and the light of my eyes went out, and I said 'surely this was not the gate of hell, but hell itself,' and for comfort, I turned away to the 9 acres of crowded graves, and I said, here at last was rest, and this to them was the gate of heaven."[26]

With aching hearts the company began their appointed task. The work itself was not difficult, for the records had been well kept and graves were clearly marked. "I find the graves can be identified perfectly," Barton wrote in some sat-isfaction. "My plan is practical *again.*"[27] Headboards were lettered, fences built, and walkways laid out, while plans were made to turn the crowded graveyard into a national cemetery. Nearly thirteen thousand graves were properly marked; only some four hundred carried the words "Unknown U.S. Soldier." Barton never lost sight of the fact that thousands of hearts mourned for these young men, and this collected suffering sanctified the spot for her as could nothing else. Late at night, in the little canvas tent erected for her outside the prison bounda-ries, she half wrote a poem, expressing her feelings.

140

Well Mothers I am here—here with your darling ones
Before me lie the narrow graves that hold your martyred sons
And sisters pale with weeping close clasp one another
Here lies the tribute wreath I've turned for that lost and noble brother[28]

Her sorrow and bitterness were heightened by the continuation of difficult relations with Captain Moore. She believed he purposefully blocked her work and misrepresented her in his reports to the War Department. When a series of falsified letters, purportedly from Clara to an "Uncle James," was published in several prominent newspapers, she accused Moore of being the author. The letters were mild enough, but they portrayed Barton as a highhanded old maid and frequently spoke of Moore in laudatory terms. It was the act of forgery that irritated Barton most. "I never had an 'Uncle James,'" she wrote angrily, "and wrote *no* letters home for publication."[29] As for Moore's reports, they did not mention Clara at all, save a scanty reference to her help nursing some of the men who fell sick.[30] The real trouble was that he ignored her in person, as well as in his reports, refusing to consult with her or pay her the homage she believed was her due. "I was shown no real consideration or respect," Barton stated to the secretary of war upon her return.

> I do not speak of those little attentions which in ordinary life gentlemen are wont to render to ladies, I have learned to dispense with these very easily, but I had not expected to be systematically ignored during the whole expedition. . . . My opinion was never asked on any question of taste or fitness. No word of consultation ever passed between Captain Moore and myself, and so forcibly was I impressed from the first by his silence, that I was never once betrayed into making an inquiry or suggestion.[31]

Moore, Barton believed, was jealous of her fame and resented her supposed influence with the War Department. She maintained that the entire expedition had been her idea and that he hoped to take the credit for it. Moore certainly does not seem to have respected Barton's opinions or catered to her in any way. His own office at the War Department was, in certain respects, in direct competition with her bureau. But it is unclear whether he was truly anxious to keep entire control of the government's effort at identifying the Union dead or was simply exasperated at the cumbersome presence of a woman. In Barton's mind he became a bitter enemy and remained so for the remainder of her long life.[32]

Barton's work at Andersonville was finished early. While the workmen completed the cemetery she spent her time chiefly in nursing the sick. One young man died, amid a scene of tears and prayers, which she recorded in her diary with Victorian sentimentality: to her he was "the last martyr of Andersonville."[33] She wandered the acres within the stockade, collecting relics left by the poor inmates—drinking

141

cups made from shells, soup plates fashioned from a gourd, a post office made from a beehive.[34] A few local people made their way to her tent and expressed disgust with the actions of the prison authorities, but Barton was by now so cynical that she assumed their motive was entirely political.

Far more affecting to her were the scores of ex-slaves who often walked twenty or more miles to see this Yankee woman and ask her questions about the government's new policies. Many had been duped into believing that with Abraham Lincoln's assassination the Emancipation Proclamation was no longer valid. The former masters were inclined to cheat a good many of their former bondsmen, and the blacks had few people to turn to for honest information. On August 13 she recorded in her diary, "Few know the worth of such a day, over 100 colored people have been to me for counsel and curiosity. I have essayed to satisfy both—old men, strong men, young men & young women and husbands, all anxious to know the law." The visits strongly reinforced the concern for the freedmen that Frances Gage had instilled in her, and when it came time to use the political power that she had amassed, she would use it for this group before any other. The circumstances also did a great deal to further her animosity toward Southern whites. Before the war she judged the slaves as "worthless in any country, only as subjects fit for missionary labors and candidates for eternity"; now it was the masters she condemned.[35]

By mid-August the work was completed, and the laborers packed their tools for the long journey home. On August 17 the cemetery was officially dedicated. It had been a trying and emotionally draining experience for the entire crew, and it was with dry throats and respectful silence that they watched the solemn ceremony. Barton's role in the cemetery's creation was officially recognized when she was chosen to raise the United States flag over the prison grounds. The passionate words and disjointed sentences of her diary entry show that her strong emotions had still not left her when, by candlelight, she sat down to record the events of the day.

> Dressing early—Capt. called me to go and run up the stars & stripes—and this at Andersonville! Where sleep those 13000 martyrs—where the flag of the country no flag had floated in four dark years. . . . I advanced . . . and ran it up amid the cheers of the beholders—Up and there it drooped as if in grief and sadness, till at length the sunlight streamed out and its beautiful folds filled—the men struck up the Star Spangled Banner and I covered my face and wept.[36]

After the ceremony, Barton parted company with Captain Moore and took a roundabout train route through Kentucky and Ohio rather than stay on board the government transport with the man she so detested. She was upset about the events of the expedition and worried that Moore would return before she did and poison every influential mind against her. She had been unable to find the origin of the falsified letters, and she was only partially mollified when several newspapers printed, at her insistence, a retraction. Barton arrived back in Washington exhausted and tense, grimly determined to continue her work with the missing men but without the wherewithal to do it.[37]

Barton scarcely had time to formulate her plans before another whirlwind of anxiety cut a swath through her life and threatened to destroy every bit of credibility she had sought so long to establish. Late in August, Dorence Atwater was arrested, on charges of larceny, for the theft of the roll of the Andersonville dead. He had persisted in his belief that the government had paid him only for the privilege of copying the document and had pressed continually for the return of the original. When the War Department refused to release the list, Atwater made up his mind to repossess it by any means he could. The roll had been taken on the expedition to Andersonville, and Atwater had frequently handled it in the course of his duties. At the end of the expedition he kept the paper in his tent, and as the official party packed to leave, he simply put it in his trunk, and locked the lid securely. Though Barton had not associated extensively with Atwater in Georgia, she listened to his story and saw in it a question of justice. She thought also that Moore had had a hand in the controversy over the list, though in fact he had not. It was with Barton's encouragement that Atwater boldly reclaimed his roll of the Andersonville dead.[38]

To her horror, during the court-martial Atwater was thrown into the Old Capitol Prison, which until recently had been used to detain notorious rebel spies. The implication of disloyalty incensed Barton, as did the prison's grim conditions. It was a crumbling old coop, built around a festering courtyard, and the food was so bad that a number of the more colorful inmates had chosen to subsist on dry bread and an occasional peach—illicitly obtained—rather than brave the daily mess of gray beans and moldy cornbread.[39] Barton did what she could to supply Atwater with food and money, but she could not alleviate his worries about the court-martial. It commenced on September 2 and lasted two days. Colonel Samuel Breck, who had made the original arrangements with Atwater, testified that they had mistrusted the former prisoner's intentions from the beginning and had never promised officially to give him a personal copy of the death list, that, indeed, the government had had the right all along to simply seize the document without offering compensation. Atwater did not testify, but submitted a written statement somewhat at odds with Breck's version of the story. Moore, completely outraged at the loss of the rolls, which were under his custody, was a strong witness for the government. The War Department, he allowed, had shown every courtesy to the soldier and had been greatly wronged at his hands. In the end Atwater was convicted of larceny and "Conduct to Prejudice of Good Order and Military Discipline." He was dishonorably discharged and sentenced to eighteen months in prison and a three-hundred-dollar fine.[40]

By begging favors, Clara managed to obtain a transcript of the proceedings. She thought them outrageous, accused Moore of packing the jury, and assumed that Atwater had not testified because he was not allowed to. She saw little sign that Atwater had been properly defended and was heartsick that the maximum penalty had been imposed in a situation that she characterized as a misunderstanding at worst. When she heard that Atwater had been taken in irons through the streets of Washington, en route to Auburn Prison in New York, she was appalled that in such a controversial case he would be treated as a dangerous criminal. Yet for all of her heightened feelings, Barton was reluctant to come overtly to his defense. Her own name had not been dragged into the court-martial, but she was apprehensive lest the final blame for the theft be put on her; already she knew that several officials blamed "unwise advisers" for Atwater's behavior. Torn between guilt and the fear of personal consequences, she would make discreet inquiries and try personal influence but would not entangle her name in the case by taking decisive action on his behalf.[41]

Barton struggled that fall against the return of demoralization and dwindling resources that threatened the collapse of her work. While she was still at Andersonville her name had finally been struck from the registers of the Patent Office, and she now had no income at all.[42] She dipped into her pocketbook, then finally began to liquidate her modest assets. By early November her last resources were gone. To her diary she was sanguine enough to write that "it is not the first time in my life that I have come to the bottom of the bag—I guess I shall die a pauper yet, but I haven't been either stingy nor lazy and if I stand I shall not be alone."[43] But Barton could not help but be worried, and her neatly penciled accounts of household expenditures show that she lived on less than fifty cents a day for months at a time. Too proud to accept charity, she was livid when acquaintances tried tactfully to help. Even as old a friend as Henry Wilson could not assist her. When, in late December, he tried to give her twenty dollars as a "Christmas gift," she refused to even consider accepting it and recorded the incident in her journal with shock and sorrow.[44]

Clara needed little to live on; the cruelest consequence of her lack of funds was that her little bureau was forced into a period of inactivity. The government would publish her rolls and give her franking privileges and transportation, but they would not pay for clerks or office space. Barton continued to receive letters from the nation's sorrowing mothers and was inundated with bags of mail from charitable agencies and stacks of correspondence over which the War Department had despaired. October 3, 1865, found her with thirty-five hundred letters unanswered and her conscience heavy over the dashed hopes that those unopened envelopes represented. "The poor mothers of the land, how can I give them up and do no more for them, will no one come to their aid, must I give up my search?" she asked herself.[45]

There was a false glimmer of hope when Benjamin Butler promised to use his influence to have the office made an official part of the War Department. He was in a poor position to wield power, however, for since his dismissal a year earlier he had become more a brunt of inside jokes than a revered former leader. Butler quickly found that the War Department wanted no part of Barton's work; they believed that their own department, headed by Captain Moore, was quite adequate. Indeed, the department would not consent to even allow her to use their records, a decision General E. D. Townsend affirmed in a rather terse message that December. "Experience has never failed to demonstrate the fatal effects of allowing irresponsible agents, for whatever purpose, to have access to information contained in the records of this office," read the letter, "and it is most strenuously recommended that it not be granted to Miss Barton, since it would be sure to place persons, through her agency, in possession of official data which they ought not to have."[46]

Barton believed to the end of her life that James Moore had done all in his power to sully her name and take over in his own office the work she had tried so hard to establish. Moore's part is left unclear by the records. He may well have been jealously guarding his territory, and his evident dislike of Barton could have caused him to spread gossip. Yet Clara did much to mar her own reputation during this time. Her part in Atwater's misappropriation of the Andersonville lists may have been simply poor judgment, but she brought herself little credit by writing hotheaded letters aimed at discrediting Moore. When Moore was chosen over her to testify at the trial of the Andersonville prison officials, she took it as a personal affront and wrote an astonishingly vindictive note to Senator Wilson. "I can *think* of *nothing* in this matter that *I have done* why I should be so *humiliated* and *trumped over*," she stormed. "I believe I have acted nobly, and well for my *country*, and *humanity* . . . and why the *jealousy* of a little *worthless* petty officer should be allowed to trample me *speechless* in the *dust*, I *cannot* understand." She acted childish and dull around those officers whom she felt had snubbed her, and she further discredited herself by pairing off with Butler, the current War Department buffoon.[47]

Barton's efforts to free Dorence Atwater were as frustrated as the attempts to attach her office to the government. She petitioned Henry Wilson and Secretary Stanton, but both were too busy with reconstruction policies to pay much attention to such detail. In October she made a flying trip to New England with hopes that Joseph Sheldon, a lawyer and husband of a girlhood friend, could advise her. Sheldon took an interest in the matter, as did a cousin, Robert Hale, newly elected to Congress from New York. Neither could divine a sure way of obtaining a pardon for Atwater. When, after two months in prison, he was released, it was not through Barton's efforts but because of an order by President Andrew Johnson requiring all military offenders not held for assault to be freed.[48]

There was little at this time that worked to alleviate Barton's depression. Jules Golay called often, as did other acquaintances, but it mattered little. She half-heartedly attended a few parties and lectures, but spent most of the autumn in her cheerless room, which was stacked on all sides with boxes of letters and ledgers representing "the coinage . . . of aching hearts."[49] She worried about the cleaning woman, her financial plight, Sally's health, and the fact that her hair was falling out. Her diary began to read as it had during the worst days in Hightstown and in the years of inactivity between Patent Office jobs. "I woke this morning with the deepest feeling of depression and despair that I could scarce remember to have known," she recorded on December 17. "I could hardly find it in me to rise and dress, and did not for some time, it seemed to me that the whole horizon was overcast and the clouds shut down all around."[50] A week later she endured the bluest Christmas she would ever spend: "not merry, not even happy . . . but like all these days so much to be done, so little aid, so much disappointment and vexation."[51]

Clara faced the New Year, 1866, still mourning the deaths of Stephen and Irving and with shaken self-confidence. She was scared of noises in the hall, unable to determine her future, and so lacking in self-esteem that she declared she had never felt herself "to be of as much consequence as a whole pie."[52] She was greatly relieved to find, therefore, that her beloved Aunt Fanny, with all of her wisdom and moral courage, was coming to visit that month. When Gage arrived, late in January, Barton was so distraught that she threw herself at her visitor's feet, crying, "what shall I do, oh—what can I do?" According to Gage, the older woman replied, "You can lecture. Tell the world as you told me the suffer [ings] of our brave boys in blue."[53] It was not the first time Barton had considered the option of going on the lecture circuit; indeed she had spent much of New Year's Day attempting to put together a lecture that would be both dramatic and eloquent.[54] She mistrusted her abilities as a writer and speaker, however, and harbored a conventional concern that public lecturing was not the proper sphere for a gentlewoman. Gage, herself a popular lecturer before and during the war, did much to offset these worries. Moreover, she pointed out that the benefits of lecturing were great. Before the American people Barton could publicize her work, vindicate her actions (and those of Dorence Atwater), and at the same time earn considerable money to sponsor her foundering office.

Barton also prevailed upon her mentor to write several newspaper articles endorsing her and her efforts on behalf of the missing men. "This is a great work, requiring many hands, and hard steady labor," Gage reported to the *New York Independent.* "Friends must be patient, thankful for what has been done, and trusting for the future." More significantly, Barton and Aunt Fanny devised a petition to Congress, asking for an appropriation of fifteen thousand dollars to enable her work to continue and expand. The memorial maintained that Barton had spent a private fortune of twelve thousand dollars during the war. That amount was to be reimbursed, and the rest was to go to the costs of keeping up the correspondence concerning missing men. The petition itself was thick with emotional prose, which lauded the brave soldiers and sorrowing families of the nation, as well as Barton's part in alleviating their distress. "Oh, my countrymen! . . ." wrote Gage. "Which of you would not give a hundred times two dollars if the case were yours to know the fate of a son or a brother and is the heart of a loving wife or mother less tender than your own?" The petition was granted in mid-March.[55]

Its passage was aided by Barton's appearance, on February 21, before the Joint Committee on Reconstruction. Hers was the only female testimony during months of hearings; indeed she may have been the first woman ever to testify before Congress. Such a public appearance was still looked upon by the vast majority of people as too intellectual, and therefore unladylike, for a well-bred woman. Barton seems to have had no such personal qualms. She adamantly told the anti-Southern politicians exactly what they wished to hear: that white Southerners had no respect for the government of the United States; that they were disposed to cheat their former slaves; that the conditions at Andersonville had been worse than inhuman. The junket to Georgia had embittered her, and she vented her opinions with dramatic intensity.[56]

Despite Barton's strong endorsement of the prevailing political opinion and the nobility of her project, the petition in her behalf did not sail through Congress without some raised eyebrows. Many women had sacrificed as she had during the war, and some legislators questioned why she should be singled out. Others were sensible of the rumors at the War Department and intimated that the Office of Correspondence with Friends of the Missing Men of the United States Army was more of a hindrance than a help to the government. More serious were the queries about the exact nature of her finances, questions that would periodically return to haunt her. She had kept no record of the twelve thousand dollars she allegedly spent, and it is difficult now to see where she could have raised that sum. Her own resources had been strained to the limit between 1857 and 1860 (she had been unable even to pay for her board the latter part of the period), she had earned only three hundred dollars before she left the Patent Office in 1862, and her father's legacy amounted to only four hundred dollars. Later in Barton's career a rumor circulated that a former suitor had left her a gift of five thousand dollars and that she had touched it only when the necessities of the war had made it seem right to do so. No records have ever substantiated this story. Yet even this would make up only half the sum she claimed to have spent.[57] Late in life she would be accused of dishonesty for accepting the money, and even at the time there were snide remarks from the formerly loyal press. "She had made a very profitable thing out of her speculation, and traded upon her patriotism to a good purpose," the Boston Post commented. "Her operations were purely of a speculative character, and exactly upon the footing of a pardon broker or a claim agent, and she is entitled to no more consideration than those classes."[58]

Barton herself seems to have felt no guilt over the congressional appropriation. The fifteen thousand dollars, given to her in the form of government bonds, made her financially secure for the first time in her life.[59] She hired Atwater and Jules Golay as clerks in her office, acquired furniture, and went about her work with a renewed spirit.[60] Barton had induced Atwater to donate his

Andersonville list to the press as a sign of his sincerity of purpose in repossessing it, and that spring several newspapers carried the roll, before the War Department had time to publish their own version. This action, which she believed to be a triumph over Moore, pleased her.[61] Her professional satisfaction was further enhanced by the home life she enjoyed that spring and summer. Jules and Dorence lived with her in the rooms on Seventh Street, which were furnished plainly, with utilitarian chairs and desks, an old rug, and a few pieces she had inherited from her mother.[62] They lived in a comfortable, casual style, ignoring the foibles of fashionable society and boarding out at a neighbor's house. Barton admitted that she owned only two dresses and found that quite adequate. When Cousin Vira wrote to say she was planning a visit, Clara reassured her about their informal ways: "You haven't to appear at table among a parcel of critical boarders at all—we walk in and eat with shawl on and take it off as we please."[63]

Despite the renewal of her office activities, in the fall of 1866 Barton began contacting publicity agents with the hope of scheduling a series of lectures for that winter season. By October she had been accepted for a rigorous tour in New York State and New England. All through a damp November and December she traveled this familiar territory, delivering her lecture, entitled "Work and Incidents of Army Life," in lyceum halls, churches, town halls, and overcrowded schoolrooms. In December she returned home for a short rest before departing for another strenuous series of appearances in the western part of the country.[64]

Her lectures were well received. Barton's instinctive sense of drama may have led her to use loaded adjectives and to harp on pathetic scenes, but the finished lectures spoke exactly to the tastes of her audience. Now far enough removed from the terror and privation of battle, the country longed to be sentimental about the war. She thrilled crowds with stirring descriptions of charge and retreat and intimate portraits of dying soldiers whispering last thoughts of mother or sweetheart. "It was as if this gifted woman found our heartstrings and was skillfully playing a sad minor hymn upon them," rhapsodized one small-town reporter.[65] Occasionally she used the lectern to promote Atwater's case or build sympathy for the freedmen and the destitute families of men who had been killed or crippled. They were frankly partisan talks, delivered only in the North and geared toward Union sentiments. More than once she used her impressions of Andersonville, not merely to evoke pathos, but to consciously foster animosity toward the conquered South.[66]

With pleasure she read and clipped the little newspaper notices of her talks, for they were overwhelmingly favorable. Clara had surprised herself with her speaking ability. She always dressed in black silk, and her small figure had a natural dignity that hushed skeptical audiences as easily as it had the unruly boys she had faced in the schoolroom. Her own musical voice was a tremendous asset, at once expressive and theatrical. "Miss Barton is gifted with extraordinary powers of description and eloquence and as a lecturer carries her hearers with her with a remarkable power," stated one newspaper.[67] Only rarely were the comments negative. One western reporter thought them devoid of any deep intellectual thought, and a few complained of her stance against many of the Union officers. Almost apologetically the *Syracuse Daily Standard* remarked, "we must respectfully suggest to Miss Barton that M-y spells My, and B-y spells By—not Me and Be. My and By are good strong Saxon words. Me and Be are stage monstrosities and should be discarded by so perfect a mistress of good English as Miss Barton."[68] Despite such comments, the lectures were a great success. Even when competing with such revered speakers as Frederick Douglass and Mark Twain, she spoke to packed and enthusiastic audiences.

The lectures were advantageous to Barton in yet another way—they gave wide publicity to her name and work. Many women, North and South, had sacrificed and struggled to aid the armies, but they had been content with a little local fame or an inner feeling of satisfaction. Barton's appearance on the battlefield made her war service unusual but not unique. That her work became legendary was due to the opportunity the lectures gave her to tell her story. Before the lecture series of 1866–68, Barton was little known outside of Washington, D.C., and the sewing circles of her home town. After the tour, her name was a household word, synonymous with humanitarian sacrifice. In her later relief work the fame was to be a tremendous boon in fund raising and securing official support. In the late 1860s it served chiefly to temper her altruism with an appetite for applause.

Unfortunately, ability and inclination do not always coincide, and Clara maintained a hearty dislike of lecturing. She never got over her stage fright, and she suffered greatly from fatigue and illness on the lengthy railroad journeys between cities.[69] "All speech making terrifies me," she would write; "first I have no taste for it, lastly I hate it." She told one friend that she worked better than she talked, and wished she were home attending to her correspondence regarding missing men.[70]

Yet for almost two years, between 1866 and 1868, Barton booked a schedule of lectures that was formidable by any standards. Her timetable for a single month of 1868 reads like a roster of major midwestern cities; it included fourteen lectures at such stops as Pittsburgh; Cleveland; Toledo; Burlington, Iowa; and Adrian, Michigan.[71]

Though to friends she maintained that she was "not naturally . . . ambitious of gain," it was clearly the enormous economic rewards of lecturing that kept her going.[72] After some initial hesitation about how much to charge, Barton received $75 to $100 per lecture, fees that were equal to those of male lecturers.[73] She sometimes gave speeches for the benefit of soldiers' funds or local charities, but the vast majority of her earnings she pocketed herself. Her expenses were far below her income; in November of 1866, for example, she spent $49.12 while earning nearly $1,000.[74] The money ensured the continued functioning of the office in Washington, but it also catapulted her into a position of near independent wealth.

The years for Clara thus wore on, the days melding into something of a hazy continuum, much as the scenery blurred through the train window: "this traveling nights gets me confused and I don't separate the days," she complained.[75] Occasionally an incident made one town, or a particular lecture, stand out. At New York's Steinway Hall, in the spring of 1867, she gave a benefit talk to a crowd of over five hundred veterans. The stage was decorated with an army tent, a stack of muskets, and a small howitzer. Across the back of the podium ran a banner with a scroll bearing the word "Grant." A drum corps announced her entrance while the band struck up the "William Tell Overture." Pleased as she was to give this lecture, which benefited the widows and orphans of her valiant "boys," she did not like such trappings, and the experience made her wary of other large gatherings. Another town was firmly fixed in her mind since it was the site of a train crash that nearly cost Barton, and Atwater, who was accompanying her, their lives.[76] Yet one more notable evening was spent in a remote town west of the Mississippi. From the stage she began to regale her audience with stories of Antietam, focusing halfway through, as she always did, on the surgeons' gratitude for simple articles, such as candles, with which she supplied them. During her lecture she spoke of one doctor, too overcome on that awful day to express his thanks. Suddenly a man sprang to his feet and ran to the stage. "Ladies and gentlemen," he exclaimed, "if I have never acknowledged that favor I will do it now. I am that surgeon."[77]

On the last day of November 1867, while changing trains in Cleveland, Barton met Elizabeth Cady Stanton and Susan B. Anthony, the two celebrated feminists, who were also engaged in a lecture tour. This is the first recorded instance of their meeting, which marked the beginning of a long and productive relationship, especially between Barton and Anthony. By 1867 Barton no longer had any doubts about the need to expand women's political and social rights. Reactionary observers might maintain that it was a pleasure to watch this feminine woman stand at the lectern because she had not "laid aside her womanhood when consenting to speak in public, and whose claims to favor, defend on a record of charitable ministrations . . . appropriate to her sex, and not on a masculine crusade against abuses, if not wholly imaginary, greatly exaggerated by a captious disposition." But these observers were wrong. She was at this time ready to declare her "own entire—earnest—heartfelt—ever before and ever-after sympathy and cooperation . . . to the thousands constantly going up for the early and complete enfranchisement of my sex, and the admission of women of whatever race to all the rights and privileges . . . which as an intelligent human being belongs to her."[78]

It was natural that she should eventually align herself with these crusading women, for her background reflected so many of their own concerns: her scanty education, and the slow and painful efforts to make up for it; the late development into physical womanhood and the shock of recognition that her intellectual proclivities made her different, indeed cast her out of her accepted sphere; her struggle to earn a living wage in a world that offered only a handful of possibilities. Nonetheless, it was her wartime service that gave rise to her dedicated feminism—and illustrated her greatest hope for her sex. The war, she maintained, had proven the sincerity of women who wanted to contribute to society, had shown them as a political force in every soldiers' aid society and abolitionist rally. And the war had marked woman's worth. "Only an opportunity was wanting," she declared in an emotional lecture, which was unfortunately never delivered, "for woman to prove to man that she *could* be in earnest—that she had character, and firmness of purpose—that she *was* good for something in an emergency. . . . The war afforded her this opportunity." [79] Further, it was not only men who had been convinced of female competence during the years of bloody conflict but the women themselves. They had a new appreciation of their capabilities now, a new understanding of their ability to command a situation. Whatever their prior frustrations, the war had given them *experience*, a fact emphasized by Barton in her best poetic effort, "The Women Who Went to the Field":

'Twas a hampered work, its worth largely lost;
'Twas hindrance, and pain, and effort, and cost:
But through these came knowledge,—knowledge is power.—
And never again in the deadliest hour
Of war or of peace, shall we be so beset
To accomplish the purpose our spirits have met. [80]

Dating from this time, a symbiotic relationship developed between Barton and the more radical feminist leaders. Anthony advertised Barton's lectures in her publication *The Revolution,* and Clara was eagerly sought after to speak at women's conventions, take part in rallies, or simply grace a gathering by her presence on the stage. [81] Barton's struggles to establish herself as a lecturer, and later to organize the American Red Cross, were actively sustained by leaders of the women's rights movement. For her part, Barton began early to rally support for female suffrage from all the spheres of her influence, most notably among the country's veterans. Using her strong emotional bond with them, she cried, "*Soldiers! I have worked for you*—and I ask of you, now, one and all, that you consider the wants of my people. . . . God only knows women were your friends in time of peril—and you should be hers now." [82]

She did not always play to the soldiers, however. Indeed, her first strong public defense of feminist principles resulted from a misguided attempt by a veterans' organization to portray her as a patriotic, but not "strong-minded," woman. Arriving in one small town, she found herself billed in the following manner:

We can promise our citizens a rare treat of patriotic eloquence, such as is seldom listened to, and we can assure them that there will be no cause for disappointment; they will not have thrust upon them a lecture upon women's rights after the style of Susan B. Anthony and her clique; Miss Barton does not belong to that class of women.

151

Outraged that she should be described thus, Clara nonetheless marched to the hall and delivered her lecture to a packed house. At the end of her talk, however, she slowly read the offending paragraph aloud to the audience and then gave this rousing endorsement of women's rights:

That paragraph, my comrades, does worse than to misrepresent me as a woman; it maligns my friend. It abuses the highest and bravest work ever done in this land for either you or me. You glorify the women who made their way to the front to reach you in your misery, and nurse you back to life. You called us angels. Who opened the way for women to go and made it possible? Who but that detested "clique" who through the years of opposition, obloquy, toil and pain had openly claimed that women had rights, should have the privilege to exercise them. The right to her own property, her own children, her own home, her just individual claim before the law, to her freedom of action, to her personal liberty. Upon this, other women claimed the right and took the courage, if only to go to an army camp, and drag wounded men out of a trench, and try to save them for their families and their country. . . .

No one has stood so unhelped, unprotected, so maligned as Susan B. Anthony, no one deserves so well; and soldiers, I would have the first monument that is ever erected to any woman in this country reared to her.

Summoning all of her strength she called out, "Boys, three cheers for Susan B. Anthony!" As she later noted with satisfaction, "the very windows shook in their casements."[83]

Barton's dedication to the feminists was genuine, but throughout the forty-odd years that she would work for the movement, Barton never allied herself too closely with it. She kept a conservative view of the proceedings, favoring advancement for women in all areas of life, and fearing that too much emphasis on the vote would retard social breakthroughs. Barton refused to allow her name to be listed as an officer of any organization, and she once stopped an entire press run of handbills, paying for them to be reset and printed rather than have her name appear as "vice president" of the National Woman Suffrage Association. Having always identified with men, Barton frequently spoke of the burdens men carried because of their subjugation of women, and she admitted that she often thought ladies deserved their reputation as frivolous, unintelligent creatures. Personally, she refused to make suffrage the driving crusade of her life; there were too many other, more glaring, needs to keep it in perspective. "When I stood month after month & year after year among the wounded & slain *men* of my nation . . . I forgot in the great privilege of going to minister to their wants that any privileges had ever been denied me. I forgot that I was a woman," she proclaimed in 1868. "When I raised the flag on 13,000 sleeping martyrs of Andersonville, I forgot that I could not vote."[84]

Her moderation on women's issues was never more evident than in 1868, when a rift developed among the feminists over the proposed Fifteenth Amendment to the Constitution, which forbade denial of the vote on account of "race, colour, or national origin." Some women, notably Anthony, were incensed that the opportunity to include the word "sex" had not been seized. Others, believing that the Negro had suffered far greater wrongs than women, feared that the protests of the feminists would jeopardize passage of the amendment in any form, a tragedy that would render sterile the entire hideous experience of the war.[85] Like Gage, Lucy Stone, and Mary Livermore, and like Frances Harper, who emotionally declared that her wrongs had been so great as a Negro that she had scarcely known she suffered wrongs as a woman, Barton chose to step back, if need be, and let the Negro's grievances be redressed first. In late 1868, at the request of Susan Anthony, she addressed the Universal Franchise Convention, where, to everyone's surprise, she spoke forcefully, not for women's rights alone, but for priority of the Negro.

> No person in this house could be more rejoiced than myself if it could be decided to admit at the same moment to a voice in the Government all persons and classes of persons naturally and properly entitled to it; and not now so admitted. But if the door be not wide enough to admit us all at once—and one must wait—then I am willing.
> . . . I am willing to stand back and see the old, scared limping slave clank his broken fetters through before me—while I stand with head uncovered—thanking God for the release.

She could not believe, Barton said at the conclusion, that the Negro, whom women had helped for so many years, would shut this door in their face.[86]

Aunt Fanny's teachings and her own contact with blacks in Georgia had, of course, greatly influenced Barton's championship of the Negro. Important, too, was a close acquaintance with Josephine Griffing, a fellow resident of Washington, D.C. Griffing was a cultivated and hotheaded woman who had come to the capital in 1865 to fight for the needs of newly freed slaves. She was instrumental in the establishment of the Freedman's Bureau and diligently promoted the idea that surplus government goods could be used to give the blacks a new start. Barton liked Griffing and her two dour daughters, despite their self-righteous and intolerant attitude toward anyone whose views did not coincide with their own. She spent several afternoons in avid conversation with them. Their discussions centered on the old barracks the Griffings used to temporarily shelter the ex-slaves who swarmed into the capital, and the Griffings' method of aid, which involved teaching the freedmen to themselves repair, refit, or sort the surplus army supplies at their disposal. These methods would have a good deal of influence on Barton's relief work with the Red Cross. At the time, however, they merely reinforced her sense that something must be done to bolster the flagging spirit of the freedmen.[87] So taken was Clara with the Griffings' enterprise that she petitioned Senator Wilson to have the crumbling Lincoln Hospital refitted as an industrial school for freedmen—with her at the helm. The plan never materialized—there were too many others clamouring for projects of a similar sort.[88]

The proposal was indicative of Barton's need for a new endeavor by this time. The work with missing soldiers was dwindling and could be easily handled by the clerks she had retained while she ran from pulpit to platform. Now only a few letters trickled in, evidence of the country's declining interest. Her lectures, too, had stopped. While speaking in a small Maine hamlet in the spring of 1868, the accumulated tension and fatigue sapped her strength and her voice failed. The well-known signs and symptoms of her nervous prostrations were there: the dimmed eyesight, the faltering voice, the inability to move or eat. She recovered slowly and was still too ill a year later to accept an invitation to speak at the twentieth anniversary meeting of the first feminist convention.[89] Somehow she managed the strength to move from her "old rookery of eight years and launch out into the world" to a large house on Capitol Hill, but she collapsed again shortly thereafter.[90] Barton made a month-long trip home to North Oxford to consult a doctor and found to her horror that her Washington physician had been prescribing a medicine laced heavily with morphine, which had added greatly to her sluggishness and muddled intellect. Reliable old Doctor Fuller amended the directions to a simple guarantee of good cheer—one glass per day of a prescription that read: "1pt of Bay Rum, pt 1/2 alspice."[91] When she told him that she merely picked at her projects, unable to concentrate on any effort, he further advised a trip to Europe.

For six months Barton readied her affairs, preparing for the trip, which she expected would take years. She wrote her will, leaving small legacies here and there but giving the bulk of the estate to her sister Sally. To the Congress she sent a final statement of the Office of Correspondence with Friends of the Missing Men of the United States Army. She wished to close the office, since all those not identified at that date she presumed to be dead. With dramatic words she reiterated their accomplishments: 63,182 letters received and answered; 22,000 men identified. Of these, the great majority had been on Atwater's death roll. To some it seemed a mere drop in the bucket, less than 10 percent of the total missing, and these identified at a considerable cost. Yet, it was 22,000 more than might have been discovered, and to the few she helped her work was a godsend. "If to enjoy the gratitude of a single heart be a pleasure, to enjoy the benediction of a grateful world must be sweet," wrote a man whose family had been helped by the four years of frustrated and sporadic work. Satisfied herself, Barton made no apologies in her final petition but turned in her record with quiet pride.[92]

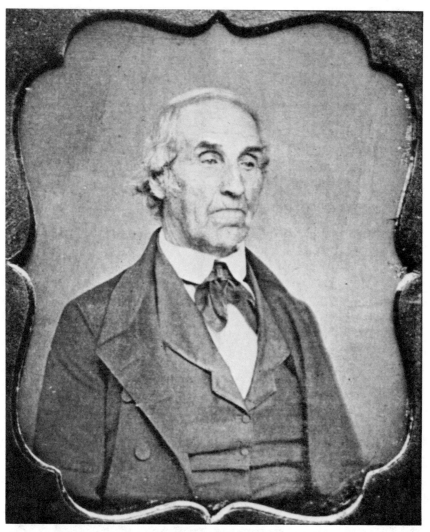

Captain Stephen Barton, father of Clara Barton. His love of military adventure and strong philanthropic bent greatly influenced his youngest daughter. Clara Barton National Historic Site.

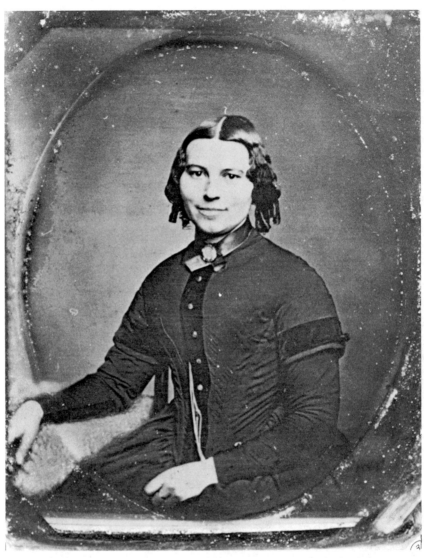

The earliest known photograph of Barton, this daguerreotype was probably taken while she was a student at the Clinton Liberal Institute. Clara Barton National Historic Site.

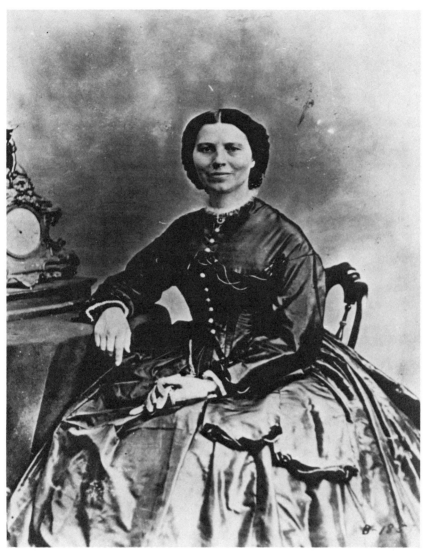

A Mathew Brady portrait of Barton, taken around 1865. Her face radiates the confidence she had gained during the Civil War. Note also the strong capable hands. National Archives and Records Service.

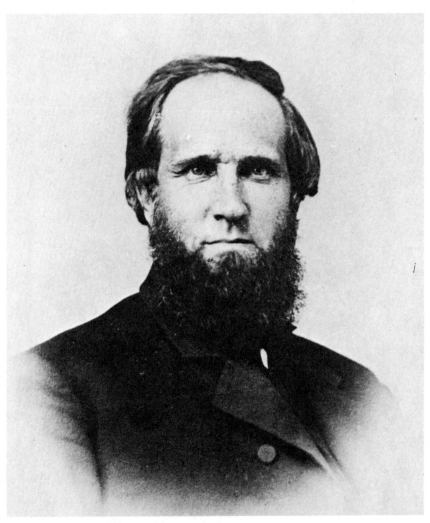

General John Elwell, one of the great loves of Barton's life. The hours they spent to-gether, she wrote, were like "golden threads in the warp and weft of my life." Library of Congress.

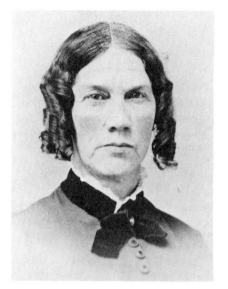

Frances D. Gage, Barton's mentor and friend for over twenty years. This picture was the one Barton kept in her photograph album. Library of Congress.

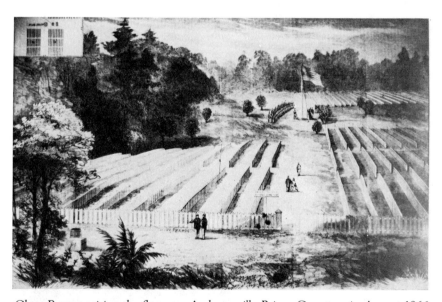

Clara Barton raising the flag over Andersonville Prison Cemetery in August 1866. "Surely this was not the gate of hell," she wrote of the prison, "but hell itself." This drawing first appeared in Harper's Weekly Magazine. *Andersonville Prison National Historic Site.*

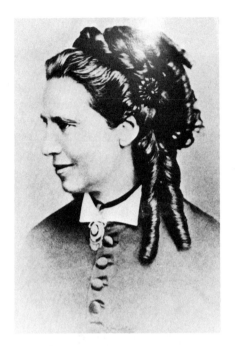

According to Barton's earliest biographer, this photograph was taken in Paris around 1871. The pin at her neck is her father's masonic emblem, which she wore for luck throughout the Civil War. Clara Barton National Historic Site.

Dr. Julian Hubbell, who devoted his life to Clara Barton and the American Red Cross. This portrait was taken around 1890. Clara Barton National Historic Site.

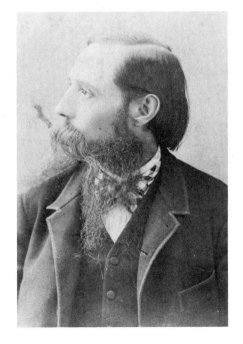

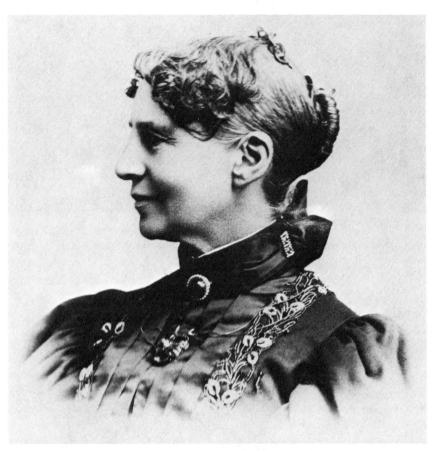

This photo was taken during a lecture trip to Chicago when Barton was 76. She is wearing the amethyst pansy and smoky topaz brooches given to her by the Grand Duchess Louise of Baden. Library of Congress.

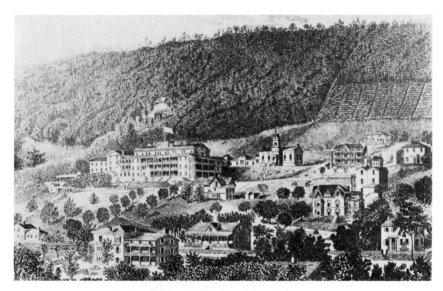

A pre-1882 drawing of Dansville, New York. Clara Barton's home was the small white house in the lower right-hand corner. The large structure in the center is the Jackson Sanitarium. Clara Barton National Historic Site.

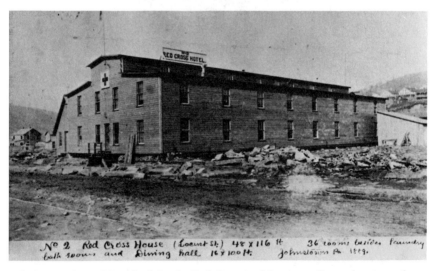

The Locust Street Hotel built by the Red Cross in Johnstown, Pennsylvania, to house flood victims. The structure was later dismantled and became the basis for the Red Cross headquarters in Glen Echo, Maryland. The notations are in Barton's hand. Library of Congress.

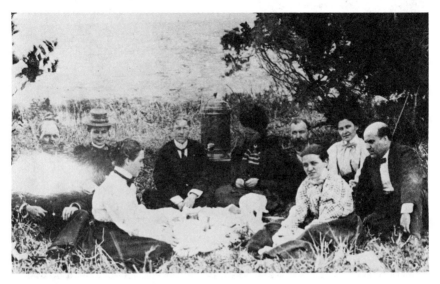

Barton and her Red Cross staff on a picnic in Tampa, Florida, while waiting for permission to go to Cuba in 1898. George Kennan, Red Cross vice-president, is on the left. The bearded man to the right of Barton is Dr. E. Winfield Egan, Red Cross general surgeon. American National Red Cross.

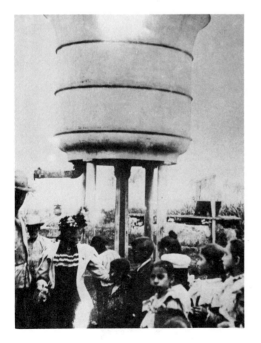

Barton visiting with Cuban orphans on her tour of Red Cross projects, April–July 1899. Library of Congress.

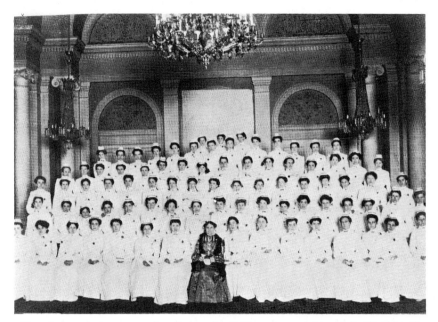

Clara Barton with a group identified as the 1902 graduating class of the Blockley Hospital School of Nursing in Philadelphia; the identification has been questioned. Barton spoke at a number of such gatherings, though she denied that she herself had ever been a nurse. "My work has been chiefly to supply 'Things,'" she wrote. Clara Barton National Historic Site.

This photograph was taken in Cuba, 1898, during Red Cross relief just prior to the Spanish-American War. Barton wears the official German Red Cross field badge, her amethyst pansy pin, and a Red Cross pin commemorating the Armenian relief work. American National Red Cross.

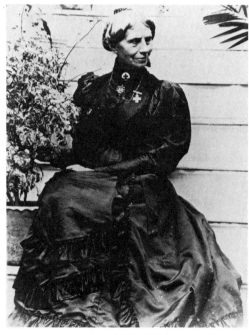

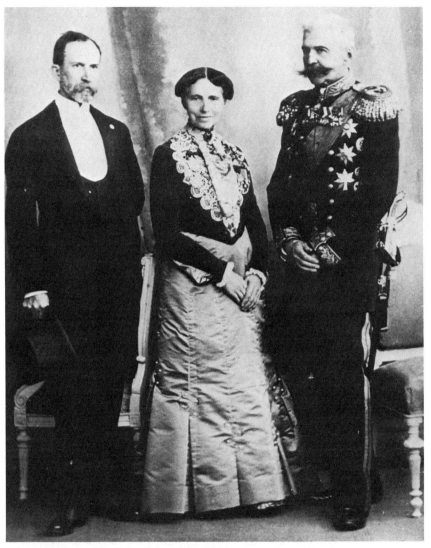

Clara Barton with B. F. Tillinghast and Russian Admiral N. Kaznakoff at the International Red Cross Conference, St. Petersburg, 1902. This is the last such conference that Barton, age eighty-one, would attend. Library of Congress.

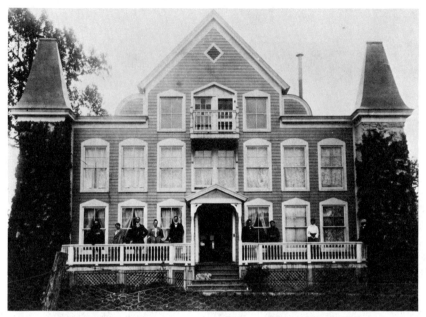

Barton, second from left, and "loyal" Red Cross members at the Red Cross head-quarters in Glen Echo, Maryland. The photo was taken on May 14, 1904, the day she resigned as president of the American National Red Cross. Clara Barton National Historic Site.

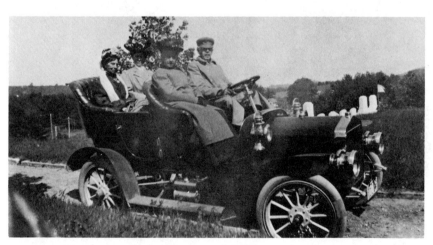

Clara Barton and her relatives driving to the North Oxford cemetery in 1910. Always forward-thinking, she welcomed innovations such as the automobile, gramophone, and electric lights. Clara Barton Birthplace.

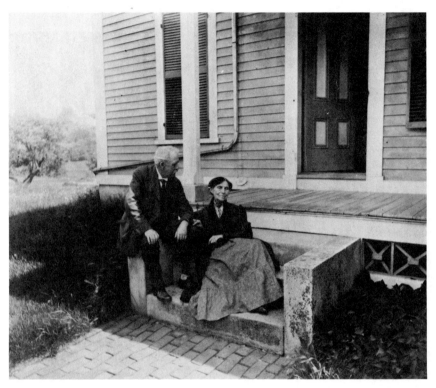

Stephen E. Barton and his aunt on the back stairs of her home in North Oxford, Massachusetts. Between 1905 and 1911 Barton spent her summers in this house. Library of Congress.

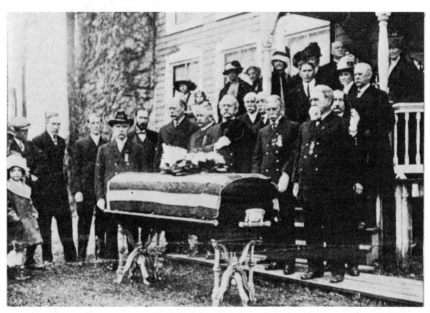

Senators, veterans, and friends pay their last respects to Barton on the steps of her Glen Echo home. Funeral services were held both there and in North Oxford, Massachusetts, where she was buried. Library of Congress.

ten

The customs officers who scanned the lines of people trooping off of the *Caledonia* at Glasgow probably failed to notice a woman of forty-eight, plainly attired in black silk and accompanied by her sister. Her passport, too, gave little reason to pay her special attention. It described her without flattery as five feet five inches tall, with brown hair, brown eyes, a prominent nose, large mouth, broad chin, sallow complexion and oval face. Barton was tired and sick after the two-week ocean voyage and in no mood for a grand tour. The doctors had ordered her away from the scenes that fretted her; at best she would refer to the trip as "my sentence."[1]

To her surprise Clara liked Scotland and England. To be with Sally and wander "among its bloom and heather, its lakes and mountains, its classic old cities, its towns and castles," was to relive the pleasures of her childhood, when together they had cherished Sir Walter Scott's romantic tales. Unfortunately—for this would be the most pleasant phase of her European trip—it was a whirlwind tour of only two weeks. Sally left her at London, and Clara stopped briefly in Paris, then traveled on to Geneva.[2]

She had plans for a lengthy stay in the Swiss city, where she could find friends, and hopefully health, in the bracing mountain air. Charles Upton and his wife, whom she had known in both Washington and Massachusetts, were now serving as American diplomats in Geneva. Jules Golay had written to his family in Switzerland, and they welcomed the opportunity to repay the hospitality Barton had shown to their son. Thus, by late September she was settled in with Papa Golay, his wife, and daughter Eliza. Amidst the genial company and Geneva's early autumn beauty, Barton believed she might find rest and strength. "Contrasting my physical condition with that of last winter I am well," she told a friend in Washington, "but comparing it with the years ago there is yet room for improvement—but I believe myself to be gaining."[3]

The hospitality was warm at the Golays', but the winds that whipped across the lake grew ever colder as the months wore on. Like Mark Twain and other American travelers, Barton thought European homes strong on outward displays of luxury but lacking in practical comfort. Her dark and chilly room faced north, and she found herself commiserating with Byron's "Prisoner of Chillon" as she tried to stay warm and cheerful. "I was so nervous & discouraged that I could scarce get through the day," she wrote one November morning when she had to huddle in bed to ward off the chill. "I cried half the time and could not help it."[4] "It will be a great day for Old Europe," Barton would write a little later when her spirits were restored, "when some wise man is born into it, who can construct a chimney."[5] Shortly before Christmas—a day she chose to spend sweeping her room in self-pity—she left Geneva for the small Mediterranean island of Corsica, hoping for sunshine and diversion.[6]

There had been one occurrence during the cool months Clara Barton spent in Geneva that would have a lasting effect upon her and upon American philanthropy, though she did not recognize it at the time. It was a formal visit from a party of soberly dressed businessmen, a courtesy call, the implications of which were not apparent until later; at the time it did not rate even a notation in her journal. The delegation was headed by Dr. Louis Appia, a man of fine classical features and great presence. He and his associates were representatives of the International Convention of Geneva, more commonly called the Red Cross. They were familiar with her charitable activities during the Civil War and, assuming her interest in philanthropic matters to reach beyond her own work, had come to ask why the United States had never acceded to the articles of the Geneva Convention. Astonished, Barton told the men that she had never heard of the organization or the treaty and asked them to give her more information.[7]

She was fascinated by the story the gentlemen told her. In 1859 a young Swiss man named Jean Henri Dunant was caught on a business trip near the scene of a terrific battle between French forces under Napoleon III and Austrian troops. Forty thousand men were killed or wounded on this, the battlefield of Solferino, Italy. Towns and villages nearby were hastily turned into open-air hospitals. Dunant, horrified at the lack of food, water, doctors, and medical supplies, set about recruiting the help of local peasants and procuring bandages and food. For several days he labored there, then returned, exhausted, to the home of his well-to-do parents in Geneva. Though physically removed from the suffering he had witnessed, his mind lingered over the scenes until he became convinced that he should take action against similar distress in the future.[8]

The horrible remembrance of men dying for want of the simplest care inspired Dunant to write a vivid account of the battle and its consequences. The book, published in 1862, was entitled Un Souvenir de Solferino. Straightforward and compassionate, it indulged in few of the standard concessions to the glory of the battlefield. Glory, if there had been any, belonged to the good-hearted peasant women who treated both sides alike, murmuring "tutti Fratelli [all are brothers]" while binding the wounds of the hated Austrians. This generosity of spirit caused Dunant to formulate a radically new concept of charitable action. It was a simply expressed idea, practically hidden among the grisly battles scenes he depicted. "Would it not be possible," queried Dunant, "in time of peace and quiet, to form relief societies for the purpose of having care given to the wounded in wartime by zealous, devoted and thoroughly qualified volunteers?"[9]

Un Souvenir de Solferino created an immediate sensation in Europe. Among the thousands who were moved by its vivid scenes was a prominent fellow-citizen of Geneva named Gustave Moynier. Choosing not to view Dunant's question as idle rhetoric, he set about turning the dream into practical reality. Moynier put together a committee that included influential doctors and army generals and began making plans for an international convention to discuss the treatment of the wounded in wartime. His organizing skills meshed neatly with Dunant's great talent as a promoter. An exceedingly handsome man, with dignity as well as charm and social poise, Dunant was able to inspire both widespread public acclaim and indispensable royal patronage for his ideas. By February 1863, he and Moynier had garnered enough support to call a convention of sixteen nations, which would have been unthinkable five years earlier.[10]

Eighteen months later the Treaty of Geneva was drawn up and signed by eleven countries; by the time Barton learned of it thirty-two nations had joined. It provided that ambulances and field hospitals, and the personnel employed with them—both professionals and volunteers—should be treated as neutrals. The wounded should be cared for whether they fell in hostile or friendly territory. The treaty also included preliminary accords for the treatment of the permanently disabled and prisoners of war. Finally, it established a badge to distinguish those neutrals aiding the wounded. In honor of Jean Henri Dunant's homeland, the sign chosen was that of the Swiss national flag, but with the colors reversed. From this time a red cross on a white field would be a symbol of impartial help for the distressed.[11]

Barton was amazed to hear from Appia that although the United States government had been approached three times, it had always refused to sign the treaty. When the committee asked why, in her opinion, this had been the case, she was at a loss to explain. She could only reply that she had never heard anything about the Geneva Convention and was "sure the American people did not know anything about it or ever heard of it." The little committee thanked her cordially, left an armload of Red Cross literature, and said that they hoped she would give the matter her consideration and support. As Clara read over the pamphlets and a copy of the treaty, she recognized how strongly she identified with the goals of the organization and marveled that the United States could have "carelessly stumbled over this jewel and trodden it underfeet to the astonishment of all the world, and in its young American confidence never dreamed that it·had been doing anything to be remarked on."[12]

Within a few days, Barton had shelved these thoughts, however. En route to Corsica, birthplace of her longtime hero, Napoleon I, she put everything out of her mind but her hopes for sun and rest. But in her edgy and demanding state of mind she found neither peace nor strength there. She moved from pensione to pensione as she found one too dirty, another with food so greasy that she was forced to subsist on olives, cheese, and wine, and yet another filled with suspicious characters, who she believed tried to rob her. The hardship of the Union army, she commented dryly to her journal, had been nothing compared to this. She felt keenly the disadvantage of being a foreigner and a lone woman.[13] Yet a friend who visited her briefly characterized her situation as a very pleasant one: a turquoise sea and sunny landscape, groves of orange trees, and merry bands of children who accompanied her on her walks.[14]

In January Barton moved to the Hotel Swiss, more expensive and less colorful than the pensiones and filled with English gentry. Though she eliminated some of the coarseness from her life, she was scarcely happier here. The English snubbed her, and in her loneliness Clara bitterly regretted that Sally had not accompanied her longer. She wandered alone through the gray-green olive groves, admired the native sheep and goats, and visited both Napoleon's birthplace and Millele, one of his favorite haunts. Finally, when her lonely wanderings were ended by the intervention of John Hitz (an old friend from Washington, now the Swiss consul in Corsica), it was too late. Her social life improved but her neglected health caught up with her. Despite loud protests from Hitz and his wife, she made plans to return to Geneva as soon as she could be welcomed by warm weather.[15]

It was a mild and beautiful spring in Switzerland. Clara stayed for a time with the Golays, then moved on to the Upton house, on the outskirts of Geneva. Charles Upton and his wife had formed a deep attachment for the renowned Miss Barton and offered her hospitality so luxurious that she was more than a bit embarrassed. "It burdens me just as it does in America to think how I shall ever repay so much kindness and attention," she wrote to her brother.[16] Ironically, she could not relax and regain her strength in such a leisurely atmosphere, for she felt aimless and beholden to her hosts; the long hours on her hands virtually guaranteed melancholy. Her great desire was to "be accounted worthy once more to take my place among the workers of the world." She contented herself as best she could by adopting every sad looking stranger that came her way, busying herself with collecting a subscription for a woman whose husband had left her, finding rooms for a distressed lady traveler, and nursing a young woman named Minna Kupfer, who had been left to die of pneumonia.[17] Yet still she could not shake her agitation and wrote that she had "lost all courage for both the present and the future."[18] As the "useless days" stretched into weeks, Barton became more despondent and more firmly convinced that she would never again be productive or truly well. She could not foresee during this spell of depression that only three weeks later she would again give crucial service during the terror and upheaval of battle.

On July 18, 1870, France declared war on Prussia and its German allies. Although the declaration was made on a flimsy diplomatic pretext, the war was actually caused by French insecurity over the changing power structure in Europe. For a dozen years the Germans had been challenging the undisputed supremacy of France in such clashes as the Seven Weeks War of 1866. The year 1870 found them in a strong position to prove their power: German military establishments, blessed with ambitious and forward-thinking leaders, had kept abreast of the industrial innovations of the time, whereas the French had not. Within a few months, by taking advantage of the initial confusion in France, the allied Germans were able to make decided inroads into French-held Alsace-Lorraine.[19]

The war acted as a tonic to Barton's sour disposition. She had followed the fermenting situation only casually, but now she watched the political and military maneuvers with a practiced eye and intense excitement. She wrote a letter to the Red Cross volunteering her services and was simultaneously petitioned by General Hans Herzog to give aid to the neutral Swiss armies should they need it. A few days later Louis Appia and a band of workers going toward the front visited Barton. Buoyed by the challenge and forgetting her broken health, she decided to join the Red Cross workers. On July 30, she hastily jotted: "start for the field if I can reach it."[20]

The first leg of the journey brought her to Basle, where the huge Red Cross storehouses were located. What she saw of the thriving organization in Basle convinced her, as words from Moynier or Appia never could, of the utility of the International Red Cross. At the storehouses she was amazed to see contributions from all over Europe, sent under neutral banners and to be used by whichever belligerent most needed them. It was, Barton wrote,

a larger supply than I had ever seen at any one time, in readiness for the field at our own sanitary commission rooms in Washington, even in the fourth year of the war . . . and trained authorized, education nurses stood awaiting their appointment, each with this badge upon the arm or breast, and every box, barrel or package with a broad, bright scarlet cross which rendered it as sacred and safe from molestation . . . as the bread and wine before the altar.[21]

Aghast that America had failed to join the organization and had therefore fostered so much suffering, she later told a group of Civil War veterans that she had stood in awe of "the work of these Red Cross societies in the field, accomplishing in four months under their systematic organization what we failed to accomplish in four years without it . . . a whole continent marshalled under the banner of the Red Cross."[22]

The International Red Cross, progressive as it was in some areas, mirrored the U.S. Army's ideas about the proper role of women in battlefield relief. Initially Barton had trouble convincing Gustave Moynier that she could be an effective worker on the field in France. At one point, despite their impressive display of goods and personnel, she became so irritated at those who blocked her way that she pronounced the committee at Basle "heartless and soulless," and determined to seek other patronage.[23] At last Moynier agreed to let her go, not alone, but accompanied by another woman, who also wanted to be a battlefield nurse. He introduced her to Antoinette Margot, a twenty-seven-year-old Swiss citizen whom Barton described as "fair-haired, playful, bright and confiding." From the beginning Barton and Margot were a well-matched team. The older woman needed fidelity and a certain adoration. Her French and German were rusty, and she therefore required a companion who would ease the language difficulties they were sure to encounter. Antoinette was insecure and appreciated Barton's larger experience and confident approach to war work. She suffered from a strict and stifling home atmosphere; for her Clara became a catalyst for leaving the confines of her village life and expanding her aspirations.[24]

On August 6 Barton and Margot set off in the direction of Mulhausen, on the border of France and Germany, where an evacuation station for the wounded had been established. It was not exactly the battlefield, but in Clara's imagination she saw herself repeating the work she had begun nearly a decade before: "'the front'—That expression was very strange after a lapse of five years, and I had thought never to hear it again in connection to myself." After entanglements with local peasants and several straggling army units, Barton and Margot made their way to the city via a broken-down railroad. They inspected several hospitals, found that their services were not needed, and from there traveled north toward Strasbourg. This ancient fortress town in northeastern France was under siege at the time of their arrival, and the Swiss, who were attempting to evacuate some of the more helpless families, put Barton in charge of an omnibus full of cringing, tearful evacuees en route to Hagenau.[25]

For several days she shepherded the stunned refugees, with growing impatience, for it was at the battlefield that she really hoped to work. Tremendous battles had taken place at Saarbrücken and Wörth, involving numbers no American battle, save that at Antietam, could equal. She and Antoinette went resolutely toward these fields, despite a dearth of wagons or other transportation and continued refusal by both German and French officers to allow them to pass through the lines. Even when they were able to find the scarce combination of driver, draft animals, and wagon, they discovererd that the wagoners were disposed to cheat or rob them. Many of the peasants thought they were spies and reacted with appropriate hostility. The very soldiers they were supposed to aid often ridiculed or endangered them. A drunken set of Germans mistook Barton for a barmaid, and when she, dignity affronted, flatly refused to pour a glass of beer for one soldier, he pinned her to the wall and held her there with the tip of his sword resting on her breast. The Red Cross badge might be respected by governments and armies, but it was scant protection against the unbridled peasantry.[26]

On August 26, they had still seen nothing of the thousands of wounded who were rumored to be in western France, and an irritated Barton exclaimed: "These days wear very hard. It is not like me, nor like my past, to be sitting quietly where I can just watch the sky reddening with the fires of a bombarded city, and neither have anything to do in or with it, nor be able to go near enough to see the shells which set the fires." In the end, Antoinette became ill, and at Brumath—the closest they got to the fighting—they were forced to turn back to Switzerland.[27]

Her inability to reach the men at the front, and to again be a part of the thrill and tragedy of war, was a disappointment that Barton did not take lightly. Indeed, although her diary and other contemporary papers show conclusively that she did not reach any battlefield in 1870–71 (Margot herself stated that "the front was out of our reach and so we saw no battlefield at all"), she frequently denied her frustration and claimed to have served with the fighting men.[28] It is difficult to know just why Barton consistently exaggerated her hardships and accomplishments. Certainly the truth would have brought strong enough accolades. Yet throughout her career she embellished the already dramatic saga by inventing titles, ovations, and perils. At times she jeopardized her good name with these stories. Antoinette Margot recalled that, after the battles of Hagenau and Wörth, Mrs. Fischer Saracen, an influential British woman, and several other ladies came to hear of their work. "Miss Barton was speaking to one of the ladies and I to the other," wrote Margot. "I told the truth and I do not know what Miss Barton said as I did not hear it, but when I saw Mrs. Fischer Saracen the next day she told me that our accounts were widely different and so asked me if we had separated at any time as she seemed to have done wonderful things but I told her we had not. She would not speak to her at all, was not even polite. I was very sorry but I could not help it."[29] Such scenes, great and small, eroded Barton's credibility until even such loyal friends as Margot did not know what to believe. At times, Barton's exaggerations brought only social snubbing but by the end of her life her personal integrity would be publicly questioned.

Much of the impetus for embellishing her accounts was supplied by Clara's own dramatic sense, her strong imagination and verbal ability. She had, too, a strong desire to please, to tell an audience what they wanted to hear, and both friends and strangers were hungry for the life-and-death scenes she could so vividly portray. Sometimes her motives were financial. It took strong words to create strong support, and, as she was increasingly to discover, there were few contributions to causes for which the need did not appear immediate and dire. Perhaps most important was the pressure she felt to justify her actions and to explain her presence in scenes of war and desolation. Public service of any kind was only beginning to be accepted as an appropriate sphere for gentlewomen. Most of society was still ready to brand an ambitious or altruistic female worker as an adventuress or worse. They were, of course, even more critical of a single woman, traveling through army lines without an official mandate. The name *camp follower* was only a flimsy disguise for the supposition that such a woman was a prostitute, or other kind of huckster, who preyed on the men. When outside circumstances prevented Barton from being an effective relief worker—such as at Hagenau—she was faced with the likelihood that her motives or actions in following the army would be misunderstood. Admitting that she had been useless, that valuable time and money had been spent crisscrossing the French countryside without any concrete benefit to either army, would cause raised eyebrows and the reflection that, after all, she was not really needed. In overstating her successes, in drawing a perhaps too-vivid picture of the suffering she met, Barton was affirming that she was indispensable. She had few examples with which to illustrate the good a lone woman could do amidst sickness and destruction. If she was to continue in philanthropic work she would have to create her own niche by convincing people of the great need and of her own exceptional ability to meet it.

In one area Barton could hardly overstate the terrors and privation she saw. The desperate plight of the French people in the fall of 1870 was a distinct shock, even to her calloused eyes. For all of the horror of the American Civil War, she had seen little civilian suffering. (The notable example of such destruction in that conflict, Sherman's march through Georgia, had not touched her at all.) Now she saw firsthand the tragedy of modern warfare: that it magnified the horrors seen by armies in the field and brought them to the populace as a whole. In their travels, she and Margot had encountered thousands of terrorized peasants, who had seen such unspeakable suffering that they pleaded with the two women to turn back. "Sometimes one would be so earnest as to come to the heads of our horses, to urge us to return . . . , each spoke from his heart," recalled Clara. "The ideas associated with war in the minds of these people is [sic] something beyond description."[30] What supplies she had went to these destitute civilians. Just as the work of Frances D. Gage and Josephine Griffing had influenced her during the Civil War, these experiences enlarged her conception of war and its victims. The military at least tried to look after its own, but the peasants had been left, as had the freedmen in America, to pack up their scanty belongings, uproot their lives, and trudge, unaided, toward a new and frightening life.

As she pondered these scenes and restlessly considered the next move she should make, a telegram arrived from Carlsruhe, the capital of the Duchy of Baden. It was an anxious note from the Grand Duchess Louise, the daughter of Kaiser Wilhelm, requesting that Barton come to Baden and work in the Red Cross hospitals. Louise, who had a lifelong commitment to philanthropy, had actively encouraged the role of women in disaster relief and had herself promoted the establishment of several nursing schools. In addition she had taken an early interest in the Red Cross and is generally credited with being the founder of its German branch.[31]

The grand duchess had learned of Barton while researching the work of female humanitarians from other parts of the world. When they finally met on September 17, 1870, they formed an almost instant friendship. Louise in 1870 was a delicate middle-aged woman, with a thinly lined face that here and there showed evidence of her once famous beauty. Her knowledge of literature and art was as rich as her regal gowns, and Barton saw in her a gentle companion and kindred spirit. Together they toured the Badisch hospitals, which Clara found large and airy, filled with Turkish nurses, and, surprisingly, dedicated to copying every detail of American hospitals, which she privately believed inferior. The military hospitals she found less efficient: "not as good—*Discord & Dirt,*" was her terse comment. Louise was on the point of installing Barton as head of the hospitals when word came that proud Strasbourg was at last about to fall to the army of the grand duke of Baden. She hastily gave Barton a pass for the railroad and sent her to survey the needs of the beleaguered city.[32]

Barton liked to recall that she entered Strasbourg the day after its surrender. Her diary shows, however, that it was on October 2, four days after the ramparts had crumbled, that she climbed "over the moats at one of the demolished gates," passing through the "most burned part of the city."[33] She was part of a delegation composed chiefly of members of the Comité de Secours Strasbourgeois, a local relief group. To her distress, a tour of the city the next day consisted of "Beer garden—ride a little—more beer—a little further—more friends & more beer—till at length we get back. . . . I am disgusted with 'do nothings.'"[34] Their attitude was all the more deplorable because the condition of the city was truly desperate. It had been under siege for nearly two months, during which little food came in and increasingly large portions of the town were burned or demolished. Many of the citizens who stood in the streets on September 29 had been crowded in dark cellars and had emerged suffering from famine, epidemics of typhoid fever and smallpox, and vermin-infested clothing. Over six thousand people were homeless. "I came suddenly into the midst of such an accumulation of woe—want & misery that there was not a moments [sic] time for anything besides attempting to relieve it," Clara wrote.[35] In addition to the civil distress, the hospitals were filled with scores of people wounded by the firing. Strasbourg had been less a military plum than a chance for the Germans to demoralize the French by coldly bombing women and children, and Clara saw, for the first time, military hospitals filled with female casualties. She both pitied and admired the women, whom she believed to be as brave as any fallen man she had helped but whose future was far less certain. The heroism of the patients made her decide to concentrate her relief work on helping the city's women. A few days later, she took a train back to Carlsruhe to tell the grand duchess of her plan.[36]

She had initially stood in the courtyard of a former prison, Barton told Louise, and handed out soup to those begging assistance. But she soon perceived that what was really needed was remunerative employment, which would rejuvenate the local economy and ease the victims' mental suffering. The bombardment had reduced them to want, she said, but handouts of food would "make of them permanent beggars and vagrants, thus doing for their *morale* all that the bombardment had done for their physical condition."[37] What she proposed was a workroom that borrowed its ideas largely from Josephine Griffing's rooms in Washington. Sewing was an almost universal skill among women, Barton noted, and clothing was desperately needed. Cloth and materials could be given out to the women, who would do the sewing in their own homes for a fair rate, and the resulting garments could then be given out to the really destitute. Louise thought it an admirable plan, volunteered an initial donation of materials, and proffered the services of a court governess named Anna Zimmerman. Encouraged by this support, Clara returned to Strasbourg in late October to begin her work.[38]

Like Antoinette Margot, Anna Zimmerman was a shy young woman who came to worship Barton. Her photographs show a plain face with hair pulled severely back and dark eyes set close together. She was a brilliant and articulate girl with, as Barton described her, "all the fire of Anna Dickinson with twice her ready knowledge and ten times her scholarship." She suffered from a home life so strict that she was not allowed to study lest she detract from her less intelligent brothers, and she quickly adopted Barton as a one-woman tutor and family, affectionately calling her "Mamma."[39] Barton, too, felt a quick bond with the young German, and within a few days pronounced "Miss Z. a treasure."[40] They spent a month together finding rooms, hiring a professional dress cutter, and publicizing their work. They were disappointed that the Comité de Secours wanted no part of the operation, preferring to view them as well-meaning but incompetent society ladies. Undaunted, they plunged ahead with greater hope than resources. On November 14 they began to cut cloth, and Barton could record with satisfaction in her diary "the commencement of our work rooms."[41]

The plan was an immediate success. Each Thursday the town's women would bring market baskets filled with finished garments to the large, curtainless room, receive two francs for each well-made piece, and take home additional items to sew. Other women worked in the rooms, sorting the clothing and seeing to its distribution. From the beginning, wrote an admiring observer, Barton was clever at "encouraging, sustaining and guiding them with the tenderness of a woman and the firmness of a man."[42] To one woman she gave such encouragement that although only three stitches in two entire skirts had been worthy of note, the following week the woman had taken care to make each stitch as perfect as those that had been praised the week before.[43] "To create something out of nothing— to bring life and light and order to a state of things entirely chaotic, to raise a perfect organization . . . had been the character of this work," wrote loyal Anna Zimmerman.[44] Barton also received warm praise from the duchess of Baden, and the grateful glances of her seamstresses so bolstered her spirits that she could write jocularly of the work to her old dressmaker, Annie Childs. "Wasn't that the last thing you would have thought of, that *I* should come to Europe and set up dressmaking," she teased, "and *French* dressmaking at that? . . . Well, you should have seen the patterns!" She ended the letter, however, on a note that shows how serious was her regard for the Strasbourgeois: "It was such a comfort to see them, week by week, grow better clothed."[45]

164

Kind words and grateful glances were food for the soul, but they did little to keep the workrooms in operation. Within a few weeks Clara was in serious need of money. Her lifelong method of relief was to establish a project before funds for its continuance were available and to beg, borrow, or steal afterward. Sometimes the plan worked very well. At other times, such as in her work with missing men, the money never did materialize and the project could be only partially continued. At Strasbourg she fell into the same pattern. The early gift of the grand duchess was soon exhausted, and Barton found that she would once again (and to her regret) have to couple the role of fund raiser with that of ministering angel.

It was not a job she particularly relished, and she found that she again had to resort to dramatization and public appeal to keep the work going. Louise and the Red Cross, after much cajoling, gave some additional support to the workrooms, but it was not enough to keep them in operation indefinitely.[46] In her diary on December 1, Clara noted, "Think our work will end here soon, we have no way to get the funds designed for us, it all goes to others."[47] In desperation she wrote a pleading letter to Otto von Bismarck claiming that support for the workrooms would further the German goal of winning the Alsacians to their side, then signed it with rather theatrical humility: "But pardon my boldness Honored Count. I am neither a Diplomatist, nor political Counsellor; I am only a maker of garments for the poor."[48] When a polite note—but no funds—came in response to this, Barton threw herself on the generosity of the public. She composed dozens of letters of appeal to American and British newspapers, conjuring up images of disease and wasted cities in her most descriptive manner.[49] She tried to get Horace Greeley of the New York Tribune to send a reporter to Strasbourg. When he demurred she took it upon herself to write an "objective" account of her work. "It is perhaps not generally known in this country," began one of her "anonymous" pieces, "that Miss Clara Barton, scarcely removed from the fatigues and indispositions resulting from her arduous and useful duties during the War of the Rebellion, was found again formost [sic] bestowing her care upon the wounded which charactized her among the suffering armies of her own country."[50] The articles had some of the desired impact, though contributions were sporadic. For the remaining six months of Barton's association with the workrooms in Strasbourg, she would daily wonder if they could continue.[51]

Some help came when, in January, the Comité de Secours merged their relief work with Barton's and the workrooms tripled their output. Sixty-seven women had been employed in the fall of 1870. Now over two hundred came each week to deliver fifteen hundred garments of every description. Dresses, coats, vests, and underwear were made in nearly a dozen sizes. Neither a minute nor a scrap of fabric was wasted—"we have the custom of making caps and mittens . . . so that no piece larger than the size of a child's hand need be left unused," Barton boasted.[52] Careful accounts were made of each woman's work, and as the Strasbourgeois became better clothed, the garments were sent to villages in the surrounding countryside that had also been devastated by the armies.[53]

When enough financing had been secured, at least for the short term, Clara could breathe a relieved sigh and settle down to something of a routine. Antoinette Margot and Anna Zimmerman were with her, so she did not lack for companionship. "I have a little home here, some small pretty rooms in which are Miss Margot and myself," she told Sally, "and in which she will doubtless keep old maid hall."[54] She enjoyed the simple fare of bread, butter, and fruit that was available in Strasbourg and basked in the adoration of the grateful seamstresses. On Christmas evening she opened her door in answer to a loud knock and saw a lovely Christmas tree, ablaze with lights, the gift of those she had helped. "It abounded in fruit & flowers, & mosses, and some little nice things which their good hearts had dictated for my comfort," she wrote in appreciation.[55] Her association with the court of Baden also gave her an introduction to the higher society of the city, and she received invitations for carriage rides, tea, and dinner parties from such local potentates as the mayor and his wife and Countess von Bismarck.[56] Her friends in America were hardly astonished to hear that the work and admiration she enjoyed in Strasbourg had cheered her soul and made her forget, at least temporarily, her ill health. "I am so rejoiced," she told Josephine Griffing,

> to be once more *at work*, once more accounted worthy a place in the vineyard, that I must sometimes, in the fullness of joy, speak of it. Perhaps no one ever knew so well as you how soul killing were the days when I was compelled to look idly on and see others work and you know well how gracelessly I bore them. I would *never, never* that they return.[57]

Barton's letter to Griffing, and her self-laudatory press reports, convey a sense of her continuing need to justify her work and to give purpose and value to her "exile." Barton still believed that the American government had turned its back on her when it had refused to support her work for the missing men. Moreover, she felt that her homeland had failed to provide her with a meaningful way to support herself. "I cannot describe how painful and tiresome I find it to work *here*, abroad, among these strangers," Clara complained to a fellow Bostonian, "with *every thought* and *sympathy* and *energy* turning and rushing 4000 miles across the sea."[58] In another note, almost angry in tone, she told the readers of the *Revolution* that she felt she had certainly served a long apprenticeship abroad, "and unless exceedingly stupid must have acquired some skill by practice." Could not America find some use for her?[59] The grand duchess of Baden, and even Otto von Bismarck, might visit her sewing room and laud her efforts publicly, but such honors made little impression when pitted against the meaningful silence at home. Even her family was loath to praise her: they let her know they thought it unladylike for her name to be continuously in the papers. From Sally she received only a crisp note that advised: "I think that you have done enough such work."[60]

Barton was hungry for American approval, but also for American faces and American conversation. She disliked the French, among whom she lived, calling them dirty and vulgar and adding, "There is no French in my character."[61] In a letter of appeal that she drafted in 1871, she pictured herself as "an old worker, often weary, and sometimes lonely, for the want of communication with the good brave generous hearts of my native land."[62] Dorence Atwater came to visit her in March and April, and her great delight in seeing him, as well as their ease of conversation, pointed up the oddity of her own social situation. Though Louise and the other court ladies were infinitely kind and admiring, Clara met them at their pleasure and in a manner appropriate to a "woman in a plain black gown without even a ring on her hands to address . . . a Princess." Barton was not free to confide or take liberties at court, and, speaking neither French nor German well, she was shy among those who could talk gaily in several tongues. In her relationship with Margot and Zimmerman the roles were reversed; they frankly adored her and obeyed her every whim. These relationships were, in her own estimation, those of a mother and child, and precious though they were, they could hardly supply the real friendship she desired.[63]

Clara Barton closed her work in Strasbourg on June 1, 1871, leaving it in the hands of the Comité. She felt she had served that city long enough to remove the edge of panic and hoped to follow the rumors of suffering to towns still requiring assistance. Paris was the center of most of the worst reports. The war had actually ended the previous February, but the people of the capital, in their confusion and anger over the German victory, had turned to the revolutionary government of the Commune, a self-styled citizens' group, which through incompetence, had facilitated the spread of hunger and fear in the city. Barton thought it best to go there, for Strasbourg was recovering nicely and her help seemed lost on her well-organized seamstresses. Though the colorful press reports of the Parisian sufferings were often exaggerated, the poorer people of the city were undoubtedly in a straitened condition. When a telegram arrived that detailed the Parisians' desperation, she offered her services.[64]

Thus she set off on the train, via Metz, to the capital. Her relief funds had been augmented by donations from a group of Boston citizens whose leader had become too ill in Paris to distribute them; their generosity was embodied in a single check which Barton anxiously carried with her. At some stage of the journey she must have been uncharacteristically indiscreet, for she came close to being robbed. A young Frenchman overheard two men making plans to steal the funds from Barton. Evidently having no way to warn her or the attendants, he spent an uncomfortable night hanging from the guardrail between the two cars that held Barton and the thieves, until he could catch the attention of a lineman in a remote station. The would-be felons were apprehended before Barton awoke. The next morning, to her astonishment, she found that the young hero was a soldier she had befriended in a hospital in Saarbrücken.[65]

The train would not take her all the way into Paris, and no cabs were available, for the horses had all been butchered to provide meat for the besieged city. She therefore walked the last seven miles, making plans as she went. The city now had a hollow, scavenging look. In the space of a few months, Paris had seen desperate and bloody fighting and terrible destruction by homemade firebombs; cynicism now replaced the romantic enthusiasm of a proud people. "I saw Paris when the Commune fell and the army of Versailles shot down its victims on the streets by the ghastly flare of blazing palaces," was Barton's own description. She offered her help to the mayor, who gratefully donated a house from which to distribute her monies. Then she set to work on the difficult task of helping the Parisians.[66]

Six months earlier Louis Appia had written to Clara, indicating a need for relief in Paris and suggesting a plan by which four stations in diverse parts of the city could be set up to dispense food, money, and clothing. It was this plan that Barton tried to adopt when she first arrived in the stricken city. She found it a difficult undertaking, however. Paris was not Strasbourg, where the city fathers knew the poor individually and could direct her to the worst cases. In Paris, ruffians and charlatans mixed with the really needy, and it was impossible to obtain true information about their situation. Barton and Margot constantly faced the danger of harassment or physical harm. There were only the two of them to assess the situation, find food and clothing, and distribute their money. They quickly realized that they could not even begin to undertake the kind of relief needed to materially change the condition of the city's poor.

Moreover, they found that their Red Cross badges were not respected in the French capital and that their supplies were frequently in jeopardy of being confiscated or stolen. Compared to the Sanitary Commission, the Red Cross had seemed to Clara an example of exceptional foresight and inexhaustible means. During the hostilities of 1870–71, however, the organization not only lacked cohesiveness but was not widely known. The medical authorities, jealous of their prerogative, chose largely to ignore it; civilians often viewed it with suspicion. One doctor, an American who had volunteered to work on a Red Cross ambulance during the war, wrote that he and his fellow workers had so little idea where they were needed that "while the majority of ambulances were wandering about the country, signal services were rendered only by the few which blundered into usefulness." Such wasted effort only made critics look further askance at the Red Cross and convinced many private citizens that the volunteers were merely spies, traveling across country under the guise of good Samaritans. Far from being guaranteed protection, Barton and Margot frequently had to defend themselves because of their Red Cross association.[67]

With these handicaps in mind they decided to concentrate their relief on three groups: the families of prisoners of war, the families of ship crews, and the many Alsacian refugees who had flocked to Paris rather than live under German rule. The latter especially interested Clara, and she tried to devise a systematic way of resettling them in southern France—a plan which came to naught. For two months she sporadically distributed small sums of money and the forty thousand garments she had brought with her from Strasbourg, but overall she could accomplish little. The government alternately thwarted her or demanded her services; the money and clothes were quickly claimed. As Margot admitted, "there was nothing at all that we could do in Paris."[68]

Perplexed by the magnitude of the problem, Barton retreated, spending much of her time sewing—for she had no summer clothes and was sweltering in the heat—and gratefully socializing with the large American community in Paris. She visited Ambassador Elihu Washburne, an old friend from wartime Washington, and was so anxious for company that she uncharacteristically frequented parlor meetings on Sunday nights to sing hymns and native songs.[69] Both she and Margot were ill with influenza in the late summer. The weeks in bed made her fret about lost time and the unspent funds from Boston. Anxious again that her motives not be misconstrued and the funds repossessed, Barton concocted a lengthy press release filled with embroidered accounts of their work. She tried to hide the report from Margot, but in the end her young assistant obtained a copy. Margot found, to her distress, that Barton had falsified accounts and included details of the work that, when compared with her own journal, proved utterly untrue. She wrote in disdain: "At the date we were in bed coughing with grippe she had reported that we were looking for the Alsacians in the station with warm food as they arrived train by train." Still, unable to abandon her mentor, Margot said nothing and allowed the report to be published.[70]

Barton stayed in Paris until August, when she went to Lyons for a short visit with Antoinette Margot's parents. Although she enjoyed seeing the city's silk industry, it was not an altogether pleasant visit. The Margots mistrusted their daughter's reverence for the Barton she "so inexpressably loved," and they treated Clara with ill-disguised hostility. Her mind was still continually preoccupied with worries over distribution of the Boston committee's money. It had arrived too late for use in Strasbourg, and she had not the spirit left to start another such large-scale project. Finally she decided to return to the Franco-German border and give small sums of money directly to the most destitute cases in cities that had been left especially needy during the war.[71]

After some cajoling, Barton persuaded Antoinette's parents to let her continue to help with the relief work. They traveled together to Paris first, staying for a leisurely month. As they were about to leave, they were met by a French gentleman who persuaded them to go to the area around Besançon where, he maintained, there was great want. He reinforced Barton's opinion that help was urgently needed that autumn, before the cold weather began, and encouraged her in her view that direct donations of small sums of money would most benefit the destitute civilians. This would enable the poor to buy the comforts they needed for the winter, which would in turn help to support the local merchants. Though unused to giving money directly to the poor, Barton had hoped that this plan would help revive the local economy.[72]

Besançon, Belfort, and Montbéliard were old fortress towns that had fiercely resisted siege by the Germans. Both armies had crossed and recrossed the area, destroying crops, killing cattle, and leaving towns and farmhouses in ashes. Of the three, Belfort had suffered the most. Though slowly starving, the proud citizens had held firm week after week, behind the medieval walls. Not until two months after the treaty ceding them to Germany had been signed did her citizens capitulate. But Besançon had also had its share of trouble, and when her people finally emerged from their long ordeal, they were gaunt, ill, and filled with suspicion and hatred. By the time Barton arrived they were on the point of riot. The night she entered Besançon, she soberly noted that, but for the skeletal figures from Andersonville, they were the most desolate people she had ever seen.[73]

Barton's work was beset with problems. The citizens, wary of her and her intentions, refused to take anything but specie, an article difficult to acquire in that devastated country. Ignorance and suspicion were so prevalent that even Barton was surprised. "They are largely Catholic, exceedingly ignorant, only a small, very small proportion even pretending to anything beyond an X for a name." She worked with the city administrators to distribute her riches, patiently sitting, day after day, filling out receipts on flimsy blue paper for the small donations. Privately, she still felt doubts about this method of charity, so opposed to her belief that work and dignity were what an overwhelmed people needed most.[74] In early November she wrote in her diary, "I am so unhappy, cannot settle in my mind what I ought to do," but she determined no satisfactory course of action. It was almost an embarrassment of riches, a seemingly endless supply of money, and yet she had no energy to devise a means of utilizing it effectively.[75]

The greatest hindrance of all was Barton's own waning stamina and growing demoralization. She had failed to care for herself during the difficult months in Strasbourg. It was the exhilaration of a new project that had kept her going, not a vigorous constitution. Now the face of suffering, which had never before made her shudder, began to play upon her nerves in Besançon. "I can endure the sight of almost any suffering that falls to the lot of the middle-aged and strong, but the weak, that *totter*, either old or young, that is *too much* for me . . . ," she complained, "[I] have been so hard at work among these wretched ones that I could not really stand it longer."[76]

She left Besançon for a bit, then in mid-December steeled herself for a tour in Belfort. She was shown every courtesy by the mayor, including the use of his house for her distributions. The citizens of Belfort were, however, in no mood for a polite show of appreciation. In their anxiety to partake of her charity they stormed the official residence, refusing to calm down until Barton emerged, said a few soothing words, and with the strength of her presence forestalled the riot. Antoinette Margot was "amused" to see Barton "*protecting her policemen*"; nonetheless the situation caused one more strain on Clara's weakening nerves. It was with difficulty that she arose each morning to record the little sums that were put into the wrinkled palms. She could stand only a week in Belfort before the anguish overcame her. Though she had failed to distribute all of her funds, she could not bring herself to stay and hurriedly packed up Antoinette. Not knowing where else to go, they headed back to Strasbourg.

In later years there would arise questions about the manner of relief given to the citizens of Belfort and Besançon. Some criticized Barton for leaving the area when the need was obviously so great. Antoinette Margot, who had sat with Barton day after day, handing out the money, stated that the sums given had been two or four francs; when a few years later she saw the stacks of receipts a zero had been added to the figures, so that it appeared that the villagers had recieved ten times that amount. Margot had no explanation for the discrepancy, but was greatly disturbed by it, especially when she found tracing paper, used to trace the signatures of the recipients, in Barton's possession. It seems unlikely that Barton, by now financially secure, was pocketing funds meant for the sufferers of France. But she felt acute embarrassment over her inability to finish the job of giving out the monies sent from Boston. As time passed and her health did not improve, she lost the opportunity for distributing the remainder of the funds.[77]

The forgery may have been meant to cover up the use of funds for a large party that Barton gave for her Strasbourg seamstresses. Having failed to see concrete results for her work in Paris, Besançon, or Belfort, she was happy to return to the scene of at least one success and toast those who had labored so hard with her. The party, held on December 30, 1871, turned out to be a great occasion. (Barton was so cheered by it that she wrote three lengthy letters describing the scene.) She decorated the workrooms with fir trees, paper snowflakes, and holly berries, and bought tiny wax candles and huge iced cakes. The trees were covered with change purses holding a few coins, one for each woman. Barton presided over the festivities, greeting every guest, cutting the cakes, and leading the singing. Afterward she recalled how "they *did talk,* and laugh and cry for joy— and *such* a time some hundreds of poor women almost beggars I think never had—'It was worth going a mile to see.'"[78] This was Clara Barton as she liked best to picture herself: the Lady Bountiful, sowing dignity and hope to the afflicted, reaping loyalty and love in return.

The party was to be the high-water mark of Barton's stay in Europe, for when it was over, she collapsed. Unable to cope with caring for herself, even with the help of Margot, she accepted an invitation from Grand Duchess Louise to stay at Carlsruhe. She and Antoinette rented rooms near the royal palace and attended a few splendid dinners and the formal opening of the Badisch Parliament, but she could not shake the depression and searing backaches. Her symptoms were now predictable: loss of sight (so painful that her eyes were bandaged from the light), anxiety, and an almost paralyzed state of mind that left her unable to relieve her situation. News of the death of Josephine Griffing, and a strange and sudden note that broke forever her friendship with Anna Zimmerman, did not help her mood. Every friend, from the grand duchess to Aunt Fanny at home, worried and clucked over her plight; invitations poured in for her to recuperate in America, to rest in London, to tour the Continent and forget her woes. But not until her dear friends, Abby and Joseph Sheldon, actually came to Carlsruhe in the winter of 1872, snatched her away to Paris, and persuaded her to join mutual friends, the George Taylors, on a trip to Italy, did she find the courage to make a change.[79]

Despite her bandaged eyes, Barton kept up with her cherished correspondence, finding it even "funny to write with my eyes shut, as if I were playing blindman's bluff."[80] Most of the letters were written to female friends, and a growing number of them dealt with feminist issues. The sad plight of most of the world's women, which had sparked the political activities she had so tentatively embraced in the late 1860s, was brought home to her daily in Europe. She was shocked by the condition of women on the Continent and saw what she had never seen in America: women harnessed to carts, driven like dogs, working a full day in the fields, then "dragging home the tools at night while he walks at his leisure." To her horror she discovered that among the peasantry women were beaten as a matter of course.[81] After witnessing a scene in which a woman was repeatedly attacked and insulted by a group of soldiers, she walked home, sat down, and wrote emphatically in her diary: "Heaven save the mark and hasten the *good work* in America that a little of the leaven fall into this dead old lump of European dough."[82] Even her two young protégées, both from privileged backgrounds, had had to fight to be taken seriously in their hopes to be educated or to follow a career. Barton could only applaud at receiving a "long, strong, logical letter" from Anna Zimmerman that began, "To the devil with the housework."[83] Under these conditions Clara saw woman's plight with new eyes. She felt a strong bond with the struggling feminists in America—"although the waves and the years roll, our spirit hands are still clasped"—and eagerly awaited news of their victories and tribulations.[84]

Barton continued her copious letters on the six-week trip to Italy, dutifully noting the "trainloads of Titians and Raphaels" (which she, guiltily, found boring), ancient cities, and old monuments. Her eye was caught only by the Milan Cathedral—on whose roof she charcoaled the names of Josephine Griffing and Frances D. Gage—and Mt. Vesuvius, which she climbed with gusto. Always stimulated by physical danger, she was pleased to read that it erupted only a few days later. The Taylors were genial companions, and they accompanied her back to London where she rejoined the Sheldons in late May.[85]

For a time Barton thought she would be content in London. The early summer days were soft and radiant, and it was so good to be among English-speaking people again. "We are a merry house full, I do assure you, and say a great many funny things in the course of the twenty-four hours," she wrote happily to Sally.[86] Horse shows and acrobatic troops occupied her evenings, letter writing her days. She enjoyed a wide circle of acquaintances, among them literary figures, such as John Chapman, editor of the *Westminster Review*. Such friends encouraged her to renew her own efforts at verse, though she attempted little beyond some jolly rhymes for home consumption.[87]

Despite her high spirits Barton was miffed that she was not asked to be a delegate to an international prison conference being held in London that July. She was only partly mollified by Abby's observation that no one had known she would be there, and by her own opinion, gleaned from a visitor's seat in the gallery, that the women were badly disorganized. Though living only a few blocks apart, she avoided visiting Florence Nightingale, who also declined a meeting with the American heroine whose work had been so like her own. Remarkably similar in personality and aspiration, neither could brook a competitor. Barton, who since 1862 had been continually called "the Florence Nightingale of America," noted with annoyance that no one was referring to Nightingale as the "Clara Barton of Britain," and was loath to put herself in a position requiring any sort of obsequiousness. Instead, the two followed proper Victorian etiquette by exchanging a few notes, then literally taking to their beds to recover from the strain.[88]

In September the house party, which now included Antoinette Margot, set off for the Isle of Wight. They had homey rooms and long conversational dinners, but Barton was beginning to be bored. It should have been a danger sign for her, for boredom led to depression and, ultimately, physical breakdown. She became disgruntled and difficult to please, declaring, "Nothing makes me so sick of life as to feel that I am sacrificing it—and it is sacrificed when one is pursued by a shadow from which they cannot escape."[89] A few weeks later she developed a chronic cough and a serious case of bronchitis. By Christmas Eve she had broken down completely. "I am so confused an[d] nervous that I can neither sleep nor rest," she noted sadly in her journal, "pass a poor night and am so nervously weak in the morning that I cannot walk straight."[90]

Clara's family sent Mamie Barton, David's young daughter, to be with her, but the presence of her niece and Margot only troubled her further. The bronchitis had robbed her of her voice, and she now sat in bed, too weak to move, while the two young women tiptoed mournfully around the house. It made her "feel herself such a restriction, such a detractor from their happiness . . . ," and she begged them to "have the same chatty day that Auntie knows they would have if they were in their own room by themselves, laughing, singing, doing nonsense."[91] In an effort to cheer the girls she sent them out on excursions or wrote out playful ditties that poked fun at her own misery:

If I were a bat, or a rat, or a cat,
It were all very well I am sure,
But as I am not that, nor that, nor that,

It is a difficult thing to endure.
In speechless blue I am the day through
Never reading a page, or a line.
But only keep winking, and thinking, and thinking
Till the thoughts are worn powdery fine.
As soon as a light, appears in sight
They're shutting and weeping with pain,
And I'm sitting and scowling, and knitting
My brow till it disappears again.[92]

Her efforts to lighten the dismal household mood were made in vain. News that Sally Vassall was ill of stomach cancer weighed heavily on every mind, and Clara, still weak in March 1873, worked herself into a frenzy in an effort to return to her sister's side.[93] The gloomy English weather did not help the situation. Clara likened the unending gray of the sky to the lead sheet of a coffin with the top closed and screws turned down, concluding, "I like old England well enough, but evidently she doesn't like me."[94] Even a visit from the grand duchess, and the arrival of the Iron Cross of Germany, which she had been awarded by a grateful Kaiser Wilhelm, could not rouse her from the doldrums. The coveted honor was never before or after awarded to an American woman, and of the twenty-odd decorations Barton would receive in her lifetime, this would be her most prized. But at this time it only reminded her that she needed work and purpose, and that she had no way to find them in the foreseeable future.[95]

Clara wanted desperately to return to her own country, nurse Sally back to health, and settle herself down at last. Yet she feared that America offered only more boredom and idleness. She had no clear project in mind, would not consider joining wholeheartedly a cause that she herself had not founded, and could not even consider retiring, at fifty-one, as a respectable, if somewhat eccentric, old maid. Thus the summer passed, with many determined bookings on ocean liners and an equal number of cancellations. Finally, hearing from Bernard Vassall that Sally was in real danger, she boarded the S.S. *Parthia* on September 30, 1873. Settling into her comfortable berth and summing up her unfamiliar roommate with words "crotchety enough," she prepared for the two-week voyage.[96] One evening, as she contemplated what her return, after three years, would mean, Barton took up her pen and composed a poem that spoke of the fear with which she awaited the homecoming:

Plow on, old *Parthia*, steady and true,
Each plunge of thy prow brings them nearer to view;
Brings me nearer the days that shall settle the doubt
If they've kept me within—or have left me without.
. . . .
Have ye place, each beloved one, a place in your prayer,
Have ye *room*, my dear countrymen, room for me there?[97]

eleven

Seasick, worn, and more than a little anxious, Clara stepped from the *Parthia* to pier 59 of New York's bustling harbor. To her surprise, it was crowded with friends and well-wishers. Eyewitnesses on the pier reported that Barton looked so well that her friends banished their fears that she had become a tottering old woman and welcomed her back into their productive midst.[1] Before she left New York she was honored at a "brilliant reception" given in the Fifth Avenue home of Clarence Lozier, a prominent doctor whose wife was on the board of the Woman Suffrage Party of New York State.[2] Barton's worries about being forgotten seemed but self-pitying illusions in the face of this acclaim. She journeyed on to New England filled with new confidence.

For six weeks she lingered and visited, first with the Sheldons in New Haven and then with Bartons, Vassalls, Stones, and Learneds in North Oxford. Clara was pleased to see David, at sixty-five still attending steadfastly to his farm chores; Vira, tirelessly carrying on the business of the local post office; and the bevy of young nieces, nephews, and cousins growing up around them. Only Sally's poor health left her saddened. During her illness in England, Clara had written in detail of every cough that seized her and every sleepless night, but Sally had answered with only hazy allusions to her own illness. It was now apparent that her condition was grave. Clara did what she could for Sally, but, realizing that her sister's death was not imminent and unable to stand the cold weather of New England where Sally was again living (or her sister-in-law Julia's cold shoulder), she moved south to Washington.[3]

Barton may have expected to enjoy the furious whirl of the capital's social season, for she indulged in some enthusiastic dressmaking about this time—so enthusiastic that it led her romantic nieces to speculate that their aunt was involved in a love affair.[4] But though her new wardrobe included a heavy white satin gown, there was no romance in the air. As it turned out, even her expectations for pleasant sociey were unfulfilled. Clara, despite the benefits of a more southerly latitude, again collapsed in sickness, a victim of her old complaint, bronchitis. Notwithstanding her doctor's best efforts, it plagued her all winter. In retrospect, those efforts seem woefully inadequate. He forbade her to live in her house on noisy, polluted Capitol Hill and admonished her to drink cherry juice, cream, and Jamaica rum for her cough. When the strain of yet another illness made her weak and weepy, he recommended hot baths of two to three hours duration, during which she was to continually drink glasses of warm water. Finally, removed from friends, adequate care, and even the comforts of her own home, she was obliged to enter Dr. Thompson's new Columbia Hospital for Women. There her condition was diagnosed as nervous prostration, and she was solemnly told that the disease was the result of "heated blood."[5]

Barton concurred with the doctor's belief that nothing was wrong with her but shattered nerves and admitted to Sally that she seemed unable to cope with even the everyday irritations of life. "I am weak and get 'in a state' as the fashionable girls say, at nothing at all, and much less than that," she wrote home.[6] In the attractive new hospital, built of light-colored brick in a Mediterranean style, she slept, wrote letters full of surprising good humor, and voraciously read nearly a book a day. Despite the discomfort she felt in being patient instead of nurse, Barton was at long last allowing herself the care that she needed. Had she remained there any amount of time, she might well have rested her frayed nerves and avoided the years of sickness that were to come.[7]

But the news from Massachusetts kept her restless and jumpy. In the spring of 1874, Sally's cancer was making its final inroads. The almost daily bulletins she received from Fanny Vassall and her nephew Stephen E. Barton—Stevé, as she fondly called him—left Clara in despair. Her last sister, the treasured teacher, "lovely as an angel," who had read geography lessons with her in bed and who soberly stood with her in the Baltimore and Ohio railroad station when the arrival of the wounded Massachusetts Sixth Regiment changed the course of Clara's life, was dying, and her own health would not permit her to tenderly care for Sally in her last hours.[8] In agony, Barton made several attempts to leave the hospital for North Oxford. About "once in two weeks [I] would have orders given to take me to the depot and on to Worcester," she was to write sorrowfully, "but before the train could come around I would be on my bed more dead than alive . . . and so wretched in mind that I would have given all I ever had to *stop breathing* and *yet feared I should*—it would take two weeks to get over this and repeat the effort."[9] Friends and family urged her not to make the trip in the bad spring weather, both because of the risk to her health and because there was really nothing to be done. Even Sally did not want her. "Mother's exclamation when she heard you were coming was 'I'm sorry,'" Bernard Vassall told Clara. "'She can do me no good, and it will make her sick to come here and be with me, it will make us both worse.'"[10] Ultimately, after the receipt of a gloomy telegram from Stevé that predicted that Sally could not last the week, Clara rallied every bit of strength and boarded a northbound train. The eight-hour trip left her exhausted, and she tarried for a day before continuing on. The next day, May 24, she made the final leg of the journey.[11]

She arrived too late. Her 4:00 P.M. train had missed Sally's last painful breath by ten hours. Prostrate with grief and guilt, she could not bear even to gaze upon her dead sister's face and was unable to attend the funeral.[12] "It was too much," Barton later wrote. "Body and soul were stricken."[13] Within days she suffered a complete nervous breakdown, the culmination of years of emotional problems and mismanaged health. "I . . . turned neither to the right nor the left," she told a friend, "but walked straight forward on the precipice and crashed on the rocks of its yawning chasms below."[14]

For two years Clara remained a helpless invalid, seeming to lack the resources needed to revive her intellect and energy. Her hair, once her sole point of vanity, dramatically turned white and thin, as if symbolizing the death of her spirit. During the first year she was almost entirely at the mercy of others. She could not be moved, could not eat, could not sleep, write, talk, walk, or see, could not do anything, in fact, but lie miserably whimpering in her bed. Like a feverish child she would sob and cry over trifles and knew not how to stop. She thought she saw mice running over the corners of the tables and screamed at any sudden noise.[15] Clara spent most of the time at the Vassalls' house in Worcester worrying about the extra care she required, later writing that she felt "good for nothing, worse than nothing, and a trouble to every one."[16] Joseph and Abby Sheldon came to see her with plans to remove her to their spacious Connecticut home, but they concluded after the visit that her condition was beyond the care they could give her. Instead Barton wrote—in a rare letter during these years—to Minna Kupfer to come to her from Switzerland. The tables were turned now and Kupfer, who had relied so on Clara's nursing at the outbreak of the Franco-Prussian War, was only too willing to help her old friend. Her kindly, religious spirit and her decisive, even-handed manner did much to aid Barton in these long months.[17]

By October 1874 Barton was well enough to do a little sketching in bed, but it was not for another six months that she could change her residence. Then her family moved her to a large country house belonging to Jerry Learned in New England Village (now Grafton), Massachusetts. She still refused visitors and seldom left her room, since she suffered from chills and was given to periodic "nervous attacks." A single fit sometimes lasted ten hours, leaving her "cold and wet as a fish every minute of the time."[18] But she could do a little embroidery, write simple letters, and dress herself. In July she began to receive a few callers and to direct some business affairs, including the selling of her small Massachusetts farm, purchased from her father in the late 1850s. Yet the gains in physical strength belied the slow recovery of her morale. "I am weak and ill, and *cannot* rally from it, and I have almost concluded it is of no use to try," Barton complained. Stacks of letters from concerned friends and resolutions offering "heartfelt sympathies" from GAR posts and the New York Woman Suffrage Society seemed to make few inroads on her depression.[19] A decade later, she would compare the collapse to death, the extinction of her spirit from which she would have to be reborn. "I have never to this day been able to calculate correctly how many more hundred times easier it would be to die of it than to live through, and get up, out of the condition. I did the latter but I have always felt that the world owed me a *pension*." The days of complete helplessness had "maimed her for life," concluded Barton.[20]

In early November the death of her beloved friend and protector Henry Wilson further tried her nerves. Wilson, who had been elected vice-president in 1872, had suffered a stroke that fall. Though he and Barton had been out of touch for a number of years, they had never ceased to regard each other with respect and affection. The account of his last hours, in which he asked tenderly about her, both eased and heightened the loss she felt at his death. He "clung to my hand and eagerly questioned me about you," a mutual friend told Barton. "Said he 'Do you know anything of Clara? . . . I haven't seen her for so long a time.'"[21] As she had at the deaths of Charles Sumner, Horace Greeley, and Abraham Lincoln, Barton bemoaned the loss of an old leader who, she believed, had guided the country through its darkest hours, and she wondered where they should find another to replace him. "How the bright lights go out . . . ," she mused. "How they fly off like sparks from a shooting torch."[22]

Barton's poor health and the loss of Wilson made her uncharacteristically irritable in company and demanding in her ways. Jerry Learned had generously loaned her the house, but she made a prudish point of buying everything else for all members of her household, flushing and remonstrating when she was offered even an apple from a neighboring tree. Money was not really a problem—she had scarcely touched the investments from her lectures of the 1860s—but the irrational fear of beggary exacerbated her unhappy mood.[23] Clara's friends were surprised to find her ungenerous and vindictive toward people. Once, when a physician acquaintance borrowed a medical volume from her and neglected to return it after a week, she flared out in a manner out of proportion to the problem. In a rage she declared that the "little Dr. has retained it through *spite*. . . . I would cheerfully let him keep it . . . if he could make it of any use to humanity, but in the first place he would never read it, and secondly could not comprehend it if he did."[24] Even a small child who lived near Barton felt the lack of warmth in her at this time. "I never *asked* Miss Barton a question," she recalled. "She told me what she wished to."[25]

Part of Barton's despair was her flagging faith in the medical profession. The years of continual illness in Washington, in London, and again in Massachusetts had made her believe that most doctors did not have the knowledge to relieve her suffering and that many did actual harm. "I must confess that my previously small share of confidence in medical aid and wisdom has not increased by last year's experience," she had written to Fanny Vassall in 1873. The trials of the following two years lowered her respect even further.[26] Barton had had no doctor since autumn 1874 and had given up on any kind of medicine save some herbal teas made with slippery elm, Iceland moss, bayberry, and the like, or an occasional nip of brandy or whiskey.[27] In desperation she made a last attempt, after her removal to New England Village, to get medical advice. She wrote a lengthy letter to Edward Foote, a New York doctor who believed, in advance of the time, that there was a connection between heredity, psychological makeup, and physical illness. In her letter Barton revealed a great deal about herself that she had never before intimated: the nervous and strange personalitites of her family; her battle to fight plumpness and tendency toward depression; the alienation from family and friends. She had been "tossed up and down" by life, she claimed, and had concluded that "the lives of us all are at best only a kind of slow suicide process." Barton then went on to describe symptoms that today would be diagnosed a combination of nervous exhaustion and bleeding ulcer. She was controlling these, she told Dr. Foote, by a rigorous diet that included raw meat and acidic fruits—foods now thought to make such a condition worse. "I submit my case to your care," she concluded. "I know you will do your best. Please tell me how to do my [part]."[28]

Dr. Foote's reply has unfortunately not survived, but soon after she received it Barton became interested in the work of another physician, James Caleb Jackson of Dansville, New York. Jackson was the proprietor of one of the largest sanitariums on the East Coast, noted for its stress on healthful diet and congenial atmosphere. An old army acquaintance, probably John Elwell, told Barton of his work and encouraged her to seek his counsel. By January 1876, she had sent letters of inquiry to Dr. Jackson and received in return several pamphlets that summarized his philosophies. She began to follow some of the advice for herself: "I weighed every suggestion and followed every advice as religiously as if the word of the Lord had spoken it," she later admitted. The results were so successful that she sent further letters to Jackson asking that she be taken on as patient.[29] When, on March 16, 1876, a young seamstress who came to help her proclaimed Dansville "the place to go to get well," the question was settled.[30] Barton spent six weeks furiously sewing, wrote a final letter to Dr. Jackson, noting with pleasure that his reply referred to her as a guest rather than a patient, assembled her household goods, then steeled herself for the two-day journey to western New York. The train went via Rochester, where passsengers stopped overnight before taking a local railroad to Wayland, the last stop. There Barton boarded a stage, which rattled along a plank toll road into the mountain valley where Dansville was situated.[31]

Barton had been to Dansville once before, on a lecture tour in 1866. She found the place little changed. It was a small, prosperous town in Livingston County, near the scenic Finger Lakes. A center for the surrounding dairy and lumber industry, Dansville boasted broad, tree-lined streets, pleasant family homes, several thriving newspapers, and the proper representation of every Protestant denomination. It was, in short, the kind of home town Americans even then cherished, and Dansville citizens were rather smugly satisfied with their pleasant burg.[32]

James Jackson had come to Dansville in 1858, bursting with ambition to start a sanitarium based on the use of the patient's mental powers to cure nervous disorders. His was a commanding personality. He had been educated in classical studies, and an admirer noted that "his resources of knowledge and thought seemed exhaustless." He had a flowing white beard, slanting eyes that gave his face a quizzical expression, and a liberal temperament that had sought an outlet in, among other things, abolition, temperance, and women's rights. Jackson read, wrote, and talked incessantly on his favorite subjects, and his articles ranged from treatises on child rearing to strongly-worded pamphlets on dress reform and sexual health. He loved to be called "father" and demanded a certain fealty from his patients. "The pride, the passions, the prejudices as well as the virtues of a strong personality were his," recalled the local newspaper editor.[33]

Dr. Harriet Austin, Jackson's adopted daughter and partner, accompanied him to New York to start the sanitarium. The building they bought had previously been a health resort but was little more than a "squalid rookery" on their arrival.[34] They built it up into a splendid facility, featuring a four-story brick building with tiered balconies, nestled among the hills and surrounded by picturesque Gothic cottages. "Guests," as the patients were called, could stay in the main building (which also contained a dining room, parlors, a large lecture theater, and other public facilities) or in the cottages on the grounds. The walls were hung with uplifting mottos advising visitors that they should "sit up straight" and not talk about their diseases, as well as refrain from taking napkins from the table. The grounds themselves were exceedingly beautiful, with graceful walks along which markers were placed every eighth of a mile so that ambulatory patients could measure their progress. The establishment overall resembled more a posh resort than a place to treat the overworked and unstrung. Appropriately, the founding doctors called the sanitarium "Our Home on the Hillside."[35]

The regimen was as attractive as the surroundings. Though the medical staff were much in evidence, the emphasis was on what Jackson called "psycho-hygiene," a combination of cheerful atmosphere and plain but abundant food, with special weight given to whole grains, exercise, and intellectual stimulation. He believed the prevalent medicines harmful in the extreme and the current dress code among women ridiculous and unhealthy. (Led by Harriet Austin, many of the female guests wore a modified version of the scandalous "Bloomer" costume, consisting of a tunic that reached below the knee and ankle-length Turkish pantaloons worn *sans* corset. The townspeople called the patients "grasshoppers" because of their exposed limbs, and little boys jeered in the streets, but many of the women admitted to a new feeling of freedom.[36]) Lectures were as liberal as the dress, with such speakers as Frederick Douglass, Susan B. Anthony, William Dean Howells, and Sojourner Truth leading the bills. Bedridden patients were allowed few excuses for not attending lectures, since cots were set up in the back of the lecture halls.[37] In addition, there were cotillions, outings, sleigh rides in the winter, and picnics in the fall. Wrote Barton: "The utmost good social humor prevails, a chatty, jolly family, with the best possible food."[38]

The food, in fact, was what Barton first noticed, and what had given the place much of its reputation. Jackson was a follower of Sylvester Graham, a Michigan doctor who in the 1830s and 1840s had popularized the notion that whole grain flours and breads were more healthful than refined wheat and that, indeed, they were the cure-all for everything from baby's croup to female complaints. Dr. Jackson himself had invented a cereal called "Granola," a kind of hardtack that was twice-baked, crumbled, then soaked overnight in a glass of milk and eaten cold.[39] At one Christmas dinner, besides the requisite turkey, "Our Home" served sixteen varieties of whole grain crackers and seven kinds of mush.[40] Vegetarianism was not required, but eating an array of fresh fruits and vegetables from the sanitarium's own gardens and fine milk products from their dairy and the surrounding countryside was stressed. "The tables are excellent and most abundantly supplied," Clara reported to Elvira Stone. If it was true that one became what one ate, she had no fears for her eventual recovery.[41]

Barton flourished in this atmosphere. She felt an immediate rapport with Austin and Jackson and willingly placed herself in their hands. She admitted that she had had little idea about how to get well and styled herself a "pupil" who was at Our Home to "learn and study and obey." Now that the day-to-day worries of life were taken from her, Clara was able, soon after her arrival, to tell a friend, "My mind is relieved from care now. I know I am surrounded by those who know a great deal more than I do and at last I can lay down the reigns and ride at my ease. I am relieved from the management of my team, and this is such a rest."[42]

Initially Barton stayed in the main building and was allowed to do little but stroll, socialize, and admire the home's famous view. Even letter writing was restricted. When she was finally encouraged to try her hand at two or three letters a week, they spoke in raptures of the comfortable atmosphere and outdoor life.[43] She shed her hastily made finery and adopted Austin's "American costume," which left her "dressed just as free and easy as a gentleman," though she was vain enough to drop it again a few months later when a visiting friend remarked that it looked silly.[44] The most tedious task for her was to learn to pace herself, for after a lifetime of relying on seemingly inexhaustible reserves of energy it was difficult to slow down. Sleep, which had evaded her since childhood, became easier, and she believed this was the secret of her returning health. Five months after her arrival, Clara could report to John Elwell that in "health I am always gaining slowly, am coming up. I don't know how high—but *surely up*. Dansville has *done me well*."[45]

Fresh air, comfortable clothes, good food, and time to stretch, relax, and take stock were the keys to Barton's recovery. Of equal importance was the delicious company at Our Home. Far from being a haven for sullen dyspeptics, the sanitarium was careful to accept only those who would contribute to the congeniality of the surroundings. About three hundred patients were under Jackson's care at the time of Barton's stay; to her delight she believed she had never seen "any group of people that combines the degrees of intellect, general intelligence, and culture as is collected here."[46] She made friends with several people who, like her, were devoted to a then-popular series of sketches that featured Samantha, a country gal of bumbling ways, and a whole cast of appealing rustics. Together they formed a "Betsey Bobbett" club, named for one of the characters, and Clara herself was nicknamed Betsey. The group wrote stories, plays, and poems, discussed dress reform and woman suffrage, and attended dinners and lectures in a tight, laughing knot.[47] Barton also enjoyed the company of Mary Weeks, then the matron of Our Home. Weeks found in Barton an older woman to whom she could pour out her heart, and Clara did much to encourage the young woman to pursue her dream of a degree in medicine. When Weeks finally broke away and went to study in St. Louis, it was Barton who sponsored her career.[48]

Barton was also attracted to Harriet Austin and developed a close relationship with her. Dr. Austin was a magnetic, endlessly cheerful person, dedicated completely to her profession, yet with a sunny and childlike curiosity about every element of life, which gave her an air of spontaneity and fun. She had, in addition, a formidable intellect and keen business sense. More than once Austin had startled the merchants of Dansville by expertly transacting the business affairs of Our Home; one hardware store owner was known to have recovered only slowly from the shock of serving "a woman dressed like a man, who does business just like a man." Barton had actually met Austin a decade earlier during her lecture tour and had been impressed then by her gentle grace and free, natural dress. Now they reestablished the friendship by discovering a shared interest in painting, women's rights, and progressive medicine. Austin paid special attention to Barton's case and sent her a long string of cheery notes, inviting her to sleigh rides, to join her for Christmas dinner, or just to observe the beauties of the day. Barton, full of admiration, recognized that Austin had an instinctive feel for the needs of her patients: "the full honest eye . . . seemed to look into your very soul."[49]

Barton made few male friends during her stay in Dansville. Indeed these years reinforced a growing tendency in Barton to draw close to women and identify more strongly with them. She had long emulated masculine tastes and pursuits, and though she had had lasting friendships with girlhood acquaintances and protégées such as Mary Norton or Antoinette Margot, the force of her character had always overshadowed theirs and the friendships had not been based on equal positions. For intellectual stimulation—and appreciation—she had turned to men: first her brothers and Lucien Burleigh in North Oxford; Samuel Ramsey and Charles Norton in Hightstown; Judge Mason and Colonel DeWitt during the Washington years; finally Henry Wilson, John Elwell, and Dorence Atwater.

Not until she met Frances D. Gage in 1863 did Barton know a woman who challenged her as men did.

What made the friendships contracted during the 1860s and 1870s so rich was the similar outlook and experience these women could share with Clara Barton. In Gage, Louise of Baden, Harriet Austin, and Susan B. Anthony, Barton found women with mature minds and dedicated careers. All, save the grand duchess, had fought for their education, place, and the privilege of earning a decent living. All had sharp, articulate minds, and hearts bent on relieving at least a small pocket of the world's suffering. They were Barton's contemporaries, her equals, and moreover, her colleagues. Far from being intimidated or threatened by so shining a group of associates, she embraced them, and in the last third of her life she drew ever closer to women. Barton herself seems not to have recognized this growing tendency and viewed herself still as a lone female traveler in the world of men. "I think I know men better than I know women," she wrote about this time; "I've always been among them more."[50] Yet for the remainder of her life she would form only one strong intellectual relationship with a man— her nephew Stephen—while embracing a group of women whose intellectual and professional tastes and accomplishments matched her own.

Clara moved out of the home after a few months to a rented house in the town proper. Here she had greater privacy and led a more normal life. Minna Kupfer came again to share the house and act as housekeeper, and Fanny Atwater, the youngest sister of Dorence, also arrived to look after her. Barton continued to take her meals at the sanitarium, for which she paid fifteen dollars a week, but she enjoyed the luxury of having her own possessions around her. The household, which came to include an ancient Atwater uncle and, eventually, Mary Weeks, got on well together. "There are among us no secrets and fortunately no need of any," she recorded in her diary on the first day of the New Year, 1877, "no jealousy, no ill feeling, and in fact although our house is generously supplied with closets, we believe there is [sic] not skeletons in any of them."[51]

The new living arrangements put Barton in greater proximity to the town, a situation about which she had a certain ambivalence. On one hand, Dansville's citizens, who were anxious to adopt the heroine as an honored member of the community, embraced and flattered Barton. She was invited to join the "Coterie," an exclusive society of the town's leading intellects, who met periodically to discuss various philosophical subjects. The library society courted her, and Civil War veterans serenaded her home.[52] On Memorial Day, 1877, the entire town spontaneously formed a parade and wound its way to her house. Children, men and women, dogs, and a band "with numerous 'flags a-floating,' made the procession gay as it moved on, led by the clergy," reported the *Dansville Advertiser.* "The Conesus brass band, taking tea at the seminary, had patriotically agreed to add to the dignity of the enterprise by their numbers and their music." Barton was entirely taken by surprise and was correspondingly moved when she realized the tribute was to her. After a few pretty speeches, each person laid a bouquet of flowers at the moist-eyed invalid's feet "till her lap was piled high and her feet buried deep in a pink and white mound."[53]

Notwithstanding such tributes, and despite her enthusiasm for Dr. Jackson's establishment, Barton was not particularly taken with Dansville and its residents, especially in the early years of her stay there. It impressed her as "nonprogressive, not over-moral, and not generous in any view one could take of it."[54] She had continual trouble with landlords and once was taken to court by a man who was trying to arrange the shady sale of a broken-down horse.[55] Clara could not even put her cat out without someone stealing it. "I really cannot form a respectful loving attachment to a place in which I find it impossible to keep a cat without her being picked up and kept for the reward I am expected to offer for its redemption," she wrote indignantly.[56]

As her nerves grew calmer and her stamina returned, Barton was able to devote more time to personal needs and long-neglected business matters. She retained cousin Robert Hale as her closest financial advisor, clearly appreciating his humor and levelheaded advice. Her first concern was to straighten the tangled ends of the finances still left dangling after the Franco-Prussian War. When she had broken down in Belfort, she had neglected to send the Boston relief committee a statement of the expenditures, and the committee had never required any account. Now she wrote lengthy and detailed accounts of the proceedings of the last years, advising the committee that during her illness she had invested the sum remaining—$3,241—and was now returning it to them. Barton had been careless in this matter, and it was with embarrassment that she now contacted the committee. To her surprise, they voted to give the money to Massachusetts General Hospital, with a provision that the annual interest should go to Barton during her lifetime. She pronounced the arrangement "perfect" and advised Edmund Dwight, her contact with the committee, that it would fulfill a longtime dream of having a backup fund to draw from when cries of distress came to her from unexpected parts. Clara had never forgotten the days after the Civil War when she had seen a need and had had no funds with which to fill it. The Boston committee's plan seemed a splendid kind of contingency fund.[57]

Another financial matter concerned Barton at this time—one less pleasant and more personal. At the time of her departure for Europe, she had entrusted about two thousand dollars in bonds to Sylvanus Gleason, who as a young man had been her student in North Oxford. While she was away, Gleason had run into financial difficulties and, without her knowledge, had sold her bonds and taken the money. Having gone further into debt, he was unable to repay Barton. This misuse of her funds greatly upset Clara, for she had always given Gleason special attention and now felt she had been duped and used. "I am less grieved about the loss than I am about the manner of his treating my trust," she explained to Robert Hale. "I was his teacher and he was one of my boys. I have always dealt straight and plain with my boys. . . . I am as square as a brick, and I expect my boys to be square."[58] Hale advised her to be gentle in her remonstrations if she wished to keep Gleason's friendship, and Barton, always prizing loyalty above any other quality, refused to badger her former pupil. She declined to take part in any bankruptcy proceedings and years later, after he had embroiled her in several other unsavory schemes, still remained his friend. The money was never returned.[59]

Barton's correspondence talked not only of money matters but much of herself during these months. It became, indeed, a time of introspection for her. While newspaper reporters and friends took care to find her face "interesting" and her mode of life "admirably modest," Clara had no illusion about either her appearance or habits. "I was *never* what the world calls even 'good-looking,'" she wrote in a lengthy self-description in 1876, "leaving out of the case such terms as 'handsome' and 'pretty.' . . . I never cared for dress, and have no accomplishment, so you will find me plain and prosy both in representation and reality." She was a modest person, Barton claimed, with unexceptional tastes and a lifestyle as "simple as a hermit's."[60] She viewed herself, however, as a woman of stature and vocation, and when Susan B. Anthony requested a biographical sketch for a forthcoming historical encyclopedia, she proudly headed the column with the title "philanthropist." After stating the numerous fields, military and civilian, on which she had labored, she ended with a melodramatic recitation of their importance. (Though she told Anthony that "an old friend" had written the final paragraph, the draft copy shows it to have been her work.) "Sensitive by nature, refined by culture," the statement began, "she has nevertheless taken unaccustomed fields of labor, walked untrodden paths with bleeding feet and opened pioneer doors with bruised fingers, not for her own aggrandisement but for that of her sex and humanity."[61]

Perhaps Barton was so anxious to praise herself because her family and the United States government still seemed so unwilling to do so. Three countries had honored her with their highest awards, but never her own. Even her family had refused to acknowledge the tremendous courage and stamina she had shown, believing it improper for a woman to become involved in projects that resulted in her name being mentioned in the newspaper. Only her niece Ida Barton Riccius seemed to take pride in her achievements, Barton wrote, sadly acknowledging that to her "it has always seemed so *unnatural* as it has been, that I could never comprehend it, and it took away all the sweet to feel that there were none but strangers to feel an interest in what came to me." The most her family had ever mentioned of her achievements, she told Ida, was to caution her that she was "in danger of being spoiled like a vain forward child and must be held in check."[62]

Barton had formerly been reluctant to express any disappointment she felt in her own family, but during these years in Dansville she frequently described her loneliness and feeling of rejection. In a revealing poem, written to a friend in the Betsey Bobbett Club in 1876, she compared herself to a swinging vine, with neither firm roots nor steady branches to hold onto.

A poor lonely maid, like a vine she has swayed.
Her tendrils onclasped, and her branches onstayed.
While the tall trees all round her waved rugged and free.
With no one to bless, to soothe or caress
No fond heart to beg for one loose flowering tress
Of the let down back hair of lone Betsey C.B.[63]

Yet she was not really unhappy, and the days passed pleasantly enough. She had energy for friendships, a bright new outlook on life, and increasing physical stamina. The marvel of Dr. Jackson's cure was that it not only helped Barton to regain her strength but taught her to maintain it and to avoid the accumulation of stress that led to nervous collapse. Only fourteen months after her arrival in Dansville, Barton could observe to a friend that she seemed "to have gotten beyond that seemingly endless liability to 'backslide' and fall back into bed again every few weeks, and have stood bravely on my feet for *almost a year* now."[64] Never again, even under the most adverse circumstances and personal crises, did Clara Barton suffer from a nervous breakdown. If she ever saw a friend "verging on to that condition," she told a nephew, "if it were given me to speak but one word, and then close my warning lips forever, that word would be *Dansville.*"[65]

twelve

Throughout 1876 and 1877 Barton's health and spirits continued to improve. Doctors Austin and Jackson still supervised her recovery. They encouraged Clara to participate in outings and programs at the sanitarium, to fill her house with congenial company, and to limit her activities to those that required little mental or physical exertion. As always, she had to guard against an inclination to overwork the minute she felt a little recovered. "I find it a difficult problem to solve, how to bring myself down to the necessary economies of my present condition," Barton admitted. "I cannot realize that a few hours, a few rods, a few steps even . . . may use up all my little capital." To prevent such backsliding she pottered in the garden or wrote chatty letters, which kept her from dwelling on more troublesome or tiring matters. But, far from resenting the admonitions of Jackson and Austin, Barton seems to have welcomed their restraining influence. "One sometimes needs to be saved from himself," she concluded.[1]

She was certainly gaining under the doctors' continued advice to rest and conserve energy as she made her final recovery. Her insomnia had disappeared, and she told the grand duchess that she had gained weight and had greater powers of endurance.[2] But as she rallied physically Barton became increasingly restless intellectually. Kept away from a meaningful employment for nearly five years, she now longed to be active again. At fifty-six she could not consider her lifework finished, and she began to look around for a new challenge, one that would test her talents and divert her mind. She found it in the International Red Cross, the organization that had so impressed her during the Franco-Prussian War.

The immediate cause of Barton's rekindled interest in the Red Cross was the outbreak of war between Russia and Turkey. In the spring of 1877 disgruntlement over Turkey's role in the Balkans sent the two countries into armed conflict. Drawn as ever to the pathos, glory, and chance for service that war offered, Clara searched for a way in which she could take part: "like the old war horse that has rested long in quiet pastures, I recognize the bugle note that calls me to my place and though I may not do what I once could, I am come to offer what I may." Remembering the enthusiastic way in which Americans had donated relief funds during the Franco-Prussian War, she hit upon the idea of forming an American Red Cross Society, which would collect contributions for the sufferers in Turkey and Russia. In her mind Barton saw many possibilities: local societies, warehouses for supplies, and a badly needed permanent job for herself. Eventually her idea expanded to include publicizing the results of the Geneva Convention and encouraging the official adoption of its principles in the United States.[3]

Thus, in May 1877, Barton wrote a lengthy letter to Louis Appia in Geneva, asking permission to promote the Red Cross in America. She deeply regretted, she told Appia, that her illness had made her "powerless to strike a blow on the great anvil of humanity, or labor one day in its vineyards"; she now longed to rejoin those working for the good of man, and she could think of no better cause than the Red Cross. She urged the members of the International Red Cross Committee to let her take up the crusade and further suggested that they appoint her "head of your noble order in this country." Barton was careful to acknowledge the efforts the International Committee had made to draw the United States into the organization. Still, she observed that few Americans understood the articles of the Geneva Convention; she could not foresee its acceptance without an enormous amount of publicity. It was, she noted, a great undertaking, and she urged Appia to reply as soon as possible.[4]

Within a month she received an answer. Appia had contacted Gustave Moynier, the president of the International Red Cross, and wrote to tell her that they welcomed her assistance. To Barton's intense satisfaction, the committee appointed her their representative to Washington, sentimentally referring to her as the "soul" of the Red Cross in America. He urged her, however, not to take too much upon herself. The Red Cross would need a body as well as a soul, and though she might be the head, she should "create immediately under that head a body, arms to write, to arrange methodically, to publish, . . . feet for running, to go, to come, to collect, to buy." Both in this and in a later letter, Appia urged Barton to make official adoption of the Treaty of Geneva an important priority, for without this an American Red Cross would have no legal standing.[5] This letter was followed by one from Moynier, reiterating Appia's pleasure that "so well qualified a person as you are should plead by your government above all things the cause that is so dear to all of us."[6]

Despite such accolades, Barton was dissatisfied with the committee's backing and insecure with her own position vis-à-vis the International Red Cross. She asked Appia for an official letter "asking in your own name or that of the International society that I do all in my power to aid you in the work and to use my power with my people and my Government—so that it can be seen here that such a want is felt, such a work needed."[7] Since the time she had been appointed an official member of the Andersonville expedition she had mistrusted any but the most formal authority for dealing with the government. The fact that most women lobbying for social reform were politely dismissed by officials (who had no need to curry favor with disfranchised females) gave justification to her need to establish herself as the legitimate representative of the Red Cross.

Both her own fragile ego and her sense that she would not be taken seriously in Washington without this rigorous backing thus prompted Barton to exaggerate; the Geneva committee must be seen to request rather than accept her services. Henceforth, to all outsiders, Barton interpreted her correspondence with Moynier and Appia as a strong appeal to her for help. She told both the Grand Duchess Louise and Harriet Austin that the International Committee had made the first overtures to her, that indeed they were clamoring for her, and that this was the reason that she was giving up her leisure.[8] She tried to gain further credibility with Moynier and Appia by accusing Charles Bowles and Henry Bellows—men who had attempted to interest the American government in the Red Cross years before—of mismanagement and indiscretion. "Bowles proved utterly unreliable and went into hopeless bankruptcy in 1873, and . . . was never worthy of confidence," she wrote. "His successor Dr. Bellows . . . accepted the position as a tribute of respect which he wears as an easy honor, and it never occurs to him that he is retarding the progress of the world in its march of humanity by his inaction. . . . But you must see that until you transfer that appointment of authority to some other person, no one can feel authorized to act, and of course will not."[9] The accusations were unjustified; both Bowles and Bellows had acted forcefully on behalf of the Red Cross. But Barton could never be secure enough in her official relationships, or in knowing she was wanted and needed.

Though wrong in accusing Charles Bowles and Henry Bellows of inaction or inappropriate conduct, Barton was correct in her appraisal of the outcome of their work. For fourteen years the Unites States had resisted signing the Treaty of Geneva. At the Second International Congress, held in July 1864, the United States had two unofficial representatives: Bowles, then European agent of the U.S. Sanitary Commission, and George C. Fogg, the American minister to Switzerland. Both wielded a fair amount of influence in private, after-hours meetings, but neither was allowed to vote. They found the problems discussed by the Geneva Convention to be similar to those then being faced in their own Civil War and urged Secretary of State William Seward to adopt the treaty. Seward, however, felt that the measures set forth in the treaty overlapped the wartime work of the Sanitary Commission and similar agencies. The United States, he maintained, had already solved the problems of utilizing large volunteer forces without interfering with military discipline, and it was unlikely to need an international treaty to validate its own practical expertise. Furthermore, Seward believed it was unfitting to adhere to such a treaty, which altered the articles of war at a time when the country was engaged in active hostilities.[10]

At the war's end, members of the Sanitary Commission, under the leadership of Henry Bellows, re-formed into an organization called the American Association for Relief of Misery of the Battlefield. The group was anxious to continue the work they had done during the war, and they kept unofficial ties to the International Red Cross. Bellows again approached Seward about becoming a signatory to the treaty, this time with formal backing from the French and Swiss governments. For two years Seward held Bellows off with evasive answers, protests that it was necessary to consult the secretary of war, and postponement of any final decision.[11] When French officials finally pressed him again for an answer, Seward replied that the United States had in time of war "voluntarily observed the principle rules proscribed in the treaty and [was] not likely to disregard them under any circumstances." He went on to reiterate the basic philosophy of the State Department, that of avoiding alliances with any other nation. "It had always been deemed at least a questionable policy, if not unwise," Seward wrote, "for the United States to become a party of any instrument to which there are many other parties. Nothing but the most urgent necessity should lead to a departure of this rule. It is believed that the case to which your note refers is not one which would warrant such a course."[12]

This philosophy, a broad interpretation of the Monroe Doctrine, which prohibited international intervention in American affairs, had long been adhered to by the United States government. Because of the policy, only a handful of treaties, chiefly those ending wars, had been signed, and the United States had participated in few formal congresses. Disturbances involving the French in Mexico in the 1860s had increased the government's resolve to enforce the Monroe Doctrine. As long as the United States kept to this philosophy, participation in the Geneva Convention, with its emphasis on the articles of war, was, as Seward wrote, "nearly or quite impossible."[13]

In spite of such unequivocal statements, Bellows persisted tenaciously in his effort to link the United States with the Treaty of Geneva. Hopeful that a new administration would prove more open-minded, he approached President Grant's secretary of state, Hamilton Fish, in 1868. But the new appointee was hesitant to break the longstanding tradition. He simply referred Bellows to the earlier correspondence on the issue, with the firm statement that he saw "no reason to change the views then expressed." Further attempts to interest the government proved futile. Their hopes for United States accession to the treaty thwarted, the American Association for the Relief of the Misery of the Battlefield quietly disbanded in 1872.[14]

Clara Barton seems to have been only vaguely aware of these activities when she took up the cause of the Red Cross in 1877; she referred to herself as "almost the only American . . . co-worker . . . and friend of the [International] Committee."[15] Dr. Appia had sent her a long outline of the method he thought would be most effective in establishing the Red Cross in America. It called for the simultaneous pursuit of a number of goals: publicity, government recognition, establishment of a national organization, and the collection of money. It was this plan that Barton chose to follow, but she stamped it with her own style and emphasis.[16] Publicity, she believed, was the most important work that lay before her. It would not be an easy task; as she told Appia, "the knowledge of your society and its great objects in this country . . . is almost unknown, and the Red Cross, in America, is a Mystery."[17] Furthermore, she sensed that without a pressing national cause or international conflict that aroused deep sympathy, in both official and private circles, the Red Cross would be seen as unnecessary. America, she admitted to Appia, "would have received it with open arms at the close of our war, when her own wounds were unhealed, and her memories fresh and tender. She will be less enthusiastic now at the end of ten years peace, and no prospect of war.[18] Its own domestic troubles resolved, America was smugly convinced that it would never be involved in another war. Barton had hoped that the conflict between Russia and Turkey would arouse enough interest that a society for collecting donations for that cause could be formed and later expanded to become an auxiliary of the international organization. But the Russo-Turkish War failed to capture the American imagination, and Barton was forced to look for another pretext on which to launch her publicity campaign.

Gaining popular acceptance was only a part of Barton's plan for promoting the Red Cross. She justly recognized that it would take influence as well as publicity to succeed in her mission. Accordingly, among the first actions Barton took, in July 1877, was to contact old friends with prominent connections in Washington. From Jonathan Defrees, the former head of the Government Printing Office, she solicited a promise to introduce her to President Rutherford B. Hayes.[19] To another old friend, General E. W. Whitaker, she sent a long letter in which she unabashedly questioned him on the current power structure in the capital. "And what I want to ask of you is to tell me how certain public men stand with [President Hayes], or with the Administration," she wrote, "for in the cause I shall be or am requested to present to him I shall require the aid of a favorable arm stronger than my own." Her most loyal allies of former days—Henry Wilson, Benjamin Butler, Benjamin Wade—were either dead or impotent with the Hayes administration, and she had little idea where she should renew ties or use her influence to gain favor.[20] At length she saw that she would have to test the political climate herself, and armed with letters of introduction from Moynier and Appia, she decided to travel to Washington.

It was not until late autumn that Barton felt well enough, and prepared enough, to board the train for the capital. A veteran traveler, she packed a picnic basket for the trip ("I . . . spread it out on my lap, and take my meal—make no apologies—pay no bills—and get *no headaches,* waiting over time, and then hurrying down food unfit to eat"[21]) and prepared to sit back and relax during the two-day journey. It had been half a decade since her last visit to Washington, and Clara noted the changes with mingled pleasure and nostalgia. Trolleys and streetlights were sophisticated additions, though muddy roads and open sewers remained. The beginning of the busy lesiglative season, when the city was filled with politicians and the entourage of socialites and office seekers that inevitably followed them, must have seemed familiar. At this season the city was, as one wide-eyed young man described it, "practically a great winter watering place."[22]

Though she carried letters from Gustave Moynier officially requesting that President Hayes promote the recognition of the Treaty of Geneva in the United States, she decided not to approach him until she had explained the organization to a number of officials and rallied some initial support for her cause. She talked with friends in the State and War departments and in the Congress but discovered, as she had feared, that there were few who were familiar with the issues. "I found the greatest difficulty to consist not in the opposition I would meet at first," Barton reported to Appia, "but in the fact that no one understood the subject, and there was no printed literature pertaining to it in the language *familiar* to the people to whom I desired to present it."[23] Consequently, she spent much of the fall translating the tracts written by Moynier and Appia and compiling a short pamphlet of her own. She gave informal talks on the Red Cross to anyone who would listen. Small groups came to evening soirées and acquaintances were stopped on the street, regaled with the Red Cross story, and urged to read the literature pressed into their hands. Clara even made a fashionable New Year's Day reception, hosted by her friend John Hitz, the occasion for an impromptu exchange of information about the Red Cross. Old friends passed along the receiving line, complimenting Barton on her many accomplishments, her restored health, and admiring a recently completed portrait; she responded with enthusiastic accounts of her new work. From as many as she could, she elicited promises of support for an American Red Cross.[24]

The response must have been encouraging, for a few days later Clara decided to broach the subject with the president. Through John B. Wolff, a well-respected businessman, she wrangled an interview with Hayes. She arrived at the White House on January 3, a bit nervous and in awe of the formal surroundings and the beautiful, laughing Lucy Hayes. To her relief both the president and first lady welcomed her warmly. Barton noted in her diary that Hayes was "cordial, knew nothing of the nature of the cause I had undertaken to bring to his notice but was willing to learn it."[25] She presented her letter from Moynier, copies of pamphlets sent from Geneva, and the articles of the Geneva Convention, and requested that one brochure, "The History of the Red Cross of Geneva," be published through the government and distributed to the citizens. Hayes made no decisions on these matters but expressed polite interest in the subject and referred her to the State Department. Barton left with the impression that the president was "both astonished and pleased to learn of its existence and principles."[26]

Heartened by the president's apparent interest in the Red Cross, Barton made plans immediately to see the secretary of state, William Evarts. "I hope one week will do all this," she wrote optimistically in her diary.[27] But she was disappointed to learn that he would not see her. Instead, the secretary turned the matter over to his assistant, Frederick W. Seward, who studied it superficially and determined that the position of the United States on the question had already been decided by former secretaries Seward (his father) and Fish. Offended by this curt dismissal, Barton was left to dwell on the power of precedents in the State Department. "This record stands in my way, and the greatest difficulty I shall have to meet, once overcome, will be this previous decision," she told Appia. "If it had never been presented at all, and I had thus no former decision to reverse, I should hope for a comparatively easy task—but *formalities* and *courtesies* stand greatly in the way of reversing or setting aside the decisions of a previous authority, and especially such authority as Genl Grant and his popular sec[y] Mr. Fish."[28] She resented not only what she considered a poor job of initially presenting the treaty to the United States government, but the easy way in which Evarts had ignored the entire concern. "I saw that it was all made to depend on one man and that man regarded it as settled," Barton later wrote indignantly.[29]

Determined to succeed where Bellows had failed, Barton spent several more months in Washington, discussing the Red Cross with senators and congressmen and continuing a series of informal talks on the subject under the sponsorship of John Hitz and his wife. Barton did not hesitate to tap the emotions as well as the logic of those she hoped to convert to the Red Cross cause and recorded one occasion on which cabinet officials were brought to tears by her talk.[30] Neither did she balk at peddling her wartime connections; an important convert, Michigan senator Omar D. Conger, was won to the cause when Barton reminded him that she had saved his brother's life during the Civil War. She made a strong appeal to the pride of the nation's representatives, telling those concerned about America's prestige that it incensed her to think that every "civilized nation on the earth *but ours,* has signed that Convention, or Treaty, we alone, class with the barbarians."[31]

Barton's work produced no startling results—there was no Senate resolution or official encouragement from the president, and no organization was formed—but she slowly gained supporters for the cause. She could not, as she admitted to Edmund Dwight, "work as rapidly in such things as I could once," but she was proud of the steady progress she had made.[32] "I have seen and *seen* people," she told Harriet Austin, complaining of the length of time it took to lure politicians away from anything but the burning issue of whether to set a gold or silver standard for the nation's currency. "I have called meetings of Congressmen. I have talked and they have listened, but if I were to pipe I doubt if they would dance unless perchance it were to the jingle of 'Silver.'"[33] By March she was rapidly tiring and felt she could make no further headway during that session. Faced with discouragement and possible illness if she stayed, Barton decided to bide her time, go home, and for the time being let "better persons run the world."[34]

Barton returned to Dansville the first week in April. She had stayed in the capital twice as long as she had intended; tired out and depressed by the many weeks of lobbying, she was badly in need of a diversion. Several recuperating friends and relatives had arrived to rest and soak up sunshine in the pleasant country-side, and Minna Kupfer and Fanny Atwater were again installed as housekeep-ers. But the house party proved to be less harmonious than Clara would have wished. She enjoyed the company of Hannah Shepard, an ailing newspaper-woman whom she had met years earlier in London and who had joined the household the previous year, but the nervous "Shepardess" became a financial burden since she increasingly relied on Barton for loans of money. Poor nephew Sam arrived on the verge of emotional collapse, with his son, a ghastly skeleton of a child, who suffered from epilepsy, and was wasted by the morphine pre-scribed to him.[35] After a week it became clear that Ira would need almost con-tinual nursing, for the result of negligence was a dreadful fit. "I am glad the poor little fellow is here, it is his *last* chance I know," Clara wrote bravely. "I am glad to give it to him but it takes the *Ease* all out of our home, henceforth we are *all watchers*. I know it is all I am equal to, but it is well done."[36] By late June, Barton had given up her own bed to yet another invalid, a Mrs. Melcher, who like the others suffered from a nervous condition. Far from being grateful for Barton's hos-pitality, Melcher joined Ira in sulking or exploded in bouts of hysterical rage.[37]

In such an atmosphere Barton found her own nerves giving way, and at the end of July she accepted a long-standing invitation to stay with her old mentor, Frances Gage, at her home in Vineland, New Jersey. Gage was now an invalid, having suffered a stroke that partly paralyzed her. Clara found Aunt Fanny "ill at ease with herself, dissatisfied," and though well looked after, disposed to feel ne-glected and useless.[38] The visit saddened Barton, who felt keenly the contrast between the vigorous woman she had tried to emulate and the shrunken, frail, and embittered being imprisoned in the house in Vineland. For Clara it was hardly an escape from the clamoring household in Dansville, but to Gage the visit was like a gust of fresh air wafting suddenly into her stifling room. "Some-times Clara do you even guess how precious you made that visit to me last sum-mer was," she wrote a few months after Barton left. "How all my life long, I shall live it over & over again—and how I long to see you suceed [*sic*] in that Humani-tarian effort which I know is engrossing your mind & energies."[39]

From Vineland Barton traveled to her former home in Hightstown for a long stay with the Nortons. This visit proved more recreational. Clara rode horseback for the first time in years, a ride she "endured & enjoyed," and sat on the shady porch talking of feminism, religion, and politics with Mary. Her recollection of those pleasant weeks was one of good conversation and a "peaceful lovely home."[40] Nearly a year later, when the strain of demanding houseguests and frus-trations of Red Cross work had taken their toll, Barton would tell Mary Norton that in that year "the last comfortable week I have known was when I was at Hightstown."[41]

As Gage suggested Barton had hardly forgotten about the Red Cross during these difficult months, but with the official doors firmly closed she was uncertain how to proceed. In early October she made a rapid trip to New Haven, Connecticut, to consult with her old friends Joseph and Abby Sheldon about the best way to promote the treaty. Once there she alternated between full workdays and the pleasure of sitting on Abby's bed gossiping and sewing as they had as school-mates. Joseph helped her complete a pamphlet entitled "The Red Cross of the Geneva Convention: What It is."[42] The leaflet gave a brief history of the international organization and stressed that the Geneva Convention was not a society but an international treaty with articles that legally bound the signatory nations. It also contained a paragraph that would have important consequences for the International Red Cross. In it Barton simply wrote that in addition to its wartime responsibilities "it may be further made a part of the *raison d'être* of these national relief societies to afford ready succor and assistance to sufferers in time of national or widespread calamities, such as plagues, cholera, yellow fever and the like, devastating fires or floods, railway disasters, mining catastrophes, etc."[43]

This concept of peacetime work in disaster relief was not entirely original to Barton. Henri Dunant, the originator of the movement, had in fact suggested it in *Un Souvenir de Solferino.*[44] But it was Barton who from this time promoted and expanded the idea of Red Cross disaster relief. Convinced that without an immediate practical application the Red Cross would never succeed in America, she began to portray the treaty as something more than a guarantee of neutrality for volunteers and supplies in wartime; it was an organization that would rescue ordinary citizens from crippling natural and man-made catastrophes. As early as September 1878, when an epidemic of yellow fever broke out in the Mississippi Valley, Barton was publicly lamenting the refusal of the government to sign the treaty, for she believed the infected region would have been an excellent proving ground for an American Red Cross.[45]

Bolstered by this new approach and a strengthened conviction that accession to the Treaty of Geneva concerned "if not our safety, at least our honor," Barton decided to try again to summon some interest in Washington.[46] She was there by mid-December, hoping to promote her cause in the Congress when it reconvened in January. But the trip proved to be short-lived and disappointing. She cajoled the president into writing a letter to the secretary of state, introducing her and asking him to "give her a hearing and such encouragement and aid as may be deemed by you fit." Despite this, and similiar backing from Attorney General Charles Devin, Evarts still refused to see her.[47] "I had nothing to hope for then," Barton later recalled, "but did not press the matter for a third refusal. It waited and so did I."[48] For a short time her hopes were rekindled when the House of Representatives and the Senate jointly proposed a resolution directing the president to "make formal and official recognition of the Geneva Convention as asked by Miss Clara Barton." Unfortunately, however, the resolution was referred to the Committee on Military Affairs, and after a few weeks it died.

Unhappy, and concerned about the expense her project was incurring, she made the tiring return trip to Dansville.[49]

Her failure with the Hayes administration caused Barton to debate whether or not she should continue the promotion of the Red Cross. "Sometimes I fancy it is better to let it go, keep to my present bounds and not extend my labors, or cares beyond my own *personal* limit," she told Mary Norton. She saw little benefit from pushing the treaty in Washington as long as the same men remained in power. After considering an alternate plan to promote the Red Cross with the governors of nearby states, who could exert their own influence in Washington, she admitted this would require "travelling, absence from home, the using up of vital power and the disbursement of private means "—factors that added to her ambivalence.[50] At length she decided to concentrate on making the work of the Red Cross known to the general public, for if public pressure grew strong enough the government would have to respond.

The work of publicizing the Red Cross was done, on the whole, from Barton's new home in Dansville, which she described as a "fine old place with a well-furnished house of twelve rooms, large gardens and an acre of entire fruit, from the small summer berries to the apple, peach, cherry, plums, pears and grapes." In addition, the property boasted stables, proximity to the town and sanitarium, and lovely views of the surrounding mountains and rivers.[51] Although she owned a house in Washington, in many ways this was the only real home Clara had lived in since her childhood, and for once she could arrange things to suit herself, relieved as she was from the pressures of being a guest or traveling constantly. After six months of enthusiastic domestic activity she told a niece that no one could have predicted how much she would love it. She planted a huge vegetable garden and enjoyed putting up the produce, making pies and jams, and keeping her cellar well filled. She acquired Tommy, a black and white kitten who became "pretty much the master of the house" and was shamelessly indulged; he ate raw steak for breakfast and "real *tea* with a *little sugar,* and a *good* deal of milk, and a *small plate* of *crackers*" in the afternoon.[52] In short, a visitor wrote, her house was "filled with almost everything that adds to health, comfort, and happiness."[53]

Clara had no desire to enjoy these surroundings alone. Minna Kupfer and Fanny Atwater continued to live with her. Hannah Shepard was virtually always there, and occasionally Barton took in a boarder. Sam and Ira had left, though the little boy's condition was no better, a situation that caused Clara some discomfort, but she urged others to take their places. Her brother David, whom she had been inviting since 1877, finally came to stay in 1880; he pronounced the house a "mansion" and declared that his youngest sister was "very attentive to me."[54] Clara was fond of reading literature and poetry aloud, and neighbors, especially children, were welcome to come and listen. "I have wished that I could run over to Miss Barton's and sit by the kitchen stove in the twiylight [sic]," recalled one young woman, who especially treasured "the memory of those evenings when we used to fill your cozy rooms and listen to your readings."[55] Patients from the sanitarium, Austin, and other staff members were frequent guests. Prominent townspeople coveted her invitations. Wrote newspaper editor A. O. Bunnell: "an evening spent with Miss Barton is a rich intellectual feast."[56]

None of the visitors left without hearing of the Red Cross and having a little brochure given to them at the door. Those who knew Barton at this time liked to recall her in her "commodious, pictoral study" writing persuasive letters or reworking speeches.[57] She drafted a new lecture on her role in the Franco-Prussian War; she dreaded delivering it, but welcomed the opportunity it afforded to speak of the Geneva Convention.[58] And she tried to give everyone with whom she came into contact a basic understanding of the organization. An enormous undertaking, it was sometimes delegated to those living with her. Even children were pressed into service. A niece, Myrtis Barton, who was staying with Clara at this time, remembered hearing the Red Cross speech so often that she memorized it. "I drank in every word . . . ," Myrtis wrote; "when she found how thoroughly I had learned my lesson, there were occasions when she was so pressed with work that she could not see every caller, and I was delegated to receive them and tell them the story they wanted to hear. I remember so plainly how she shook hands with some callers, and then had to excuse herself to get back to her desk, saying she left them to the care of her little niece."[59]

Among the groups Barton entertained or addressed was the faculty and students of the Dansville Seminary, a private school with classrooms near her home. It was through this institution that Clara met the man who would come to be her most loyal supporter. Julian Hubbell, a small, shy man with eyes like a frightened deer, was a science instructor and co-principal at the seminary. As a boy in Iowa he had idolized the legendary Clara Barton, and it was with great excitement that he discovered she was a neighbor when he moved to Dansville in 1876. Hubbell relished the literary evenings at Barton's home and was an early convert to the cause of the Red Cross. He enthusiastically built a tin can telephone between Barton's office and his seminary room and begged his heroine to let him help her with her work. After some consideration she told him that she needed the help of a physician (an idea proposed by Louis Appia), and if he wanted truly to aid her in the Red Cross he should get a medical degree. Anxious to please, the young man began studies with a local doctor and later enrolled in the medical school of the University of Michigan.[60]

That Hubbell was willing to suddenly change careers is indicative of both Barton's persuasive nature and his own evident need to subordinate himself to a stronger personality. Just as she needed to command, Hubbell looked to her to define his life. With a childlike dependence he called her "Mamie"—and referred to himself, usually in the third person, as "her boy." In Barton's service he found a way to fulfill his desire to help humanity without calling attention to himself, a role that suited them both admirably. Throughout Barton's long Red Cross career he worked loyally, and apparently ably, at her side. Yet he never challenged her authority or questioned her policies. He seems, in fact, to have been extremely uncomfortable whenever she approached him for suggestions. "Mamie must not estimate his ability to help her as high, he does not want her to, he is afraid he will be the cause of her making mistakes . . . ," Hubbell once told her; "he wants M. to always consider his suggestions as no more than a child's, and never to act upon *any* of them until they have passed her careful judgement."[61] He followed Barton with devotion and in every way gave his life to her. For Clara's part, she appears to have been fond of Hubbell, but she very quickly took him for granted. Rarely is he mentioned in her letters or diary, and he became neither a significant intellectual companion nor a confidante.

During the years in Dansville Barton took time to reestablish her ties with several feminist organizations. Under the influence of Harriet Austin, her interest in their work, which had lain dormant during her illness, again was aroused. Her proximity to New York City and Rochester, where a number of the leaders had headquarters, made her more accessible, and she was continually called on to speak at conventions, write endorsements, or donate money. Before Barton committed herself to the Red Cross, Susan B. Anthony had, in fact, hoped to persuade her to make women's rights her new crusade. "I am so glad you are gaining strength," Anthony wrote in September 1876, "& hope you may yet like to do as much for women's emancipation as you did for the slaves & the soldiers—How gloriously our movement would go on, if it had the like of your hand, brain & heart to organize, systematize, vitalize & marshall its forces—do get well, my dear, & come to the help of the weary & worn in the service of woman."[62] Even after it became clear that her time was taken up by the Red Cross, suffragists clamored for Barton's help. "Give Washington and the Red Cross a month's vacation, if need be," pleaded the secretary of the New York Woman Suffrage Association. "You can work all the better when you are enfranchised."[63]

Busy as she was between the years 1876 and 1882, Barton accepted many of these invitations. She contributed letters and articles to a number of feminist publications, enthusiastically subscribed to *The Woman's Journal,* and publicly endorsed the work of the suffragists whenever possible. Barton, with Hannah Shepard, attended the National Suffrage Convention of 1878 in Washington, D.C. (though she had a "miserable seat" in the back of the room, she was recognized and brought to the platform amid cheers).[64] On Decoration Day, 1879, she added a staunchly feminist paragraph to her praise of the nation's soldiers. "American women: how proud I am of you; how proud I have always been since those days to have been a woman," she declared. "Abraham Lincoln said that without the help of women the rebellion could not have been put down, nor the country saved. Since that time I have counted all women citizens."[65] (The next year, having been honored by the privilege—unheard of for a woman—of reading the Declaration of Independence at the Dansville Fourth of July celebration, Clara sat and fumed while the keynote speaker railed against woman suffrage for forty-five minutes, ending with the proclamation that women should keep to "the sphere to which nature and nature's God has assigned them.")[66]

Despite her many feminist activities and the pressure to participate even more, Barton held herself aloof from a leadership role with the suffragists. As she had in the late 1860s, she wished to keep her own counsel rather than adhere to the political aspirations of any one group. Once she was committed to the promotion of the Red Cross, she also became sensitive to the dangers of having that organization indelibly connected with the women's rights movement. Determined to have the politicians in Washington assess her proposals without prejudice, she hesitated to link her name too prominently to a cause that was unpopular with congressional and administration leaders. Her own interests also leaned more toward practical, social benefits for women, rather than the ability to vote. Thus she applauded the acquaintance who undertook to run a farm by herself ("she *farms*, she doesn't *play* at it, it is *her* hands that go into the dirt") and went to a great deal of trouble to encourage young women to pursue professional careers.[67] Nonetheless, many feminist leaders were disgruntled that she did not make suffrage work a priority, and a few, among them Lucy Stone, even questioned the sincerity of her commitment. To such women, Barton replied with firm (and quotable) statements. "And you modestly ask 'if I am so much interested in the cause as to come,'" Barton replied to Stone. "I did not suppose that to be a matter of doubt. If on the occasion to which you so kindly invite me, there shall be in your assemblage one woman who doubts this, say to her for me, . . . Sister you do not know me."[68]

Though determined not to align herself too closely with the feminists, Barton did go to considerable lengths to court favor with organizations she thought could help her and the Red Cross. One of the most useful allies she cultivated was the Associated Press. The AP began in 1847 as a loose union of telegraph operators who had organized to transmit news by the recently invented wire system. Originally it was conceived as a simple agreement to share the expense of newsgathering. As the one unified news agency in the country, with a vast network of contacts and a wide readership, it had become immensely powerful. By the late 1870s the AP had a large staff of reporters, numerous regional bureaus, its own system of telegraph operations, and subscribers in more than 350 cities.[69]

The Washington AP office was run by Walter Phillips, a dynamic young man who had invented a telegraphic code that facilitated sending pre-edited news copy to the member papers. A creative and likable person, with an eye for human interest stories, Phillips also had a strong personal commitment to philanthropy. Barton met Phillips and his assistant, travel journalist George Kennan, during her lobbying work with the Hayes administration. Since her days of working with the Union army's missing men, Barton had had a shrewd understanding of just how crucial effective publicity could be; she also saw that the power wielded by the third estate had, if anything, increased since the Civil War. To her satisfaction, Phillips and Kennan were easily persuaded of the importance of the Red Cross, and they began to actively publicize Barton's efforts. Both journalists would become charter members of the American Red Cross, and their influence helped give Barton the benefit of a remarkably favorable press. Indeed, Barton once remarked that during this period the press never issued "a word of blame, never a criticism from those whose right and whose business it is to discriminate and criticize if need be; but always the gentle, aye, tender respect that a sister might look for at the hands of noble, proud and loving brothers." [70]

Barton also cultivated the acquaintance of reporters not connected with the Associated Press. In Dansville, A. O. Bunnell of the *Dansville Advertiser* became a valued ally. She helped a number of young women with journalistic aspirations, including Hannah Shepard, who wrote under the name "Buckeye" for several newspapers. The reward was a bevy of articles that promoted her and her cause. A piece in the *Providence Daily Journal,* for example, admonished the State Department to sign the Red Cross treaty for the memory of Miss Barton's work in the Civil War, if not for its own merit. "Let not our own Florence Nightingale have continued reason to feel that a republic is less grateful and less sympathetic than a monarchy," the author concluded. [71] Anxious to keep the favorable reports coming, Barton fed information to reporters and flattered them whenever she could. During the summer of 1879 she attended a convention of the New York Press Association, where she made important contacts and gave a gracious toast calculated to include the press in her campaign for ratification. "And how shall I reach [the government] or the people at large, but through the great national leaders and teachers?" she asked the assembled banquet guests. "And at last they sit before me here tonight in hundreds, aye, thousands and listen to my poor words. Their quick intelligence will take the subject in, they are wise and will judge it well; they are powerful and will speak in their own good time." [72]

Of equal importance was Barton's association with the Grand Army of the Republic. The GAR was an association of Union army veterans that had been founded in Illinois soon after the end of the Civil War. Originally meant as a friendly club of former soldiers, it grew with great rapidity to include branches in virtually every county of the northern states. As early as August 27, 1865, the *Chicago Tribune* stated that the "Grand Army organization is very strong . . . having drawn to its ranks almost every discharged soldier in the country and now holds the balance of power." [73] Many of the members had joined more for the influence the GAR enjoyed than for the camaraderie it offered, for the frankly political organization was staunchly Republican in sentiment. In every election since 1866 the veterans had used their collective votes to ensure the victory of their chosen candidates. Not overly pleased with the administration of Rutherford B. Hayes, the members of the GAR took an early interest in the candidates for election in 1880. [74]

From the beginning Barton had enjoyed a special relationship with the GAR. It was composed, after all, of her "boys," and they recognized her as the ultimate heroine, who had braved bullets and gossip to aid them during the war. She was made an honorary comrade of the local GAR post in Worcester and was a valued member of the female auxiliary of the organization, known as the Women's Relief Corps. In Dansville the local chapter renamed itself the "Clara Barton Post" after she moved there. Constantly sought after as a speaker at reunions, picnics, and Memorial Day festivities, she tried to attend as many as she could and sent poems or little greetings to those she refused. One ex-soldier wrote that her attendance at the annual encampment of the Twenty-First Massachusetts Volunteers was so valued that the "inquiry at every reunion is where is Miss Barton— or before each as you meet comrades, 'Will Miss Barton be there?'"[75] Barton, of course, returned the compliment: "They know that my highest respect and my deepest devotion are theirs—that I am with them, as in the days of old and that the most kindly honor they can bestow upon me, is . . . to recognize me as a comrade who shared their perils, their hardships, and their dangers, and would now share their confidence, and live a little in their memories."[76]

After 1878 Barton began to use her contacts with the veterans to foster support for the Treaty of Geneva. Through the GAR she met John Logan, a former brigadier general with the Army of the Tennessee. An initial organizer of the GAR, Logan had served three times as its president; in 1879 he was a powerful figure in the Senate. His support was crucial if the veterans were to endorse the concept of an American Red Cross. Barton's earnest manner of speaking and prestige with the veterans persuaded Logan (and his active wife, Mary) to rally to her support, and as a result both Logans did early and important work publicizing the Red Cross. Other prominent veterans followed the Logans' example, among them Congressman R. D. Mussey and General Phil Sheridan. Barton made numerous speeches to the troops, all of which connected adherence to the Treaty of Geneva with the GAR mandate to guard the liberties of the country. She also took leaflets with her to every rally and reunion. In the spring of 1881, the Dansville chapter passed a resolution that the GAR "urge its consideration upon congress, to the end that the United States, by its official action, may aid in promoting this great charity." The following June, at a nationwide encampment in Indianapolis, the same resolutions were passed by the national association.[77]

Hoping to enhance this backing with direct political campaigning, Barton joined the veterans in their support of James A. Garfield, the Republican presidential candidate. Garfield, a brilliant, ambitious man who had worked his way up from poverty by driving mules along the canals of Ohio, was ideal from Barton's point of view: not only was he a veteran general, but he was known for both his support of Christian charities and his inability to say no to a worthwhile cause. In an evening parade, given in Dansville a few weeks before the 1880 election, Barton marched with the soldiers, then spoke to them from a balcony, amidst the smoky glow of torchlights. In an opening typical of the many speeches she gave to veterans, she told the men that she was flattered by their demand that she speak, that she stood with them as she had in 1861, and that she charged them to "defend by your votes what you saved by your arms." She then strongly endorsed Garfield, calling him a "statesman, a scholar, a true-hearted honorable man."[78] With the veterans, of course, she was pushing on an open door, and it is not surprising that that night her speech was greeted with resounding cheers. But Barton shrewdly maximized the effect of the speech by enclosing a copy in a fawning letter of congratulation, written to Garfield after his successful election. Afraid to ask directly for an audience to discuss the Red Cross, Barton protested that her missive was "objectless." But when Garfield replied with a brief, courteous letter, the stage was set for a renewed effort in Washington.[79]

Barton called on President Garfield soon after his inauguration. Once more she carried the letter from Gustave Moynier that implored the United States to sign the Treaty of Geneva; once more she told the long story of the International Red Cross. The president received her cordially and, whether motivated by her campaigning or by a sincere interest in the subject, promised to give her as much help as possible. Like his predecessors, he referred her to the State Department, but this time with the pledge of a genuine hearing. He advised her to deliver Moynier's letter in person to the secretary of state, and to it he attached a brief note: "Will the Sec'y of State please hear Miss Barton on the subject herein referred to?"[80]

Barton kept her appointment with the new secretary, James G. Blaine, a few days later. She was accompanied by her nephew Stephen E. Barton, called Stevé, an earnest young businessman with whom she had developed a new plan of publicizing the Red Cross. When, on their arrival at the State Department, Blaine kept them waiting for over an hour, her heart began to sink; it was all too reminiscent of the indifferent treatment she had been given three years earlier. As it happened, Barton's fears were unnecessary, for Blaine's personality and foreign policy were far different from those of his cautious predecessors. He was a man of stature and a popular and forceful speaker with magnetic charm. Not only ambitious for himself but for his country, he saw foreign policy as the key to reshaping America's role in the world. Unlike Seward, Fish, and Evarts, Blaine believed that American foreign relations should be fluid, able to adapt to new conditions, not merely fixed to old credos such as the Monroe Doctrine. During his tenure under Garfield, and later under Benjamin Harrison, Secretary Blaine would ease the United States out of its long policy of isolationism. He promoted better ties in the Western Hemisphere by creating the Pan-American Union, and he convinced the Senate to ratify treaties of agreement on international copyright laws and the suppression of the slave trade. Far from viewing the Treaty of Geneva as a threat to America, he welcomed the strengthened relations it would provide with the member nations.[81]

Blaine listened intelligently to Barton's explanation of her mission, delivered, according to Stevé, in "very fine and pleasant style." He asked a number of questions, requested a copy of her brochure, and spent some time discussing which method would have to be followed to win approval of the treaty—he believed that it would be necessary for both the Senate and the War Department to concur. Blaine advised Barton to call on Robert Lincoln, the secretary of war, as soon as possible and promised to "cooperate fully with her in carrying the matter successfully through." To Stevé and Clara's delight, he assured them that he was "in full sympathy with it," and that "if it needed the action of the Senate that would be had." "The Monroe Doctrine," Blaine concluded, "was not meant to ward off humanity."[82]

The following day Barton and her nephew went to the War Department to see the secretary. When they arrived they found that he had already gone, but in a subsequent interview he listened patiently to their speech. Unabashed at playing on people's emotions when she thought it would be to her benefit, and adroit at shedding tears for dramatic effect, Clara told Lincoln that the real reason she had requested the interview was to thank him for the help his famous father had given her. Though she had met Abraham Lincoln only a few times (and then briefly), Barton told his son that she "knew President Lincoln well," and that he had always aided her with great kindness. "I felt my tears flowing before I had finished," Barton recalled, " and was ashamed that I had failed to control them, but when I glanced up at the Secretary I saw he was weeping too." (Barton still does not appear to have found this oldest of feminine wiles at odds with her public statements about the country's need for strong, courageous women; instead she gloated over the success of her crocodile tears, just as she had when similar techniques had softened up the generals in 1862.) A sympathetic tie established, Lincoln assured Barton that he would support the Red Cross if Blaine recommended it.[83]

These interviews, and similar successes with Treasury secretary William Windham and several prominent congressional leaders, gave the Bartons increasing reason for optimism. "She is sailing into Presidents, cabinets, Senators & Representatives," Stevé wrote gaily, "with her 'Cross' in one hand & I am pleased to state that her efforts are telling and the prospect of pleasing results is very encouraging."[84] Clara's friends wrote to give further encouragement: "We all felt like hurrahing when I read . . . the report of how you are carrying all before you," Harriet Austin exclaimed. "That is to say, of the fact that men of power and place are interesting themselves in your mission, and we are hoping for the complete success of your efforts."[85] Even usually pessimistic Clara was emboldened by the assurances of the Garfield administration to write a tentative victory letter to the International Committee in Geneva. "After all these years of writing, hoping, and waiting," she told them, "I want to give you and your noble society the first word of hope."[86] Indeed, it seemed as if nothing could go wrong that spring. Upon receipt of Barton's note, Moynier wrote a letter to Blaine renewing the official request for the United States to sign the Treaty of Geneva. A few weeks later, he received as answer a letter that confirmed the secretary of state's commitment to achieving that goal. Moreover, the Senate sent a formal order to Blaine requesting him to forward documents pertaining to the treaty for their consideration.[87]

With success in sight Barton made plans to establish an American branch of the International Red Cross. It was a practical move, for it was necessary to have a body to handle business matters once the treaty was signed. It would also, Barton believed, serve the purpose of keeping the movement visible until the administration took action. Until this point, she had always heeded the counsel of men like Samuel Ramsey, who advised her to concentrate on securing treaty ratification; once it was signed she could worry about establishing a national association. But she now believed that the cause should be shown to have more than one supporter, and she personally felt the need for additional advice and aid. She therefore called a meeting of those who had shown particular interest in the Red Cross. On May 12, 1881, the small group met at the home of Senator Omar D. Conger.[88]

Once more Barton explained the purpose of the Red Cross and the possibilities a national association would offer, adding that she badly needed help to continue the work. But though her listeners heartily supported the idea of an American Red Cross, this and a subsequent meeting proved inconclusive. On May 21, however, Barton made a third appeal to the group to formally begin a Red Cross organization. A woman who was present on this day recalled that all of the chairs in the room were pushed against the wall, and that the meeting was presided over by Judge William Lawrence. Barton, serene and stately, stood at one end of the room. Summoning all of her considerable theatrical power, she regaled them with stories of the horror of war, of the terrible numbers who died on the battlefield from neglect or the lack of supplies. At the end of the speech she implored them to come to her assistance, saying that she was discouraged and did not know whether or not she could keep up with the work. "I want every one of you to get up in turn and say what I shall do," she declared, vowing to drop the work if they did not support her. The first person said, "Go on with the work"; each one in the room followed suit. "Then and there," wrote one who was present, "we took an oath of allegiance to the Red Cross, and we pledged ourselves to see that the work was carried through."[89]

Twenty-two people became charter members of the American Red Cross that night. They were a diverse group, ranging from prominent politicians to old personal friends of Barton. Besides Kennan and Phillips, a number of newspapermen signed the charter, among them Richard J. Hinton, a renowned author of literature on the far west. Charles Upton, Joseph Holmes, and John Hitz were influential men with European connections. Judge William Lawrence and Adolphus S. Solomons, a well-respected businessman and philanthropist, were both important figures in Washington, D.C. Conspicuously absent, however, were any society figures or old established families. Barton, who always referred to her own background as "humble," felt uncomfortable in such circles, though she recognized the benefits well-connected men and women could bring to an organization. It was significant that at a time when the wealthy had a growing interest in philanthropy, none of the charter members of the Red Cross was listed in Washington's Blue Book; Barton never attracted this element of society to her cause.

The constitution that the charter members adopted and signed for the American Association of the Red Cross on May 21 reflected goals that were much the same as those espoused by the American Association for Relief of Misery of the Battlefield fifteen years earlier: to secure adoption of the Treaty of Geneva in the United States; to gain official recognition of the new society by the United States government; to organize a national system of relief; and to cooperate with other national Red Cross societies. The group met again a few weeks later, at which time Barton was elected president, with Judge Lawrence as vice-president, Solomons as treasurer, and Kennan as secretary.[90] When Blaine assured Barton that he welcomed the news of the organization's founding, the future of the American Red Cross seemed assured.

A few weeks later, however, President Garfield was shot by a disappointed office seeker. Throughout the summer he hovered between life and death, and the activities of the administration came to a halt while officials waited to see whether or not he would be succeeded by Vice-President Chester A. Arthur. A tragedy for the country, Garfield's assassination was a personal disaster for Barton. Not only was action on the Treaty of Geneva postponed, but Barton was uncertain whether Arthur would be in favor of ratification, or even if he would retain her mentor, Secretary Blaine. Not until September, when Garfield died, did she learn the unsettling news that Blaine would only stay on until December.[91]

As if these uncertainties were not enough, a number of small problems rankled Barton during the summer of 1881. As soon as word of the new organization was made public, she was besieged by letters from citizens who requested membership, asked to work as agents for the group, or solicited aid for their own relief societies. Barton had not expected the onslaught of mail and was ill-equipped to handle it.[92] The incorporation of the association was also a problem. Clara, and a number of other Red Cross members, hoped to get a congressional charter for the group when the treaty was passed; such a charter would give the organization official recognition and quasi-governmental status. In her euphoria over the favorable events of the spring, Barton even believed that Congress would appropriate working funds for the association—perhaps as much as 1.5 percent of the War Department budget.[93] But William Lawrence and a number of others were anxious to keep the association on a more private scale, incorporated in the District of Columbia and using government influence only to gain impressive figureheads for the group. Barton disapproved of the idea and was dismayed by this, the first challenge to her authority. In the end a compromise was reached: the association would temporarily incorporate in Washington, D.C., until congressional action was secured, and the president would serve as the head of a board of consultation, made up of both Red Cross members and people influential in government and business.[94] Hardly was this situation resolved, however, when still another problem arose. Since the original signing of the Geneva Convention, several articles dealing with naval warfare had been passed but not ratified by all of the member countries. Secretary Blaine, surveying the original treaty and the new articles, became confused, and when he questioned Barton, she was forced to admit that she did not know exactly which documents the Senate needed to ratify. With apology she wrote to Moynier asking for specific instructions about which articles to sign. Finally Moynier replied, stating that the United States need only sign the initial accords since the others had not yet been officially adopted.[95]

Barton was also troubled that summer by the growth of a number of rival groups. She had not foreseen this effect of her far-reaching publicity campaign and was now puzzled and hurt to find that she had competitors who also wished to head the new American Red Cross. One, named James Saunders, had founded an organization called the "Order of the Red Cross," which he claimed had more than two thousand members. In the summer of 1881 he had begun to publish a newsletter called the *Journal of the Red Cross,* in which he asserted that since his order had been in existence since 1879 it was a little late for Barton, or anyone else, to be talking about organizing a Red Cross. Saunders's journal, and apparently his organization, died rather quickly and quietly, but while they existed they greatly alarmed Barton.[96]

Far more serious was the formation, the same year, of the Women's National Relief Association, which came to be called the Blue Anchor after the badge the group had chosen. These women were concerned with all manner of national and international relief, but their special project was to equip and staff lifesaving stations along the shores of the United States. To Clara's discomfort, they claimed to be seeking American accession to the Treaty of Geneva. What made the Blue Anchor particularly distressing was that it had been started by Hannah Shepard and Fanny Atwater, women who had lived under Barton's roof and partaken of her generosity. Like Anna Zimmerman and so many other Barton worshipers, they had become disillusioned and had left her service with rancor. In the organization's newsletter, *The Alpha,* and elsewhere, Shepard published articles that claimed that if the Blue Anchor desired "to render aid to foreign countries belligerent with each other, it would be entitled to add the ensign of [the Geneva] treaty—the Red Cross—to its own insignia."[97] By the fall of 1881 the Blue Anchor was claiming to have outfitted fifty lifesaving stations and was forming a number of national relief auxiliaries. Worse yet, Shepard had managed to attract the support of both the press and the wives of prominent men, among them the first lady. As if this were not enough, Shepard began to contest the legitimacy of

Barton's organization. "The 'Women's National Relief Association' does not ask Congressional aid," ran one pointed comment. "It is an association of women, not an association for *one* woman. It has the claim on the people of *priority*, of successful accomplishment, of having in its membership, not one alone, but many of the blessed Florence Nightingales who served our wounded soldiers in the war." [98]

Shepard's papers do not give any clues to the reason for her disaffection, but Barton's personal hurt at these actions was acute. Hers was not a nature to welcome the advent of a group with similar goals, and Shepard's malice made it all the more difficult to cooperate. She feared that the Senate, as yet undecided on the question of the Red Cross treaty, would be swayed by the prominent names in the Blue Anchor to recognize it as the international body's official representative in America. Barton characteristically exaggerated the threat, allowing Shepard and her compatriots to rob her of sleep and make her feel persecuted and alone. Despite the assurances of Gustave Moynier and the secretary of state that their confidence was firmly placed in her and her organization, she believed Shepard's group would prevail in the end. Moreover, she came to resent the lack of concern felt by other members of the new American Red Cross and wrote in despair: "All are busy; and I am to go on with this alone, as I plainly see. . . . I do not believe any member of my Society will be of any help to me in this hard work. They are all too busy." [99]

Barton had few defenses against Shepard's attacks but to cultivate her own influential contacts and to enlarge her organization in size and purposefulness. Upon returning to Dansville in July, she took steps to attain that end. On August 22, 1881, she, along with Jackson, Austin, and other town leaders, started the first local auxiliary of the Red Cross. A loosely structured body, with annual dues of twenty-five cents, it was heralded as a "Move in the Right Direction" in the *Dansville Advertiser*. A few weeks later another chapter opened in Rochester, New York, with the help of Susan B. Anthony, who viewed it as an opportunity to get women involved in a potentially powerful organization. Similar local groups opened in Syracuse and Onondaga County, New York, during the next few months. [100]

Then, in mid-September, a disaster gave the Red Cross occasion to test the strength of its good intentions. A forest fire, the result of drought, several weeks of hot southwest winds, and the carelessness of settlers, blazed across the thumb of Michigan, causing extensive property damage and the loss of nearly five hundred lives. Great winds whipped the fire out of control—it was said that the heat could be felt some seven miles offshore on Lake Huron. Soon after she heard of the calamity, Barton sent out a broadside asking for donations of clothing, food, household articles, and money, stating that the organizing group would be the Dansville society. She was full of sympathy for the sufferers but also well aware of the opportunity this meant for her burgeoning organization. "Nothing could give our association more standing and popularity," she told Judge Lawrence, "than to issue a call upon its local societies to aid in the present emergency."[101]

Late in September Barton opened workrooms, established to solicit, sort, and crate donations for the sufferers in Michigan. After collecting twenty-five hundred dollars from the Rochester Red Cross, and more than thirty-eight hundred dollars from the Dansville chapter, as well as countless boxes of clothing, tools, and bedding, Barton dispatched Mark Bunnell, son of the Dansville newspaper editor, to Michigan to oversee the distribution. He joined Julian Hubbell, now a student at the University of Michigan, who was already near the scene of the disaster. Barton continued to solicit contributions, using the meetings to increase Red Cross membership as well as to plead for the victims of the fires. Americans had always given in a generous and neighborly way in times of trouble, she said, "but their gifts were irresponsibly received, and not infrequently wasted disgracefully or misappropriated before the suffering had been alleviated. Hence the necessity of such a systematic and reliable organization as that of the Red Cross society."[102] All of these activities—speeches, broadsides, and delegation of relief agents—were done without the consent, or even consultation, of the executive board of the Red Cross—the ominous beginning of an unfortunate pattern in Barton's administration. Hoping to soothe the ruffled feelings of officials who had not even been informed of her intentions, Barton wrote a hasty letter of apology, requesting their indulgence and defending herself with the not-too-convincing words, "I could scarce do otherwise than I did."[103]

In Michigan Hubbell and Bunnell surveyed the damage and found that there had been little exaggeration either in official reports or in the press. "Have seen much that I would not have credited had it been told me before visiting the place," Hubbell told Clara. Crops, houses, animals, even deed books and personal papers, had been destroyed. Housing, beds, and bedding were most needed, Hubbell believed, and after this cash to finance the rebuilding of farms. He and Bunnell were canvassing the area, trying to help the neediest victims first.[104]

Though Barton wrote a lengthy and dramatic account of Red Cross activity in Michigan, lauding the "help and strength of our organization, young and untried as it was," it is clear that their efforts there were minor.[105] The contributions from specific localities were generous, but they were hardly enough to completely reestablish fifteen hundred destitute families. Furthermore, Bunnell and Hubbell found that local Michigan philanthropists were not only equally forthcoming with contributions but well-organized in their distribution. "Major Bunnell has come in from the burnt district," Hubbell reported to Barton. "He is well pleased with the manner of work and says that it is so well organized that it would not be well to interfere."[106] Indeed, the local committees were competing with each other for dominance in the field; the dissension became so uncomfortable that the governor of Michigan had to appoint a formal committee through which all distributions would be made.[107] When Barton protested that the Red Cross was not getting enough publicity and recognition, Hubbell forestalled her by stressing that the dissension had only pointed up the need for a permanent organization to take over all such philanthropic work. In the end Barton had to be satisfied that the Red Cross had been one of many organizations to take a small role in the Michigan relief.[108]

Despite her success with the local societies and the modest achievements in Michigan, it was a painfully depressing autumn for Barton. She watched nervously as Chester A. Arthur, whose views on foreign entanglements were unknown and who had few ties to Barton and her supporters, took office. Walker Blaine, the son of the secretary of state, added his name to the executive board of the Blue Anchor, which seemed to be growing in size and influence. Anxious and in need of advice, she went with Joseph Sheldon to call on Henry Bellows, who did what he could to reassure her. Already, he said, she had accomplished what he could not, and despite concerted efforts by Shepard to use him as a figurehead for her group, his confidence was firmly placed in Barton's Red Cross.[109] But she continued to feel alone; Stevé was back at his business, Hubbell in medical school, and no one else seemed willing or able to come to her aid. Even the financial burden still rested with her. "I shall have to put *all* my income, every cent from *every* source into this Treaty business for *this* year," she wrote at year's end, "as I have largely for the last four years, but once it is accomplished I can *hope* for easier times."[110]

A breakthrough finally came in late December, when President Arthur, in his annual message to Congress, unconditionally supported passage of "that humane and commendable engagement," the Treaty of Geneva.[111] Greatly relieved, Barton moved again to Washington, this time with plans to settle permanently. Concerned now that the Senate was the key to acceptance of the treaty, she spent the next two months calling on politicians and securing the help of Alvey A. Adee, the new third assistant secretary of state. With flattery and hard logic Barton gained the promise of Senator Elbridge Lapham of New York to sponsor the bill. She wooed the Massachusetts congressional delegation with an elegant reception, served from a friend's valuable Count de Gras china service. Senator Conger's early support was fortified by the recent work of the Red Cross in his home state, and senators William Windom, George F. Edmunds, John T. Morgan, and George H. Pendleton—all members of the Foreign Relations Committee—seemed to be in accord. More help came from the press. Ben Perly Poore, a popular journalist, promised to secure the aid of several printers he knew; Frank Leslie, editor of one of the period's most influential magazines, wrote a lauditory editorial; Walter Phillips and George Kennan sent out frequent dispatches through the Associated Press. Even Barton's living conditions improved, as she left her cold rooms for the bustling home of the Reverend William Ferguson, a friend from Civil War days and a charter member of the American Red Cross.[112]

If it was a time of promises and expectations, however, it was also one of delay and discouragement. Having finally determined which parts of the treaty needed to be signed, government officials could not agree on the exact process required to ratify the articles. Some believed that the president need only sign it; others thought it required passage by the full Congress. Not until January 31 did the Senate Foreign Relations Committee decide that it was a treaty like any other, requiring only the consent of the Senate and the president's signature.[113] The leaders of the Blue Anchor also kept up a campaign against Barton, harassing her personally and succeeding in disillusioning at least one key senator. Distraught, Barton indulged in self-pity: "I do not care what Mrs. Shepard and Fanny do," she concluded, "if only I am not where I am confronted by them and my life spoiled by them, even they take the joy out of the sunshine for me."[114] On February 6, 1882, her strength ebbing, she knelt by her bed and tearfully prayed for guidance, vowing to lay aside the work as soon as ratification was secured. "I will try with God's help to go on faithfully to the end, with no support but His . . . ," she wrote in her diary. "This has been a day of instruction and discipline, and, I dare hope, not lost."[115]

Three weeks later, still uncertain about the status of the treaty and beginning to wonder "if I am not a crank myself," Barton called on the secretary of state's assistant. To her surprise he handed her a large, soft, unbound book, the official copy of the Treaty of Geneva. "It is not customary at this office to let unsigned papers be seen, but we do not fear to overstep in your case," he tod her. "We *want* you to see if it suits you." As she read over the familiar words, each one so laboriously translated and publicized, Barton realized at last that the treaty was really to be signed, her work of five years completed with success. She handled the soft parchment pages with emotion, tears running down her cheeks. Assured that the treaty would be signed "*any time now*," she hurried to the White House to make sure that when at last it passed the Senate, the president would sign it with dispatch.[116]

In fact, it was to be three more disheartening weeks before Senate ratification was finally achieved. On March 10, Senator Lapham informed her that it had passed the committee and would be sent to the full Senate shortly. Then, on March 16, a day that had been all "tears and sadness" for Barton, came another message from Lapham. "*Laus Deo!*" it read, and Lapham informed her that that day the Senate had unanimously ratified the Treaty of Geneva. Exhausted, emotionally and physically, Barton took only a moment to jot the news in her diary. "*Treaty Ratified,*" she wrote in red at the top of the page, and then added honestly: "So it was done at last and I had waited so long and got so weak and broken I could not even feel glad, but laid down the good letter and wiped my tired head and eyes."[117] Though she hastened to tell Phillips, the American press took only scanty notice of the Senate's action. But that night, as Barton later liked to recall, when the cables she sent to Moynier were received, there were bonfires in Geneva, Berne, and Paris, and the Europeans pierced the night with the cheer, *Vive l' Amerique.*[118]

The ratification of the Treaty of Geneva was an enormous triumph for Clara Barton. She lobbied against a bureaucracy that was convinced any agreement with a foreign nation was not only unnecessary but meant compromising America's autonomy. That she persevered to erode this antiquated opinion was a test of her own determination and tenacity, more so because she worked alone; though she could never believe that "someone would not rise up for its help," no one ever did.[119] She labored in an exclusively male world, among politicians and diplomats who had no reason to even consider receiving a disfranchised female. Yet Barton was received, and listened to, and her treaty was considered—a testament both to the respect she had inspired with her Civil War work and to her self-possession and formidable powers of persuasion. Her success is to be measured not only against the goals of humanitarians—where it stands as a stunning achievement—but also with the work of diplomats, for with the passage of the Treaty of Geneva the United States shed its young timidity and began to define the ideals it held in common with the other nations of the world. The American Red Cross stands, one hundred years later, a monument to Clara Barton's foresight, courage, and perseverance.

thirteen

In the early spring of 1882, amidst piles of telegrams, letters, and cards congratulating her on her unparalleled achievement in bringing the United States into the Red Cross, Clara Barton sat contemplating her future and that of the fledgling society she had formed. Having "worked so hard and done so much for y[our] country, as well as for the benefit of all others," the Grand Duchess Louise had proudly written, "must have given you great happiness."[1] This is hardly how Barton would have characterized her mood. She was only too aware that the struggle to keep alive her ideal had scarcely begun. Financial difficulties, rival societies, an indifferent government, and her own shaky health threatened to turn the signing of the treaty into an empty victory. Too drained financially and emotionally to continue the work, too fearful of failure to quit, she pondered the best course for her future, and that of the American Red Cross.

At sixty Barton was at the height of her personal powers. "If she had belonged to the other sex," Henry Bellows wrote about this time, "she would have been a merchant prince, a great general, or a trusted political leader."[2] Those who described her noted a magnetism in her bearing and a self-possession in her voice that spoke of experience and confidence. "Miss Barton's face shows power," commented a reporter, who went on to mention that "her voice, so low, sweet, yet fine and tensly [sic] toned, has musical timbre in it, which when its possessor is roused can become clear and resonant with deep controlled notes, and tones having marked oratorical effects."[3] The face that had been so homely at eighteen and "full of interest" at forty had now taken on an ageless quality and would change little for the remaining thirty years of Barton's life. Art and nature had combined to ease the lines of time. Her hair was dyed, but arranged in "an old-fashioned way, crimped over her temples." Most people who met her thought that she looked fifty. Even someone as close to her as Elvira Stone was astonished at how little she had changed in middle life and exclaimed, "Does time stand still with you?"[4]

Though the physical changes were minor, in some respects her personality had hardened, sobered, grown more weary with the years. The commanding presence had a harsh, authoritarian tone to it now. Admirers from an earlier time had called her "my precious angel"; now even the most loyal co-workers would refer to her as "the Queen" or the "Great I Am."[5] Though in public she kept her opinions in check, in private she wrote sharp, censorious words about anyone who differed with her. From her own point of view the worst change was her loss of humor: "I am always afraid I am not as jolly as I was thirty years ago," she told a former pupil. "Somehow a *good many things have* happened in the time and some of them with sober natures, that I fear stole a little of the merry ring out of the clear laugh that my *own* ears remember." The cares of her life crowded out the hours of merriment. "I laugh," she concluded, "when I don't forget it and *have* time."[6]

Barton's mature personality was a complex combination of insecurity and forthrightness, rigidity and flexibility, and was frequently at odds with itself. Though possessed of immense personal magnetism—at times an almost charismatic charm—she herself was never convinced of the love or esteem of others and continually sought compliments from friends and praise from the public. She had, however, "a just and accurate estimate of her ability to master a situation," as one friend attested.[7] It was this face of the fearless, self-possessed, rational, and even-tempered leader that she preferred to show the world. Underneath bubbled emotions she found difficult to manage. Timidity still plagued her and caused her to shrink from new situations and new faces, though she controlled it so well that few ever guessed she was so shy. She was intensely loyal to her friends and in her multitudinous correspondence kept up with an astonishing range of people: her father's former hired man, half forgotten pupils, distant relatives, and kindred spirits, such as her beloved Aunt Fanny. Barton so cherished these friends that she was anxious lest they not reciprocate her love, and jealousy and self-pity appear frequently in her diary. Outwardly stoic, calm, and deliberate, Barton covered the turmoil she felt within.

Behind the shyness and fears of rejection was a strong sense of solitude and of not quite fitting in with the ways of the world, for she had been the odd man out since childhood. Both the estrangement Barton felt from her relatives in Massachusetts and her choice of a single, career-oriented life had cut her off from the usual security and fellowship of a family. Once, feeling hurt at the indifference her family had shown to her accomplishments, she told a niece that it has been so "*unnatural* . . . that I could never comprehend it, and it took away all the sweet, to feel that there were none but strangers to feel an interest in what came to me. . . . I think you can have little idea of what a strange world this has been to me."[8] At numerous times during her life Barton tried to make up for the lack of a family by "adopting" people, such as the Nortons of Hightstown, or by creating her own unofficial family where she lived and worked. But in Dansville, as later, these parties of fellow spinsters, Red Cross workers, and fond nephews did not, somehow, bind themselves into the close and supportive unit for which she longed. In the end, despite abundant friends, she would turn again to her diary or letters and write of her isolation. November 30, 1881: "The way has been wearisome, often dark, and always lonely";[9] the following January: "I am to go on with this alone I can see, and I shall make up my mind to let all go and strip myself to the neck, and go on with it myself."[10] The loneliness sometimes overshadowed even her greatest achievements, leaving her alienated and unfulfilled. When a friend complained that she had done little but raise a family, Barton wrote back sorrowfully, "Still you have your children which are all *your own*—I have had nothing."[11]

Barton had always turned to work, not only to force her mind away from chronic introspection, but to fill the lonely hours and help her gain the recognition she so desperately needed. In the years to come she would increasingly cite her work not only as an escape but as a substitute for a family. She spoke of the Red Cross as a child and of her own responsibilities in a maternal fashion. "Like other children, I suppose the Red Cross must have its natural enemies . . . jealousy, calumny, and misrepresentation," she wrote in one of many examples of this metaphor, "and its mother must stand by the child till it is safely over them, but you will not wonder that she sometimes feels that she watches alone in the dark."[12] To her brother she wrote defensively, saying she could well imagine him thinking that she had nothing worthwhile to do, "Not a chick nor a child to look out for and dont need to work very hard." But, she told him, the Red Cross filled quite enough of that need; indeed she saw her responsibilities as so close to those of a family that she could half boast: "I don't quite keep clear of that chase myself."[13]

At the same time Barton began to feel that the work was not merely a self-created measure to consume her energy and restless emotions but a kind of divine appointment. If others had been given a home, children, and accepted place, her lot had been to embrace all of humanity. She came to view herself as "a tool to do His work in this particular direction" and prayed that God should find her "equal to the task, made up of the right material of the true and suitable metal."[14] By believing that God had placed the Red Cross in her trust, Barton in a sense withdrew her own responsibility for deciding to remain with the infant organization. "You have no power to judge the work you are doing," she advised a namesake, Clara Barton Knittle, "if it is given you to do and you do it faithfully you are only to lay it finished in the Master's hand—and he will judge it."[15] If God had placed this trust in her, she declared, he would tell her when to lay it down. Early 1882 was decidedly not the time.

For these reasons, and because she saw such initial problems for the Red Cross, Barton chose to stay on as president in the early years of its existence. But, compelled as she was to remain with the organization, the decision, in numerous ways, went against her better judgment. She was right when she declared

214

that the Red Cross had "not been a pampered child" and had had no "doting Godparents" to shower it with gifts.[16] Barton had borne the entire costs of securing treaty ratification. Now she must initially finance the organization until help could be obtained from the government or from private patrons. Within a year she would have to dip into capital to pay personal expenses and keep the Red Cross running, and she was forced to write an embarrassed note to her bankers explaining that she was "not becoming extravagant as the years go on" but that Red Cross expenses were heavy and she was "anxious not to . . . overdraw."[17] The work was also dangerously close to overdrawing on her emotional assets. She was tired and ill and came to believe that the Red Cross was exhausting every bit of her strength, indeed was hastening her death. Barton cursed the struggles that caused her so much unhappiness and longed to escape to a house in the country to "live an out of doors, quiet, restfull [sic] life, and get acquainted with nature—books, myself."[18] But the work was her calling, her handle on life. For the next twenty years she would remain the president of the American Red Cross.

Several initial problems pressed the organization in the months following ratification of the Treaty of Geneva. Most crucial was the need for money. Barton's own purse and the dollar or so that members contributed could not sustain the Red Cross indefinitely. She was even buying stamps out of her own funds, and her remark that it was time the Red Cross "got out of the one woman's little pocket where it has been so long" was fair.[19] Barton hoped to persuade the Congress to appropriate an annual sum to run the association, a move that would securely establish the Red Cross both financially and in its relationship with the federal government. She was conscious, however, of the dissent caused by the fifteen thousand dollars given to her after the war, and she was loath to have her name attached to the petition or to have such a bequest appear to pay her a salary. But the attempts to obtain government funds, first as a standard appropriation of 1 percent of the War Department budget and later as monies appropriated each year as needed, were unsuccessful. Congress saw the Red Cross as a private organization merely acting on principles set down in the Treaty of Geneva, and they feared setting a dangerous precedent if they too willingly funded such a charitable body. The most Barton could muster was the promise of one thousand dollars worth of free printing, taken from the State Department budget.[20]

Without overt governmental support, Barton had nowhere to turn but to the business community. In the early months of 1882 she sent out several appeals for help in the form of broadsides, and she utilized the press as much as possible to convey the urgent need she felt. "I still want to stand in the gap as well as I can until someone of more abundant means comes to understand the import and importance of the movement sufficiently to make some donation . . . ," she told a reporter from the *Woman's Journal*. "There are a thousand men in this country who, if they knew this opportunity, and realized what it would be, would not sleep till they had done it; but as it is, each will go on endowing some musty old college,

215

and think he has done a wise thing."[21] These and future attempts to tap private sources were too sporadic and undirected to elicit much response. Despite a large influx of money whenever fire, flood, or pestilence threatened the nation, Barton was never able to project the urgent need for office space, secretaries, and paper clips.

Barton's hope for government funds was coupled with a pressing need for formal recognition of the American Association of the Red Cross as the official representative of the Geneva Convention in the United States. As she soon found, it was imperative that some sort of formal relationship with the government be established before her group would be accepted by the International Red Cross Committee. "It is important that we be able to certify that your government is prepared to accept your services in case of war . . . ," Gustave Moynier wrote from Geneva. "We would be placed in a false position if you failed to obtain for it a privileged position by a formal recognition of the government."[22] To her intense frustration Clara found the Congress as slow to create an authorized relationship as they had been to appropriate working funds. She did the best she could to give the organization an official look by persuading the president and every cabinet officer to stand as members of a "Board of Consultation," and by arranging for an official proclamation of the treaty and its ramifications by President Arthur. She contacted the new secretary of state, Frederick T. Frelinghuysen, explained the problem, and after an agonizing round of bureaucratic notes, which sent her running from Congress to the War Department, then to the White House and back to the State Department, finally succeeded in fastening "the ends of the work I have been knitting up, stitch by stitch, these five years."[23] Amidst an impressive array of seals and ribbons, official recognition of the American Red Cross was sent to Geneva. On June 9, 1882, the International Committee formally accepted the organization, and Barton could breathe a long sigh of relief.

Barton's anxiety to secure official approval for her group was exacerbated by the continued rivalry she felt with the Blue Anchor association. Hannah Shepard's attacks on Barton and the Red Cross had not ceased with Senate ratification of the Geneva Convention. Newspaper articles that bore the unmistakable imprint of her malicious hand continued to surface, and personal letters from Shepard to Barton followed, full of petty accusations and insinuating remarks.[24] More serious was the fact that Shepard's undeniable ability to attract socially and politically prominent people to her side slowed for several years the congressional action Barton so desired. When, in March 1882, a Blue Anchor benefit was held for the victims of floods in the Mississippi Valley—victims the Red Cross was also trying to help—several influential senators attended, thousands of dollars were contributed, and the whole event threatened to overshadow the modest efforts of the Red Cross.[25]

Gustave Moynier assured Barton that the International Committee would deal with her society alone, and he willingly offered to help undermine the rival.[26] Friends and fellow Red Cross workers were equally supportive. "What

216

care you for these Pigmeys [sic] that soulessly [sic] try to irritate you?" asked Frances Gage indignantly. And Walter Phillips, seeing that Shepard's bark was far more venomous than her bite, simply scoffed at the whole conflict. "Really it seems like loading a howitzer to kill a gnat," he wrote of Clara's attempts to foil Shepard. "I can ignore her with complacency. If I liked I could grind her to powder by quoting her own words. . . . But she isn't worth it."[27] Barton was hardly in a mood to be jollied out of her concern, however, and continued to agitate over the situation. Always thin-skinned, she exaggerated Shepard's attacks and chose to view them as the representation of an ungrateful nation. "There is no spite they do not glory in towards me—I do not think that they would at all hesitate to kill me if they had the good opportunity any more than if I were a beast," she cried.[28] Finally, with the aid of Mrs. Francis Blair, an early Blue Anchor member who had come to believe that Barton was being maligned by Shepard, Clara succeeded in discrediting the society in the eyes of the government. As Walter Phillips had predicted, it gradually lost its audience, and after a few more months of sporadic activity, the Blue Anchor ceased to exist.[29]

The turmoil caused by Blue Anchor contributed to the despondency and self-doubt with which Barton struggled during this period. Part of this feeling was the letdown which was a natural accompaniment to the completion of a major project. Ironically, Barton's depression was heightened by the receipt, in the summer of 1882, of the highest medal given by the International Red Cross. It was, Gustave Moynier wrote, "a simple memorial to the most meritorious of our assistants."[30] Still struggling to achieve a basic recognition of her role from the American government, Barton sighed and questioned again why foreigners continued to laud her while her own countrymen chose "misrepresentation and slander." "I shall certainly come to feel that I want to escape them . . . , I should never want anything more of this country nor its people," Barton wrote heatedly.[31] But, as in every crisis to come, there was enough emotional release in threatening to leave the United States and start anew on foreign soil to keep her from actually doing it. Instead of making real plans to leave the country, she again took up her pen, thanked the International Committee for their decoration, but said that she would not accept it—not until she saw the Red Cross firmly and irrevocably established in America.[32]

Barton performed her early work from headquarters at 947 T Street, a modest row house in northwest Washington, which still stands today. She had bought the place in 1878 for fifteen hundred dollars on the advice of General Whitaker but had rented it out for five years. She preferred to stay at the Fergusons' spacious house on I Street, which was not only more convenient, since it was closer to the center of town, but filled with congenial company. She traveled only a few times a week to the T Street house, where, with odd bits of furniture, she had set up business. Barton later referred to the building as "the first Red Cross warehouse," and it is probable that many of the rooms were used to store the clothing, bandages, bedding, and other contributions, which poured in at the first news of a disaster. An early photograph shows a two-story ivy-covered house, with a decorative frieze, topped by a large red cross, which was probably added around 1884. Here she began work to solicit funds, organize local societies, and establish the Red Cross as a truly national organization.[33]

In these early years Barton pictured the Red Cross as a loosely organized, decentralized body. She desired to keep the parent, or national, society small and manageable by allowing as members "only a limited number of experienced and active workers."[34] This group would officially represent the United States to the International Committee and oversee the activities of the local auxiliaries, which were, in turn, responsible to it. Local societies, the backbone of the organization, could be founded, with unlimited membership, in every community. There would be no state organizations to add to the confusion, but rather a small committee assigned to regulate the relief activity in each state. Barton hoped to persuade the governor of each state to serve on the state's committee, a move which would lend the Red Cross prestige and official sanction.[35]

Barton's dreams of a widespread network of societies were slow to materialize, however. Several new chapters, such as those in Chicago, New Orleans, and Madison, Wisconsin, joined the early local auxiliaries in Dansville, Syracuse, and Rochester, New York. But effective publicity was still needed before she could attract large numbers of members to the Red Cross. To this end Barton began expanding and revising her 1878 pamphlet, "The Red Cross of the Geneva Convention—What It Is." The booklet was distributed widely but failed to inspire many local societies. As Hubbell noted, it needed "personal work to interest people in the work—many who had received books had not looked at them—and yet seemed greatly interested as soon as the subject was understood."[36] Speeches, especially those Barton delivered personally, also helped to spread the Red Cross story. Still, there was a limit to what even Barton could do by way of such personal advertising. No one else was working full time for the organization, and she was juggling too many other matters to devote all of her energy to publicity.

She was, in many ways, ill-equipped to undertake the organization of what was an enormously ambitious project. Barton had the habit of command, but although devoted friends would hail her "executive ability,"[37] she was a poor administrator. Accustomed to working alone, she preferred to keep records, plan projects, and oversee relief work personally. She felt suspicious of fellow workers and annoyed employees by incessantly looking over their shoulders or giving advice while they worked.[38] With laudable humility, she was willing to undertake even the most menial tasks alone, but all too often this overtaxed her strength or distracted her from administrative duties that desperately needed her attention. In a revealing sketch, Dr. Hubbell described Barton's work habits:

> She never considered any kind of work beneath her, and if there was need of help in any department of the household either of her own or wherever she might be that part

she always filled whether it were in the line of nursing, of advice . . . sanitary matters, chamber maids work, washing room, cleaning house, dishwashing, gardening . . . in all places she did the actual work herself. She never gave commands never gave orders, but always worked in all things with her helpers and always took the most difficult part of the task herself.

After she had begin [sic] a task she always wanted to finish it herself no matter how disagreeable or minimal it might be. If it were a task that *belonged to another* who had neglected it that person must leave it alone . . . after she had taken it up, and not offer to *help finish* what really belonged to him to *do entire*.[39]

Within the first year, Barton dismissed the possibility of finding anyone with whom she was able to collaborate in the Red Cross. "Decide that I must attend to all business myself . . . ," she wrote in her journal, "and learn to do all myself."[40] It was understandably difficult to direct societies eight hundred miles away, and she was bewildered by the petty troubles they brought to her to solve. She was as amazed by the strong personalities of the Wisconsin and Chicago societies, who wanted authority to act in emergencies without the permission of the national body, as by the timid souls of the New Orleans chapter, who refused to make a move without her direction. Barton knew that the local auxiliaries did not "seem to clearly comprehend the relation they bear to the Parent Society." She would not, or could not, recognize, however, that it was her own quixotic nature that was sending the confused signals.[41]

Another problem that hampered the growth of local Red Cross chapters, which Barton recognized at the outset, was the absence of a sense of urgency about relief matters. The Sanitary Commission had grown rapidly into an extensive national network because there had been a perceived danger and a corresponding desire to contribute to the war. But in time of peace the same complacency that had made Barton's initial introduction of the Red Cross in America so difficult now hampered the organization's growth.

It was during two natural disasters in the first year of the Red Cross, therefore, that the most enthusiastic new converts were found. In the spring of 1882, and again the following year, the Mississippi River flooded, the consequence of heavy rains and the runoff from melting northern ice. Barton, anxious that the Red Cross prove itself indispensable, dispatched Julian Hubbell, still a medical student, to the stricken area. In 1882, Hubbell traveled to New Orleans, where he heard reports of widespread destruction. Few had died in the flood, but many had lost their homes, the newly planted crops of cotton and sugar, and all of their clothing. Fifteen thousand persons were estimated to be in need in Arkansas alone, and the governor had sent out an appeal for help, to "prevent suffering, if not actual starvation."[42] Hubbell found a number of small relief societies earnestly at work, as well as a government transport, which was distributing army rations to those most severely hurt. He joined one of these transports and dili-

219

gently took notes on the devastation and the relief efforts. Everything, he reported to Barton, was under water save some ancient Indian burial mounds, and the banks of the rivers were "so high as to hide the smokestacks of steamers." Relief consisted mainly of army rations and occasional handouts of clothing.[43]

Before the area had recovered from this disaster, it was inundated again in May by a flood that wiped out the newly replanted crops. Hubbell again accompanied the government transports, handing out donations of twenty-five dollars to the neediest cases from a hastily solicited Red Cross fund. He saw that meat, meal, and fodder for animals were the most urgently needed items, along with seeds to replace those borne away by the murky waters. From Rochester, New York, came a godsend: ten thousand dollars worth of seeds, donated by a local nurseryman. The distribution of these seeds was the organization's most significant work in 1882.[44]

Hubbell, in fact, had found embarrassingly little to do. Local organizations seemed competent to handle local relief. The government had undertaken, through the army, all emergency feeding and the rescue of those who were stranded. It was of little use to publicly criticize the president for sending in the military rather than putting relief services in the hands of the Red Cross, which was begging him for an opportunity to be tested. As in Michigan, Hubbell was concerned lest the new organization appear to be taking over work already cherished by local philanthropists. "Of course, I suppose, there are isolated cases in [need of] looking after . . . ," Hubbell wrote rather forlornly from the lower Mississippi, "but I have not heard of any more than exists in any community of equal extent." Determined to avoid conflict, Hubbell satisfied himself that relief was being tendered and kept a low profile for the Red Cross.[45]

He saw also, however, that much of the disorganization, last-minute collecting of goods, and duplication of effort could be eliminated through one central relief network; that the Red Cross purpose was not at odds with these local enthusiasts but could help to streamline their activities. There was a gap, too, between the time a disaster occurred and the hour government aid arrived, which the Red Cross, by preparing ahead of time, could help to bridge. It was on these points that Hubbell sold the Red Cross to local leaders throughout the Mississippi Valley with considerable success. Red Cross chapters were formed in New Orleans, Vicksburg, Natchez, and Memphis as a result of his trip. So effective was his work that when a cyclone ripped through Louisiana a year later, the New Orleans chapter handled the relief with only minimal help from Barton's national body.[46]

Ten months later Hubbell faced much the same situation. This time the citizens along the upper Mississippi and Ohio rivers suffered, and the floods began as early as February. Barton sent out an immediate call for help, collected almost five thousand dollars in money and goods (including three thousand dollars from the German Red Cross), and again plucked Hubbell out of medical school to tend to its distribution. This time his tour took him from Toledo to St. Louis, with stops in Cincinnnati, Dayton, and Louisville.[47] He found streets and houses covered with five inches of sediment, crops of winter wheat washed away, and scores of anxious faces. Worst hit were the small farmers, who, though free of debt, had virtually no funds with which to rebuild their farms. The flood was hardly a major disaster; Hubbell in fact had difficulty finding victims to aid and told Clara that "the urgency for help does not seem very urgent."[48] Most of the suffering was, again, caused by failure to anticipate and prepare for the flood. Citing the need for preparation, Hubbell organized mayors and businessmen into effective Red Cross units, capitalizing on the present need and their struggles to cope with it. Louisville, Cincinnnati, and St. Louis all formed chapters. Hubbell and Barton were heartened by the strength of the Red Cross organizations of New Orleans and Memphis, which sent donations to their stricken northern affiliates only a year after their own devastation. Though the Red Cross had again found little to do, Barton was pleased with the work. She characterized Hubbell's six weeks in the field as "quick, short, sharp work, and yet the most brilliant and successful field work the Red Cross has approved. We are constantly gaining, both in usefulness and appreciation."[49]

This earliest relief work was important for its ability to publicize the Red Cross name and to rally support for it. But it had a further significance, for much of the Red Cross philosophy of charitable action was formed at this time. The seeming uselessness of the Red Cross at these fields was not lost on Barton, and she was thereafter careful to enter only those areas in tremendous distress or of national import. Despite pleas from some influential southern Red Cross members, she did not want the national Red Cross to be part of the work in a yellow fever epidemic of 1882, which already involved several prominent southern relief agencies, including the famed Howard Association of New Orleans. Rather than react to every small misfortune, Barton wrote, "we must hold ourselves *dear* and *rare*, gather and husband our resources, and be ready to move like the winds when the true moment comes. . . . I think we should *never* move until the need or shock is so great as to annihilate *political* considerations, which are of all things the greatest abomination."[50] Henceforth, the Red Cross would survey the damage first and then decide whether or not to give relief.

Hubbell's observations also confirmed the view that a judicious reticence should be used in giving outright charity. In most cases, food, fodder, clothing, and seeds were more effective donations than money. While the former could be put to use immediately, money too often relieved nothing—since there was frequently nothing to buy—or was used to drown sorrows in whiskey. Indiscriminate handouts merely encouraged indolence, noted Hubbell, and in many cases, he believed, the greater need was for lessons in thrift and industry. From Louisiana he wrote: "While *every body* is giving—while the papers are making sensational reports—telling what had been done . . . it is rather hard to stand by and not fall in with the popular tide and *give*—but while every body else is giving is just the time to stop. . . . I think of *but one* donation that is *needed* in any part that I have yet seen and that is frugality."[51] These views matched (or perhaps reflected) Barton's own opinions. She had never seen the Red Cross as an agency devoted to long-term relief. Its purpose was to fill the gap between disaster and

221

recovery, much as her place on the battlefield had been between the bullet and the hospital. Thus Red Cross relief would be given to only the immediately needy, and would be of the kind that reinforced the longstanding New England virtues Barton and Hubbell held so dear: hard work, thrift, and self-sufficiency.

While Hubbell was assessing the damage in the Midwest, Barton was pondering another problem. She spent New Year's Day, 1883, at the home of Abby and Joseph Sheldon, where she had hoped to find peace and rest on an extended Christmas visit. There she received a letter from Benjamin Butler, requesting her to undertake the superintendency of the Massachusetts Reformatory Prison for Women. The position, he told her, wanted "a woman at once of executive ability and kindheartedness, with an honest love of the work of reformation and care of her living fellow creatures." It required residency in Sherborn, Massachusetts, the site of the reformatory, and paid a salary of fifteen hundred dollars per year.[52]

Butler had been elected to the governorship of Massachusetts in 1882. He almost immediately lost his popularity, having managed within a few months to insult nearly every political group of consequence in the state. Among these was a body of reformers—always cherished in Massachusetts—who had fostered an interest in the Massachusetts female prison. The prison was progressive, not only in its methods of reforming the inmates but in the fact that it was run by women. Butler had loudly proclaimed his dissatisfaction with the institution, which he believed to be costly and ineffective, and had threatened to impound the prison's funds. He did not believe that women could run such an establishment and bedeviled the superintendent, Dr. Eliza Mosher, until she finally resigned. By January 1883 his office was rocked by loud protests from prison reformers as well as critics of the reformatory and feminists. Forced to reply to questions on all sides, Butler began to look anxiously for a woman who could manage the prison, and whom he could trust to give him a candid report on the expenses and requirements of the institution. Barton, as a native of the state and a nationally known philanthropist, who had been the general's confidante for twenty years, seemed perfect for the part. Moreover, as Butler was well aware, Clara owed him more than one favor.[53]

On January 17, Barton traveled to Boston to speak with Butler about the subject, then continued on to Sherborn to look over the prison. She was less than enchanted with the prospect of undertaking the job. For one thing, her health had been poor for over a year, so precarious that she had spent a good deal of the previous summer in Dansville suffering from "symptoms too unmistakable to be disregarded."[54] She was, furthermore, dedicated to the Red Cross and desirous of devoting what strength she had to its development; a tour at Sherborn would retard the work and possibly cause her to lose her control over it. Last, the prison was heavily involved with an established philanthropic community, whose reactions to her were unknown. She had never received support from the professionals—be they doctors, statesmen, or generals—with whom she had worked, and she had little desire to reencounter them now.

Yet Barton was hesitant to turn the job down, chiefly because it was Butler who offered it. "I remember that of the many requests I have made of you, you not only never denied me one, but never listened indifferently,"[55] she had once told the general. That knowledge stung her conscience now. Although she was preoccupied with writing a speech on Fort Wagner, to be given at the Connecticut State GAR encampment, and with the details of her return to Washington in early February, Butler's proposal preyed on her mind. In the end she felt she could not accept, but it was with mixed feelings that she sent Butler a letter declining the position: "That *you* General, offer it, gives it all its value and importance, and my grief is, that there should come a moment, when you should again invite me to stand and do service under your banner and I am not free to render it acceptably."[56]

A friend told Clara that when Governor Butler received her letter "he sat back in his chair in a sort of despairing way and says 'well, I don't know what I shall do.'"[57] What he did do was to refuse to let the matter drop. He contacted Barton again and persuaded her friends to convince her to take the superintendency, at least temporarily. In March, when Butler was in Washington, he did Barton the favor of accompanying her to the White House to talk of Red Cross appropriations and pressed her again on the Sherborn matter. She nervously consulted a trusted friend, Sarah B. Earle, and nephew Stevé, and with great reluctance noted in her diary that she felt "more [and] more that the prison impends."[58] Finally, on the condition that Butler's enemies accept her wholeheartedly and that she keep the job only for six months, Barton relented. On April 11 she was formally and unanimously confirmed by the state legislature as superintendent of the Woman's Reformatory Prison of Massachusetts.[59]

She traveled to the post via North Oxford, where tragedy had struck the family. Stevé's little daughter Lauretta had been killed by a heavy wagon; his wife had sunk into a desperate gloom. Clara arrived to find the blinds lowered, "little Retta laid out in the parlor," and herself greeted with an inexplicable coolness. She bustled about, trying to help, but retired to her room when it was made apparent that Stevé's family felt she was interfering. Thus it ever was for her at home. If she had offended anyone she did not know how, and she had to get through the time as best she could. She left Stevé's house as soon as she could after the funeral. To her diary she commented dryly, "I don't think I shall *long* to go again."[60]

Barton took the oath of office in Sherborn on May 1. She was timid and uncertain, and somewhat overwhelmed by the enormity of her undertaking. The huge prison complex—so large that for the first few weeks she could not find her way without a guide—the questioning faces of the convicts, and the isolation of the spot, all worked to sap her confidence. "I might as well be in the desert of Sahara for *human* companionship," her predecessor had written on her first night at Sherborn, and now Barton felt much the same loneliness and intimidation. "Took my place at table to preside at my own board," she wrote that night in her diary, "seemed very new and I felt diffident [and] timid—all beautiful, kind—but I am so strange [and] bashful I don't think I can do it right."[61]

In the ideology of prison reformers of this time, the notion of domesticity was paramount. A homelike atmosphere was thought to foster thoughts of the highest spiritual order and to bring out the gentler aspects of a woman's nature. At Sherborn, therefore, cells were more like pleasant dormitory rooms than depressing cages; recreation rooms, library, and halls were spotlessly maintained, and women with infants were allowed to bring them to the reformatory. Indeed the iron bedsteads and white linen were a cause for complaint by those who criticized the prison. Not only were the sleeping conditions superior to those in most private homes, but the food served the highest class of prisoners was believed to be "pleasanter and the table better spread than those of the best class of mill operatives, and is about equal to that of the average mechanic." In light of the amount of money spent at Sherborn, the *Boston Herald* complained, those who had studied its record were "not particularly jubilant" over the results.[62]

Yet those most interested in prison reform looked to the Massachusetts Reformatory for Women with great expectations. Already it embodied many of the changes crusaders such as Elizabeth Fry and Dorothea Dix had fought for during the previous half century: an emphasis on reform, female guards, industrial training, and restraint in the use of physical punishment. By the 1870s these ideals had been strengthened by feminists who believed that most of the prisoners were simply the victims of men and a society that offered little opportunity to honestly earn a living. The reformatory at Sherborn, with its sympathetic female matrons, physician, and chaplain, its stress on the superior virtues of women, and its training in sewing, baking, and other marketable work, offered a significant opportunity for feminists and prison reformers to justify their theories.[63]

One of the experiments that pleased zealous reformers most was a merit system for rewarding and controlling behavior, instituted by Barton's predecessor. It was a complex method of classifying the inmate according to seniority and conduct. A woman entering the prison was interviewed, then taken to a sparsely furnished solitary cell and left alone to meditate and adjust to the prison for one month. At the end of the time she was dressed in a plain, dark blue gingham dress, white stockings, and low-heeled shoes, and was allowed to join the other level 4 prisoners, who shared each other's company, the prison's drabbest costume, and the plainest board. Several months of exemplary behavior, including quiet talk, devotion at chapel, and industry in the prison laundry or sewing rooms, could boost her to level 3. Here she donned a frock boasting a hairline check of white (evidently symbolizing the tiny spot of purity in her otherwise tainted nature) and moved to a room without barred windows. Level 2 brought greater freedom (and a larger white check) and level 1 included the privileges of better food, permission to post pictures in her room (now a large outside chamber), and a chance to work outside the prison as a domestic servant. Demerits brought a lowering of status and haughty glances from fellow inmates. More serious punishments, which included placing a prisoner on a diet of bread and water, working at the most exasperating tasks in enforced silence, or, in extreme cases, solitary confinement in one of the prison's few dungeonlike basement cells, were rare. Mosher and other reformers felt that through this system they had found a way of promoting initiative among the women. At the same time, they removed them from temptations they could not yet resist.[64]

"My family is large—," Clara wrote Mary Norton after taking over the prison, "you want to know how many—well about 240 inmates and abt 30 other women."[65] On optimistic days she praised the prisoners' cleanliness and attempts at self control; at less cheerful moments she saw herself as buried in a "smelling yeasty mass of human sin."[66]

Overall the misdeeds of the women did not seem to her very great. Only a handful were sentenced for theft, assault, or other high crimes. The remainder had been arrested for disrupting the public order or offending its moral code. Charges ranged from "stubborness," and vagrancy to illegally practicing abortion and abandonment of a child. More than one-fifth of the women were in Sherborn for "offenses against chastity," which included prostitution, adultery, and "lewdness." By far the most common crime, however, was drunkenness, for which half of the women had been sentenced.[67] Many arrived at the prison suffering from alchoholism; they were dreadful apparitions given to tremors, delusions, and hysteria. This in itself kept the house physician, Dr. Lucy Hall, busy, but she also treated the quarter of the women who were syphilitic and dealt with childbirth, diabetes, and measles.[68]

Eliza Mosher had been interested in the background of these criminal women and took care to record their personal histories and to compile statistics on the successes of the reformatory. They were a young group, with over half under thirty years of age. Only one black prisoner was at Sherborn; the majority were from Irish families. (Whether this reflected the poverty of this immigrant group, social custom, or the prevalent anti-Irish bias of many officials is not clear.) A majority of the women were married, but the group almost uniformly came from disordered or tragically impoverished homes. The determinist theory of crime, which maintained that social or environmental forces, not genetics or the human will, influenced a person's destiny, had recently been embraced by reformers, and the statistics Mosher compiled were used to bolster it. Because of this, those watching with interest the progress of the Massachusetts Reformatory for Women advocated stricter sentences for the women, who they believed could only benefit from the hygienic and idealistic atmosphere of the prison. They argued that a year (the average sentence) at Sherborn was too little to change lifetime habits. When the prisoner reentered her old environment, she would simply revert back to the patterns of her past.[69]

Barton was inclined to agree with the proponents of strict sentencing, for she felt that her charges were there for salvation, not punishment, and that more than a few were jailed for protection against themselves. The youth of the inmates, their impoverished backgrounds and precarious futures, distressed her. She knew too well the limited opportunities that a woman who would work faced in the world and the scanty protection that that world afforded her; she had, after all, herself faced "the fearful odds." Barton's pragmatic feminism balked at laws that would send a woman to jail in punishment of deeds that a man could not even be tried for, and at the courts, in which women were still not allowed to testify or sit on a jury. Inevitably she came to the conclusion that the inmates, if weak, were nonetheless victims of society, and especially of the men who deluded and preyed on them. In righteous indignation she told the state commissioners that the real culprits were to be found at the State Prison for Men at Concord. Those at Sherborn were "more often weak than wicked; more often sinned against than sinning."[70]

Unlike the prison chaplain, who thought the women "vicious," Barton had little but pity for the majority of inmates. Some she thought had been shockingly treated by the state. Her sense of justice aroused by one woman in particular, Barton spent much of her own time researching the case. Convinced that the woman had been wrongly condemned, that indeed she did not even understand the crime she was accused of, Barton began to fight for her release. "I could not hold this heartbroken woman under me," she wrote. "I could not live in the prison with her and see its hard rules bear upon her; I could not go and leave her to the cold mercy of another, I could not claim a new trial—there was but one recourse left—to beg executive clemency and beg her pardon." Governor Butler, trusting as always Barton's judgment, readily complied with her request and the woman was released. Still, Clara was haunted by the memory of that inmate, for the "poor wronged woman went out with the additional degrading injustice heaped upon her of having been pardoned for a crime never committed nor attempted nor even comprehended."[71]

Barton was at Sherborn less to change conditions than to observe and report on them to Butler and other state officials. Thus she kept most of the day-to-day routine of the reformatory intact. The inmates still attended chapel each day. This was a lengthy, moralizing Protestant service, which made no attempt to serve the half of the inmates who were Catholic. (Only one Mass was offered each week.) From chapel the inmates walked to the sewing rooms, where they spent the day at sewing machines making shirts for a large New York firm, or leaning over washtubs doing laundry on a tariff basis. A quarter of the women were illiterate; these attended school for a portion of the day. Barton also found the food "wholesome and plentiful." Its emphasis on grains and vegetables, and corresponding lack of meat, met with her approval and she left the diet alone. In the evenings there was exercise and recreation. Barton's only suggested change, instituted by her successor, was that the large acreage be turned into a farm and orchard, which would supply the tables and employ more women in healthy out-door work. [72]

In her round of duties, Barton had little contact with the prisoners. She arose early, supervised the purchase of the prison's food and supplies and oversaw the kitchen. Fifty plumbers and carpenters, employed to lay new pipes and a fire alarm system in the building, came under her supervision, as did the thirty-eight female staff members. Barton arrived to find one hundred letters on her desk, and the amount of correspondence—with concerned relatives, doctors, and re-formers, and the State Commission on Prisons—did not abate during her tenure. Also under her care were the reports and record-keeping that the state required. Added to these daily cares was the burden of inadequacy she felt in managing an institution that differed so radically from her other experience. "I entered that prison feeling myself so ignorant of all that pertained to its line of work and methods and thought . . . ," she told a group of philanthropists a few years later, "that it seemed to me positively *wicked,* to waste my own time and that of the community and those who must come under me, in the strengthless, thoughtless vacancy of my attempted work—I seemed to myself a kind of empty baloon [sic]." [73]

The prisoners were devoted to Barton, despite her infrequent meetings with them. Once a week she addressed the women in the chapel. Rumors of her he-roic activities had circulated long before she ever set foot in the prison, and the inmates were impressed and honored by her interest in them. Barton's personal magnetism and great dignity of bearing further awed them. Her control was so great over the prisoners that a reporter once watched her calm a hysterical woman with one withering glance and a few well-modulated words. She was far from imperious with the women, however, and her personal kindness made her a shining example to everyone at Sherborn. "She was a perfect inspiration to the prisoners," said the prison's doctor. "She would tell them of her work and in our own war and in the wars abroad, and they were fascinated." With such stature she had little need to preach. As Barton recalled nearly twenty years later, "I did not weary them with advice, they had had a surfeit of that a long time before, nor correction—they were having enough of that, Heaven knows, as the weary days dragged on. I told them stories of the lives of other persons and left them to draw their own inferences." [74] One improvement she initiated at Sherborn also increased her popularity. With so little time available to really associate with the prisoners, she decided to communicate with them in the way she knew best: by correspondence. To this end she had two boxes posted outside her office into which any inmate could drop a suggestion, complaint, or request. One box was addressed to Barton, the other to the state officials who ran the prison, and no one but the addressee saw the notes. To Barton, whom they frequently addressed as "Dear friend," they sent tear-stained pleas for release, for protection against drunken husbands, for help in court cases. Barton did not always grant their requests (she replied to a petition to allow windows to remain open on sultry summer days, for example, by saying that prison meant locked windows and a loss of fresh air, in order to protect the community), but she answered every note with uniform kindness.[75]

Though sympathy and control were Barton's keys to operating the prison, she also showed a respect for the prisoners that they deeply appreciated. In little touches—such as the suggestion boxes or her way of addressing the inmates as women rather than girls—she made it clear that she was not shocked or offended by her charges, that they were still human beings with feelings and hope. If ever they were to be reformed, she declared stoutly, "it must come under some such elevating influences and conditions of self-respect, self-reliance, honor, love and trust; penalties, degradation, distrust, disgrace, never yet reformed any human being and never will."[76] But her unwillingness to look down on the women of Sherborn had not only to do with theories of reform; it sprang from an inner fear of the similarities between herself and the inmates, and an identification with their temptations and troubles. With her unstable background, memories of Dolly's insane and murderous ravings, her brothers' and cousins' unlawful pursuits, and her own tendency to despair and falsehood, she could so easily have crossed the line overstepped by these women. She was greatly disturbed throughout her time at Sherborn by the thin veil of morality that separated those who walked free and those incarcerated. On days when she left the prison, when the inmates sobbed and kissed her hand, she thought it all wrong that she was the keeper and judge of these women, who differed so little from herself. "Surely," she worried, "we must be too near alike, if not akin or they would never have clung to me with that pitiful love."[77]

The inmates were thus easily won over to Barton and her notions. State officers were a distinctly more challenging group. Much of Barton's time was spent juggling the differing priorities of Governor Butler, the legislature, and the prison commission. Barely four weeks after her arrival she hosted a delegation from the legislature, who came bent on ferreting out overspending and inappropriate leniency toward the prisoners. They found neither. Barton guided many other groups through the institution in the next six months and wrote numerous reports, with similar success. She had found little to justify the charge of overspending and contended that ten cents per woman each day was the minimum decent expenditure. The grounds, Barton acknowledged, might be more productive if they were farmed or used to pasture dairy cattle. The building, too, was underutilized, and she began tentative arrangements to turn the old nursery and maternity wards into a separate center for the insane prisoners of the state.

228

(This plan ultimately was dropped because it was thought it would interfere with the high moral tone of the prison.)[78] The system, she advised the chairman of the state prison committee, was "admirable in its designs and execution, nobly and humanely conceived, patiently, faithfully, carefully, and laboriously administered."[79]

Barton made one major change during her tenure. In June 1883 she recommended that the offices of steward and treasurer be abolished and put under the jurisdiction of the superintendent. The move, which would save several thousand dollars a year, was speedily approved. To the surprise of Butler, Barton posted her own bond when she took over the job, in the form of railroad securities left from her fifteen-thousand-dollar congressional appropriation. Barton won the acclaim of feminists for her abolition of the two offices because, under the theory that women could not arrange financial matters, they had been previously held by men. Equally pleased that she had acted with so much dignity in posting her own bond, advocates of women's rights pointed to Barton with pride as, in late July 1883, she took up the books at Sherborn.[80]

Barton proved immensely skillful at placating the politicians and satisfying the demands of the prison board. She had the willing ear of Butler and a sympathetic ally on the board in an influential woman named Ellen Johnson, but it was her own forthright personality that did the most to ensure the continuation of the prison system. So well did she defend the institution that when she returned to Dansville in June to gather a few of her belongings, the remaining staff felt immediately threatened by her absence. The old complaint that women could not run the institution was being bandied about again. Dr. Lucy Hall reported this news to Clara and urged her to return quickly. "We keep hearing that Gov. Butler is growing angry and worried and is going to do desperate things generally," she wrote anxiously to Barton, "and then we think of your protecting wing and can hardly wait for its blessed shadow again to cover us."[81]

Having so competently calmed the bureaucratic furies, Barton was consequently annoyed to find her effort tossed about in the political meetings that commenced that fall. A harsh campaign for Butler's defeat was being fought, and at every opportunity the governor took the credit for placing Barton at Sherborn and even for her excellent administration. Though Butler's words were laudable and the opposition dared not criticize her, Barton was incensed that her name was allowed to be dragged into political speeches and her own actions possibly interpreted in the light of intraparty promises. She feared, too, that she would not be free to leave Sherborn after the election, that she would become part of campaign pledges or lose needed support for the Red Cross with the victors if she left at the end of Butler's term. "I have held more than silently and still, through all the rabid campaign which has gone on these last months," she wrote indignantly that November. She had not brought herself to quarrel over the matter with Butler personally, but she resented his action after her sincere efforts to uphold his reputation in the eyes of the citizens and the prison board.[82]

Because of this politicism, Barton's last few months in office were not pleasant. And she had further to contend with a nasty bit of infighting among her own staff. The chaplain, Susan Harrold, with whom she had already differed over the "sinful" nature of the condemned women, had taken exception to Barton's management at Sherborn and had begun reporting separately to the prison board. Barton, who so prized loyalty above other traits, was livid when she discovered evidence of what she called "sly 'toadying,'" and feared that scandal would be the result. She accused the chaplain of poisoning several of the matrons against her and encouraging them to carry out contradictory orders.[83] Barton worried that Harrold, who had the most personal kind of access to the women and who controlled their probation, would begin to influence even the inmates against her. She began to feel personally persecuted, accusing the chaplain of spying on her quarters and writing negative reports about her authoritarian manner to the state prison board. She would not be calmed, even by Lucy Hall's best efforts. What the chaplain's real complaint with Barton was, whether it stemmed from desire for power or from disapproval of the superintendent's notoriously authoritarian methods and need for complete personal fealty, has gone unrecorded. Clara saw no solution to the problem but to be honest with the board and break the chain of secret correspondence. "If they ask you if you think Miss B. has realized or felt this state of things . . . ," Barton told Dr. Hall, "you can tell them that you know that there have been months of bitterness and ashes on this very account—that she has seen and lived it all, that she has gone timidly, through her own halls, dreading the scrutiny of the critisizing clique she knew [and] felt was there to meet her."[84] Her warning was enough to give Dr. Hall doubts about the desirability of the position. Although Barton asked for and received Butler's word that he would have Lucy Hall made superintendent at Sherborn, when at length she was offered the job she declined it.[85]

Occasionally Barton could joke about the situation. She once wrote to a friend that after her "conduct during the last two or three years, what else could be expected, than that my tricks would be discovered, and due punishment overtake me." But it had been a depressing year for Clara, and she later referred to her superintendency as the "most foolhardy thing [I] ever did."[86] She had left the prison only twice—once to bring back her possessions from Dansville and once, late in October, to deliver an address at the International Woman's Congress in Chicago—and she felt as isolated and alone after six months as she had at her arrival.[87] Her Red Cross work had been neglected and her strength overtaxed. It was with relief that she resigned from the position soon after Butler's defeat in November. She had said she would remain for half a year, and her time had been up the first of that month, but Butler begged her to stay out the calendar year and she reluctantly agreed.[88] She left the prison with "a burden of thoughts," caused by her association with the unfortunate women, a renewed sense of the disadvantages with which women had to struggle, and a new opposition to alcoholic beverages. She was not, however, convinced of the success of either her own influence or the system in general. Barton knew she could control the prisoners and manage the institution but doubted that she, or anyone else, could truly reform people. The best chance, she came to believe, was to set a fine example, to instill hope, to promote good resolutions.[89]

On the last day of the year she gave a party for friends, staff, and prison board in the superintendent's house. The next day she walked out of the house, shut the door firmly, and left the Massachusetts Reformatory Prison behind her. "I went out from the prison walls of Sherborn next morning," she mused a few years later. "I have never seen a face there since. I have never returned and have no desire to."[90]

fourteen

Of course the American Red Cross suffered while Clara Barton was managing the prisoners at Sherborn. She had been concerned about this when she reluctantly agreed to take the position, and the problems of the emerging organization continued to nag at her throughout 1883. Yet she could not bring herself to give up its leadership, even temporarily. Soon after her arrival at the reformatory she decided she would not "neglect it, but simply . . . add this charge to it, and conduct the two."[1] Barton obtained permission from the prison committee and Governor Butler to hire John Hitz or someone else to help her with the Red Cross work, but, for undisclosed reasons, this was not done. The burden was eased only once, when faithful Julian Hubbell came to Sherborn for a few weeks to help with correspondence.[2]

What Red Cross work Barton could do was hastily completed in the small hours of the morning, and this, understandably, was inadequate.[3] Those addressing the national headquarters were likely to receive a note from Hubbell explaining that Miss Barton was occupied at Sherborn and would reply upon her return. Communities interested in forming local Red Cross societies were puzzled to find their requests for membership unanswered. One group of eminent citizens and physicians in Philadelphia came to believe that the American Red Cross was completely defunct and wrote directly to Gustave Moynier in an attempt to revive the work. This naturally alarmed and embarrassed Barton, who hastened to reassure both the doctors in Philadelphia and the International Committee in Geneva that the American Red Cross still existed. It was with relief that she contemplated a return to Washington and the Red Cross in January 1884.[4]

Clara had scarcely begun to pick up the confused bits of undone business when a disaster occurred that would prove both a challenge and a boon to the American Red Cross. In early February 1884, the Ohio River again flooded. Barton was quickly informed of the situation and was equally quick to respond. On February 9 she left for Pittsburgh to personally survey the damage, stopping only to visit with precious Aunt Fanny, now near death.[5] Though Pittsburgh had suffered much less damage than other cities on the river, Barton was shocked at what she saw, and immediately sent out an appeal for donations. Once the checks, barrels of clothing, and gifts of food began to arrive, she left for Cincinnati in hopes of finding the worst of the destruction and to determine the most urgent need.

Barton had become accustomed to exaggerated reports, so she was surprised at the truly terrible conditions along the Ohio. The river was rising half an inch every hour, and towns like Lawrenceburg, Indiana, were entirely swept away, re-placed by swirling masses of debris. Cincinnati lay under seventy-one feet of water. Chicken houses and railroad ties floated by, mingled grotesquely with dead pigs, rumpled clothing, and the everyday treasures of private life. There had been few deaths, but property damage was extensive. Barton had had no intention of staying on the scene—she wanted too badly to handle the pressing business of the Red Cross—but found herself "surprised and captured." Sensing that this was a challenge equal to those of the old war days, she lost herself in the business of saving lives. It would be more than three months before she would return to the national headquarters.[6]

Congress appropriated $500,000 in relief funds for the area, money earmarked for the recovery of missing persons and for distribution of emergency rations. The American Red Cross had no desire to compete with the federal government; in-deed it could not have done so. Instead it sought to supplement the government's work. It was still midwinter, and warm clothing, fuel, bedding, and feed for the animals were desperately needed. All were items that the army boats, plying the rivers, neglected to carry. Barton also found that the government transports con-centrated on the larger towns, or those with easy access, and that many a stranded farmer or out-of-the-way village was neglected. "My agents are looking the ground over very carefully . . . ," she wrote on February 22, "seeking among the *smaller* towns, the *little people,* who are likely to be over-looked, what their necessities may be."[7] She initially set up warehouses in Cincinnati, but when a tornado struck the lower Ohio a few weeks later, she hastily moved her head-quarters to Evansville, Indiana, where there was more immediate need. After some frustration she rented a large steamer, the *Josh V. Throop,* and hired a crew to load and unload her "precious freight." She also assembled a small staff, which included Hubbell; Enola Lee, an ambitious young woman from Evansville; and Mahala Chaddock, a loyal friend from Dansville. When a local blacksmith ham-mered a large cross out of metal and painted it red, Barton had it hung between the smokestacks of the ship and made ready to depart on her twelve-week odyssey.[8]

The *Josh V. Throop* headed toward Cairo, Illinois, zigzagging its way down the river. At precarious landings it threw off fodder, shoes, thick woolen blankets, and coal. Small items such as scissors, needles and thread, and writing paper were also handed out. Indeed, Barton had come to feel that the supplying of such items, often overlooked in the larger want, was the mainstay of her work. "My work was, and chiefly has been to get timely supplies to those needing," she would write in 1908. "It has taught me the value of 'Things.'"[9] At many places the ship edged up to tiny points of land where the outstretched hand of a staff member released a bundle before they hurriedly steamed away. Where they could, however, the Red Cross workers visited the destitute families in order to assess the situation and more effectively give aid. In this way they foiled both those hoping for handouts and those too shy to ask for help. At larger towns Barton entrusted the stores to a few citizens who knew the area and would see to their equitable distribution. For the demoralized families, who rowed out in skiffs or frantically waved handkerchiefs from the boggy shore, a sudden visit from Miss Barton and the *Throop* was an unforgettable experience.[10] As one victim of the floods wrote:

> At noon we were in the blackness of despair—the whole village in the power of the demon of waters—hemmed in by sleet and ice, without fire enough to cook its little food. When the bell struck nine that night, there were seventy-five families on their knees before their blazing grates, thanking God for fire and light, and praying blessings on the phantom ship with the unknown device that had come as silently as the snow, they knew not whence, gone, they knew not whither.[11]

Barton was aware of the mystique surrounding the boat, believed that it had a certain value, and at times actively cultivated it. She enjoyed appearing out of the sleet and mist like a miracle or apparition; the sense of being an answer to a prayer, of arriving unexpectedly when hope was gone, gave her the same gratification that her startling appearance on the battlefield had twenty years earlier, and she knew it also lent drama and prestige to the burgeoning Red Cross. When the *Josh V. Throop* nudged up to the shore, she saw relief, thankfulness, and *interest* in the faces of the needy. As they steamed away she noted with satisfaction that they left on shore "an astonished *few*, sometimes a *multitude* to gaze after and wonder who she was, whence she came, what that strange flag meant, and most of all, to thank God with tears and prayers for what she brought."[12] Once they learned the meaning of the Red Cross flag, few of these people would ever forget it.

Barton was not the only one to see the dramatic appeal of this mission. From the moment of her arrival in Evansville, the press covered the journeys of the Red Cross on a daily basis, with lengthy feature stories, supplemental background articles on the organization's history, and interviews with its indefatigable president. The Associated Press made it a "standing rule . . . to handle all Red Cross matters liberally."[13] The *Chicago Inter-Ocean* installed a reporter on board the *Josh V. Throop* to get firsthand coverage. Barton further encouraged press reports by having staff members write glowing accounts of the work and send them to newspapers around the country. Thus the *Evansville Courier* commended the relief efforts of the Red Cross, done with "flying colors and willing hands."[14] The *St. Louis Democrat* eagerly announced Barton's arrival in that city.[15] And day after day the *Chicago Inter-Ocean* praised the work. "Of all the schemes for the relief of sufferers along the course of the lower Ohio," an editorial proclaimed on March 22, "none have been so thoughtfully planned and so wisely executed, none have been so careful and painstaking to its details and so beneficent in its results as the relief expedition of the Red Cross."[16] Nothing, of course, could have pleased Barton more than this widespread publicity. With one great rush it had accomplished all she had been trying to do since 1877. The press coverage had, as she told Joseph Sheldon, "*tied the knots* in a warp and web of seven years."[17]

Barton hoped the publicity would show her organization's professional and businesslike face to the world. But she also shrewdly took advantage of the romantic temper of her day by encouraging reporters to stress especially pitiful cases or those that radiated the strength of human courage and hope. One notable story was written by Barton herself and widely published under the title "The Little Six." Six children in Waterford, Pennsylvania, had given a variety show, the proceeds of which—$51.25—were donated to the Red Cross. Barton chose to keep the contribution separate, to be used for a family whose progress could be reported to the children and the press. All along the Ohio she kept the sum in mind, and when the *Throop* came upon a widow with six children, living in a corncrib near Shawneetown, Illinois, she saw an ideal spot for the contribution. "There was misfortune, poverty, sorrow, want, loneliness, dread of future, but fortitude, courage, integrity and honest thrift," noted Barton. The Red Cross workers listened to the woman's story with misty eyes, told their own sentimental tale, then left her with boxes of clothing, fuel, and the gift of the Little Six. Hearing the story, the donors were delighted and advised the Red Cross president that "sometime again when you want money to help you in your good work, call on the 'Little Six.'"[18] Such stories were satisfying to readers, who wanted to believe that their donations were going to worthy victims, and they gave a more human picture of the suffering than did statistics on damage or record water levels. In addition, pieces such as "The Little Six" justified the work of the Red Cross by highlighting activities that were beyond the scope of government relief.

As a result, contributions and requests to join the Red Cross poured in. On returning to Evansville after the first trip up and down the river, Barton was surprised to find the small town inundated with checks, crates, and boxes of every sort. Whereas Hubbell's modest excursions on the Mississippi in 1882 and 1883 had raised only $8,000 and $18,000 respectively, the Red Cross in 1884 solicited contributions of over $175,000.[19] The Chicago Red Cross chapter alone sent more than $5,000 for distribution. For years Barton had been used to thriftily checking every dollar and finding the funds still short. On this mission she could write with relief: "We have always enough."[20]

In late March, Barton heard disturbing reports of flood conditions in the lower Mississippi Valley, and believing the distress to be greater there than on the Ohio, she changed her field. With difficulty she found another boat—the *Mattie Belle*—and a crew willing to brave the still treacherous Father of Waters. On board were Hubbell, "Hail" Chaddock, Andrew Leslie, who was president of the St. Louis Red Cross, and his secretary, Octavia Dix. John Hitz joined the party as they set off on April 2.[21]

Much the same work was done along the Mississippi as had been done on the Ohio. Barton and her staff found the people more impoverished and more difficult to reach. At time the *Mattie Belle* became stuck in the shifting Mississippi sand bars, and Barton had to don long rubber boots and wade through the mud to reach the needy.[22] Stranded and starving animals were an especially acute problem. Clara's love for dumb creatures, and her realization of their importance for the rehabilitation of farming areas, prompted her to be especially attentive to their rescue and feeding. It was a tricky business to care for stock when people were known to be starving, but she managed it so well that one press report, critical of other aspects of her aid, acknowledged the vital contribution she made in this area.[23] In order to reach the most people in the shortest time, she adhered to the pattern she had followed aboard the *Josh V. Throop*: find a landing, "visit the worst places, stay long enough to learn the real needs, and supply them. . . . This is the original *style* & spirit of real Red Cross work."[24]

Whenever possible Barton entrusted the distribution of supplies to local people, frequently taking care to include blacks on the committee to ensure that no one would be overlooked. The items she brought were the bare essentials—salt, meal, meat, nails, lamps, fodder, and clothes—but, after all, the needs were basic. She knew that the Red Cross could not replace losses but only offer people a boost until they could manage their lives again.[25] Rarely did she give cash. Frequently there was no place to spend it, and if there was, she, like Hubbell, had found that the victims "would never take the money and purchase that *needed* article, and half the time they would never know what they did get with it."[26] Money, at best, involved a long delay in order to change conditions.

The voyage of the *Mattie Belle*, like that of its predecessor, was highly emotional. "Never a day that did not bring us incidents to be remembered, sometimes sad and touching, sometimes laughable or ridiculous," Clara would recall. Local women or little girls brought flowers on board at every landing; military and government boats saluted the little steamer; tearful blacks knelt by sacks of grain and declared Miss Barton a messenger from God.[27] Little boys on rafts fought swirling waters, waving a bandana handkerchief as they poled away with kerosene, coal, or chicken feed. People clambered on board the boat when they heard Barton would talk on the Red Cross, and when the decks were full they lay on the roof above to hear a bit through the cracks in the boards. Astonished families watched the workers unload lumber, nails, and shingles, and assemble a makeshift house, the only shelter some had seen for a month. "But the most touching of all," remembered Barton, "was the honest gratitude which poured out on every side." [28]

Added to this daily emotional upheaval was the strain of shipboard relations. Most of the staff were old and ardent supporters of Barton, but in Andrew Leslie the company found a professional skeptic. He recognized the necessity of the trip but found gaps and omissions that disturbed him. "The truth is I have been considerably disappointed," he wrote confidentially to a friend. He saw that long distances were passed without explanation. Expenditures seemed less than the distribution warranted, and he could find no accurate accounting scheme. "I suppose the matters will not be scrutinized very closely this time," he concluded, "but it should not be repeated." [29] Alarming, too, was Barton's habit of keeping only her own counsel and her growing fatigue at the end of the journey. Toward May she directed matters from a day bed, though she was anxious that this not become common knowledge. [30] Barton and her supporters believed Leslie to be merely a troublemaker who amused himself by poking fun at the Red Cross president. On one occasion, when Barton spent an extraordinarily long time ashore and Leslie declared that those remaining on the ship were "waiting there for the old lady to die," several men threatened him with physical violence. [31] They later had him censured for his "discourteous conduct towards the president of the Association ignoring her position, judgment & Executive ability," and his "irregular usurpation of power." [32] Loyal as they were, however, some of Barton's aides also worried about her indecision and poor health. Between Hubbell and Chaddock ran a note that questioned whether "Miss Barton was losing her mind, or that she is getting too old to know just what she wants to do." With ears to the ground for any hint of criticism, they covered her mistakes, kept certain information from her, and defended her devotedly, but they privately discussed ways to persuade her to resign. [33]

Tired as she was, Barton elected to join the last leg of the relief expedition. In late May, her work along the Mississippi completed, she again hired the *Josh V. Throop* for one last trip down the Ohio. In the spring sunshine she observed the progress that had been made in the three months since she had first seen the devastated area; with pride she noted her accomplishments. It was all she could have hoped for in field work: government cooperation, abundant funds, personal contact, tangible results, and acclaim by press and public. [34] The Red Cross had proven itself, and this pleased her enormously. "We have tested its power and ability to sustain and encourage," she bragged to Adolphus Solomons. "We have proved that the Red Cross can start instantly, in small funds, without procrastination . . . sustaining itself through the heaviest campaign . . . and come out firm financially and socially with unblemished confidence and undisturbed integrity." [35]

In early June 1884, Clara returned to Washington, more exhausted than she cared to admit. Her head remained clear enough to enable her to tackle the mountain of letters that had accumulated in her absence, but she was confined to her bed for several weeks.[36] With a look, she quickly silenced those who suggested that the relief work took too much out of her, and she insisted that the bed rest was just a selfish indulgence. Sensitive about her age and her record of poor health, she was afraid that others would find her unequal to the task of directing the Red Cross. When she traveled to Dansville that summer, therefore, Barton took pains not to alert the press or to advertise her weakened condition to other members of the Red Cross.

She did reveal her condition, however, to Gustave Moynier and her longtime Senate supporter, Omar D. Conger. Both men were urging her to attend the Third International Conference of the Red Cross, which was to take place in Geneva at the beginning of September. Barton, though anxious to cement the role of the United States in the international organization, felt too weary to undertake such a responsibility. "I have not got my usual strength back again," she told Conger, "and am still weak for such a journey under *favorable* circumstances."[37] But when Secretary of State Frederick T. Frelinghuysen insisted that she was the only American who could properly represent the country at this conference, she reluctantly consented. With hesitation she thus accepted the first appointment as a diplomatic representative ever offered to a woman in the United States. Adolphus S. Solomons, long recognized for his philanthropic work both in and out of the Red Cross, and Joseph Sheldon, now serving as counsel for the organization, were also appointed. After much ado, involving dressmaking and the finding of appropriate companions, the group sailed for Europe.[38]

The conference began on September 1. American journalists, reporting on this type of international gathering for the first time, were dazzled by the opulent entertainments and the array of distinguished representatives, all of whom seemed to sport splendid decorations, ceremonial military uniforms, or colorful diplomatic sashes. The eighty-five delegates represented twenty-two countries; officials of another dozen nations observed the proceedings. Eight-course dinners and lavish receptions, given by the city of Geneva, the Swiss state, and individuals such as President Moynier, took place every night and all day Saturday and Sunday. Fireworks and military parades were interspersed with the more formal functions.[39]

More sober were the proceedings held during the day. Morning assemblies considered such topics as the position of the national organizations in peacetime, the role of ambulance drivers, and the garnering of supplies for use in war. Barton, motivated by her experience at the close of the Civil War, led a discussion of the methods used to identify the dead and wounded in war, and Judge Sheldon gave a well-received address that detailed the achievements of the American Red Cross in disaster relief. The conference was impressed with the job Barton and her associates had done at the time of the Ohio and Mississippi floods, and with the expanded vision of Red Cross work that she had espoused in America. After hearing of their work, of their hopes and plans for making the American Red Cross an organ of peacetime relief as well as a military accessory, the conference voted to adopt these principles as part of the international treaty. The amendment provided that "the Red Cross societies engage in time of peace in humanitarian work analogous to the duties devolving upon them in periods of war, such as taking care of the sick and rendering relief in extraordinary calamities, where, as in war, prompt and organized relief is demanded." In a lasting tribute to Clara Barton, this addition to the treaty of Geneva was entitled the "American Amendment."[40]

In the afternoons, demonstrations were held that highlighted various surgical techniques, new designs for hospitals, ambulances, and medical stores, and improved methods of military field work. Barton, whose philanthropic career had, after all, begun with an interest in battlefield relief, was a keen observer at these demonstrations. She was particularly impressed with the portable field hospitals, which could be transported long distances, came equipped with their own surgical supplies, and offered better shelter than the flimsy army tents. Most spectacular, however, was the afternoon spent displaying the uses to which the newfangled electric light could be put in clearing the battlefield of dead and wounded. Clara, like many others who had seen firsthand the terrors of warfare, came away saddened by memories of the men who had frozen to the ground or lain for three days without help on the battlefield of Virginia, but stimulated with hope for the "humanization" of warfare.[41]

The American delegation was more than welcomed at their first international Red Cross conference: they were fêted and honored wherever they went. Joseph Sheldon's speeches were attended with much greater interest than the usual cursory respect shown the speakers, and the humanitarian work of Adolophus Solomons was acknowledged when he was elected a vice-president of the conference.[42] Above all, the convention became a personal triumph for Barton. Everywhere she went she was in demand; at every reception and committee meeting her opinion was sought. The *New York Daily Graphic* gloated:

> Scarcely had the American representative, Miss Clara Barton, arrived, in Geneva before she became a centre of attraction, and I might almost say homage. Her perfect inobtrusiveness yet dignified appearance, her manifest good will, and deep interest, yet also the evident ease with which she deported herself in so distinguished a deliberative assembly constituted her at once as if by common consent the peer of the foremost members of the conference.[43]

With the greatest of esteem the company singled her out for public honor. As the conference came to a close, the Italian delegate sprang to the platform and proposed that Clara Barton was deserving of the highest praise and thanks of mankind for bringing the United States into the Geneva Convention.[44] At another point in the midst of a speech, the assembly broke out in a cheer at the mention

239

of Barton's name. "For her especially it was a triumphant success," Sheldon acknowledged, "and if she should ever go to another such meeting she will be certain beforehand of a reception fitting and due to her."[45]

Barton turned these personal accolades into a larger triumph for women. Four other women were representatives at Geneva, but she was the only one to participate in all of the proceedings as a complete equal of the male delegates. It was in many ways a difficult role. In a society in which women were still discouraged from participating in public affairs, in which they were booed from speaker's platforms and denied access to government leaders, the simple fact of her presence aroused curiosity and comment. "To see on the platform a woman who represented the government of the United States was to this audience . . . a novelty," admitted the New York Tribune.[46] But as she had broken the barriers at the Patent Office and had persistently changed the opinions of senators and cabinet officers, so did she pass this test with courage and poise. Her simple attire and unassuming manners charmed the delegates, and her well-known achievements in the United States and numerous foreign decorations filled them with admiration. Barton's connection with the German court also aided her, for the Grand Duchess Louise had instructed her delegates to assist Barton in every way. "How it smoothed and opened the way for me, a woman alone, to take a man's part among so many men," Clara wrote in thanks.[47]

All of her life Barton had broken traditions, not by verbal protest but by determined action; she expected fair treatment and allowed no person to deny it. Now, in 1884, she made it plain that she saw herself the equal of the other national representatives. At the same time, by her own excellent example, she smoothed the path for other women, who could now point with pride to the dignity she had brought to the United States as its official representative. Antoinette Margot, who watched the proceedings from the gallery, was overwhelmed with the thought of what Barton's actions meant for the social emancipation of women:

> I have in the last weeks looked on to see her sitting in one of the grandest assemblages of men that could be gathered . . . acknowledged as possessing every right and privilege belonging to any delegate in that assemblage, no less a national Representative than any. . . . This had been an instance of acknowledged women's rights, never before seen in these countries, and as I believe, never known in the world.

For women everywhere this was not an isolated event but a beginning, a promise of change. "Miss Barton has not proceeded to batter down opposing walls with a sledge hammer," Margot concluded, "but has quietly and skillfully opened a door with a well-turned key; it will never be closed."[48]

The convention lasted only a week, but Barton stayed on in Europe for several months. Before leaving the United States she had been selected by a private group as delegate to the Universal Peace Union, to be held in Geneva immediately after the International Red Cross Conference. She remained for this and for private meetings with Moynier and Dr. Appia.[49] She tarried to visit with Antoinette Margot's family and to revisit Strasbourg, where so many sad and productive days had been spent. Upon the receipt of an invitation from the grand duchess, she arranged to go to Baden to meet the Empress Augusta and bask in the honors of that court—"a boon," Barton wrote, which she would "prize all the days of my life." At this meeting the empress awarded her the silver Augusta Medal, given for outstanding humanitarian work, a huge and heavy decoration that was highly regarded in Germany. Laden with honors and charged with renewed enthusiasm for her work, Barton finally sailed for home near the close of November.[50]

Eighteen eighty-five proved to be a lackluster year. Barton's tour in Europe stimulated her to a high level of excitement and energy temporarily, but in the longer term it eroded her already precarious health. When she returned to America she was once again confined to her room, suffering from a lame back, weak bowels, and overwork.[51] As soon as she gained a little strength, she made a long trip to New Orleans to complete a task she had undertaken for the German Red Cross. The Crescent City was, that year, the site of the Cotton Centennial Exhibition, a world's fair and trade exposition that was expected to attract millions. The German Red Cross had persuaded Barton that this would be the perfect place to publicize the organization's work and had made her their delegate to the exhibition. Barton arrived in New Orleans late in December, surveyed the fair and conferred with leaders of the New Orleans Red Cross chapter. They hit upon an eye-catching idea for an exhibit and persuaded exposition officials to set aside one day for a Red Cross celebration. The exhibit was to consist of large silk flags from every signatory of the Treaty of Geneva, arranged in a spectacular pattern over the main archway of the exhibition buildings. Barton enthusiastically launched into a campaign for procuring the flags and official greetings from the participating countries. Ill-health tempered her activity, however, and she was forced to remain confined, unable to leave New Orleans until the late spring.[52]

Barton had, as usual, left no one in charge in her absence, and she had no secretary to help her with the never-ending mail, which collected and worried her. She felt herself growing depressed at the thought that she would never get beyond the everyday routine and be able to tackle relations with the government, reorganization of local societies, or protection for the Red Cross insignia. She knew not how to dispense with the correspondence, felt every piece should be answered, could not bring herself to delegate the work to others. Yet she yearned to find "time for better thought than I can get with a mandatory mail pouring in upon me *five* times every day of the week. . . . I want more time, and some good help toward thinking out the reorganization of the Red Cross, if indeed it is to be put upon a living basis."[53]

Though the New Orleans exhibition was a success—crowds flocked to see the flags and the press gave the Red Cross significant attention—it could not justify the precious hours Barton had expended on its organization.[54] The American Red Cross was still badly in need of funds, publicity, and new, energetic blood; nods of approval and good intentions from society leaders who visited the display were of little value to her. Despondent, she made plans to go to Dansville for a quiet summer. Barton's single solace was the news that Antoinette Margot was coming from France to work as a secretary in her household. Memory, fealty, and the fact that Barton needed her help and companionship had influenced Margot's decision. Clara's expectations for the visit were high, as were her hopes for the season at Dansville. Mentally she planted the old garden and renewed her acquaintance with Harriet Austin and other friends.[55]

But Dansville was also to be a disappointment. The journey was uncomfortably long and tiresome, and Clara found Doctors Austin and Jackson preoccupied with their own projects. Her house was in an unsettled state, and Margot, upon arrival, was diffident and silent. There was trouble, too, about a family who had been subletting the house from her, and for whom the community felt she was responsible. Local talk reached an uncomfortable pitch, and a court case ensued. The whole situation caused Barton to become increasingly defensive and unhappy. For months the case dragged on, as she "waded through perplexity, malice, injustice and danger." Finally, early in 1886, with a pretty little speech and amidst the fanfare of the town, she gave up her long beloved home and left Dansville for the last time.[56]

Barton's removal from Dansville was one of many changes that took place in her personal life during this decade. It was something of a transitional period, in which old influences and sources of strength disappeared and new friends and opportunities appeared to replace them. Longtime friend John Hitz became embroiled in a scandal involving the Swedenborgian church, and Clara reluctantly saw him leave the Red Cross fold. The strain between Barton and Margot was another such painful change, and its impact was the greater because neither woman had expected it. Margot found the "noise and confusion" of Clara's erratic household disturbing, and Barton thought the younger woman silly, self-indulgent, and overly charmed by the Catholic faith: "one of those unsteady unbalanced minds that must be controlled."[57] Like so many other once-zealous admirers of Barton, "beloved Kitty" would leave her service with a certain rancor.

Thus Barton was left without a protégée, and at the same time she lost her mentor. Frances D. Gage, so long a prisoner of her paralyzed body, had died in November 1884. The news was so painful that Barton could neither speak nor write of it for nearly six months. When she did, it was to express deep sorrow and pity: "her faithful, strong loving letters full of faith and trust come no more—No friend loved me as well or trusted me as much—capable faithful, grand strong loving Mother."[58] No other woman had been such an inspiration to Barton, and no other would serve as her model in the future.

Worse yet was the loss during these years of the last of her immediate family. On March 15, 1888, David Barton died on the family farm at North Oxford. Stevé wired the news to his aunt, then sent a long letter that shocked her. Though Clara destroyed this missive, and all other evidence, there is a strong indication that David committed suicide. For some years he had been in financial difficulties. Stevé and Clara had tried to help in 1881 by buying his farm and allowing him to stay on it, but from time to time he had still had to face the indignity of asking his younger sister for a loan.[59] His wife had reported him to be "figity & nervous" and given to hypochondria.[60] But it is Clara's own words that point most directly to a tragic end to David's life, for her reaction was far from the sad acceptance that should have accompanied the natural death of an eighty-year-old man. "I know the worst," she wrote in distress to Stevé only five days after David's death. "I have no words! It is all so dreadful, so shocking, so pitiful. To what misery he must have been driven. God pity him, and pity us, and save us." She worried about the effect on David's sensitive daughter Mamie, who lived near the scene, and on the reputation of the family. "How *will* they endure it at home? It is enough to kill them all. How frightened shocked and timid they must be." She wanted desperately to help but for once found herself hesitant and afraid. "I have not written Mamie. I don't know how to," she confessed. "I feel a kind of fear to communicate where so awful a thing has transpired."[61] Clara did not attend the funeral (if indeed there was one, for there was no announcement in local newspapers) and, as she had with Stephen's robbery, Dolly's mental illness, and her mother's neurosis, kept the dark knowledge a secret in her heart. She was nonetheless filled with a profound sense of isolation. "This was the last of my family proper," Barton sadly told a friend, "no brother, nor sister left: one feels very much alone. Am almost timid to be in a great world like this—all alone."[62]

New faces appeared as the old ones passed into memory, some of them to be only temporary anchors, others to remain steadfastly in Barton's life for her remaining twenty years. Increasingly it was to women that Clara turned for trust and love, though several young men became valued friends and assistants. Dr. Lucy Hall, the ambitious physician at Sherborn prison, flattered the Red Cross president by viewing her with much the same respect that Barton had felt for Aunt Fanny. Now a staff member at Vassar College, Hall wrote affectionate letters to her "Ma" and included Barton in every feminist or medical activity that came her way. Hall's fealty was shared by Enola Lee, with whom Clara had worked during the Ohio floods in 1884. The Red Cross activities filled a gap in Lee's life, and she was converted completely to Miss Barton's work. When she married Dr. Joseph Gardner of Bedford, Indiana, a few years later, she brought him into the fold, and for years the two were among the most active Red Cross workers and the closest of Barton's personal friends. They in turn introduced her to a brilliant, creative young man named John Morlan. He would have a far-reaching impact upon her life. Morlan was hard-working, handsome, and possessed of the dash that so often caught Barton's eye—and was so often her undoing. In many ways he exemplified the new friendships made by Barton during this time. Each one was based as much on a commitment to the Red Cross as on a personal understanding, and in each case loyalty was prized over companionship, or even integrity. The 1880s thus marked a changing of the guard among Barton's friends. Where memories—of North Oxford, Clinton, or the Civil War—had been the cementing force between Clara and her acquaintences, future hopes now proved to be the bond.

Against this backdrop of mercurial personal relationships, Barton carried out, as best she could, the work of the Red Cross and the responsibilities impressed upon her by the status of public philanthropist. The various duties weighed upon her heavily. At the same time that she was called upon to survey and help people at numerous sites of unforeseen disaster and to maintain crucial ties with the government, she was besieged by requests to speak at conferences on women's rights, prison reform, religious charity, and professional nursing. Ever mindful of the great need to find sponsors and widespread public support for the American Red Cross, Barton rarely turned down an opportunity to speak on its behalf. She became something of a roving ambassador in the years following the Third International Red Cross Conference. Her name, more than ever a household word, was enough to draw large crowds, and her astonishingly broad career touched on areas dear to many new organizations. To various groups at various times she personified individual initiative, the triumph of the determined woman, Christian charity, or the more romantic side of the Civil War. Between 1884 and 1890, most of Barton's time that was not actually spent in field work was taken up with an exacting round of writing speeches, traveling, and addressing eager audiences.

Yet there was still no one to really take her place in Washington; while she traveled the painstaking work needed to build a strong, truly national network was attempted in little fits and starts. Predictably, the national society failed to gain the momentum it needed to create and interact with the diverse and widely separated local auxiliaries. Barton patiently explained the history of the Red Cross movement to hundreds of audiences, but her own colossal personality tended to overshadow her words. The public held tenaciously to the notion that the Red Cross was the personal charitable organ of Barton, that it was well endowed, and that it was to be commended but needed little material help. The effort she took to popularize her cause thus turned against her with sad irony: while she was away from Washington the necessary groundwork could not be laid to expand the society, and as she spoke enthusiastically of the Red Cross, she found the audience cheering her own achievements with such fervor that they had left for the Red Cross only a few polite claps.

Almost immediately after Clara left Dansville in 1886, she embarked on an extensive tour of the western United States. While there she alternately lectured, was honored, and vacationed among the California mountains. In July she stopped first at St. Paul, Minnesota, to address the delegates of the National Conference on Charities and Corrections, then backtracked a little to Chicago to open a nursing school named after her and to enjoy a few pleasant hours with a protégée, Dr. Mary Weeks Burnett. From there she took a spectacular train trip across the western two-thirds of the United States. She was headed for San Francisco and the National Encampment of the GAR, and she traveled in the private railroad car of the post commander of Massachusetts, adorned with the title of honorary commander of the Massachusetts Women's Relief Corps.[63] In San Francisco she was fêted and fussed over, awarded the gold and diamond pin of the National Relief Corps, and listened to with rapt attention as she nostalgically reminded the company of the glorious war days. "They showed me wounds they said *I* had helped to heal, and stumps of limbs they said *I* had tried to save, and they clustered around me like loving boys and I—I cried and they cried too," Barton sentimentally recalled.[64] After the encampment she encouraged prominent San Franciscans to form a Red Cross society, then set off for a camping trip with friends in the High Sierra.

It was a beautiful, if strenuous, excursion. Dressed in "dark strong calico . . . some immense straw hats, some wide plain ribbons and several yards of veiling," she traveled forty miles a day on foot and horseback to Webber Lake. There she and her friends hunted and fished, supped on venison and wild honey, and reveled in a "sky as clear and blue as indigo could have made it." A few years later she would acknowledge that the "memories of the little camp up among the pines grow sweeter every month."[65]

Before August gave way to an early mountain winter, Barton left California. On her way east she heard of an earthquake near Charleston, South Carolina, that had reportedly left the town in ruins, and she consequently changed her travel plans to go by way of the shaken city. She arrived several days after the quake to find many buildings demolished, the city virtually cut off from outside help, the inhabitants dazed and demoralized, and army and government support inadequate. Barton surveyed the area, visiting an orphanage, an old folks home, the city hospital, and, on what proved to be a haunting visit, the home for Confederate veterans. At each of these institutions she left her best wishes and a crisp one-hundred-dollar bill. In all she expended only five hundred dollars (donated by the Chicago chapter of the Red Cross). It was the tiniest fraction of what suffering Charleston needed, but it was all she felt capable of giving at the time. From the point of view of the Red Cross, the Charleston disaster was, as one observer noted, "an object lesson as to its limitations at the time."[66] Barton and Hubbell were too tired, and too busy, to take charge of the situation, and the Red Cross coffers were nearly depleted. Charleston revived, owing to the generosity of those in neighboring states, but the monies were not distributed through the Red Cross, as Barton had hoped all such relief would be. It would be a long time before the American Red Cross would become the organization that first came to mind in time of disaster.[67]

The situation was repeated a few months later, when the Red Cross was called upon to aid the victims of a twenty-month drought in central Texas. Two crops had been lost, and many people were leaving the state; one source estimated that in Eastland County alone there were close to three thousand destitute people. Reports of the dire conditions had been coming out of the state steadily, but the stories were conflicting and often fantastic, and little had been done to relieve the sufferers. A well-meaning clergyman with the evocative name of John Brown had taken it upon himself to publicize the problem and lobby for its relief. Unfortunately, he had a style that relied more on flair than fact, and government officials and newspaper editors paid him little attention. In January 1887, when he arrived in Washington and sought the help of the American Red Cross, Barton decided to go to Texas herself and assess the situation.[68]

The three-day trip by train, boat, and carriage was made at her own expense and in the company of Dr. Julian Hubbell. They arrived in the dusty countryside around Albany at the end of January, where they soon found that nature was not the only uncooperative force at work. Longstanding battles between cattlemen and farmers, prejudice against foreign immigrants, sniping local politicians, and poor farming methods complicated the effect of the unfortunate weather. The people were not actually starving, as some reports had claimed, but they were in want and had lost hope and the willpower to remedy the situation. "I have no time to tell you how it is," Clara wrote in a note to Fanny Vassall, penned hastily between the jolting drives by horse and buggy, "but can you be sure it is bad enough."[69]

The great need was not for simple handouts but for a future-oriented program that relied on seed, tools, and the determination to begin again. The Red Cross, with its pragmatic bent, was the ideal group to undertake the relief, and Barton was anxious that it should, but she had no more resources to offer than she had had at Charleston. From the Red Cross warehouses she sent what stores she had collected, but she admitted that "they were no great quantity."[70] "What it would be now to have the facilities at hand which the Red Cross should have," an associate lamented. "A corps of experienced workers with ample stores to draw upon? In the absence of these we must give them all the brains we can." With reluctance Barton and Hubbell declined to undertake the field, though in their statement they stressed not the unpreparedness of their own association but the local nature of the disaster. (In fact it was more national in character than many they were to relieve.) As compensation they formulated a plan by which they hoped the disappointed Texans would be able to help themselves.[71]

With the aid of the Reverend John Brown, Barton drafted a report to the Texas state legislature, detailing the suffering and stressing that she had personally observed the damage. On the strength of this and the prestige of Barton's name, the legislature voted that a hundred thousand dollars should be sent to

246

the most devastated counties—not enough to eliminate the distress, but a good beginning. Barton then contacted newspaper editors in Austin, Dallas, and other major cities and asked them to run articles about the drought and to begin a fund, which could be collected through the daily journals. She lent her own name to the drive and contributed the first twenty dollars from her private purse.[72] Reciting the emotional story of the Little Six, she appealed to the children of the state to help, and when President Grover Cleveland vetoed a ten-thousand-dollar congressional appropriation to the area, she held it out as proof that the proud state must rely on its own resources.[73] In early March Barton and Hubbell returned to Washington, where they tried to arrange for donations of seed and free train transportation for goods shipped to the stricken area.[74]

Clara often pointed to the Texas situation as evidence of the cautious approach the Red Cross took in determining which areas needed disaster aid. This was brave rhetoric; in reality, her experience in the Lone Star State sobered and depressed her. "A long hard journey . . . ," was how she characterized the trip in her diary, "without a dollar of help or return, much strength lost, and time given up that was needed at home."[75] She knew that the Red Cross had not helped in the way that it could have, and as it became increasingly evident that the hundred-thousand-dollar appropriation was inadequate she became ever more despondent. "My heart is sore over these things and has been every day since I left Texas," she wrote.[76] The newspaper campaigns failed to collect much money, and she had to report that she had had a similar lack of success in raising funds along the eastern seaboard. Even her attempts to send boxes of clothing were foiled by ruinously high freight tariffs. In the end it was the timely arrival of the rains, later that spring, that brought hope and renewal to central Texas, not Clara Barton.[77]

Fortunately, each disappointing field seemed to be matched by an initiative that showed the strength of Barton's reputation and drive. As she was musing over the sorry mess in Texas, an opportunity arose to exhibit the Red Cross in Washington in a practical way and cement its relationship with the armed forces. The National Drill and Encampment of the GAR was to meet in the federal city in June 1887, and Barton, ascertaining that the city was poorly prepared to handle the crowds, volunteered the services of the Red Cross for any emergency that might occur. "This is the first opportunity the Red Cross has had to exhibit itself in its true relations, viz as an aid and a part of the military forces of the country," Barton wrote excitedly to the local chapter in Philadelphia. "It will also be the first 'object lesson' the military has ever had and cannot fail to make itself better understood and comprehended by the class of persons for whom it really exists."[78] She convinced surgeons and nurses to come from that branch, obtained tents, supplies, and stewards from the War Department, and set up a model mobile hospital that effectively treated nearly two hundred cases of illness in six days. It was a resounding triumph and caught the eye of the more influential city fathers.

The loud praises of the press were nectar enough, but the week was sweetened further by the fond attention which "her boys" showered on Barton. "The week of the camp was one continuous ovation to Miss Barton," Hubbell proudly announced. "It was difficult to get to her through the throng of persons that had waited years to grasp her hand, get a look at her face or waited just to listen to her."[79] Senators and generals called at her home, and veterans from the ranks lined up to greet her at the Red Cross tent. Said General Dennis: "the Queen of England could not have received greater attention had she been there."[80]

During the same period Barton took pride in another short but glorious field. On February 19, 1888, a tornado struck Mount Vernon, Illinois. Though there was only a small loss of life, the little town suffered great destruction of property through the tornado itself, torrential rains that followed it, and fires that broke out from overturned grates and exposed electrical wires. For unexplained reasons, and with most unfortunate results, the press almost uniformly reported that there was little suffering. A collection was begun by a local committee, but when, after several weeks, their efforts proved fruitless, the local fathers·appealed to Clara Barton for help. Anxious to restore the credibility of the Red Cross, she undertook the work.[81]

Barton's first act was to fetch Dr. Hubbell and set off for Mount Vernon. She stepped down from the train to find wretched weather exacerbating the already bleak conditions. The Red Cross president immediately sent out a series of emotional press releases. "The destruction, loss and needs, are far greater than is realized by the public," she wired the United and Associated presses. "Everything is needed, every aid welcome, and should be rendered."[82] The next day she sent out an appeal that was eloquent in its dramatic simplicity: "The pitiless snow is falling on the heads of three thousand people who are without homes, without food or clothing and without money."[83] The response was immediate. Within two weeks the public sent donations totaling over eighty-five thousand dollars. Money was welcome, but as always it was the familiar items of everyday life that were most useful at such a time. Barton found nearly every family needing something; "*nothing* could be amiss *there*, from a bedstead to a nutmeg grater, or a paper of pins," she informed a donor.[84]

Red Cross activities in Mount Vernon also included caring for the sick, helping to rebuild homes, establishing a school in a large storeroom (the damage at the schoolhouse was declared too vast to be repaired), and organizing societies to carry on the rehabilitation after Barton and her co-workers left. Enola Lee and John Morlan were there to help her, as well as Hubbell, and the work progressed easily. After two weeks they had cleared up the worst of the debris, seen that each family had at least temporary shelter and food, and assured themselves that the city was over the first shock of the misfortune. Feeling that the townspeople were now able to take care of themselves, the Red Cross workers, "with their blessings ringing in our ears," quietly departed.[85]

Before she left Illinois, Barton wrote a letter to the chairman of the relief committee of Mount Vernon. In it she explained her reasons for leaving the field after so short a time. To stay, she maintained, would be to do more harm than good, for continued relief would be "unbearably burdensome, and perplexing, to those peoples who must serve them; inculcating a spirit of dishonesty, and instituting a system of beggary in the place of industry."[86] Not only at Mount Vernon but in all of the work of the Red Cross, this was Barton's essential philosophy. She expounded it before nursing students and ministers, as well as philanthropic leaders, at the Conference on Charities and Corrections in St. Paul in 1886. Professional colleagues at the annual Social Science Conference nodded their heads in agreement when she declared that handouts of food or money did little real good. Instead they caused expectation and dependence. She had come slowly to the conclusion that there was a significant difference between philanthropy and charity, Barton told her audiences. She had, moreover, seen the distinction reluctantly, for it went against all of the precepts of Christian charity and her own impulse to help every miserable creature she saw. But she had found that her good intentions had produced little lasting good. In the 1850s alcoholics had sold her gifts of bread to buy a drink. Two decades later destitute families had depleted her loans without the least concern for economy or future needs, and the children she helped showed a preference for continued beggary to the confinement of the classroom. Her experience at Sherborn solidified the impression that indiscriminate charity stifled initiative and thrift. "Nothing leads more directly to crime, nothing offers so fair and safe opportunities as the temptations that come of beggary."[87]

The Red Cross system was thus set up to aid but not pauperize. Barton clearly differentiated between two periods in disaster relief—the initial stage, during which immediate need is felt and direct help is often needed; and the secondary stage, in which the community is again functioning and the help needed is more educational than material. She frequently saw in disaster relief the opportunity to teach the skills of thrift and financial planning, and these she considered among the greatest benefits her organization could offer. Close observers of the young American Red Cross frequently agreed. "The Red Cross has become a grand educator," ran one commentary, "embodying the best principles of social science and that true spirit of charity that counts it a privilege to serve one's fellow men in time of trouble. The supplying of material wants . . . is only a small part of its ministry."[88] Barton also mirrored the prevailing philanthropic theory by advocating the disposal of funds on the basis of justifiable need, ascertained by the philanthropic organization rather than determined on the strength of an individual's requests. Therein she saw the difference between relief and beggary. She especially deplored those who sent their children to ask favors of the Red Cross, and consistently refused to help those whose condition had not been inspected by one of her workers. "Let it not be said," Barton announced stiffly, "that any child ever learned to beg at the doors of Red Cross."[89]

This idea of reserving help for those who were not only needy but struggling humbly on their own was not too far from the old Calvinist concept, upheld by Barton's family, of aiding the worthy poor. Psychology was only beginning to enter the field of social work, and few professional activists of the time believed that environment, heredity, or ignorance could influence an individual's ability to become a productive member of society. Barton certainly did not. She viewed questions of cleanliness and economy in moral terms, and saw a person's inclination to work as the arbiter of his virtue or degradation. With pride she pointed to an editorial that praised the Red Cross for guarding "zealously against lazy, whining frauds, who shun work (and soap and water) as they would against the deadly Upas tree."[90] To Clara all individuals were accountable for their actions, had control over their destiny, and were responsible to some degree for the social good. "Has the woman, who gossips and drinks away her time, neglecting her children till they suffer, a right to demand that you sustain her home and keep up her family relations?" she asked. "Have the couple who never had seven dollars ahead in their lives but *have* seven little children without food or shelter, and no visible means of support no responsibilities?"[91] She doubted that the family who saw no means of help would continue in indolence and allow itself to starve. Charity, Barton proposed, needed to be divorced from sentimentality and put upon a pragmatic and unemotional basis.

Barton's vision of the Red Cross, however, was viewed with ambivalence by the social theorists of the day. Dedicated charity workers had long realized that there was a need for combined resources, organized methods of action, and well-recognized figures of authority to whom the nation would naturally turn in times of trouble. This was exactly how Barton saw the Red Cross, as an organization whose purpose was not so much to "increase the *amount* of charitable work done, as to *systemize* what we have, and bring some *order* out of our past chaos of irresponsible unorganized and unsystemized work in that direction. It has been in everybodies [sic] hands long enough," maintained Barton. "The Red Cross essays to bring it into *sombodies* [sic] hands, and make that somebody responsible for the manner in which it is done."[92] This desire to cast the nation's humanitarian efforts under a large and hospitable Red Cross umbrella was, however, at odds with other cherished notions of the philanthropic community. While many social workers applauded any effort to systematize their profession, they also greatly respected the traditions of community responsibility and believed that local citizens often knew best how and where to dispense relief. Many of the problems the early Red Cross encountered were due to confrontations with old and well-established local agencies, which resented outside interference, especially when it showed signs of self-righteousness. Increasingly, Barton also ran into conflict with professional zealots who wanted to eliminate charitable work done by any who did not have academic training and scientific motivation. However scanty her early credentials, Barton's own role had long ago been accepted by her cohorts, but she often had trouble justifying the bumbling actions of the volunteers who surrounded her. She made sincere attempts to interest doctors, nurses, and social workers in the Red Cross, but, for the most part, her own efforts were fleshed out with the very amateurs who, in the current trend of professionalization, were despised. Though agreeing in theory with the need for more skilled workers and greater system in relief work, Barton necessarily found herself having to praise workers with little training and to defend those whose judgment she could not always trust.[93]

One reason Clara was so interested in attending conventions and speaking to her colleagues was her ever-present concern with maintaining the reputation she had fought so hard to build and with placing herself among the professionals of her field rather than with the benevolent-minded ladies' sewing clubs. It was for this reason that she undertook the representation of the American Red Cross at the Fourth International Red Cross Conference in 1887. Tired and moody, she had little inclination to go, even though it was to be held in Carlsruhe, the seat of her beloved Grand Duchess Louise. She did not volunteer her services, but instead "kept very quiet with a kind of childish hope of not being observed."[94] The grand duchess begged her to come, and the secretary of state appointed her, however, so in the end she felt she could not refuse. The conference was held during the final days of September, amidst a court resplendent with the confidence and wealth of the newly unified German state. Doctors Hubbell and Lucy Hall accompanied Clara but saw little of her once they arrived in Carlsruhe. Barton was made an official guest of the palace and spent much time tête-a-tête with Louise and her other friends at court.[95]

"It was a presence not to be forgotten, that body of nearly one hundred and fifty delegates from the governments and countries of the entire civilized world," Barton wrote enthusiastically after the first day.[96] The company discussed many of the same problems they had spoken of in Geneva, with an emphasis on medical techniques, and refinements to the portable hospitals, which were increasing in popularity. The question of relief to nonsignatory countries was hotly debated, and methods of reducing losses in naval warfare took up an entire day. Barton's contribution was a speech on behalf of protection for the international emblem, which was being cheapened by manufacturers who used it to legitimize and sell their products. "Thus we are met by 'Red Cross Cigars,' 'Red Cross Brandy,' 'Red Cross Whisky,' 'Red Cross Washing Machines,' 'Red Cross Playing Cards,' 'Red Cross Churns,' 'Red Cross Soap,' and 'Red Cross Dog Collars,'" she told the convention. To her gratification they unanimously passed a resolution requesting the various signatory powers to pass laws restricting the use of the sign.[97]

The noble subjects of the daytime discussions were no match, however, for the brilliant entertainments offered after hours. The gentlemen once again appeared in dazzling outfits, and Barton did not hesitate to compete by covering her chest with medals. (Several new royal jewels graced her bosom, including an extraordinary amethyst, two inches across, carved in the shape of a pansy and suspended from a pearl and diamond pin. It was to become Clara's favorite among her jewels, and she was rarely seen without it.) Even Barton was over-whelmed by the "state receptions—royal dinners, excursions, royal operas, and theatre, musical entertainments, mainly within the palace, where our royal Host and Hostess were in constant attendance." Impressionable Lucy Hall could do little more than gush. "Shall I ever see another reception which will not appear tame after that 'wondershönes' one which was our last in Carlsruhe?" she asked Clara a few months later.[98]

When the conference closed on September 30, Barton received an invitation from the royal family to spend a few days with them in Baden-Baden. There she met the aging Kaiser Wilhelm, who recognized the Iron Cross he had awarded her fifteen years earlier and asked anxiously after the German immigrants that had settled in America. Otto von Bismarck greeted her, too, and these scenes, offering again the kind of recognition that she felt she had never received in her own country, touched her deeply. After leaving Baden she stopped in London, where she looked up old acquaintances and contacted one she could have gladly foresworn—the inevitable English bronchitis. At the end of October she arrived home, tired, sick, but with her spirit rekindled by the conference.[99]

Barton's presence at these conferences was by now so accepted that although she and Hall were the only women allowed on the floor, little fuss was made over them. Political feminists were, nonetheless, anxious to harness her expertise and prestige. The conference marked a turning point in her relations with the suffragists, since for the previous four years she had participated in only a few of their activities. There had been a number of reasons for this: ill health, pressing Red Cross business, and some unfortunate misunderstandings with major figures in the movement. Barton was also still anxious that the Red Cross not be allied too closely with the political aspirations of the women's rights organizations. Again and again she was compelled to point out that the Red Cross was not "some or other organization of *interested women*, endeavoring to do what good they can, like e.g. the WCTU, or WRC, or AAW or any other arrangement of the alphabet," and that, unlike these groups it had "legal confines beyond a constitution and By-Laws of its own conception and making."[100] When, in addition, Barton tried to make it clear that she had neither the time nor the energy to devote herself full-time to the feminists, she was often misunderstood. Several women's rights leaders began to question her loyalty to their ideals. Kate Gannett Wells went so far as to state that Barton did not really believe in woman suffrage; Clara answered acidly that she had shown a great deal of reticence in not telling the movement's leaders how to run their organization. Suffrage, she continued, was something that might as well be restricted as expanded, and though she could "see no good reason why that restriction should be made along the line of sex," she told a horrified Wells, she "should be likely to be found upon that question . . . in favor of *discriminative* rather than universal suffrage."[101] This letter, and her reluctance to expend all of her spare energy on suffrage issues, kept her on probation with the women in Boston and Syracuse for several years.

Another incident further divided Barton from the suffragists during these years, and caused personal heartache as well. In 1885, at the request of Alice Stone Blackwell, an editor of *Woman's Journal*, Clara sent a series of dispatches, purportedly from the Dakota Territory, stating that the time was ripe for a vote there on woman suffrage and that the territory seemed to favor it. This was a delicate subject, for similar referenda in other states had uniformly failed, partially because of poor timing. When, after a space of several months, it was discovered that Barton had never set foot on the western prairies, there was a sharp reaction. The feminists were anxious to legitimize their work, and it was just this sort of shady statement that they believed kept them from being taken seriously.[102] At the time of the discovery Barton was in Texas. She was shocked and humiliated that Susan B. Anthony had publicly criticized her, going so far as to question whether her dispatches from Texas were of the same sort as those from Dakota. Barton hastened to write her old friend an apologetic, indeed obsequious, letter. "I was pained for what it implied and for the manifestation of your opinion in regard to my reality and sincerity," Barton told Anthony. "I was still more grieved for my own loss, that of the rest one feels in the loving confidence of a friend unshaken by suspicion; one is sorry to lose such out of life." Eventually Barton and Anthony were reconciled, but it was several years before Barton would appear publicly with the suffragists.[103]

When, on the platform at suffrage conventions, Barton claimed, "This is not my place. It is not my right. I have not toiled as you have toiled," she was saying less that she had no interest in the ballot than that her aspirations for women had a broader horizon.[104] To her the vote remained an issue, but only one of many challenges for women to face. In her own life she would happily have sacrificed the vote for educational opportunity, fair employment standards, fair pay, and fair judgments by a society that often did not even try to understand her. Without these, Barton believed, the ballot would be a shallow privilege. Thus she encouraged countless young woman to "put by your embroideries and your laundry . . . and commence your studies," and she rejoiced when they heeded her advice.[105] Clara applauded the growth of women's organizations such as "Sorosis" (a New York society of which she was an honorary member) because they allowed for an exchange of ideas and the chance to learn the principles of organization and cooperation. In response to a social invitation from Sorosis she penned a charming rhyme that illustrated her belief that such gatherings offered women more than a chance to gossip.

Sorosis my child was a pioneer
When pioneers were rare
Among the matrons prim and staid
And the maidens shy and fair.

When Pater familias due at his club
Was never in the lurch;
And the women sat demurely
In vestry and in church.

Sorosis, my child, was a pathfinder
And the track was oft doubtful indeed;
But with forehead erect she bore on her way,
And the weaker grew strong in her lead.[106]

Barton found proof of the expertise gained in such organizations at an 1888 meeting of the Woman's Christian Temperance Union. She was extremely impressed with the attending women, whom she found to be competent, organized, and skilled in debate. She noted wryly (and she was in a position to know) that the gathering was decided superior to many meetings held by men, which frequently degenerated into evenings of drinking and carousing.[107] Women, she concluded, were coming of age; they were breaking out of the historical confinements with astonishing speed. "There have been great women in all ages, but never an epoch when *all* women were so great . . . ," she wrote proudly. "Women begin to *dare* to do, aye, dare *be*, even, for the time has been when the ordinary woman scarcely felt that *this* belonged to her. . . . Think of a 'Woman's Club' fifty years ago: of a 'Woman's Council' where women could have met with ideas worth expressing, and have had the social liberty and the courage to express them."[108]

Nonetheless, Barton gave renewed emphasis to the question of suffrage at the conventions and rallies she attended in the late 1880s. At meetings of the New England Woman Suffrage Association, International Woman's Congress, National Woman Suffrage Association, and American Woman Suffrage Association, she lent both her formidable powers of speech and her noted reputation to the cause. In 1888 alone she spoke at seven different suffrage rallies. Always she emphasized women's intellectual and moral equality with men, and ridiculed the idea that she should go begging, hat in hand, for treatment that should be fundamental to every human being. "I have never been able to see any difference between [men and women] and have never held them, their rights, interests or privileges in any manner distinct, the one from the other," she proclaimed. "The state and society has need of both and the same law that restrains or binds the one should, I fancy, do the same for the other."[109] Later, in one of her most effective feminist speeches, she put the matter even more clearly, and the result was a statement that reflected the strength of her intellect and foresight.

Whenever I have been urged as a petitioner, to *ask* for this privilege for women, a kind of dazed, bewildered feeling has come over me. Of whom should I ask this privilege? Who possessed the right to confer it? . . . Virtually there is no one to give her the right to govern herself, as men govern themselves, by self-made and self-approved laws of the land; but in one way or another sooner or later she is coming to it. And the number of thoughtful and right-minded men who will oppose, will be smaller than we think; and when it is really an accomplished fact, all will wonder, as I have done, what the question ever was.[110]

So busy was Barton with speech making and other public appearances that even her relief work seemed at times to be wedged in between bouts of conventioneering. In August 1888, in the midst of an usually heavy lecturing season, disaster again struck and Barton volunteered the services of the Red Cross.

The crisis this time was yellow fever, a recurrent threat in the southern states. In 1888 it had grown to epidemic proportions in the area near Jacksonville, Florida. The New Orleans chapter of the Red Cross reacted at once, since many members had experienced firsthand the perils of the disease. In cooperation with the Howard Association, an old private charity founded to aid victims of yellow fever, they offered to supervise the relief. Barton was inundated with hundreds of applications from nurses who wished to go to Jacksonville, but, anxious that the nurses themselves be immune to the disease, she allowed the Red Cross in New Orleans to pick their own candidates from among those who had had wide exposure to it. Early in September a band of thiry nurses, white and black, male and female, left New Orleans for the stricken city to the east.[111]

Leading the group was Colonel F. R. Southmayd, a one-armed former Confederate officer and at that time the energetic secretary of the New Orleans Red Cross. For years Barton had corresponded intimately with this man, who not only held her in the utmost admiration but was bursting with enthusiastic ideas for the promotion of the Red Cross. As Clara once told him, "no one comprehends the spirit of our work as you do, no one has or can work as effectively as you, next to you is my inestimable young friend Dr. Hubbell but he has neither your views nor experience and probably would never develop your organizing power."[112] Not immune to yellow fever herself and determined to fulfill her previous engagements, Barton forwarded money and instructions to Southmayd and firmly placed the entire supervision of the nurses in his hands.

The trust proved, as it did with so many of her confidants, to be misplaced. Southmayd was, in Barton's euphemistic phrase, "a man of quick impulse and intense feelings."[113] He arrived in Jacksonville to find several groups competing for control of the nurses. Moreover, he believed the accounts of yellow fever were exaggerated and the martial law established to provide order in the area confining. Though the relief organizations, under Surgeon J. Y. Porter, were made up of "earnest, warm-hearted workers," they were badly in need of organization, a task Southmayd took upon himself to attempt. This attitude, though possibly justified, was certainly resented. Southmayd soon found himself in confrontations with both the army and local doctors.[114]

Far worse were the scandals caused by his own nurses, whom he had evidently picked without determining any qualifications other than their resistance to yellow fever. On arrival in Jacksonville, he had let them loose with only minimal supervision. Several of the nurses were charged with drunkenness, one having snatched an alcoholic medicine from the lips of his suffering patient. Another nurse appropriated Red Cross funds for his own use, then disappeared, and several of the female nurses were branded as prostitutes and ordered to leave town. On September 16 and 17 the New York World carried long descriptions of these problems under the headline "Drunken Red Cross Nurses," charging that they had come to Florida to "prey on the sick." Sputtering with rage, Southmayd contended that the charges were false and provoked fights with newspapermen, doctors, and other nurses until he himself became the chief liability of the Red Cross. Finally, on September 22, Dr. Porter sent a dispatch to Barton, requesting that she "confer a favor on me by withdrawing Southmayd. He is a hindrance to me in my official capacity." Barton readily complied with the request, then sent Hubbell south to investigate the situation.[115]

The publicity of the New York World cast a long shadow on Red Cross activities. It was the organization's first experiment in actual nursing services, and the conflict tarnished its reputation in this area for many years. (During the Spanish-American War, for example, two Red Cross nurses assigned to Jacksonville were not allowed to work under the society's badge, because Red Cross nurses were considered "women of the town."[116]) Sadly, it also meant that much of the good service done by the Red Cross in Florida was overlooked. At MacClenny, a small town some thirty-five miles from Jacksonville, ten nurses jumped from a moving train when they found that the town had been cut off because of the rampant yellow fever. It was not yet known that the disease was carried by mosquitoes, and all traffic—and help—coming to MacClenny had been halted. The nurses arrived in a dreadful rainstorm, shed their wraps, and proceeded to work for seventy-two straight hours, many of them without food, to bring comfort to the distressed families. Yet far less coverage was given to these heroic workers than to those who drank, pilfered, and wenched.[117]

The effect of the adverse publicity was evident, too, in the dissatisfaction Barton felt about the role her subordinate had taken. Never again would she allow a relief field to be directed by another, even when it meant the sacrifice of pressing Red Cross business matters. Her conviction that she must do everything herself had heretofore held back the expansion of the Red Cross. For the next ten years, influenced by the poor experience in Florida, she would continue unswervingly in that path.

Clara was bitterly disillusioned by Southmayd's conduct, which she came to think of as a personal betrayal. A year later, after the first shock had worn off, she viewed him as nothing but "a bag of tricks, full of conceit, and not too straight, the less attention he gets the better for his case, for all he is after is notoriety and the gratification of the most stupendous vanity."[118] These comments were made to close personal friends, however; her public declarations carried quite a different tone. "I stood by him when all the world left him," Barton admitted.[119] Unable to acknowledge her mistake and afraid that the government would withdraw from its affiliation with such a notorious organization, Barton defended both Southmayd and the nurses. She claimed that the nurses had been "more troubled than trouble" (which had in a few cases been true) and that most of the excitement had been caused by the resentment whites felt in dealing with black nurses.[120] She gave orders for Red Cross workers to keep mum about the matter, in fact to deny any knowledge of the affair.[121] But in the end, after Red Cross solidarity had been demonstrated and the guilty parties recalled, she could only sit back and wait for the public to lose interest. "We drew a long breath of relief when the frost came and it was over," she wrote in retrospect, "and thanked fortune it was no worse."[122]

The "great yellow fever Epidemic, scare and farce combined," as Hubbell termed it, left Barton wondering what direction the Red Cross should next take.[123] So many problems still beset the association, problems she had not the money, staff, or time to solve effectively. The national organization still had no professional staff to carry on the work, and the local societies needed supervision. Philadelphia's medically minded group had become strong and independent by neglect; Milwaukee's had turned into a social club that sponsored dances and outings instead of philanthropic works. The national office had lost control not only of these groups but also of the ones that proceeded "to 'form a society' adopt its insignia, or in short set up a Red Cross of their own, never realizing that they are treading on the grounds of an international treaty."[124] Finally Clara gave in to the feeling that new regulations were needed for the local auxiliaries, and she completely suspended the formation of new societies until they were devised. To those who criticized this move she pleaded pressing national and international work and the folly of too-rapid expansion. "Long life. Slow growth," she told one who questioned the matter. "You have seen the difference in the growth of an acorn and a squash seed. The Red Cross is an acorn."[125] Barton's personal impressions were not so sanguine. Without grassroots support, she doubted that the Red Cross would survive in the United States, either as a popular movement or as a branch of the government.

She was also desperately anxious to strengthen her ties with the government. The Red Cross needed financial support, a stronger commitment from the military, and protection for its insignia. The Red Cross brandy and Red Cross dog collars about which she had complained in Carlsruhe were still appearing on the market, and her attempts to obtain a patent for the badge had come to naught.[126] Abroad Barton had been able to see the full favor the Red Cross held with the European governments, and the experience had been frustrating. "In no other country does the organization of the Red Cross stand as an ordinary benevolent association, in all others its relation to the govt is pronounced and its prestige assured," she wrote angrily.[127] She saw that the Cleveland administration was largely indifferent to the treaty and rejoiced when a Republican, Benjamin Harrison, was elected in 1888. She knew, however, that it would take more than a new administration to secure the concessions she wanted. Skillful lobbying, "some good friends at court," and a credible reputation were necessary.[128] In sum, as she told John Hoyt, the governor of Wyoming, in a remarkable letter, the Red

Cross could no longer continue on its present disjointed, hand-to-mouth basis: "'here and there,' 'now and then,' will not establish it any more than it would make a success of *any business* operation. And it must take up the same methods, if it would live and be of use to the world." [129]

It is significant that Barton saw so clearly, at this early stage, the pressures on the Red Cross. Often, for the sake of propriety or out of fear of criticism, she denied the perplexities that beset the organization. The questions she outlined so directly to Governor Hoyt were the very ones that would haunt her in 1904, when detractors from within and without judged her to have been oblivious to the real needs of the Red Cross. In reality she was all too aware of the defects and weaknesses of her self-proclaimed "child," but she felt unable to overcome them herself and was reluctant to let others take over the task.

Yet no one was more eager than she to lighten the burden she had undertaken. Barton's personal correspondence, diaries, and private notations for the years 1884–89 are filled with references to her weariness, periodic ill health, and financial strain. "One thing I think I make clear," Clara announced to a group with whom she was discussing reorganization, "viz. that I alone carry it *no further.*" [130] She was working nineteen hours a day, and still the correspondence piled up, the requests for lectures poured in, and every area of the country seemed to beg for help. Her private purse was being depleted at an astonishing rate. She alone had paid the nurses at Jacksonville their four thousand dollars in salaries, had sponsored the Red Cross activities at the National Drill of 1887, had even paid for the meals on board the *Josh V. Throop* and *Mattie Belle.* Barton complained to nieces and friends that the world pulled her "in every direction," that it made her "'feel old and grumpy.'" [131]

Yet she hesitated to relieve herself of the burden—or the honors. That she should give up the titular head of the association seemed unthinkable. "I am never certain if I should continue the active work of the Red Cross," she wrote candidly in her diary. "That I will hold the National Presidency, & the International relations is not a question." [132] Barton hoped to find someone who would carry on the day-to-day work of the Red Cross, but her subordinates disappointed her, and no one strong enough to lead yet willing to remain in her shadow ever seemed to come to her attention. With a sigh, Clara made some moves toward a reorganization but inwardly resigned herself to the status quo. To Enola Gardner she pleaded forgiveness for her inaction, saying that she felt like "a horse which has fallen in the harness, and either *can't* get up, or thinks he can't, without help. I fancy how he feels lying there still, till someone unbuckles the harness and helps him up. But as no one comes to my aid, yet I expect to lie where I am." [133]

Barton planned to discuss reorganization and other matters at the annual meeting of the American Red Cross on June 8, 1889. Before the meeting could take place, however, a disaster of such magnitude occurred that all of Barton's worries and hopes were eclipsed by the need to hurry again to the field.

Johnstown, Pennsylvania, located at the junction of Stony Creek and the Conemaugh River in the southeastern portion of the state, had often endured spring floods. But in May 1889 the rains were unusually heavy, and after a week much of the city lay under water. Then, discomfort turned to tragedy when a dam, used to create an artificial lake for a gentlemen's sporting club, broke ten miles away. A wall of water and debris thirty feet high rushed down to kill nearly three thousand people and destroy millions of dollars in property.[134]

In Washington Barton waited just long enough to confirm the almost unbelievable reports, then made hasty preparations to depart. She rounded up a few nurses and wrangled a pass aboard the first train allowed into the city. She was in such a state of excitement that when several medical students offered her and a young female nurse their place in the sleeping car, she uncharacteristically accepted rather than face the next day with jangled nerves. The area surrounding Johnstown had also been inundated with water, and the train's progress was slow. Finally, on June 5, five days after the disaster had occurred, Clara arrived at Johnstown. Barely had she stepped off the train when she commenced work—work that would continue nonstop for almost five months.[135]

The scene that awaited the Red Cross workers was so ghastly that at first they could not take it all in. Barton's disjointed recollections of the town were of pouring rain and upended houses and the "half-clad poor," who stood staring with dazed eyes at the spots where they had last seen relatives and friends. Determined as always to personally assess the destruction, Clara made a reconnaissance tour her first priority. "I cannot lose the memory of that first walk on the first day," she wrote as she left the field the following November. "The wading in mud, the climbing over broken engines, cars, heaps of iron rollers, broken timbers, wrecks of houses, bent railway tracks, tangled with piles of iron wire, bands of workmen, squads of military—the getting around bodies of dead animals, and often people being borne away. The smouldering fires, and drizzling rain."[136] Along the way she found the Pennsylvania Militia officer in charge of the terrified city, a General Hastings, and informed him of the arrival of the Red Cross. To her annoyance, he had never heard of the organization but waved her on with a certain skepticism.[137]

Hastings might well have been confused. The chaos at Johnstown was created as much by the huge numbers of outsiders who arrived to gawk, speculate, or help, as by the rubble and rain. One group of foreigners, which came to be called "the Huns," settled into Johnstown expressly to loot the dead bodies as they washed up. The undertakers who had been brought in from Pittsburgh to supervise the grisly business of identifying bodies found that they did not like each other and decided to go on strike. Many relief agencies spent more time feeding themselves than the starving Johnstown citizens and frequently counted among their ranks professional thieves who "relieved" the poor of what little they had left.[138] The chief of police, in exasperation, finally issued a statement aimed at eliminating some of the charitable people who had flocked to Johnstown: "There are too many relief committees and not enough workers. There are more relievers than sufferers. Almost every man you meet here has on a lot of yellow ribbon. A lot of dudes came down here and think more of filling their stomach than relieving the poor." [139]

Fortunately the Red Cross, though little known, was held in suspicion for only a short time. Barton set up headquarters in a tent, with a packing case for a desk, and began soliciting supplies, sending for workers, and answering the mountains of requests that came her way. The Philadelphia chapter sent doctors and nurses and proceeded to establish the area's only official hospital. When, after a week, carloads of lumber, clearly marked with a Red Cross, began to arrive (a donation from the citizens of Iowa), the local officials decided to take Barton and her workers a little more seriously. [140]

Disease had been one of the gravest fears of town officials; under such conditions of decay and overcrowding they thought it likely that an epidemic of measles or typhoid fever would break out. This fortunately did not happen. Food was also less of a problem than had been anticipated. It was shelter and clothing and hope that the victims needed, and in the early days it was the latter that was desired most. Few families had escaped without the death of a beloved member, and ninety-nine families were wiped out altogether. [141] Barton looked with pity on these people whose grief was so great that they had not yet begun to feel their material wants. "Their every thought is turned upon the heaps of debris which possibly contains [sic] some member . . . of their family," she told a clergyman who wished to know what the people needed. "They do not know if they are hungry or naked; they watch and wait the blasts of dynamite that throw up the ground, and then rush to the spot to see what it reveals. . . . These poor people do not yet realize that they are not in their own homes as fully as they will later." [142] As the depressed families began to pick up the pieces of their lives, Barton sent Red Cross workers to their camps and homes to find, on an individual basis, the best route to recovery. The rich had suffered as well as the poor, she noted, and were often less able to function with only the necessities of life than their less privileged neighbors; Barton did not, as did a number of relief organizations, ignore this class of citizens. In all, the Red Cross contacted and aided twenty-five thousand people, the largest number of any relief organization present. [143]

Of the Red Cross initiatives, the most significant was its plan to provide temporary shelter for the homeless. "This is the first great want leading all others," Barton observed. [144] With the lumber donated by the state of Iowa, they erected a "Red Cross hotel" and then, when it was filled within a few days, proceeded to build two more. The design, contributed by Hubbell, consisted of a long central hallway, flanked by suites of rooms. Communal activities, such as eating and socializing, took place in the central well; privacy was offered in the adjoining rooms. The walls were raw pine, the furniture a hodgepodge of crates, castoffs, and pieces salvaged from the heaps of debris. But to families who had been living in waterlogged tents or the living rooms of friends, the surroundings seemed palatial. The first hotel was opened on July 27. Recognizing that the people of Johnstown were as hungry for conversation and relief from their anxiety as they were for scarce fresh vegetables, Barton gave a modest tea party to celebrate the opening. The tables were set with white cloths and wildflowers, and the guests, so accustomed to sad thoughts and sad pursuits, found to their surprise that they could still laugh and talk. "As the sun went down we found them still there," remembered Clara, "reluctant to break up a party so novel and grateful." After the opening the management of the hotel was given over to a local woman, who was allowed to charge no more than twenty-five cents per day but could keep any profit for herself.[145]

So the summer went, with the Red Cross distributing goods, building houses, fitting clothing, and forming committees to carry on the work after their departure. Fifty workers were with Barton, including John Morlan, Julian Hubbell, and the Gardners. They prided themselves on their ability to work well with everyone; there would be no repeat of the mess at Jacksonville. The army and the Children's Aid Society found them congenial, and even when the Philadelphia group complained that Barton was "dictatorial, inefficient, and much too old," she smilingly left them alone to do their medical work and continued to supply "things."[146] Barton was enormously proud of this work, which she termed "phenomenal and exceptional." At Johnstown, she knew, the Red Cross had made an awesome contribution, one that had significantly touched the lives of thousands of people.[147]

She was frustrated, therefore, that the press—which was ravenously collecting every tiny fact about Johnstown—had not given her work the coverage she believed it deserved. The country still remained ignorant of Red Cross aspirations and achievements, and this glorious opportunity to educate it was being woefully ignored.[148] Barton invited not only her nephew Stevé but other members of the National Red Cross to observe the work, and she urged congressmen and senators to examine the Red Cross in the field. Disappointed when she received no reply to these invitations, she desperately prodded some influential members of the central committee. "In Heaven's Name, De Graw," she wrote in exasperation, "as a charter member of the Red Cross from its very night of birth *can't* you set something better than this on foot?" No one, from the humblest reporters to the president of the United States heeded her call, and Barton was left to deplore the "*self-imposed* and *self-permitted ignorance of my country people.*"[149]

By the end of September, Johnstown was beginning to undertake some of the activities of a normal town. Stores were open, schools in session, churches functioning, and the people clothed. "The town is improving wonderfully," Barton wrote a friend. "The hammers are so busy that one is troubled to hear what another says. All the houses come up like mushrooms in the night."[150] Under such circumstances the Red Cross stuck to its principle of leaving before its help demoralized the citizens. At the end of October the remaining workers packed their bags and prepared to depart.

If the national press had forgotten to praise Barton, the townspeople of Johnstown would never forget her. The forty thousand dollars she had expended had been utilized so skillfully that the governor of Pennsylvania believed "not a single case of unrelieved suffering is known to have occurred in all the flooded district." Moreover, the destitute had been treated with such dignity that "the charity of the Red Cross had no sting, and its recipients . . . [were] not Miss Barton's dependents, but her friends."[151] The women of Johnstown bought her a local "medal," a fine pendant of gold and platinum, encrusted with diamonds and sapphires. "To her timely and heroic work, more than to that of any human being," wrote the *Johnstown Democrat*, "are the people of the Conemaugh Valley indebted for whatever may be their favorable circumstances and condition of to-day."[152] The *Johnstown Daily Tribune* preferred to express the people's feelings more poetically. "Hunt the dictionaries of all languages through and you will not find the signs to express our appreciation of her and her work. Try to describe the sunshine, try to describe the starlight. Words fail."[153]

fifteen

Barton's arrival in Washington was greeted by a cheering throng, which had gathered at the Willard Hotel to honor her. But though the applause for Red Cross activities at Johnstown ended after the November 2 reception, the work did not. For nearly a year Barton was pressed to answer requests for information, work out financial details, and finish the packing of supplies.[1] The stickiest problem involved the three Red Cross hotels. Once the organization had built the hostelries and turned them over to private landladies to run, Barton considered its role finished. But the location of the buildings, rumors of excessive fees and drunken brawls, and the accusation that the presence of the hotels was holding back the local construction business caused them to be unpopular. Only a month after she left Pennsylvania, Barton began to receive letters of complaint. "I hear that the popular name for it is '*the bummer's retreat*,'" wrote one influential man of the Locust Street hotel.[2] Barton had hoped to keep at least one hotel standing as a permanent monument to the Red Cross relief work, much as the temporary clinic started by the Philadelphia auxiliary became the foundation for a permanent hospital. She had an emotional tie to the Locust Street hotel, for it had been the first and best building erected by the Red Cross at Johnstown, and, she told Dr. Hubbell, "it is *not* without pain that I give the order to blot it out of existence before it shall have even sheltered one body from the blasts of the coming winter."[3] Under pressure from local leaders, however, she did give the order to dismantle the buildings. Furniture, supplies, and several freight cars of boards were shipped to Washington.

The boards were sent to three lots on Kalorama Heights in northwest Washington. Barton had purchased the land in 1890 out of her own funds, with an eye to building a large new headquarters and warehouse for the Red Cross. The property, which overlooked Rock Creek and bordered on the city's most fashionable section, was an important investment; for this reason she became increasingly hesitant to build anything at Kalorama that might jeopardize its future value.[4] As she debated the question to herself, an offer came for some land in Maryland, near the old Chesapeake and Ohio Canal. Two brothers, Edwin and Edward Baltzley, were building a residential and social community at a site they called Glen Echo, some seven miles from Washington. The plan included buildings for a branch of the national Chautauqua, a popular movement that promoted education and productive recreation in an atmosphere combining the more pleasant elements of a summer camp and a country fair. The Baltzleys hoped to attract a cultured—and monied—elite to the community, which they titled "the new Washington Rhine." The presence at Glen Echo of a body as well-respected as the Red Cross, they believed, would give a kind of sanction to the project and promote sales. The brothers therefore carefully explained their plans to Barton and offered to donate land and workmen if she would move there at an early date. The cultural tone of the development appealed strongly to the Yankee in Barton, as did the offer of some free land. Even when it became apparent that the Baltzleys were in financial difficulties, that lot sales were moving slowly, and that the brothers were looking to her for financial support as well as prestige, she remained pleased with the entire idea. To Cousin Delia Robbins she wrote effusively, "I am a *solid* Barton as you know and not *apt* to get enthusiastic but really *this* thing does make its way to my heart."[5]

Dr. Hubbell made plans for the building, along lines similar to the Locust Street hotel. It was to be a combination of office, home, and warehouse, larger and more solidly built than the houses at Johnstown, but with the same design of a central hallway with rooms and storage space opening onto it. Throughout the spring, teams of workmen labored on the huge building, and in early June Barton and her household made arrangements to move. The area surrounding Glen Echo was still decidedly rural, and Clara looked forward to a summer in the countryside and the expanded facilities she would have. "I think I shall like my new large fresh rooms among the trees," she told Cousin Delia. "For once, I hope to have *space* enough to work live & move in. That is *all* I crave in a house."[6] Her plans for a peaceful life at Glen Echo, however, were premature. It turned out to be a "rough and tumble" existence in a half-finished building with a leaky roof, inadequate bedding, and insufficient cooking facilities. To make matters worse, Barton, in her enthusiasm, had invited Stevé's delicate wife, Lizzie, to stay for the summer. Clara, who turned seventy that year, could stand (and in some cases relished) the spartan style, but Lizzie was shocked at the crude life. The episode created bad feelings in the family, and as a consequence Clara felt a good deal of remorse. "I should have *known* I could not make an elegant family comfortable where I could not be comfortable myself and should have had the wisdom and firmness to have said so," she apologized to Stevé.[7] Bitter memories, inadequate shelter, and inconvenience—for it took half a day to reach Washington—drove her away from Glen Echo. During the fall of 1891 she decided to use the entire space as a warehouse and moved to a hotel in the city.[8]

Not the least of the reasons that Barton was so interested in securing larger quarters was her desire that the Red Cross appear to be a large and flourishing organization. The poor little rooms on Vermont Avenue gave the Red Cross the appearance of being a kind of garret association, run on a shoestring by a small band of aging zealots. This was, of course, not far from the case. But Barton had not forgotten her pre-Johnstown plans to examine and restructure her organization, and she was now anxious that it appear to be as she envisioned it: an important international body, with strong links to the government, solid financial footing, and the patronage of, in her words, "the best people."

The key to this status was the passage by Congress of two bills, talked of so long and still so far from reality. The first would incorporate the Red Cross as a national body, with sole and absolute authority to aid the military in case of war and an annual budget commensurate with its official position. This was no more, Barton argued, than was outlined in the treaty, and far less than most of the other signatory powers provided for their societies. The second bill called for protection of the insignia from commercial or unauthorized philanthropic use. Red Cross whiskey and Clara Barton cigars had now been joined by a Red Cross brewery and the use of the international badge on the medical products of the burgeoning Johnson and Johnson Company. Far more threatening was the adoption of the symbol by various charitable organizations, which were not at all associated with the treaty. It was imperative, Barton maintained, that the Red Cross badge be used only by the official organization, so that in time of war its neutral status would not be undermined. The two bills were prepared during 1890 and 1891, with the legal assistance of Judge Joseph Sheldon, and were presented to Congress late in 1891.[9]

Because they followed closely the Red Cross success at Johnstown, the bills were expected to be passed without hesitation. Nearly every cabinet officer appeared to favor the legislation, and President Cleveland was solidly behind it. Furthermore, after a decade of service to the country, the Red Cross was no longer a stranger to the members of Congress.[10] Senators, Barton informed Judge Sheldon, now took occasion to say they had watched her work with "grateful respect"; "none of them speaks to me now, as if he were conferring a favor, he comes out of Executive Session, sits down, and says he is '*honored by the call.*'"[11] She and the rest of her executive committee were surprised and disappointed, therefore, to find that the Congress was in no mood to speedily pass either bill, but sent them to committee for review, where they eventually died. The society's troubles, which Barton had hoped would be swiftly resolved, were thus prolonged indefinitely.

At the same time Clara was moving to change the structure of the national organization. She consulted actively with her closest advisors; then in May 1893 she held the first meeting in nearly ten years. Reports were given, somewhat tardily, on the various fields of relief, then discussion was opened about the relation of the local societies to the national body. It was decided that the executive committee should be small and permanent and that its members would not be elected but appointed by the president. Half were to be charter members, half to be prominent government officials. The local societies would have no autonomy; their existence was solely for the aid of the national organization. Dues were discussed, as was the possibility of two classes of membership—one for "the high grade people," the other for the ordinary interested citizen. Action was taken on a few of these issues and a new constitution was drafted and approved. At this time the name was changed to the American National Red Cross. [12]

Barton was determined to straighten out these administrative matters before she became bogged down in another project that would rob her of time and energy. Dedicated as she was to disaster relief, she saw that it was drawing the Red Cross away from its primary purpose of providing aid to the military. There was danger in being associated too closely with domestic philanthropy, for it made the Red Cross appear to be just one of the many selfless organizations that labored without the prestigious backing of an international treaty. It was time to turn slightly away from disaster relief (which Barton admitted was "*not* a legitimate part of the treaty work of the International Red Cross, but rather a pasttime [sic], a kind of 'knitting work'") and make a concerted effort to establish the correct relations with army and Congress. [13]

Thus, where disaster relief had been a priority in the 1880s, the early 1890s saw a drive away from field work and entangling projects. Funds were sent to victims of a great fire in Milwaukee, but no Red Cross workers arrived on the scene. [14] Barton made a few trips to survey damage from drought in South Dakota and storms in Kentucky, and she assigned John Morlan and Julian Hubbell to do the same in Texas and Iowa. In all cases the Red Cross made token contributions but undertook no extensive field work. [15] When New Orleans requested help from floods as damaging as those of 1884, she replied that they had not the staff to send to the area, but that (in a phrase that indicated the degree of separation then existing between national and local societies) they certainly did appreciate the New Orleans chapter's "loyalty in referring to us for leave to act after all this lapse of years." [16] Other works were also shelved. Plans to begin publication of a monthly Red Cross journal were dropped for want of energy, and all calls for speeches and interviews were politely declined. Even when Barton was approached, indeed, positively begged, to prepare an exhibit for the World's Columbian Exposition in Chicago, she held back. "We can see nothing but loss, labor and disappointment in tearing up where we are and transporting to Chicago," she told Morlan. "It would entirely break up our summer leave us poor in purse, probably vexed and disappointed, and all for what? . . . A very small part of what would be required to exhibit at Chicago, would make and keep our Headquarter's [sic] here." [17] In the end Barton did put together a small exhibit, consisting chiefly of the flags she had collected in 1885, but only because she feared that the public would believe the organization defunct if it did not make a showing.

It was with difficulty that Barton kept the Red Cross from reacting to every small crisis that beset the country. She had briefed the press so well that at each calamity the Red Cross was flooded with requests for attention—and corresponding criticism for inattention. Inevitably, the organization succumbed to some of the pressure. Late in 1891, the press began highlighting an issue that finally became impossible for the Red Cross to ignore.

For several years the grain harvest on the Russian plains had been poor; in 1891 it failed completely. Disastrous weather conditions were the immediate cause, but the weather only complicated the notoriously backward agricultural techniques and crippling taxation system, which left little surplus for lean years. The devastated area was the richest section of the Russian Empire, the "bread basket" that supplied much of the rest of the country. Fifteen of its twenty districts experienced total crop failures. As a result there was want far beyond the stricken region; it was estimated that some thirty-five million people were starving. The Russian government and several individuals, notably the author Count Leo Tolstoi, were attempting to help, but poor transportation and the sheer magnitude of the problem foiled them. From St. Petersburg the American minister wired: "The present famine is one of those stupendous catastrophes which almost baffle description." [18]

All over the United States, relief societies and subscription funds to help the Russians began spontaneously appearing. By the 1890s the country was less isolationist than it had been thirty years before, and its citizens were far more confident of their ability to aid others without jeopardizing their own security. *The Northwestern Miller*, under the direction of editor William C. Edgar, declared that there was enough grain on the floor of every mill in the United States to save a starving peasant. In Iowa, the *Davenport Democrat*, under the leadership of Benjamin Franklin Tillinghast, started a campaign that culminated in a veritable crusade to send corn from the state. The Citizen's Permanent Relief Committee of Philadelphia, and that city's Red Cross, launched a most successful program to buy and transport wheat to the famished Russians. The *Christian Herald* started its own appeal, and the governors of eight states called for donations. In New York a group of influential businessmen and Washington officials formed the Russian Famine Committee of the United States, which raised a record forty-five thousand dollars under the slogan, "Grain from the West, Money for the Cost of Transportation from the East." [19]

It was Barton's association with Tillinghast, a longtime supporter of the Red Cross, that got her involved in this work. Iowa farmers were pledging corn in abundance, and local railroads had provided free transportation to the east coast, but shipping overseas was less certain, and the donors needed assurance that the grain would be distributed fairly in Russia. The Red Cross, with its international charter to which Russia was signatory, seemed the logical solution. It was a bad time for Barton to undertake the work, and she was hesitant for reasons beyond her wish to concentrate solely on the congressional bills. She had often pondered the role a national branch of the Red Cross should play in international wars or disasters. The German Red Cross had sent funds to the sufferers of the Ohio River floods in 1884, but Barton had refused to go to Greece during the Balkan wars a decade earlier and had given only a passing thought to sending aid to starving Serbia a few years later. Such aid, she felt, was beyond the scope of the organization's charter.

What changed her mind in 1891 was the popular clamor for Red Cross involvement, for she still felt that the organization should not go to an area unless specifically requested. She also had a hunch that if the Red Cross were officially designated to deliver and distribute the American grain, it would be a round-about method of gaining the recognition she sought. Congress was debating a bill that called for the use of U.S. Navy vessels to carry the grain.[20] Should these boats fly the Red Cross flag as well as the stars and stripes, Barton surmised, it would be tantamount to a government proclamation that the Red Cross was "its own, and its *only* recognized and authorized agent for such service." For the Red Cross, she wrote wistfully, it would be "everything for it, the grateful summer shower on the parched and dying plant—the food to the famished like those we seek to rescue, for it has worked many a year with small recognition, slender purse, weary head, faint heart, and tired feet."[21]

But the Fifty-first Congress was finding, like so many others before it, that philanthropy was a much more complex business than a simple desire to help others. Many members doubted whether they were authorized to use federal funds for such a purpose and feared political repercussions if they did. Far graver questions were raised about the appropriateness of supporting a country universally thought to have an antiquated, repressive government. Stories of peasants being sentenced to a lifetime in prison for stealing a few turnips and of the anti-Semitic policies of the Russian government were circulated widely, causing congressmen to have serious misgivings about American aid.[22] "Why should we spend our strength and give our money to prolong the wretched lives of these poor miserable creatures . . . ," asked Alexander Johnson, the secretary of the Indiana State Board of Charities. "Every dollar we send to Russia means a dollar given to help support the worst possible government in the world."[23] In its first debate on American humanitarian aid, the Congress thus found itself mired in the same questions plaguing every decision concerning foreign aid that followed: To what extent should the ethical and political beliefs of the recipients enhance or hinder the humanitarian gestures of individual Americans? To what degree does such economic aid bolster a type of government repugnant to the United States? In the end, though the aid bill signified only a small gesture by the government, and despite support from the president and the Senate, the more politically motivated House failed to pass it. If it wished to relieve the sufferers in Russia, the Red Cross would once again have to work on its own.[24]

Upon hearing that Congress had failed to pass the bill, Barton wired Tillinghast that the Red Cross would "set immediately to secure transportation for the Iowa Corn." For five months she collected funds, contacted shipping companies, and arranged for Red Cross representatives to be in Russia when the food arrived. With so many separate bodies working for the relief, there was a good deal of confusion about where to send money or grain. Barton was suddenly faced with the news that the nation's stationmasters were being overwhelmed by crest-fallen farmers, "who in some way got the marvelous announcement into their journals that the fixing of a red cross tag upon any package . . . would insure its *free* transit to New York."[25] Barton received a continual stream of letters from Tillinghast, who worried incessantly about details such as whether the corn should be shipped shelled or on the ear, or whether the Russians knew how to grind it. Others were concerned that the Russians would starve rather than eat corn, which most Europeans considered food fit only for pigs or cattle. "This is no time to educate the people to the use of food they do not understand," wrote Robert Ogden, a rigid and humorless, but generous, Philadelphia philanthro-pist.[26] To ease the pressure on herself, Barton put John Morlan and Samuel Goodyear (a noted accountant and Hubbell's brother-in-law) in charge of finan-cial arrangements, and set Hubbell and Tillinghast to the task of finding a suit-able ship.

Donations of money were disappointingly slow. Many, of course, had already given to the relief organizations in New York and Philadelphia, but even Barton was surprised at the small sum they were able to raise. Tillinghast had secured the use of the S.S. *Tynehead,* a ship of British registry, for $12,500, but after several months it seemed doubtful that the ship would sail. A last-minute dona-tion of $700 from the Elks Club, and some deep digging in Clara's pocket, finally made up the balance; Barton would later recall how large the Elks' donation seemed compared to the checks for ten dollars and crumpled five dollar notes that the Red Cross generally received. Finally, early in May, 229 carloads of corn and flour from Iowa were loaded on the *Tynehead* in New York. It was not the first nor was it the largest of the relief ships to leave the country (the Philadelphia Red Cross and the *Christian Herald* had sent two ships, with cargoes worth $100,000, and the *Northwestern Miller* had dispatched the *Missouri* carrying 5.5 million tons of "sweepings" from its constituents' floors). But it sailed off proudly, amid a flurry of "waving flags and cheers from thousands."[27]

Three weeks later it arrived in Riga and was met by Julian Hubbell, who was already in Europe attending an International Red Cross conference in Rome. More lusty cheers greeted the ship, and Hubbell reported that the local steve-dores vied with one another for the privilege of unloading the precious cargo. Hubbell, in the company of Count Tolstoi, escorted a portion of the grain to its destination. It was sometimes greeted by the benumbed peasants with wild ec-stasy, other times with passive disbelief. Always, Hubbell noted, it was accepted; the Russians seemed to have few problems growing accustomed to the unfamiliar food. Many wished to know the exact names of the people who sent the food, and in some cases women stitched elaborate embroidery on the grain sacks and sent them as a thank you to their benefactors. "From the highest prince to the lowest peasant, all Russia is deeply touched by what has been done by the United States for her hungry people," wrote the *Moscow Gazette.*[28]

269

It was estimated that Red Cross relief fed seven hundred thousand people for one month. This was, of course, only a gesture to a country in which thirty-five million peasants were starving over a period of years. Barton's organization was still too small to be able to harness the immense wealth and energy of the country, and in many ways the Russian famine relief served chiefly to point up the acute problems of the American Red Cross. Compared to the efforts in Philadelphia and New York, the work of the national body was small indeed. The Philadelphia auxiliary would not work with Barton—"her judgment was so poor, her methods so loose and her statements so inaccurate that cooperation was impossible"—and thereby further severed the tie between national and local groups.[29] Barton's faulty judgment led her to delegate financial responsibility to Morlan, a young, inexperienced worker several hundred miles away. A longtime friend named Louise Thomas persuaded Barton to secure special passports for travel to Russia, then through mistake or design announced that she was an official Red Cross representative and traveled throughout the stricken districts with escorts from the Russian government. She came home to complain about the role of the Red Cross and embarrass Barton with her presumption of status and accusations. Because of these factors, whatever small success the Red Cross had had in Russia was matched by a growing public concern about the administration of the national organization.[30]

The political character of the Russian famine relief kept Clara in Washington during most of 1892. She was, in fact, resigned to using the house at Glen Echo solely as a warehouse, for its distance from Washington isolated her at any time that speedy communications were needed. Working from a hotel room, however, was hardly feasible for any prolonged period, and she was still dedicated to the idea of a suitable headquarters for the Red Cross. Barton therefore began to rent a house on the corner of 17th and F streets, about two blocks from the White House. The house was a large, rambling structure, the design of which casually combined elements of several architectural styles. It was known locally as General Grant's old headquarters, because during the Civil War that gentleman, and several other prominent military men, had kept offices there. Naturally, this gave the house tremendous appeal for Clara. It was, as one Barton relative recalled, "a house in which to remember half forgotten stories and bits of history, each and all suggested by the rooms themselves or their contents."[31]

Barton took this somewhat hallowed structure and embellished it with her own vast collection of memorabilia. It came to look something like a museum, as did every house she would inhabit thereafter. She owned few pieces of furniture and her personal life was so simple that she had little desire for the plush chairs, carved tables, or fussy antimacassars so dear to her Victorian counterparts. Barton covered the walls with the huge flags gleaned from around the world, and filled every bare space with photographs of herself and her associates, or souvenirs picked up throughout her remarkable career. There were bunches of wild rice gathered and dried at the siege of Fort Wagner, portraits of the grand duchess, and sketches she had made while convalescing in Switzerland in 1870. Some "curious and beautiful" leather pillows, the gift of the Russian government, graced one reception room, and in another were displayed the pitifully crude utensils she had collected at Andersonville Prison. Her own room was "plain, simple, and devoted entirely to business." The same could be said for the official Red Cross offices.[32] Not one to remain behind the times, Barton had acquired a Remington typewriter, a stenographer who could write shorthand, and a gramophone with which she could dictate letters. The latter alternately amused and frustrated her. "I think this talking into a funnel is the funniest thing I ever heard of," she told a friend with whom she commiserated about such matters. "How did it seem to you when you first did it? How did your own voice sound to you? Mine sounds like some grim old croaker with a *horrible* cold."[33]

A feature of the house that Barton found especially nice was the group of large reception rooms, which could easily accommodate hundreds of guests at a time. For too long, she believed, the Red Cross had been on the receiving end of invitations. It was time the organization played host to those who had helped it and made itself more visible by competing for social as well as political attention. Washingtonians, transient or otherwise, still found socializing an effective way to make contacts, reinforce formal ties, and make under-the-table agreements, and thus the city ran in a breathless whirl of gaiety every winter. "From the first of January to the first of March or the beginning of Lent there is one uninterrupted series of parties day after day," wrote Red Cross vice-president George Kennan.[34] With the acquisition of the headquarters at 17th and F streets the Red Cross stepped briskly onto the merry-go-round.

As one of the grand old ladies of philanthropy, Barton had long been sought after for receptions, balls, teas, and cotillions. She had been a special guest of the president at the inaugural ball in 1889, and she wrote with enthusiasm to her curious nieces about the decorations and supper: "We saw so many nice people, we did not get home till three o'clock in the morning."[35] Invitations to the White House poured in during the sympathetic Harrison administration, as they did from the medical society of Washington and the newly formed Daughters of the American Revolution. She was invited to meet the princess of Hawaii when that young woman visited Washington and to attend a dinner given in honor of Susan B. Anthony's seventieth birthday. Every GAR reunion or visit by a former general brought a flurry of social obligations. Now added to this were the large receptions Barton herself gave. Volunteers from the Homeopathic Hospital, feminists, and a group of ladies who wished to start a kindergarten in the capital all enjoyed her hospitality.[36] A "brilliant" New Year's reception followed, as did a large banquet given for the "Survivors of the Union Army." "I have been in a perfect round of receptions of late," wrote a weary Barton in February 1893, "and if I can hold together long enough I am to have one more and 'quit.'"[37]

This final reception of 1893 was held on February 24. It was a large and lavish affair, and as Clara proudly noted, it was an enormous success. Despite several competing diplomatic receptions and a night session of Congress, over two thousand people attended. Barton stood at the head of the receiving line, resplendent in pearl satin and pink brocade, her bosom covered with foreign medals and royal jewels. Next to her were the charter members of the Red Cross, several senators, Dr. and Mrs. Gardner, and her nephew Stevé. For four hours, she reported, "the throng passed me like a moving panorama." Not trusting a caterer, Barton's own household concocted the refreshments—sandwiches, ice cream, orangeade and lemonade, salads, and cakes—which young girls served.[38] Barton was especially pleased that she had room to seat most of the guests at once and was happy to find that there was food enough and conversation enough to make it a memorable occasion. "It was said," Dr. Hubbell wrote with relief, "that no attention was lacking."[39]

The "lions of the evening" were Joseph and Enola Gardner, and the grand scale of the reception was largely in honor of them. Though Clara had contemplated such an event for some time, her plans were hastened by the desire to announce to the public the "princely gift" the Gardners had made to the American National Red Cross. For many years Barton had hoped that the Red Cross would receive an endowment that would enable it to meet operating costs and ensure its future. In early 1893 there were signs that the moment might nearly have come. In February she received a letter from Dr. Gardner stating that he wished to donate a 782-acre tract of land near his home in Bedford, Indiana, to the Red Cross as a "thank-offering to humanity." The land contained a village, a large quarry of first-rate limestone, stands of timber, and abundant fertile farmland. It was near a railway and had river frontage and several buildings. Gardner stated that he was giving the land to Barton because of his belief in her ability to "make small amounts of money do the work of large ones," and because he believed that the gift would encourage other potential donors to give money or property to meet the steady demands of the organization. He and John Morlan would oversee the running of the farm, Gardner told Barton, "thus relieving you of troublesome details that could as well be delegated to others."[40]

It was not the first charitable gift Dr. Gardner had ever made, nor the first time he had taken a fancy to a cause or unusual pursuit. Born in 1833, he pursued an interest in medicine, receiving a degree from the University of Louisville in 1861. He practiced throughout the Civil War and was one of the first Americans to accept the microbic causation of disease. As shrewd in business as he was in diagnosis, he made a number of spectacular real estate deals and by the 1880s was independently wealthy. Now free to follow his own whims, Gardner pursued his scientific avocations with fervor. Those who encountered him in Bedford noted his distinguished figure, classic features, and trim pointed beard, but shied away from his booming confidence, which frequently appeared authoritarian. The earliest and gravest of the mistakes Clara Barton made in regard to the property, which came to be called Red Cross Park, was to give him too much authority over the acreage.[41]

Barton's second mistake was to allow the deed to be made out, not to the American National Red Cross, but to her personally, and with virtually unlimited powers. She should, the deed stated, "have absolute control of the hereinbefore described lands . . . [and] shall thereafter have full power to govern and manage this trust against all comers, under whatsoever guise, claim, or pretext such comers shall appear." The intent of this passage was to stop those who, through greed or misdirection, might try to use the land for commercial benefit. In the end, however, the deed would be used as proof that Barton had used her office in the international organization to receive valuable gifts, and that she had become incapable of distinguishing between her personal resources and those of the Red Cross.[42]

Gardner had not stipulated a purpose for which the land was to be used, but his bequest fired the imaginations of Clara and her associates. She grandly envisioned the park as the "one piece of neutral ground on the western hemisphere, protected by international treaty against the tread of hostile feet." It would be a sanctuary against invading armies, she wrote; later she pictured it as a kind of wild game park, where buffalos and rare animals would "have a little world of their own—with no guns to molest." Dr. Gardner came up with a number of what he called "castles in Spain," including the establishment of an orphanage, a hospital, a Tired Women's Rest, and a camp for Junior Red Cross societies. Until funds could be collected to build such establishments, however, it was decided to use the land as a farm, the fruits of which would help stock the Red Cross larder against the next disaster.[43]

John Morlan, the youthful worker who had caught Barton's eye in Mount Vernon and Johnstown, was put in charge of the farm. He moved there in March with the intention of raising blooded stock, especially horses, on the property. The idea appealed to Barton, who was still fond of horses, though she had long ago given up riding. From the earliest stages she knew of Morlan's intentions and praised his ability to muster support by "a lot of tall begging," which, she glibly noted, he was "inclined to do in an elegant way."[44] As time went on the young man's enthusiasm became uncontrollable. He pictured the park as an extension of his own interest in racing and race horses, with stables of champion thoroughbreds and a well-equipped race track. Part of the park he thought could be given over to pasture for older horses, a sort of Tired Horses' Rest, complete with a cemetery for the dignified burial of the once noble steeds. Though Barton raised an eyebrow at some of the notions, in the end she gave them her endorsement.[45]

Some of the trappings of Morlan's scheme were already in place when she and Hubbell visited Bedford in May 1893. By this time, Morlan had bought a great deal of furniture, stock, and equipment at Red Cross expense—almost twenty-five hundred dollars worth, it was later found. He had thirteen registered trotting horses on the property, as well as some equally pedigreed dogs, and was building a stable to house them.[46] The news that Morlan was taking the horses around the countryside to races and pocketing the money seemed not to bother Barton at all. On July 4 she accompanied the farm manager to some local festivities. "A trotting race," she recorded in her diary, "Morlan's Jefferson Clay trotted, won 2nd get 30."[47] Barton was in raptures over the possibilities she saw in the farm. A garden and orchard were flourishing and she wandered over fields of wheat, oats, and sorghum "in such quantities it makes one dizzy."[48] In all of this she saw a Red Cross future that was secure, established, financially at ease. "I don't think you ever conferred so much happiness before, as when you thought out that Park and gave it," she told the Gardners.[49]

But it soon became evident that the Gardners had also had personal interests when they gave the land to the Red Cross. On her return from the Midwest, Barton was surprised to find a hasty letter from John Morlan stating that a portion of the property known as the Yocky tract had not been paid for, and that the twelve-hundred-dollar debt must be settled immediately or they would forfeit eighty-four acres of land. It seemed that Gardner had been anxious to get the property off of his hands and that he had planned to sell it piecemeal at a loss if the Red Cross had not taken it. Clara, who had known nothing of these matters, now found that the doctor not only refused to speak about the subject but claimed that his property was encumbered and could not be used to raise funds, and that he was unable to get a loan because of the financial panic which had hit the country earlier that year. From her personal funds Barton therefore paid the mortgage but penned a sharp note to Morlan. "It was a very unexpected call and but for a peculiar precaution which had fortunately been taken might have been most embarrassing, in fact, impossible, considering the situation all around and the times. . . . *Will you please learn positively from Dr. Gardner if there are other liabilities which I may learn later,*" she implored.[50] The chief liabilities, as she would indeed learn, were John Morlan and Joseph Gardner.

Barton's trip to the Midwest had encompassed more than a simple reconnaissance of the Red Cross Park. She had spent a good deal of time in consultation with Gardner and Hubbell about the new Red Cross constitution, the best method of extending local societies, and publicizing Red Cross activities. She visited Chicago to make a brief appearance at the World's Fair, met with the GAR in Indianapolis, and visited with old friends Minnie Kupfer Golay, Mary Weeks Burnett, and Frances Willard. She was tired out by the time she returned home, and her fatigue was heightened when she encountered Morlan's letter and the messy business over the Yocky tract.[51]

For this reason, and because she was still firmly convinced that the Red Cross must concentrate on organizational matters, Barton tried to refrain from any relief work. But late in August 1893 a call came that, like the Russian famine, was impossible for the Red Cross to ignore. The disaster this time was a hurricane off the coast of South Carolina. It was a dreadful storm, one which still held records for death and destruction seventy-five years later. Five thousand people were killed outright as it swept across the low-lying Sea Islands, and buildings, crops, gardens, and boats lay in ruins. The plight of the remaining inhabitants was worsened by the contamination of all fresh water, the loss of their crops just when they were to be harvested, and rains that continued relentlessly for two weeks.[52]

It was initially thought that the entire population of the Sea Islands had been killed, and that there was therefore no need for relief. Then, day by day, the news came in that by clinging to a tree here, a piece of floating timber there, many of the inhabitants had managed to save their lives, if not their property. There were said to be some thirty thousand destitute people, many without even clothing, for the storm had literally ripped the shirts from their backs. When Barton was approached about aiding the victims, she demurred, stating that the work was too much for her small organization; this was a field for government aid. But the state of South Carolina begged off with a plea of poverty, exacerbated by the hard times created by the financial panic, and Congress, which had generously given aid during the Mississippi and Ohio floods of 1884, proved equally recalcitrant. In desperation Governor Benjamin R. Tillman and Congressman M. C. Butler of South Carolina asked Barton to inspect the area and, if possible, give it what help she could.[53]

Barton found the region desolated and the population utterly demoralized. She had no heart to reject their call for help, especially as she was incensed to find that they had been largely ignored because of their race. She had learned well from Frances Gage and Josephine Griffing and had never denied aid to any needy person, black or white. Now in South Carolina, she was ashamed of the government, which turned its back on the blacks. There at the Sea Islands, the very place at which Aunt Fanny had opened her heart to their condition, Barton was all the more determined to assist these forgotten people. She ignored the "discouraging, not to say appalling" messages from local citizens and fellow philanthropists, which warned that she "did not know the negro that he never did nor could be made to work where any free rations, or feeding were given, or in sight, that if provided for he would become at once demoralized and lazy and worthless and probably uncontrollable." Her own experience denied these predictions, and she set about disproving those who claimed that Red Cross methods "would not answer and . . . must fail.[54]

It was not because of racial prejudice, then, that Barton was reluctant to take the field, but because of monetary restrictions and a bone tiredness in her seventy-two-year-old frame. The Red Cross treasury was virtually empty, and her own accounts were depleted by the recent demands at the Red Cross Park. The grave economic worries of the country made once-generous people unusually tightfisted, and her energetic auxiliary societies were either alienated or defunct. Faithful Julian Hubbell and a few others could be rounded up to assist her, but she could count on no large party of relief workers. With the future of the Red Cross in a precarious position before Congress, Barton could not very well withdraw her support from the Sea Islands. Yet after a call for money, tools, clothing, and seeds for the area, she found that her total resources were something under thirty thousand dollars. From the beginning it had been evident that this would be a prolonged work, for it was necessary to provide for the people until their next crop could be harvested, nearly a year later. Thirty thousand people and thirty thousand dollars meant there would be only one dollar per year per person. "The Red Cross . . . has accepted the control of this relief, with both misgiving and reluctance," Barton wrote shortly after the work began,

> and solely because it saw no other source in the entire country, from which these help-less wards of the nation might hope for continued care through the . . . months of desolation, enforced idleness and unsheltered hunger which must at best be their sorry lot. I know that the people here, who understand the situation stand aghast at the burden we have assumed. . . . It only remains to say that such a body of helpless humanity cannot be safely left to chance, or some winter morning the reporter of some enterprising *newspaper* will wake the country and the world up to a 'national disgrace'—*a famine in the sea islands of the United States of America.* It will then be too late to save ourselves; it is for this as well as humanity and duty that the Red Cross stands in this 'forlorn hope' today.[55]

To a reporter who visited the islands she stated the matter more succinctly: "I feel that we are standing on the edge of a volcano."[56]

The familiar topography of the islands, even in their disheveled state, brought back a flood of memories to Clara. Aunt Fanny's rose-trimmed garden, the terrible blood and sand of the siege at Fort Wagner, and the golden moments with dashing John Elwell all seemed very near here. "I suppose you have been in my thoughts many times everyday . . . ," ran a nostalgic note to the old quarter-master. "How could I have charge of Hilton Head and Morris Island and all that lies between them . . . and direct such shipping and boating as was necessary, and not think of the chief quartermaster? If you could know how I have longed for you."[57] Little incidents whirled her back thirty years: a group of veterans of the siege came to pay a courtly call; one old black woman, remembering Barton for three decades, walked thirty miles to see her.[58]

She had little time to be sentimental, however. The islands stretched one hundred miles southward, a huge field to cover, even with good transportation, which Barton unfortunately did not command. Skiffs and small boats were all that enabled the Red Cross workers to reach those in need. Upon their arrival it appeared that everything needed to be done immediately; it was difficult to make priorities when the demands for shelter, clothing, food, and medical care were vying for attention and "30,000 to 35,000 people were knocking, knocking, knocking at our doors beseeching and imploring us in the most heartrending tones to be saved from starvation and perishing from the cold."[59] Surveying the desolation with a trained eye, Barton concluded that although this field would see little of the publicity with which the Red Cross was surrounded at Johnstown, it was in fact a disaster of much greater proportions; indeed she believed that there had not been such necessity for philanthropic work since the wartime efforts of the Sanitary and Christian commissions.[60] Frightened and alone, the Red Cross workers took inventory and prepared to open their doors on October 1. "Tomorrow will be the first day that we shall stand in this great work," Clara wrote in her diary that sleepless night, "all by ourselves, with no help, no funds back of us, and no one to *create* them. It is a perilous situation—if we fail we are lost."[61]

Food, it was decided, was the most immediate problem. From Red Cross rations they could afford to supply only a peck of corn and a pound of bacon per week to a family of seven. The people were encouraged to supplement their rations with fish and to plant winter gardens from the turnips and cabbage seeds that had been donated. The climate was ideal for growing foodstuffs, but the inhabitants were not accustomed to growing their vegetables, and much of the early work involved instruction in planting and cultivating a vegetable patch. Barton insisted on this plan despite skeptics, and no rations were issued to families that did not plant at least a small plot.[62]

As ever keeping a check on the dangers of pauperizing disaster victims, the Red Cross required a family to present chits in order to receive the meal and bacon, and the chits were obtainable only by work. To prepare the land for planting, nearly three hundred miles of drainage ditches were dug with tools that were loaned by the Red Cross and returned each night. One million feet of lumber went into the construction of new houses. Extra work was rewarded with double rations, and the Red Cross found that, contrary to the pessimistic forecasts, the people worked with a will. Organized in teams, generally around a parish church, the men went on to help their neighbors after their own cabins were completed. It was immensely gratifying to Barton and her staff to find that, far from expecting free assistance, the people asked for work.[63]

Nowhere was this more apparent than in the "clothing department," an establishment set up under Enola Gardner and several local women. Donated garments came in every guise, but most often they were torn and dirty, or unsuitable—castoff ball gowns being a favorite donation. To make the clothing usable, island women were recruited to cut, shape, sew, and clean the garments, and to distribute the items to the families most in need. The women were paid with a hot meal and the satisfaction of self-support. The plan, modeled on Barton's sewing rooms in Strasbourg, was similarly successful. The community took pride in its self-reliance and acquired skills useful in less troubled times.[64]

At the field were Barton, Julian Hubbell, the Gardners, John Morlan, and George Pullman, who had joined the Red Cross staff as financial secretary the year before. New to field work, Pullman spent the majority of his time in the trimly appointed, whitewashed office that he shared with Barton, attending to financial details and correspondence. Also among the workers was Dr. E.

Winfield Egan, newly adopted as one of Barton's "boys," who took charge of the medical activities. This skeletal force was fleshed out with a few local volunteers who came to help sort seed potatoes, supervise work forces, and oversee the distribution of clothing. When Joel Chandler Harris, the beloved author of the Uncle Remus stories, visited the islands, he thought the small force personified a marvelous lack of bureaucracy. "Its strongest and most admirable feature is extreme simplicity," he wrote. "The perfection of its machinery is shown by the apparent absence of all machinery."[65]

Beneath the calm surface, however, there were a few staff frictions. John Morlan and the Gardners were, ominously, barely on speaking terms, and Morlan believed Egan was poisoning Clara's mind against him. Indeed, the young man appeared to have a nervous breakdown during the mission, for he fell to weeping uncontrollably and goading the other workers into fights, while begging to be allowed to return to the Red Cross farm. "However courteously disguised for my sake," Barton acknowledged, "the bitterness was everywhere evident."[66] Feelings were further strained by a martyrlike attitude Barton adopted for most of the mission. As always, no matter what the quality or quantity of assistance, she felt that responsibility for the work fell completely on her shoulders, that she worked "alone and unaided."[67] She tried to make up for what she considered slack work by intermittent bursts of supervision, during which she watched her subordinates' activities with such a peering scrupulousness that they were left drained and resentful. "When I think of the *farce* we used to go through down in the packing room," one assistant recalled bitterly, "sitting round all Day & then at night stand with a smoky lamp in one hand & a Barrel Head in the other waiting for the Old Lady to muse over a lot of second hand pants, stockings & Boots it makes me *cuss* yet."[68] Several members of the staff were also disturbed that Barton carried so little weight in Washington that, despite several trips there during 1893–94, she was unable to raise any government monies.

What help the government did provide was in the area of medical service. Doctors Egan and Hubbell had set up a clinic designed for the poorer citizens of the islands; they were anxious not to alienate the area's doctors by luring away the patients who could pay. Malaria was the most common problem they found, with over two thousand cases recorded. On the average the clinic treated seventy-three people a day. But the doctors were handicapped by an inability to get out to the farthest islands to visit those too sick to travel to Hilton Head. Thus the permission Barton gained from the secretary of the treasury to have the revenue cutters *Boutwell* and *Morrill* distribute supplies and to take medical officers to assist the sick greatly enhanced the excellent record of the Red Cross in the area of health care. At the end of the Sea Islands' relief, boasted Barton, not one death from illness was recorded.[69]

"This field of relief work is a strong *steady pull*, without excitement, or urging, rest or relaxation; everyone from leaders to wheel horses pulling for all they are worth," Barton wrote in January 1894.[70] By early spring the effort was beginning to pay off. Gardens had begun to flourish, and the families were raising chickens and hogs and collecting wild berries to supplement their diets. Those who had doubted they could get through the winter had depended "*on God and Miss Barton*" and were now talking hopefully of the next year's cotton crop.[71] With immediate want eliminated, the Red Cross could concentrate on securing the future for the island people.

To do this, Barton first insisted that they continue to plant the fine-quality long-staple cotton for which the islands were famous. The seed was difficult to procure and local merchants were urging the people to plant ordinary cotton. Maintaining that "nothing could be more damaging both to the islands and islanders" than to plant an inferior quality of cotton, Barton wrote to the secretary of agriculture to obtain the special seed. By some fast bargaining she got it, and the quality of that important cash crop was assured.[72] At the same time, Red Cross workers began systematically to educate the Sea Islanders to the necessity of staying out of debt and to help them learn to use the community as a basis for self-help. "I told them that I had desired to do more than merely make a gift for distribution," Barton said of her work in South Carolina. "I wished to plant a tree. I could have given them their peach, which they would eat, enjoy, and throw the pit away. But I wished them to plant the pit, and let it raise other fruit for them."[73] The result was a virtual renaissance of self-reliance for the islands. Not one in twenty contracted a debt in the years following the disaster, and the cotton yields per acre had doubled. When the Red Cross officially closed its doors on June 30, it was with the certainty that the islanders were in a better condition morally, financially, and physically than ever before.[74]

Of the major relief fields undertaken by Barton's Red Cross, the Sea Islands was undoubtedly the greatest. With inadequate provisions, a tiny workforce, and against a skeptical press, they sustained thirty thousand people through a precarious year. Hope, incentive, and courage were given more freely than bread or meat. No kudos rang out as they left the field, there were no congratulatory receptions, and no shining medals arrived at the State Department. The thanks of the islanders, their shy offerings of eggs and strawberries as Barton left, and their determination to help the Red Cross when the time came were the only monument to the year's toil. Of all the national correspondents clamoring for a story, only Joel Chandler Harris seemed to take notice of the work. But Barton herself recognized its importance and believed her organization had proven itself once again. "It is probable," she wrote with pride, "that there are few instances on record, where a movement toward relief of such magnitude, commenced under circumstances so new, so unexpected, so unprepared and so adverse, was ever carried on for such a length of time and closed with results so entirely satisfactory to both those served and those serving, as this disaster."[75]

"The paths of charity are over roadways of ashes; and he who would tread them must be prepared to meet opposition, misconstruction, jealousy and calumny. Let his work be that of angels, still it will not satisfy all."[76] So Barton would write in 1898. With such a philosophy it should hardly have been a surprise to her that various papers charged the Red Cross with ignoring white victims for the less worthy blacks, with demoralizing the blacks by giving them handouts, and with extracting onerous sums for Red Cross supplies. But Barton had never grown used to criticism, and she was shocked and hurt at the unfair reports, especially when Governor Tillman, who had begged her to come to South Carolina in the first place, began to use the organization's troubles for his own political ends. She claimed stoicism, but in reality Clara burned, and she misguidedly tried to answer each accusation with detailed reports of the work. Advisors told her to ignore the criticism, but she could not erase the rough words from her mind.[77]

This kind of petty sniping, however, was a great deal easier to bear than the criticism that had begun to accumulate from businessmen, government officials, and other philanthropists. What had started as small in-house gripes about the lack of reports, financial disarray, and Barton's highhanded methods, had grown into a loud and public protest. Much of the criticism came from local societies who had either failed to receive direction or had grown to be so rich and independent that their size and influence rivaled that of the national body. The head of the old and prestigious Rochester society heard so little from Washington that he began to think that "the parent society is a myth."[78] And the powerful Philadelphia branch, which had found Barton impossible to cooperate with both at Johnstown and during the Russian famine, began to communicate directly with the International Committee in Geneva and to consider conducting an investigation of Barton's activities. "I have never looked into the standing of this Society, nor tried to get its account," wrote one of the many influential members of the Philadelphia auxiliary, "but I have heard from others by inquiry . . . that it is a difficult thing to investigate. It seems to me that at some future time when there is no burning question to consider it would be well for the matter to be looked into."[79] The dissatisfaction of the gentlemen in Philadelphia, who had powerful connections in business and government, formed a very real threat to Barton's group.

Many complaints centered on the organization's lack of accountability. Gustave Moynier repeatedly called for accounts of the American society's proceedings and despaired of their inaccuracy when he did receive them. His faith in Barton began to falter as he glanced through correspondence filled with partial and inconsistent information. "I will tell you for example about page 24, which is absolutely fantastic and contains no words of truth," Moynier wrote of one dispatch.

> I cannot explain how this can be possible, but I believe that this lack of historical truth may greatly harm your cause. The procedure is not only reprehensible, but moreover if your rivals in Philadelphia perceive it that will furnish them with a very powerful force against you. As for the International Committee, that would render its relations with you very delicate I fear . . . when they have seen your pamphlet and what it contains they will doubtless say that they will no longer be able to hold entire

faith in the communications of Washington, whose veracity will be suspected by them. I am personally greatly troubled.[80]

Barton's countrymen felt a similar frustration. Even the national members heard no report of Red Cross activities between 1882 and 1893. In March 1894, while Barton was still at the Sea Islands, *The Review of Reviews* printed an article that, for the first time, stated these objections boldly—and publicly. The author, Sophia Wells Royce Williams, did not mince words when she called for greater systemization of the Red Cross organization. "It has been of great service to suffering humanity," she declared,

> but when one asks for detailed reports, for itemized statements of disbursements, for a careful recapitulation of its labors, its achievements, its failures, its experience and the teaching and lesson of its work—these things either do not exist or are not furnished. . . . I asked its officers for reports. I pleaded for all of its statements and two or three pamphlets were all I could secure. Manifestly these things ought not to be. This national body ought to have a national organization, a national board, and reports which would stand as model and guide for all relief work, the country over.[81]

As Williams pointed out, financial records were also a problem. Barton kept the Red Cross accounts much as she looked after her personal finances: on scraps of paper, in miscellaneous notebooks, and with a rigid adherence to the rule of never throwing out check stubs, receipts, or bank statements. One Red Cross worker made the shocking statement that "contributions were received by Miss Barton alone and most of the Deposits were made in an old black silk undershirt of that Ladies [*sic*] wardrobe."[82] She had not been parsimonious with the Red Cross and never marked her private contributions as anything other than Red Cross funds. But the Red Cross books, for a field such as Johnstown, consisted of boxes of blue-lined receipts covered with the shaky signatures of needy persons, bank drafts signed by twenty different members of the Red Cross staff, and letter-books filled with thousands of acknowledgments that never once mentioned the sum or the item received. Official reports of the amount spent at Johnstown ranged from forty thousand to a quarter of a million dollars. Retention at some fields of Samuel Goodyear, a specialist in bookkeeping, and the hiring of George Pullman as financial secretary, seem to have done little to sort out the mess. Occasionally, serious problems cropped up. In 1895, for example, John Morlan suddenly "found" several thousand dollars that had been donated, under his charge, to relieve the starving Russians. This caused great embarrassment to Barton and others, who had promised that all monies would be expended for the purpose for which they were contributed and who well remembered their own pitiful efforts to scrape together the money needed to charter the S.S. *Tyne-head*.[83] The public grew wary of such an organization and contributions faltered; businessmen, whose aid could have influenced tremendously the growth of the American Red Cross, ignored the body and disregarded its pleas for help.

281

Such criticisms were difficult enough for Barton to bear, but sharper barbs were hidden beneath these relatively impersonal accusations. Since the organization was so small, and Clara so inexorably entwined with it, any complaint about business methods was bound to land in her lap. In painful procession the personal attacks arrived. She was too old, they began, too unused to administrative matters, too bombastic, and too dictatorial. Others believed she was entirely self-serving, that she stayed in the organization solely to meet European royalty, that she thought of her own welfare first and let the organization take its chances. One detractor wrote that "in her operations the sequence is, first Miss Barton, second the Red Cross Society, third the object."[84] More frequent—and more accurate—were the objections that the Red Cross had become so absolutely identified with Clara Barton that it could no longer function outside the area of her observation. Indeed, maintained one critic, it was "the Society *which represents her.*"[85] It was Sophia Williams, however, who once again spoke out most pointedly.

> The National Red Cross Association in this country has been Miss Clara Barton, and Miss Clara Barton has been the National Red Cross Society. . . . What the United States ought to have is a *National* Red Cross Society . . . with leading men in our great cities . . . on its board, with delegates from the Philadelphia College of Physicians and Surgeons, and the New York Academy of Medicine . . . and the Army, Navy, and Marine Hospital Staff, on its board of surgical and medical control and with a constituency representing the entire country. Instead the country has Miss Clara Barton.[86]

At times of introspection and absolute honesty with herself, Barton would agree with many of these pronouncements. "I do not manage well," she admitted to her diary, "and it is better to stop before I become troublesome to others. I have made of the Red Cross an occupation, it may have done some good. It will never go on in any lines I have marked out. It was only to be mine while I was able to manage it."[87] Her only reluctance in retiring stemmed from a desire to see that the future of the Red Cross was secure, that it was financially sound, recognized by Congress, and in the hands of those who would respect and nurture it as she had. For fifteen years Barton had carried on the work "with one hand on a tired thinking forehead and the other in a shallow pocket." As she well knew, it was nearly impossible to find that dedication in others.[88]

Certainly she did not see it in those who chose to "stand off at long range and sling discontent" under the guise of "helping" the American Red Cross.[89] She blamed the critics, not the play, for the bad reviews. When among friends, she referred to them as "enemies" or "comers" and lashed out angrily at their presumption. "Where were you during the long years of struggle that led to the founding of Red Cross and those early years when the organization was struggling for survival?" she demanded in private of one supposed expert on Red Cross matters.[90] It seemed unthinkable to Clara to hand her child over to these upstart critics who failed to supply any real support for the society, impossible to allow them to pressure her away from her life's work. At a hurriedly organized meeting of the Red Cross in January 1895, Barton rather obsequiously presented her case to her fellow members of the executive board. Stating that "whoever brings the most thought and the best work to the organization should be its head," and that she would "gladly give place to such without jealousy, and will stand by and help just the same," Clara organized a vote for new officers. The result was that she was unanimously elected "permanent president" of the Red Cross.[91]

From an organizational point of view, Barton chose to see the problems the Red Cross faced in the 1890s as public relations matters, and she chose to counter them by public relations. Rather than making substantive changes in the organization, she and her small band drew into themselves and strengthened their resolve to allow no "enemies" or unsolicited suggestions to infiltrate their camp. With some glee, Barton observed how her detractors were temporarily silenced by the sharp countering words of the Red Cross. After a particularly nasty rebuttal had been sent to one skeptical Red Cross member, Clara gloated: "I begin to fear that Mrs. Parker will arrive at the conclusion . . . that she could have occupied herself in several ways more profitably than in opening up a correspondence with Mr. Kennan, finding that he is not only an 'ugly customer' himself, but 'trains in an ugly crowd.'"[92] Moynier's complaints were met by an apologetic, almost whining letter from the charter members of the Red Cross, which asserted that Miss Barton carried too many burdens to concern herself with accurate reports, and that "her extreme modesty and humility would never allow her to make the full statement of work accomplished." (Barton and Hubbell concocted the letter, and though it was gratifying to find the members of the American Red Cross eager to sign it, it apparently had little effect on Moynier.[93]) Sophia Williams's articles were answered by an attempt to discredit her personally and an insistence that the *Review of Reviews* retract the statements.[94] These were good tactics and poor strategy, of course. They forever sullied Barton's once cherished hope of keeping the Red Cross free of the "wheels of discord." Once she had written that "whoever else differs and squabbles, the Red Cross must not."[95] Now she wrote in a much different vein, as a beleaguered combatant, disdainful of the "pigmy tricks" of her foes, naively confident of the future.[96]

Hurt and worry were an additional tax on Barton at a time when she was already fatigued and heartsore. The early 1890s combined personal sorrow with the loss of public prestige. Harriet Austin, Minna Kupfer Golay, and Bernard Vassall died, each one unexpectedly, each departure leaving an unfillable void. Even her little cat Tommy, a companion for seventeen years, purred his last and was laid away in the rose garden behind the Red Cross headquarters. Isolated and depressed, Barton questioned the value of her accomplishments: "In the great din of the life's march . . . there runs ever the one tender strain, low, weird, plaintive, *where are thine own?* A kind world approves, nay *praises* it may be, but the ears it would have fallen sweetest on are closed, the hearts that would have throbbed deepest, are still and cold."[97] Beginning to acknowledge her own mortality, she drew closer to her nieces and nephews, contemplated writing her autobiography, and, inevitably, clung tenaciously to the old friends who remained.

It was thus that she became involved, late in the mid-1890s, in a test of wills with Julian Hubbell. She was apt to take the young doctor's extraordinary fealty and deference for granted, but she would not readily dispense with it, nor would she allow it to be distracted by other loyalties. When Hubbell began to fall in love with a charming and beautiful young woman, therefore, Clara brought to bear every pressure she could to end the romance. The rival, named Mary Elizabeth Almon (affectionately called Mea), had at first been an interested Red Cross member and Barton's friend. After a time it became evident that Mea's interest in the Red Cross had hidden motives, and that the lavish gifts she sent to the organization's chief field agent were more than friendly tokens. When Hubbell began vacationing near her home, Barton took action. By a show of poor health, continual talk of the needs of the American Red Cross, and long spells of silent martyrdom, she broke the doctor down, until even Mea's open pleading could not compete with his guilt and feelings of duty. Years later Hubbell's nieces summed up the situation: "C.B.'s domination won. Like a strong-willed parent she commanded." There was, of course, a price on her victory. Hubbell remained steadfastly at Barton's side, but he was silent and detached. The romantic allegiance and strong familial ties he had once held for his heroine were replaced by the memory of Mea and his love for her.[98]

These personal losses took their toll on Barton. To relieve the exhaustion of mind and spirit during this period she began spending the summers away from the unspeakable weather and constant pressure of Washington. She spent several summers with the Gardners, in the midst of a grove of Indiana hardwoods.[99] One year she made an exciting trip to the northwestern United States, a repeat of the refreshing camping experience she had had in 1886. She wanted no part of the life of a pampered septuagenarian but looked forward to roughing it among "the real stuff—Sagebrush and alkoli."[100] With Julian Hubbell, John Morlan, and nephew Stevé and his wife Lizzie, she traveled from Yellowstone Park to Spokane, Washington, and finally to the spectacular beauty of Lake Chelan. There they settled in for several weeks of hunting and fishing: "You would think by the accouterments, rods, lines, guns, revolvers, pouches & game bags that we might be anything from a troop of mountaineers to band of brigands." She was a lively member of the party, gamely helping to set up camp, devising shovels and other implements from sticks and flattened tin cans, and relishing the chance to sleep, away from the cares of the world in "perfect *ignorance and peace.*"[101] To maintain her dignity she demanded the right to wear her favorite bonnet, even in the woods, and her nephew recalled that on the entire trip he never saw her without the little rosebud-trimmed hat, securely tied with pink satin ribbons.[102]

After George Pullman joined the Red Cross, Barton began to spend her summers at the Thousand Islands in the St. Lawrence River. Her financial secretary was a nephew of the famed inventor of the Pullman palace car, and the entire clan met every year at several islands owned by the great railroad magnate. Though there were a number of houses available to her, Clara often chose to stay in a tent, and the cool breezes and cheerful family parties did much to relieve her mind from worry and overwork. "I could scarcely walk any more and my eyesight failed me through weakness, till I could not see to read nor write," she said of her arrival at the Pullmans' house in 1894.[103] Six weeks later her vigor and spirits were restored. While at the islands she could think and plan, compose the long, chatty letters she so enjoyed writing, and converse with neighbors such as Marietta Holley, the author of the series of Samantha books Clara had read while a patient in Dansville. Lingering until the cool weather arrived in late September, she reluctantly returned to Washington and the press of business.[104]

Another salve to Barton's beleaguered vanity was the time she spent with her "boys" during these years. The cheers for her had never died out among the ranks of the GAR, and any encounter brought forth bands and handsome speeches or sentimental tears. Many of Clara's activities also centered on the women's auxiliaries of the GAR, the Potomac Corps, and the Women's Relief Corps.[105] During these years she also became a charter member and surgeon general of the Daughters of the American Revolution, a group, founded on patriotic principles, which she admired greatly. Barton frequently used her Washington headquarters, so well adapted to hospitality, to entertain these organizations. At the meetings she was acclaimed and fussed over and could speak to rapt audiences of her military exploits and those of her ancestors. She enjoyed it all hugely and could never reconcile the cheers of the veterans with the criticisms of other groups.[106]

Barton spent rather more time with the veterans than she did with the feminists during the 1890s. She was still asked to attend every congress and banquet, but she usually declined the invitations during this period, pleading lack of time and other commitments. Nonetheless, she tried to send a written message to the conventions when she could. Asked her opinion of dress reform, she spoke out against the "tyrant fashion," saying that if "the monster could be *slain* and its power annihilated, leaving women free in body and soul . . . this I should regard once well established, as a lasting and real reform."[107] A well-known journalist, Frank Carpenter, requested her opinion on the question, "If women came to Congress what would be the result?" and she answered with another series of questions, penetrating in their insight. The churches, schools, conventions, and new towns of the American frontier, stated Barton, all accepted women only after much debate: "Has their presence there been demoralizing? Have they bred discord? Have they readily entered into iniquities and tricky plans? . . . If women had not gone what would have been the result?"[108] Her name still had the power to dignify, and her pen the power to persuade. Perhaps the greatest tribute to her role in the feminist movement in these years came when a young woman, with whom she had been acquainted at Johnstown, wrote Barton to tell her how the friendship had changed her life. "To what you are as a woman—I said my first 'I am glad I am a woman,'" wrote Sarah J. Elliot. "Further, as I worked with you—as you educated me in the work of other women, I heard for the first time of those other women crying for help."[109]

Clara's enthusiasm for women's work, and for the wartime memories of the veterans, came together in a dramatic way in 1892. At a final gala meeting of the Potomac Corps of the WRC, at which tears were mingled with patriotic rhetoric, Barton was asked to give a toast to "The Women Who Went to the Field." Writing late on the eve of the banquet, she composed a poem, as she often did on such occasions, and in the strength of her emotion it rose to a standard that few of her verses attained. Thirty years after Antietam and Fredericksburg, she no longer felt any rivalry with her sisters in mercy, only a profound respect evident in every stanza. "What did they go for, just to be in the way?" she asked in her tribute to Aunt Fanny, Mary ("Mother") Bickerdyke, Almira Fales, Dorothea Dix, and others who had sacrificed comfort and reputation to help fill the desperate needs of the war. "She has smoothed his black plumes and laid them to sleep," Barton wrote at the poem's end.

Whilst the angels above them their high vigils keep:
And she sits here *alone*, with the snow on her brow—
Your cheers for her comrades? Three cheers for her now.
And these were the women who went to the war:
The women of question; what *did* they go for?
Because in their hearts God had planted the seed
Of pity for woe, and help for its need;
They saw in high purpose, a duty to do,
And the armor of right broke the barriers through.
Uninvited, unaided, unsanctioned ofttimes,
With pass, or without it, they pressed on the lines;
They pressed they implored, till they ran the lines through,
And *this* was the "running" the men saw them do.
.   .   .   .
And what would they do if the war came again?
The *scarlet cross floats* where all was blank then
They would bind on their "*brassards*" and march to the fray,
And the man liveth not who could say to them nay;
They would stand with you now, as they stood with you then,
The nurses, consolers, and saviors of men.[110]

"The Women Who Went to the Field," still powerful nearly a century later, was an immediate sensation. Newspapers reprinted it, magazines extolled its spirited message. WRC chapters claimed certain lines as their official slogans. But the poem was most memorable to those who saw Barton read it only a few hours after it was written. From the platform the small figure in stiff black bombazine had such a quality of legend to it, and her voice had such solemn depth, that the reading took on almost the character of a drama. "The air was white with the sympathetic 'kerchiefs' of the ladies," reported one newspaper, "and the imposing figure of Clara Barton, standing with uplifted arm, as if in signal for the cheers, so grandly given, completed the historic and never to be forgotten scene."[111]

It was fortunate that Clara had such emotional outlets, for still more disappointments were to come her way in the eighteen months following the Sea Islands relief. She was relying on a bill to protect and recognize the Red Cross to balance the continuing criticism, and in late 1894 she again, with a renewed commitment to its passage, had it submitted to Congress. But there was to be no such triumph. Upon submission of the bill she found a fierce and effective opposition among the businesses already using the Red Cross insignia or name, especially the medical supplier Johnson and Johnson. This company had been using the trademark for eight years, and so successful had its products been that it hired a noted jurist to lecture the Senate on their constitutional powers—which, the jurist maintained, did not include restricting the use of insignia that had not been granted a trademark by the Patent Office. Much subdued, the Senate tabled the bill. Hasty consultations then ensued between Barton's staff and the representatives of Johnson and Johnson. The Red Cross found the company willing to join them in a fight to limit the use of the international sign if it could retain the right to display the cross on its packages. To this Barton readily agreed. Unfortunately, so effective had the company's preliminary protests been, that the Senate was unwilling to back down on its original decision, making it necessary to modify the legislation once more before it would pass. This time nearly all of its clout was eliminated. Business and commercial firms could continue to use name or badge with impunity, though they were advised to request permission from the American Red Cross before employing it. Only competing charitable organizations were restricted in its use. Barton put a brave face on the matter, declaring that all along their "real & serious objection" had been to the "promiscuous misuse of the insignia . . . [by] these irresponsible and unrecognized societies." It was, however, a pale shadow of the recognition and government protection she had sought to secure by legislation.[112]

And in the end, though the bill sailed through both houses, even this poor compromise did not become law. Instead of the jubilant letter she had imagined writing to Gustave Moynier, Barton was forced to tell him that she had "reason to be heartsick"; the president had not signed the bill. By law all legislation was required to have the chief executive's signature before the end of the congressional session during which it had passed. The Fifty-third Congress was notoriously slow and argumentative, and dumped so many hastily passed bills on the president's desk in the final days of the term that Grover Cleveland decided to teach the legislators a lesson. Fifty-five bills went unsigned, including Clara's cherished Red Cross bill. "I would not be sincere with myself were I to neglect

287

telling you that my heart does *not* swell with a national pride at these things," she advised Moynier, assuring him that the bill would undoubtedly repass during the next session. Her promise proved optimistic; no protection for the Red Cross sign or name would become law until after the turn of the century.[113]

While the Red Cross bill remained in a state of limbo, Barton was understandably anxious that little of the discontent that she was facing come to the attention of Congress. She was also unwilling that any further scandal be added to the already unmanageable pile. It was with shock, therefore, that she received a letter detailing real troubles at the Red Cross Park. She had had hints of irregular activities before, in the form of anonymous letters that stated Morlan had inadequately trained his "old poke of horses" and had lost over a thousand dollars "betting or worse." Further, he had illegally rented out portions of the land and personally pocketed the proceeds.[114] Barton had chosen to ignore these accusations. By August 1894, however, Gardner was so wary of Morlan that he had dismissed him. Morlan claimed that livestock, equipment, and furnishings had been bought at his personal expense and refused to move without either the property or adequate compensation for it. Gardner, maintaining that every item on the farm belonged to the Red Cross, forbade him to touch any of it and threatened court action if he did. It was at this point that Morlan contacted Barton. If she did not help him quickly, he wrote, he would sue Gardner in a manner that would produce the worst sort of publicity for Barton and the Red Cross.[115]

Clara was at the Thousand Islands when she received Morlan's letter. It so frightened her that for a fortnight she could not bring herself to respond. A public trial disclosing the activities of a dishonest manager, gambling on Red Cross property, and a deed that gave Barton personal property as a result of her official capacity would hand her detractors the very ammunition they needed to end her public career forever. When she finally replied to Morlan, the long letter gave full vent to her bitterness and deep sorrow that this should have been the final outcome of Joseph Gardner's "princely gift." Afraid that she personally would be blamed for mismanagement of the park, she took pains to deny any involvement and begged the two men to allow her to change the deeds to the property before the matter went into litigation and involved her in the scandal. "Indeed, there seems to be no choice given me, and no chance left me," she wrote in desperation. "If you two men come into a public quarrel, before the courts, while it will entail little or no disgrace upon either of you . . . it will mean failure, shame and infamy to *me*, and death to the organization to which I have given the most useful years of my life."[116] Characteristically, Barton overreacted to the situation, and it is unfortunate that she did. Ten years later the letter would be cited as proof that she had been involved in activities so underhanded that her name would be ruined if they were ever made public.

For several months the situation was at an impasse while Morlan and Gardner lined up witnesses and documents. Then, in January 1895, Clara, accompanied by Hubbell and Stevé, traveled to Bedford to assess the matter for herself. They found the farm in a state of disrepair, the animals in poor health, and several suspicious persons apparently enjoying free quarters.[117] Morlan, whom Clara had relied on so earnestly, had, in Stevé's words, "proved to be a rascal . . . I found that he was unable to account in any way for the money he had expended in developing and carrying on the farm for one or two years." His bluff called, Morlan became hysterical. On his knees he begged Barton not to abandon him or reveal his transgressions. "I put the poor fellow to bed," reads Clara's diary, "and left him to sob himself to sleep."[118] Nor were the Gardners, as it turned out, blameless in the matter. Confronted by Morlan, they were forced to admit that their "thank-offering to humanity" had been a deal contrived by them and Morlan to secure a tidy profit on some marginal land. Gardner had expended seven thousand dollars on the property originally; the plan was to have Barton pay him twelve thousand dollars, bit by bit, for the park. A shocked Barton heard this for the first time nearly two years after her announcement of the gift and was stunned when she considered the implications. As contrite as Morlan, the Gardners begged Clara to "wipe the slate off clean . . . let nothing be remembered, and even if I said let Morlan remain, they would not say a word."[119] Morlan was dismissed, however, and arrangements were made for Hubbell to stay at the farm as manager. Too "sad and crushed to speak," Barton packed her bags and returned to Washington.[120]

For a year Hubbell remained in Indiana. He had enough success with the property that he was able to send several carloads of grain and produce to Barton for storage. He managed to conduct the affairs of the park discreetly, with no untoward activities save an ill-considered scheme to breed Russian wolfhounds. Hubbell had no real interest in the farm, however, and after a year or so his initiative flagged.[121] In January 1896 the Gardners, fearing public embarrassment, sent Barton a legal paper that severed any relations, personal or professional, with the Red Cross—"a most remarkable document," Barton wrote.[122] She disregarded the paper, and in her loyal way continued her friendship with the Gardners. Though occasionally she still thought of uses for the land, from this time the grandiose plans for "the one piece of neutral ground in the western hemisphere" were essentially forgotten.

Thus, the "gay nineties" passed by with continual tension between disappointment, thundering cheers, noble work, and sharp questioning. Nowhere were these opposing trends combined more poignantly than in a mission Barton began in 1896, this time in Turkey and Armenia. By popular acclamation she was compelled to take the work on; because of public doubt it was scrutinized, hampered, and criticized as it had never been before.

During 1894 small articles had begun to appear in American newspapers about the atrocities committed in Armenia by the Turks. A proud and nationalist people, the Armenians had long resisted incorporation in the Ottoman Empire but had been continually beaten by the fierce fighting of the Turks. The Armenians' position was worsened by the fact that they were Christians in an aggressively Moslem nation. News of a planned revolt by Armenian nationalists in 1893 again brought the sultan's troops into their territory. For eighteen months they killed and pillaged Christians in a barbarous frenzy. It was essentially a religious war; in an attempt to unify the empire, dissidents had to be either eliminated or converted by the sword. American feelings were ruffled by the brutality, but when American missionaries began to be harrassed by the Turkish government because of their aid to the victims of this holocaust, the disapproval turned to outrage. [123]

In New York a group of prominent leaders and businessmen such as Jacob Schiff, Spencer Trask, and Bishop Henry C. Potter banded together with Chief Justice Melville W. Fuller and other Washington notables to form the National Armenian Relief Committee. Its aim was to aid the Christian sufferers and bolster their rebellious sentiment, and its members took little trouble to cloak their anti-Turkish feelings. Their plans were great: they hoped to collect five million dollars and see to its allocation. The question that held them back was the proper group to distribute it. The missionaries still in Turkey were suspect and were likely to be robbed or worse, and the American groups that sponsored them had been forbidden to send any more representatives to the divided nation. The Red Cross, which had experience, an affirmed international standing, and a branch in Turkey, seemed the logical organization. Moreover, the American Red Cross had Clara Barton, whose name could be counted on to help bring in donations. [124]

"Reporters to the right of us, Reporters to the left of us. Reporters in front of us. Volleyed and thundered," wrote George Pullman from the Washington headquarters, as word spread that the president of the American Red Cross was debating whether or not to undertake the Armenian relief. "All day long our house has been besieged by newspaper men and women, messenger and telegraph boys running continuously to the house. Men and women who were anxious to go to Armenia and one 'crank' who with a small Bible in his hand wanted to 'hire out as a missionary.'" [125] Barton was in no mood to hand the reporters a hasty decision. The work was unlike anything she had previously undertaken, and she had no way of getting trustworthy accounts of the actual conditions. Remembering the pinched resources at the Sea Islands, she had little desire to start with inadequate funds—and the relief committee was being spectacularly unsuccessful in soliciting contributions. Barton was also not altogether convinced that the sultan would even allow them into the country, especially given the critical tone of the American press. "I have no doubt [the relief] will be dangerous as well as hard," she told George Kennan's wife; "I have grave doubts if it [the Red Cross] could distribute it." [126]

As she hesitated, so did the members of the National Armenian Relief Committee. Disturbing reports of Barton's behavior during the Russian famine began to filter in, particularly from Philadelphia's active Robert Ogden. In such a crucial situation, it would be wise, he advised, to find a younger and less controversial figure to take charge of the relief. "I consider the first element of Miss Barton's character to be consummate egotism," Ogden wrote confidentially to Spencer Trask, "which is combined with a lack of executive ability, and these two conditions largely limit her capacity for managing any extensive affair."[127] The committee members were nonetheless reluctant to abandon what seemed to be the only organization that might conceivably be allowed into the country. They consequently backed away from either appointing Barton as their representative or looking elsewhere for a distributor. In January 1896 Clara met with Trask and others and found it "the most *tiresome* meeting I ever *knew*. Everyone afraid of committing himself, and simply made words."[128] Finally she herself gave them a commitment: if they would unanimously agree that the Red Cross should go and would raise a sufficient amount of money, she would undertake the relief. After some dispute, the relief committee agreed to these conditions. On January 22, 1896, Barton once more set off for Europe, admist "swarms of reporters" and the cheers of well-wishers.[129]

More confusion greeted Barton on her arrival in England. She had sailed before receiving confirmation that she would be able to land in Turkey, and rumor had it that Sultan Abdul-Hamid II was angrily opposing their mission. Newspaper reports, like one appearing in the New York Tribune in which the sultan was charged with "seeking to guard his dearly loved right to murder and maltreat Christians," had done little to endear him to what he viewed as a sanctimonious body coming to feed the Armenians at the expense of his own people.[130] Barton and her company (which included Hubbell, Pullman, and an American stenographer by the name of Mason) thus tarried in London while they awaited word from the American minister, Alexander Terrell, in Constantinople. When it finally arrived they made a speedy trip across the continent, stopping only to speak with Gustave Moynier in Geneva before boarding the Orient Express for Turkey. On February 15 they arrived in Constantinople.[131]

To her dismay, Barton found that her plans had indeed not been approved by the Turks. After some negotiations between Terrell and the Turkish Foreign Ministry, Barton was granted an audience with a high-level official, Tewfik Pasha, to explain herself and her intentions. Barton diplomatically avoided any judgmental comments on the political situation in Turkey. Instead she reported simply that the condition of the starving inhabitants of Armenia had aroused American sympathies and that she was there to distribute food and medical aid to them. Despite American sentiments she would give assistance, as she was bound to by the Treaty of Geneva, indiscriminately to Moslems and Christians. In the end she strengthened her case most by assuring the press-sensitive pasha that she had not come to report on Turkey's misdeeds, only to help them in their misfortune. As Barton later recalled, she concluded the audience by saying:

Nothing shall be done in any concealed manner. All dispatches that we send shall go openly through your own telegraph and I should be glad if all that we shall write could be seen by your government. I cannot, of course, see what its character will be, but can vouch for its truth, fairness and integrity, and the conduct of every leading man who shall be sent. I shall never counsel nor permit a sly or underhand action with your government, and you will pardon me Pasha, if I say that I shall expect the same treatment in return—such as I give I shall expect to receive.

Almost without a breath he replied—"And you shall have it. We honor your position and your wishes will be respected. Such aid and protection as we are able to, we shall render."[132]

The Turkish government stipulated, however, that Barton was to work as an individual, not as the representative of any official body, including the Red Cross. The pasha's decision to allow her to stay spoke well of the impression Barton made in Constantinople and of her reputation for fair and impartial relief work. It nonetheless greatly troubled the National Armenian Relief Committee in New York, whose members began to suspect that Barton would turn their project into a personal triumph and utilize the funds in a way that would be anathema to some of the donors.[133]

From her headquarters in Pera, the European section of Constantinople, Barton began to put together the missions to the interior of Turkey. She did not plan to go herself; she knew that she was needed in the capital to deal with the government and communicate with her benefactors in New York, and, for once, she believed that the work was too rough and uncertain for a woman of seventy-five. To supplement her own staff she found willing workers among the American missionaries, most notably Dr. Ira Harris. W. W. Peet, another locally established missionary, was also instrumental in advising Barton and eliciting support from the European community in Constantinople. From firsthand accounts and vague rumors these workers learned of the most disastrous areas and began to put together teams of doctors, guides, Red Cross staff, and translators. In all, four missions—to the ransacked cities of Harpoot, Arabkir, Zeitoun, and Marash—were undertaken. By foot and by mule, with trains of supplies carried by horse or occasionally camels, the expeditions set off to aid sufferers they knew of only by rumor.[134]

They found little in many villages but heaps of dust and rubble. The families that were left were huddled in rags among the wreckage of their former lives. Many were so frightened of any strange face that they initially refused to speak to the relief workers or cooperate with them. The plunder had been so complete that even the simple tools of living—the cooking pots, sickles, water bags, and hand looms—had been stolen or destroyed, and the inhabitants were without means of rebuilding their lives. Fear and despair had made them inert. It was, in fact, one of the most important aspects of this relief field that the workers were able to cut through apathy and misery and help the survivors begin again. The idea that strangers had come from thousands of miles away to help them seemed to rejuvenate the Armenians. "One of the greatest contributions made by the benevolent men and women in distant parts of the world," wrote a doctor accompanying Hubbell, "was the assurance brought by their gifts that they cared for these alien sufferers; . . . that this afflicted people was not left abandoned of all men."[135]

With limited funds the men set about their work of rehabilitation. They donated seed, acquired draft animals, taught hygiene and sewing, and set blacksmiths to work making tools, wagon tongues, and other equipment not procurable locally. For five weary months of "rough, uncivilized life," they tutored, doctored, encouraged, and relieved until they began to feel that the people could make a harvest and take care of themselves.[136]

Their most notable contribution, however, was in health care. Soon after the caravans set off, word arrived in Constantinople that both typhoid and typhus fevers had broken out and that nearly one hundred people were dying daily. It was feared that because of the lack of food and the crowded conditions, there would be a widespread epidemic. "I have witnessed scenes of suffering both in the United States and the Orient," Dr. Harris wrote of Zeitoun, "but never to my dying day, will I be able to dismiss from my mind the horror of the pinched, haggard faces and forms that gathered about me that first day. Before we left the tent one of the doctors said: 'We will now see the place is full of walking skeletons.' This expressed fully their condition."[137] Dysentery and diarrhea were also rampant, caused in part by the unsanitary refugee camps which filled the countryside. Believing that prevention of disease was the greatest need, Harris and his counterparts in other villages stressed cleanliness, set up soup kitchens to ensure proper nourishment, and encouraged the sufferers to leave the teeming camps and sleep away from infected areas. His work, and Hubbell's in neighboring Arabkir, were remarkably successful. In five weeks they not only cured the great proportion of those suffering from the fevers but prevented the start of an epidemic that could have engulfed a large portion of the country.[138]

From the beginning it was evident that this field was quite different from the ones undertaken previously by Barton and her staff. The problems of language, converting currency, and dispelling the natural distrust of foreigners took up an enormous amount of time. A letter sent from Constantinople to the interior took six weeks to arrive—if it did arrive. Dispatches to and from America had an equally uncertain fate. "The difficulties in the way of transacting even ordinary business, here, are so great, and so tiresome—that one wears out under them," Barton complained to a friend in Washington.[139] Travel in the countryside, along rough mountain passages and through completely unchartered areas, was onerous. Any unforeseen problem, such as the death of her stenographer, Mrs. Mason, on March 15, required lengthy and frustrating negotiations. Much of the time Barton was forced to make decisions based on only the scantiest knowledge of what was happening in the interior.[140]

As if this were not enough, she began to be sharply questioned, to the point of harrassment, by the members of the National Armenian Relief Committee. They worried incessantly about delayed cables, proper distribution of funds, the staff in Constantinople, and Barton herself. Their initial hesitancy about her capabilities had tinged their relations with an obvious mistrust, which hindered and annoyed both sides. Halip Bogigian, a rug dealer who was coordinating the relief work in Boston, had been shocked by the actions of one of Clara's aides as she was about to depart for Turkey. "When I handed Miss Barton the letter of credit for $7,500 on the steamer," Bogigian wrote, "he grabbed it, as I was about to hand it to Miss Barton and put it into his pocket. The question has come to my mind since, whether one cent of that $7,500 ever went to the starving Armenians." [141] Bogigian thought that the best way to handle the matter was to send lengthy letters, heavy with advice, to Turkey, a habit that angered Barton. "Mr. Bogigian claims the privilege of being 'plain' with me," she wrote hotly in a series of private notes. "He perhaps is not able to make the distinction between plainness of speech, and impertinence." [142] The committee, having little idea of the slow paths of communication or Barton's delicate relationship with the Turkish government, could not understand what appeared to them as abrupt changes of itinerary and reckless distribution of funds. Barton, with her tendency to gloss over difficulties (not to mention failures) and to draw her cloak more securely around her organization as it came under fire, became less and less willing to explain the true situation to the men in New York. Dispatches, which began with phrases such as "What are those folks doing over there?" began to be ignored. [143]

In the end Barton, believing that the committee and she would both be better off minding their respective businesses, decided to cut her ties with Trask and Bogigian. After checking her finances and her staff, she sent a message that mocked their attempt to use censure as a form of assistance. From Constantinople she wired: "We will finish the field without further aid." [144]

This move partially relieved Clara of anxiety, but she was still held in a delicate balance between American ambitions and Turkish realities. Chief among the complaints of Trask and his colleagues was the fact that she was assisting Turks as well as Armenians, the perpetrators as well as the victims of the atrocities. A new concept had come into this field of foreign relief, one that had been foreshadowed during the Russian famine and would come to maturity in the Spanish-American war. Americans became dissatisfied with merely supplying bread to starving or neglected peoples; they wanted to supply justice, too. Politicians and philanthropists began to see that temporary relief measures would not really help the Armenians or Russian peasants except in the very short term; what were needed were political and social changes. And the changes they sought were of the most subjective kind, reflecting values that were often at odds with the precepts of justice laid out in the Koran.

This politicalization of charity impeded Barton's work. As American criticism of the Turks grew, so did her difficulties with the Turkish government. Ever suspicious that it was the Red Cross that was feeding horror stories to the American Congress, the sultan's government took care to make sure that no adverse cables were sent across the Atlantic. At the same time, American supporters of the relief work were disappointed, for they had hoped to find justification of their

294

efforts in the tales of suffering sent back from their workers. They had not wanted impartiality and were distressed when, without their consent, their monies were dispensed in that manner. Caught on a tightrope between the quest for justice and the need for relief, Barton found that no matter what her action it met with suspicion.

Of course she reacted personally to the situation, taking suggestions as insults, and criticism as treachery. After her divorce from the National Armenian Relief Committee she felt an initial burst of relief, which caused her to remark, "Since assuming the ascendancy there has not been a moment of unrest. I was never on a more pleasant field for work."[145] Barton began to fill her diary, however, with comments that belied such confidence. She believed that not only the relief committee but the American people were opposed to her presence in Turkey, and that even Stevé, who had loyally tried to defend her, was against her. Under stress Clara sought her familiar escapes of contemplating suicide and flight. "I doubt if I will ever feel the same in my country again," she wrote. "It will seem to me a fair pleasant field, with every stone heap full of snakes."[146] Perhaps never in her life, she complained to Lizzie Barton, had she felt "so near an outcast."[147] But she was too old to start again in another country, she told herself, and so she kept her dreams centered on the peaceful pleasures of death. "I must . . . withdraw within myself and close up the tangled web of a long jagged life," she scribbled during her last days in Turkey. "I need not regret to see the end coming. It has had many sore spots, and rest seems welcome."[148]

Barton revealed her inner dismay to no one and remained in Armenia to finish the field with credit to herself and her organization. Though she knew that the relief had been inadequate (at her departure it was estimated that fifty thousand people would die before spring, despite Red Cross assistance), she was satisfied that they had done the work as well as any group could have. In five months they had expended more than $116,000, giving thousands of hopeless people the ability to reshape their lives. Missionaries, as well as the Turkish government, praised her work, pointing out especially the way in which the money had been directed for specific purposes rather than scattered "here and there in an aimless way."[149] She had kept herself independent, walking such a careful diplomatic line that she managed to keep from being recalled by either the Turkish or American government. While the men in New York sat with mouths grimly closed, Barton returned home in late September to plaudits from the feminists, cheers from the GAR, and a public reception that featured an eight-course dinner and an entire evening of patriotic music.[150] At the State Department she was congratulated by Secretary Richard Olney, who handed her the second order of Shekafet, sent to the department from the pasha in Constantinople. Of staggering size and encrusted with diamonds and other precious jewels, the medal was awarded for exceptional service to the Ottoman Empire. Like so many other decorations she had won, it had never before been awarded to a woman. With it had come a message: If the United States wished to send further assistance to Turkey, they would be pleased if Miss Clara Barton was sent to administer it.[151]

sixteen

The Turkish field had not yet really closed before press and public invited—indeed required—Barton to take up a prolonged mission in Cuba.

For nearly two years Americans had trained their eyes to this neighbor some ninety miles from their shores. In 1895 the Cubans had staged a revolution against the colonial rule of Spain, but the insurgents had lost and the despotic policies against which they were fighting were strengthened. To show their displeasure and to attract the attention of the United States, the rebels destroyed property and planned guerrilla raids on Spanish military fortifications. To check the rebels the government rounded up suspect inhabitants of the countryside and herded them into concentration camps. The Spanish administrators were unable or unwilling to provide for the *reconcentrados*, as they came to be known, and the wretched people were left to starve in the filth and exposure of the camps. It was estimated that one-third of the Cuban population died in these miserable camps during the last years of the nineteenth century. Such a situation was manna for the sensationalist press of the day, and the plight of the reconcentrados became increasingly prominent in feature stories.[1]

Barton was sitting in the shade at the Thousand Islands, making plans to produce a series of Red Cross medals to be awarded to the veterans of the Turkish campaign, when the first intimation of possible American aid to Cuba reached her. She was back in Washington, clearing up the final financial accounting and writing a lengthy report of the Middle Eastern field, when requests for Red Cross aid began to filter to her. At first these pleas were editorials in the press calling for help for Americans who were among those suspected by the Spanish authorities and were therefore also being held in the camps. "The Armenian venture . . . has established the precedent that it is not necessary that two countries should be at war in order to admit of the intervention of the Red Cross in behalf of the suffering," the *New York Tribune* declared in January 1897.[2] Barton did not share the enthusiasm of the press for such a venture. There had been altogether too much criticism of her work in Turkey, too many delicate negotiations with unfamiliar governments, for her to take lightly the idea of another foreign mission. And the situation in Cuba was undeniably explosive. It involved three hostile parties and a state of quasi war between the Cubans and their rulers, which made the legal position of the Red Cross ill-defined. Moreover, Barton was far from convinced that the American public—or the American government— really knew what they wanted when they so earnestly sought her help in Cuba.

In a sense the clamor for Red Cross intervention in Cuba was indicative of the way in which Barton had become a victim of her own success. During the infant years of the American Red Cross, she had been so anxious to prove the organization's value, and to publicize its work, that she had heeded almost any call for help. Despite the remaining misunderstandings about the official relations of the Red Cross and the government, there was now a broad public awareness of the practical good work that Barton and her small staff had accomplished. But it was blithely assumed that the Red Cross was a much larger organization than it was and that its resources were vast, its ability to respond unlimited. Now Barton was nearly overrun with requests that she should fly to the scene of every disaster that befell the country. Her work in Turkey had exacerbated this situation by adding the miseries of other nations to the list of tragedies the American Red Cross was called upon to relieve. At the same time that the Cuban situation was drawing to a head, Barton was required to take action in Texas, again at the Sea Islands, and in Greece, where Christians were once more battling the Turks. To these fields she sent token amounts of money, sometimes dispatched advice, and made a polite show at rallies called to solicit financial or political support. On the whole she hoped to keep Red Cross activities regarding the reconcentrados at the same level. Only when rival organizations began to show an interest in the problem did she reconsider the role she and the Red Cross should play in Cuba.[3]

During the early part of 1897 Barton kept Cuba in the back of her mind; her more immediate concern was with the exacting process of moving her household and business out to Glen Echo. Tired of the distraction and dirt in Washington, Barton hoped to try again to establish a country home, where animals and a garden could share space with Red Cross supplies, and where she could find peace and quiet to reflect and do a little writing. But other concerns also helped shape the decision. In the summer of 1895, when she and other staff members had visited the Red Cross warehouse, they found that the building had been broken into and a number of valuable supplies stolen. They had considered moving out at that time, but the Armenian campaign had postponed it.[4] Another factor was the desperate plight of the Glen Echo developers, the Baltzleys. Poor land sales, an outbreak of malaria, and overextended credit had all eroded the reputation of the "Washington Rhine" and left the brothers embarrassed financially. Ever loyal, Barton bought some additional property from them in 1897 and determined to move the Red Cross headquarters to Glen Echo. This, she hoped, would finally give the spot the prestige sought by the developers when they originally donated the property to her. When, in late 1896, the Baltzleys convinced a local transportation company to build a trolley line linking Glen Echo with Georgetown, Barton's remaining doubts were overcome.[5]

Moving the contents of the headquarters at 17th and F streets was an enormous undertaking. Throughout the month of February, wagonloads of mattresses, books, cookware, and Clara's precious relics rumbled along the canal road to the little village of Glen Echo. The Red Cross "family," as Barton liked to refer to it, followed the goods in early March. Hubbell, Pullman, several servants, and Lily Mason, daughter of the Red Cross worker who had died in Constantinople, all fitted up their rooms in the ungainly structure at Glen Echo. It was still a glorified warehouse when they arrived, with bare pine boards for walls, no heat, and no plumbing or finished detail. As Barton noted to a friend that spring, the house needed "not repairs, but finishing."[6]

For the next eight months the house resembled an overgrown work camp, as large crews removed an "unsightly" stone facade, added running water and walnut banisters, and stretched muslin over the bare boards to make a smooth and inexpensive surface for painting. Barton planted a garden, bought a cow and some chickens, and the place began to take on the bucolic aspect she loved.[7] The house itself reflected its owner's unusual personality, melding as it did personal needs with the pressing work of the Red Cross. Parlors doubled as official reception rooms, Barton's and Hubbell's bedrooms became private work spaces, and the halls were lined with closets containing emergency supplies of blankets, bandages, and Horlick's malted milk. Stained glass windows featuring a large red cross, and a flag flying from the front gable, reinforced the house's official function. All of Clara's treasures were there, and the "museum" now included several splendid Turkish carpets, the gift of the pasha's grateful government.[8] Some visitors found the huge, tree-shaded house dark and spartan, even forbidding, but the place came to mean a great deal to the Red Cross president.[9] "She loved her Glen Echo home on the Potomac," Julian Hubbell would later write, "because of its quiet, its nearness to nature, the hills and the trees and the birds and the water, and used to say the moon seemed always to be shining there."[10]

"I am so thankful for the physical labor that has come with the making over, and up of my rough, crude country home—it has been a salvation to me," Clara wrote in a despondent mood; "there is still a little of it left and I cherish every day of it—anything to divert the thoughts and keep down the worry."[11] Thus, the daily changes in the house and the outdoor activity at Glen Echo worked to cheer Barton through an unsettled period. Her old enemy, bronchitis, struck again in the summer of 1897, bringing with it fears of another physical collapse

298

and the loss of precious work time. She was pressed by administrative problems and the need to keep an ever-vigilant eye on the situation in Cuba.

Barton rallied enough energy to attend the International Red Cross Conference in Vienna in September but was so weak and low on cash that she made the entire trip in less than a month, not even pausing to visit the venerable Louise in Baden. The conference was not the uplifting experience that the former gatherings had been. Barton, along with Hubbell and Pullman, arrived two days late and left early, declined most social invitations, and contributed little beyond a report of their work in the Sea Islands and Armenia. There were no great ovations for her, though the rooms were filled with familiar faces. Barton felt uncomfortable with questions about the apparent indifference of America's wealthy businessmen toward the Red Cross, and she found it "humiliating" to have to state that the Congress had yet to protect the organization's name or insignia. Even the journey proved unpleasant, for the rough Atlantic incapacitated the delegates on both voyages. Most distressing of all, however, was the cool reception Barton received from Gustave Moynier, who was hardly ecstatic about the refusal of the United States Congress to recognize the Red Cross as a national organization. He was also concerned with a pamphlet he had received, which complained about Barton's indifference to the Cubans. Though Barton was able to explain the situation satisfactorily to Moynier, it left her feeling anxious about her potential role in Cuba. For the first of many times she realized that no matter what course she took in the matter, it would not please everyone.[12]

Though she reacted with ambivalence to the Cuban situation, Barton was hardly indifferent to the plight of the reconcentrados. Throughout the spring and summer of that year she had followed their story and had noted the growing public appeal for the Red Cross to come to their rescue. Both the president and Congress were considering political and humanitarian aid—in fact the Congress voted in May 1897 to send fifty thousand dollars to the island to relieve American citizens being held there—and Barton felt that under the circumstances the American Red Cross should wait until it was officially requested by the government to go to Cuba. She felt, with similar conviction, that it was important for the Spanish government to understand her mission and receive the relief in the spirit of neutrality under which it would purportedly be given. But, as in Turkey, the American people were not neutral, and the Spanish government, though signatory to the Treaty of Geneva, was disinclined to accept what they considered to be support for a group of dangerous guerrillas. As early as January 1897, Barton had approached the Spanish minister in Washington, Enrique Dupuy de Lôme, suggesting neutral Red Cross assistance for the reconcentrados. His nebulous reply suggested that perhaps Barton could go to Cuba as a private individual, as she had done in Turkey. He added, however, that Spain could not guarantee safe landing for supplies or personnel sent by the American Red Cross. Meanwhile, newspaper reports kept anticipating the departure of the Red Cross workers for Cuba or demanding that Barton make some statement on the situation, "So much has been said, written and printed back and forth in regard to the Red Cross and Cuba . . . that I have not known what to say, or if to say anything. . . ," Clara would write. "One day we are expected to go, the next qualifies the expectation."[13]

The confusion in Barton's mind was over whether or not the American public should assist the reconcentrados at all; she had no doubt that if they did, the Red Cross was the proper vehicle of relief. Consequently, she viewed with alarm the advent of the "National Relief Fund in Aid of Cuba," an organization established by the wives of several senators, Supreme Court justices, and other prominent locals. Barton dubbed the group the "court ladies," politely advised them, and even attended one of their meetings, all the while trying to determine to what degree they posed a threat to her Red Cross. When she found that the women were using the red Greek cross on letterhead and receipts and bandying its name about "in ignorant profusion," she tried first to restrain them, then took the matter to President William McKinley. In a private meeting at the White House she told him she believed the situation in Cuba was one of war and in such situations the Red Cross had no authority to act but by his command. She was willing to wait his call, but she feared that in the meantime the "court ladies" and similar groups would do real mischief in their "excess of zeal, and scarcity of knowledge." The president suggested, somewhat patronizingly, that perhaps the women should "consult their husbands," and he accepted Barton's proposal that the secretaries of war and the navy examine the case.[14]

The court ladies finally faded from view, but other groups appeared in their place. Newspapers, most notably the *Christian Herald,* offered to send their own relief outfits, and congressmen continued to debate on government appropriations. "I fear by the trend of things that the breeze is blowing a little too brisk in the direction of relief for *Cuba* to be quite ready for us," Barton wrote with misgiving.[15] She was still determined that, should the relief go, it would be under her direction. Feeling that she must step on the bandwagon or be left behind, on November 30 she wrote again to Minister Dupuy de Lôme, offering the services of the American Red Cross. She also consulted again with Assistant Secretary of State William R. Day and the president, who finally urged her to go personally to the stricken island. Barton had not yet established the means of securing contributions, however, nor did the Red Cross have Spanish permission to land.[16]

Barton had avoided one crisis by appealing directly to the president, but another befell the Red Cross during these months, one she was powerless to prevent. The scandal, which involved financial secretary George Pullman, held a personal sting as well as a professional threat, and the year 1897 ended on an unhappy note. "This has been a dark year," Clara wrote gloomily; "it is still dark with me, and I *cannot* lighten it."[17]

Pullman had joined the Red Cross staff in 1892. The young man interested Barton because of his connection with the famous inventor of the palace car, but also because he was newly widowed and quite obviously nursing a "tender crushed heart."[18] Barton's attraction to anyone with even a hint of the waif about them was by now notorious, and he joined the group of former prostitutes, chronic debtors, and other misfits who from time to time filled her house. He was snub-nosed and broad-shouldered, with a dapper beard and merry eyes—a likeable, witty man. Moreover, though not particularly proficient at financial matters, he was a willing worker, capable of keeping up the official journal and light correspondence, and of withstanding the rigors of field work. Barton described him as "helpful, faithful, efficient, gentlemanly and true," and she grew increasingly fond of him through the years.[19]

Indeed the despondence Clara felt whenever Pullman was absent, her use of red ink to mark his comings and goings in her diary, and her growing emotional dependence on him hint at an attachment that may have gone beyond sentimentality or close friendship. For years she planned her vacations around the Pullman family's annual reunions at the Thousand Islands. After 1893 Clara was loath to travel anywhere without "G.P.," and when the plans to move into the house at Glen Echo were carried out, she installed him in a bedroom adjoining hers, an arrangement that was to cause more than a few raised eyebrows when it became public knowledge several years later. These actions were perhaps not significant—after all, she had treated both Hubbell and Morlan in a similar manner—but the persistent heartaches described in Barton's diary when Pullman was absent and her obsession with everything he said or did point to a sad infatuation. There was nearly a fifty-year difference in age between them, however, and Pullman, who affectionately referred to Clara as "the Queen," showed no sign of reciprocating any tender feelings.[20]

So devoted was Barton to her financial secretary that when he evidenced unmistakable signs of alcoholism she sought only to help and protect him. As early as 1893 she was giving him money and sending him to the "Keely Cure," a popular form of therapy based on a patented elixir and (to Barton's delight) whole grain mush. When there were lapses, as there more and more frequently were during the next few years, she chose to turn her head and "once more 'Give that man his chance.'"[21] But in the summer of 1897 Stevé and Hubbell could not refrain from writing to Barton of the danger the situation posed. Pullman was slipping off to Washington and New York for repeated drunken bouts, and there was some evidence that he was also undergoing treatment for syphilis. Clara would be foolish, wrote Stevé from New York, to ignore the "danger to which the good name of the Red Cross and your dear self are exposed by his presence here in the condition [in] which he has been seen, and on the business which I am told he confesses brings him here."[22] Unless Pullman could drastically change his habits, urged her two advisors, "his connection with the organization should be severed."[23]

To make matters worse, Pullman had become entangled with another of Barton's wards, Lily Mason. She was a sullen and untruthful young woman, but because her mother had died in service to the organization, Barton felt responsible for her and was loath to turn her out before she had had a chance to become skillful enough as a typist to support herself. But to her diary Clara dryly noted that "our boat was running good time & speed, but that it had 'picked up a snag' and [is] 'thumping.'"[24] It is unclear just what the actual relationship between Lily and George was, but when Pullman began showing signs of interest in another young woman, Mason became hysterical. She claimed that he had promised to marry her, that she was pregnant, then later changed her story to claim that he had already married her. None of the charges proved to be true, but fearful of the publicity, Pullman resigned from the American Red Cross on December 7, 1897. This did little to deter Mason, however. She haunted and abused Pullman everywhere he went until he was finally forced to flee to Europe. Occasionally Mason threatened to blackmail the Red Cross, and she made up libelous stories about Barton. Few believed her tales; the exaggeration only served to make her look ridiculous and pathetic.[25]

Barton could scarcely ignore Mason, however. Not only had she lost her beloved G.P., but the Red Cross was close to succumbing to the scandal of sexual excess, alcoholism, and poor judgment on the part of its president. Lily Mason had indeed set the boat "a thumping," and now there was "a hole in the bottom & all hands have to stand at the pumps to keep it afloat and moving."[26] Barton had hoped that there would never be another break in Red Cross staff like the one she had faced at the Red Cross Park two years earlier; she had wished "that *always* the goings out [are] . . . sweet, friendly and leave no sting."[27] Now she had to contact a lawyer to look into a possible libel suit against Mason, had to deny knowledge of the guilty parties, and had to sever forever her connection with the hospitable Pullmans. "I have only sorrow like your own," she told George's father, the Reverend Royal H. Pullman, "a hundred times a day the tears fall, and I cannot help them."[28]

Toward the end of the year, Barton received a copy of President McKinley's plan to help the reconcentrados. In order to satisfy the Red Cross, as well as the *Christian Herald* and private donors, he had established the Central Cuban Relief Committee (CCRC). It was to be a body of three: a representative of the American Red Cross; Louis Klopsch, the editor of the *Christian Herald;* and Charles Schieren, a prominent New Yorker. Barton chose Stevé to sit on the committee and heartily approved the plan, which called for the CCRC to solicit and collect contributions throughout the country. The goods and money would then be shipped to the American consul general in Cuba, who at the time was General Fitzhugh Lee, nephew of the famed Civil War general. Finally, the distribution would be handled by the Red Cross. Hopefully, the president added, it would be directed by Barton herself.[29]

In January 1898, the CCRC sent out, under the seal of the Department of State, an appeal for supplies and donations of every kind.[30] The response was tremendous. Klopsch pledged ten thousand dollars a month from the *Christian*

Herald if Barton would "personally take charge of the relief," and within a month the consul general wired from Havana that donations were coming in so fast that there was immediate need of a "suitable" person to oversee their distribution.[31] With the government solidly behind her and secure finances, Barton no longer hesitated. In the last weeks of January she made preparations for the care of the house at Glen Echo, hired a stenographer to attend to general correspondence, packed her grips, and set off for Cuba. On February 9, armed with a flattering testimonial from President McKinley, she arrived in Havana.[32]

Barton found conditions unexaggerated by the "yellow press," though she believed the Spanish were not being given credit for their efforts to alleviate the situation. The problems caused by herding the population into camps surrounded by barbed wire and armed guards had been increased by drought and the clearing of farmland by the insurgents, which destroyed not only cash crops but the basic food supply. The resultant suffering was terrible. Skeletal forms were huddled together in filth, with scarcely a rag to clothe them. Children and expectant mothers lay neglected and dying without even the comfort of a cup of clean water. Not since the Civil War had Barton seen human wretchedness so appalling that she could not bring herself to describe it. "The massacres of Armenia seemed merciful in comparison," was all that she would state.[33]

Misery Barton found in abundance; she also encountered an explosive political situation. The caution McKinley showed in sending aid to the reconcentrados had resulted from his unwillingness to appear as an ally of the Cuban rebels. Though personally distressed by the suffering on the island, he had little desire to commit the country to war with Spain. Both he and Barton were well aware that the public that gave so generously to relieve the Cuban neighbors wanted justice for them, as well as short-term relief. The "struggle between the two," Barton sagely observed, "held the country in a state of perplexed contradiction for months running into years."[34] Accordingly, she refused every opportunity to criticize Spain's policies, made a point of relieving both Cubans and Spaniards, and took pains to accommodate herself, whenever possible, to the authorities from Madrid.

The dangerous nature of the situation was made abundantly clear on February 15, when the U.S.S. *Maine* blew up in Havana harbor. Barton, who had lunched on board with the captain only two days before, was shocked when a "terrific burst of thunder—and the fiery balls playing in the heavens, told us that *something* had happened.[35] Not one to miss a dramatic opportunity, she wired a short message to the president: "I am with the wounded."[36] What few wounded there were—for the blast had killed 260 crew members—had, in fact, abundant care in a Spanish hospital. Clara went along anyway to take their names and hear their stories. She took some time to collect a few "charred and splintered" fragments of the ship for her relic cabinet, and a little more time to reflect upon the consequences of the event. Though no one was ever able to positively trace the origins of the blast, public opinion condemned Spain, and war seemed inevitable. As one relief worker, summing up the rash feelings of his countrymen, put it, the only way to get relief into Cuba was to shoot it in. Barton herself gave few comments to the swarms of reporters who had invaded the island. Her work, she declared, had not changed its nature with the explosion of the *Maine*. She was in Cuba to give impartial relief to suffering people, whether they were American, Spanish, or Cuban, and that relief would continue, regardless of political events.[37]

For the next six weeks she toured the countryside in an effort to change, even a little, the condition of the islanders. She was accompanied by John K. Elwell, the nephew of her old wartime flame, who had worked for years as a businessman in Cuba and thus knew the language and the best methods of storing and shipping supplies. Together they visited tiny villages and towns swollen with reconcentrados, established soup kitchens, supplied hospitals, and distributed clothing. At times they entered buildings so filthy that they were driven back by the stench. The orphanages they set up—always under the care of a local dignitary—were among the most notable of their projects. Dazed, filthy, and emaciated children were seemingly everywhere; some were in such dreadful condition that Barton could hardly associate them with live children, "which they no longer seemed to be."[38] When Senator Redfield Proctor arrived in Cuba, determined to assess the situation for himself, she led him on an emotional tour of her projects. The conditions Proctor saw shocked him, and he ultimately gave a passionate testimony to the Senate, which was to greatly influence that body's decision to fight Spain.[39] For Clara Barton he had nothing but praise. "Miss Barton needs no indorsement from me," he told his colleagues.

> I had known and esteemed her for many years, but had not half appreciated her capability and devotion to her work. I specially looked into her business methods, fearing that here would be the greatest danger of mistake, that there might be want of system and waste and extravagance, but found she could teach me on these points. . . . In short I saw nothing to criticize, but everything to commend. The American people may be assured that their bounty will reach the sufferers with the least possible cost and in the best manner in every respect.[40]

The consul general echoed these sentiments, telling Assistant Secretary of State William R. Day that he believed the distribution was effective and systematic, and Barton's work laudable in the extreme.[41]

Back in New York, however, one member of the CCRC was unwilling to take the word of Proctor. Anxious to oversee the operations himself, Louis Klopsch determined to take an active part in the work in Cuba. He was a short man, with persistently wavy hair and keen, wary eyes; his carriage radiated the confidence he had acquired in a lifetime of getting his own way.[42] Convinced of his own utility and against the wishes of the other members of the CCRC, he set off for the beleaguered isle, determined to write the final story on the tenuous situation.

Though he had, at the outset, promised Barton that it was "not his purpose nor his desire to in any way dictate or direct what [her] actions should be,"

Klopsch had hardly landed before he began to meddle in the distribution of re-lief.[43] He insisted on inspecting every warehouse and relief station and blithely commented on them without knowledge or tact. When advised by a number of doctors that there were still pockets of dire distress, he immediately wrote out checks for one or two thousand dollars, stating that this was not the time for deliberation but action. He was entertained and fêted by Consul General Lee, while a jealous Barton, who had been received only perfunctorily by the general, stood by and fumed. Klopsch dropped his original plans for a brief visit and re-mained for a month to give orders and advice, much to everyone's annoyance.[44] The extravagance of his response to the sad plight of the Cubans was matched only by Barton's own spectacular overreaction to his presence in Havana. In a letter that was overwrought, even for her, she told Stevé:

Our chances for peaceful comfortable, or respectable work . . . are nearly ruined by the poisoning of K. who was there so long, that he got his fangs in, and his slime over nearly every department and person—he was there half as long as we were, and *in* the hotel with the *Consul-Genl* and nearly all the *reporters*, and made it headquarters for all malcontents he could ingraft, and slung his money about like chips, and used us for a target day and night . . . I was probably never so maligned in my life.[45]

Klopsch's critical remarks centered largely on what he considered unnecessary bureaucracy. "Red tape and red paint will not feed the hungry," he told one re-porter.[46] But he also made unfortunate references to Barton's age and the "old fogyism of certain members of the Red Cross."[47] As the quarrel began to be front-page news, Stevé pleaded with his aunt to be diplomatic and with Klopsch to be less critical. Clara, stung to the quick, was in no frame of mind to tolerate such abuse, however. She charged Klopsch with hampering her work and confus-ing local officials by contradicting the policies of the American consul and the Red Cross. When he showed no intention of leaving soon, she made a quick decision to return his money and leave the field. "I will no longer be burdened with his gold," she told an astonished press. By all accounts her work had been splendid, yet, sadly, it had hardly begun. But Barton would not stay and work under the direction—and censure—of the forthright Klopsch. "No relief work with which I have been connected in the past has given me less satisfaction than this in Cuba," she announced on her arrival in Washington.[48]

The first thing Barton did was to request an interview at the State Department. To Assistant Secretary Day, she complained of the situation and warned him that she would not return without a complete endorsement from the government and an understanding with the CCRC that their job was merely to collect money; the Red Cross had sole responsibility for its distribution. In a massive show of will she accomplished everything she had hoped to on the journey. Klopsch, though he remained in Cuba for a few more weeks, was in the end forced to resign from the CCRC. He was replaced by Joseph Sheldon, an appointment that gave the committee a majority of Red Cross members. Moreover, as Stevé proudly noted, she "was requested to return immediately to Cuba and pursue her good work—according to her own methods, with the full authority and sanction as well as the support of the government and this Committee." Having gained these points, Barton spent a few weeks conferring with her nephew and acquiring supplies before she returned to the stricken isle.[49]

It was to prove a costly delay. While Barton was making plans to renew her work among the Cubans, William McKinley succumbed to public opinion and delivered a war message to Congress; on April 25 war was declared. He had not wanted this, but the press was clamoring for war, and hot-headed rivals, such as Theodore Roosevelt, were declaring that "Woobly Willie" had not "the backbone of a chocolate eclair."[50] The April 23 departure of Barton's newly chartered relief ship, the S.S. *State of Texas,* was therefore just a bit too late to assure her arrival in Cuba before the confusion and restrictions of war caused all American activities on the island to come under review. When, in late April, Barton, Hubbell, and a staff of nurses and doctors, including Egan and the Gardners, arrived in Florida, ready to join the ship, they found that it had been ordered to remain in Tampa indefinitely.[51]

Tampa was the departure point for American troops. As such, it was rapidly becoming swollen with soldiers and sailors, whose mood alternated between boredom and lighthearted high jinks. With admirals and generals appearing in the town daily, an active social life commenced, of which Barton was a conspicuous part. The martial spirit—which she frankly enjoyed—and flattering attention could not compensate, however, for the annoying delay in obtaining permission to proceed on to Cuba. Most "of the sufferers will be past the need of food before we can get to them," she wrote as it became clear that they would be held for more than a few days.[52] Barton called on Admiral William T. Sampson to protest their detention, reminding him that her mission was to give impartial relief to the Cuban civilians at the express wish of the president. Sampson received Barton cordially, but candidly told her that he believed her program entirely at odds with his own goal, which was to blockade the island and force Spain to capitulate. As Clara explained the matter to Stevé, "Admiral Sampson says openly and truthfully that my aim and efforts are exactly opposed to those of the government from which he takes his orders; that while my effort . . . is to get food into Cuba, his object, which is the object of the Government, is to keep food out."[53] Back in Washington Stevé tried to gain permission to resume the humanitarian work, but with equally unsatisfactory results. Not only did McKinley uphold Sampson's position, Stevé reported, but he underscored it by stating additionally that "he could not think of sanctioning any action that would put either you or any member of your staff in any danger."[54]

Thus they were kept, for nearly two months in a limbo between the expectation of departure and despair of ever obtaining permission to continue their work. The cost of keeping such a ship at anchor—over four hundred dollars per day—caused more than a few raised eyebrows in New York, as did Barton's refusal to return to headquarters to coordinate the war relief effort, which was then beginning.[55] She tried to put a brave front on the situation and to prove that the Red Cross was filling a need in Tampa. "We wish you could see how busy and hard at work our force all is here," Barton wrote to New York. The staff and crew were collecting supplies, learning Spanish, and feeding the starving prisoners of war, who had begun to be captured from Spanish prizes. George Kennan had joined the company and was writing glowing newspaper accounts of their efforts.[56] Yet tensions among the staff were increasing, and Barton had to admit that it was "a demoralizing thing to hold a shipload like this, quiet in a place near the shore, yet at sea, as we are doing."[57] In a mood of deep despondency she questioned whether any of her work, which seemed so frequently beset by similar problems, had ever had the chance to be really effective.[58]

What was perhaps most exasperating was that the government in general—and the military in particular—continued to misunderstand the Red Cross. According to the Treaty of Geneva, the announcement of war should have brought the American Red Cross into an active role with the military. The organization's reason for being, after all, was to supply the bandages, ambulances, volunteers, and organization to eliminate needless wartime suffering. Barton had worked for twenty years to relay this message to the leaders of the army, and now it was apparent that she had failed. Many military men still did not even know of the existence of the treaty or of its organizational offshoot. Others still held to their long-cherished beliefs about the need to use only military men for medical duty; volunteers were enthusiastic but untrained and liable to lose their heads under fire. "Where the medical department of the army is all it ought to be," stated one official document, "volunteer aid societies are, to say the least, needless."[59] The report went on to recommend that the Red Cross be excluded from the active operations of the army; its role, if any, was to procure delicacies for sick men. "This 'link between the civil and military element,'" it concluded, "which M. Moynier regarded as a 'necessity' is not to be found."[60] Neutrality of personnel, supplies, or action was also still an alien concept in 1898; indeed it seemed at odds with the concept of war as American military men had known it. Hence, Admiral William Van Reypen refused to have all boxes of relief goods marked with the red cross, which would have ensured their impartial use, and Surgeon General George M. Sternberg dismissed requests from civilians who wished to carry water or stretchers on the battlefield.[61] Not until June 6, after intense urging by both Stevé and Clara, did the government formally accept the services of the American Red Cross. Even then a combination of personalities and misunderstandings kept the Red Cross from working in a close or effective way with the army in Cuba.

307

The confusion was increased by the still-fragmented nature of the Red Cross organization. While Barton battled officials off the Florida coast, ambitious men and women around the country established local soldiers' aid societies, frequently using the Red Cross insignia. The California Red Cross was an early and noteworthy group; so expertly did they handle relief to the men fighting in the Philippines that Barton virtually ignored this theater of the war. In Minnesota another forceful society was founded, which concentrated on working at the crowded and fever-ridden army camps in the United States. Most formidable of all was the great New York Red Cross. It had sprung from the Red Cross hospital in New York, a small nurse training establishment that had been founded with Barton's blessing in 1895. During the hundred days of war with Spain it would grow into a powerful body with 112 auxiliaries, led by persons of such stature as John Jacob Astor and Jacob Schiff. Spurred on by news of the dreadful conditions at the army camp on Montauk Point, Long Island, they harnessed their impressive resources and established an organization that would contribute nearly three hundred thousand dollars to the medical care of the army. Each auxiliary was charged with a specific area of relief. Auxiliary No. 1 bought and outfitted ambulances. Auxiliary No. 3, which would become the greatest of the group, recruited and paid trained nurses, and No. 10 shipped so many tons of ice to the tropics to ease parched throats and burning fevers that they became known as the "Ice Plan Auxiliary." [62]

The national organization had virtually no control over these bodies. To varying degrees the auxiliaries were aware of the Treaty of Geneva and Barton's small nuclear group, but even had they desired to be responsible to Washington there was nowhere they could apply to receive their orders. The headquarters now consisted of one charming but naive young stenographer named Lucy Graves, who sent even the most innocuous messages on to Stephen Barton at the CCRC, where they were wired to his aunt. Initially, Barton showed a curious lack of concern about the mushrooming societies. They symbolized to her only that the Red Cross had at last succeeded in attracting "into its fold the men of wealth and standing and prestige" who she believed were essential to its eventual success. [63] "You are correct in thinking that this is the time to build up the Red Cross," she told one correspondent, adding that she had long foreseen that it would take a war to make Americans understand the true nature of the organization. [64] It was Steve who saw the potential confusion and rivalry with these groups and made the first efforts to bring them into an established relationship with the national body. When the New York auxiliary began using the name and badge of the international society without official permission, he contacted their president, William T. Wardwell. Together they agreed that the New Yorkers would operate under the name "American National Red Cross Relief Committee," that their role would be to garner supplies without exercising any control over relief work, and that they must submit reports to Barton at the end of the operations. [65] Only later, when Clara realized that the Red Cross the American public recognized was not her own little band of a dozen workers but the mighty network of hospi-

tals, nurses, warehouses, and societies led by the New Yorkers, did she understand how dearly she had paid for her months aboard the *State of Texas*.

On June 20, Barton heard news that the American navy was leaving the shelter
of Tampa and Key West in order to confront the Spanish fleet near Santiago,
Cuba. She applied for permission to follow them; when she received no response
she decided to go anyway. She was pleased with her staff: besides Hubbell, Egan,
Kennan, and the Gardners, there were now Dr. A. Monae Lesser of the Red
Cross Hospital, his wife (a trained nurse known as "Sister Bettina"), and four of
her colleagues from New York. After their weeks of inactivity they were as anxious as Barton to begin work again with the reconcentrados.[66]
    Despite the declaration of war, it was still civilian relief to which Barton was
committed. Her plans were to meet Elwell near Santiago, unload the fourteen
hundred tons of supplies in the hold of the *State of Texas*, and begin the laborious
process of transporting and distributing them in the interior of the island. But
the events of the campaign changed her course. On June 25, just as the *State of
Texas* was nearing Cuba, some members of Teddy Roosevelt's eager Rough Riders
rushed onto a precarious landing and engaged in a series of skirmishes that resulted in heavy casualties. By chance Barton's ship was nearby, and the Red Cross
workers hunted the shoreline for signs of the soldiers. They anchored off Siboney
and made their way to the shore, where they found Cuban and American field
hospitals side by side. What the government had tried to prevent—the active
participation of the Red Cross on the field—had happened by accident. For the
next fortnight Barton would find herself in the familiar position of making gruel
for wounded soldiers.[67]
    "It is the Rough Riders we go to," she wrote excitedly in her diary, "and the
relief may be also rough; but it will be *ready*."[68] The Red Cross was, in fact, a
great deal more prepared for battle than the army surgeons. The resources Barton
found at the hospitals near Siboney were as sadly lacking as those at Antietam
had been thirty-six years before. There were no cots, no mattresses or ham-
mocks, no clothing, and very little food. Men with fevers and flesh wounds were
lying on coarse stubble grass in the tropical sun, with "no covering over them
save such as had clung to them in their troubles, and in the majority of cases no
blanket under them."[69] Doctors who had not had the foresight to cram a few
delicacies and extra bandages into their pockets had little to offer the wounded
men. Dr. Gardner was disgusted with the plight of this army, which had boasted
of its self-sufficiency but suffered a total absence of even basic necessities. George
Kennan, accustomed as he was to reporting on the more dismal aspects of human
life, was shocked at the scene he saw in Siboney. "That it was wretchedly incomplete and inadequate I hardly need say. . . . If there was anything more terrible
in our Civil War, I am glad I was not there to see it."[70] For Barton, the horrid
condition of the field hospitals left a special sadness. It was this very situation
that she had hoped to change by introducing the Red Cross in the United States,

and through her inability to convince the army of its value, the organization had failed to carry out its primary function. She would complain that the "Government was not ready for [the war]; it was not willing to wait until it was ready, and the consequences have been short comings on all sides," but in her heart she knew that somewhere a fundamental understanding about the treaty, its advantages and its obligations, had been lost.[71] In her diary she lamented the lost opportunity to show how the Red Cross could alleviate some of the terrors of battle: "I felt that it was again the same old story and wondered what gain there had been in the last thirty years."[72]

Initially, the army surgeons would not even admit that they needed help—certainly not help from a band of women in starched uniforms. When the American surgeons adamantly refused offers of assistance, Barton and her staff politely left and tendered their services to the Cuban doctors next door. They were welcomed there, for conditions were even worse than in the American hospital. Within twenty-four hours the men, who had been huddled together on bits of rag without anything to eat for three days, were lying on cots, in a spotlessly clean hospital, enjoying the comforts of soft porridge, fresh sheets, and sympathetic words. The Americans, lying close enough to note the contrast, pressured the surgeons to allow the Red Cross to aid them. Somewhat sheepishly the chief surgeon approached Barton and formally requested her assistance.[73]

For the next weeks the dozen men and women worked almost nonstop to clean, comfort, feed, and clothe these wounded men, and those that poured into the hospital after the July 1 battles of El Caney and San Juan Hill. They had an abundance of supplies but were short of staff. Landing the goods was a considerable feat, since the tidal currents kept anything but the lightest flat boat from reaching shore, and even small craft could be landed only at low tide between 3:00 A.M. and 10:00 A.M.[74] Surgeons were desperately needed: Lesser, Hubbell, Egan, and Gardner joined the weary staff doctors to perform over four hundred operations in two days. Enola Gardner helped feed mush to the famished and stirred together a concoction called "Red Cross cider," made from stewed dried apples and prunes. They gave their best effort, but the short staff made it impossible to care for the thousands of wounded as they would have liked. That they had been able to help at all was merely an accident. "Such as it was, we freely and tirelessly gave," Barton soberly observed a month later.

> We know that it was a great deal too much when we hear it repeated . . . "The Red Cross saved the army"—we know that was not so—but that we saved much suffering and many lives, we are willing to admit. If we could have been permitted or properly called to the field only one month before the outbreak, there would have been no unnecessary suffering, no lack of food, or care, or nurses.[75]

At seventy-seven, dressed in a calico skirt and apron and energetically preparing food and applying ice to fevered foreheads, Barton was a magnificent and legendary figure. She worked sixteen hours a day to oversee operations in the field, in addition to the time she spent chasing intrigues in the military bureaucracy. "Even to us who know so well Miss Barton's powers of endurance," Dr. Hubbell reported, "it seems a marvel when we think of all the mental as well as physical strain which she has endured during the past months of Cuban work." [76] Barton herself seems to have been somewhat amused to be replaying a role she had believed forever relegated to dim memory. "I had not thought to ever make gruel again over a campfire," she later reminisced. "I can not say how far it carried me back in the lapse of time, or really where or who I felt that I was." [77]

She could not rally the spirit, however, that she had felt in former conflicts. Clara had not approved of the conflict, which she believed not only demeaning to the United States but merely the product of an irresponsible type of press coverage. Only rarely did she find herself captivated by the vision of blue and gold uniforms, buglers and solemn marchers. [78] "I am sorry for this war," she confided to a close friend, "but now that we are in it there is no way but to go through it. I never thought to see and take part in another war. It seems very strange that I should do so. Sometimes I almost think that it is not right, that too much of that kind of thing comes to me; but it is the last and must be met as it can be." [79]

"If we had had in Siboney a number of assistants, and fifty Red Cross sisters instead of six to make work easy . . . we might have been of more service," Dr. Lesser wrote in an official report of the Red Cross field work. [80] It was not for lack of trying on Barton's part that these things were unavailable. As soon as it became clear that the Red Cross was, after all, going to be at the front, she wired to Stevé, asking him to send more supplies and, most importantly, a contingent of twenty-five trained nurses. The members of the CCRC and Auxiliary No. 3 duly recruited and outfitted thirty experienced young women and sent them to Cuba aboard the S.S. Lampass. When they were refused permission to land, the ship steamed on to Puerto Rico where less finicky doctors welcomed their help in the desperately understaffed hospitals. But the army's rejection of the nurses aboard the Lampass was an ominous sign. For the duration of the war, the armed forces held fast to their prejudice against female nurses at the field. Barton and her staff were the only Red Cross personnel to work directly at the front during the entire conflict. [81]

It was Surgeon General George M. Sternberg who posed the greatest obstacle to sending female nurses to the field. He was a small, retiring man, who held firm opinions about the conduct of the army's medical department and its relation to the American Red Cross. He feared the association, which he believed would keep his department from operating independently, and he did not trust Barton and her staff with the lives of his men, opinions which were reinforced by rivals such as the DAR's strong-willed Anita Newcomb McGee. Against the use of female nurses he had particularly adamant convictions. Like his counterparts in the Civil War, he thought them liable to be flighty, demanding, and skittish. "It is not our intention to employ volunteer nurses at U.S. general hospitals,"

Sternberg wrote at the very time that men were perishing in Siboney from exposure and inadequate care. "It is the duty of the Government to take care of the sick and wounded soldiers of our army, and we feel fully able to meet this obligation with the resources at our command." So strong were his opinions that although Secretary of War Russell A. Alger and the president both advocated the use of female nurses, Sternberg's decision held for the first half of the war.[82]

Sternberg never accepted female nurses on the field, but he was eventually persuaded to allow them on hospital transports and in army hospitals in the United States. In large part his decision was due to the extraordinary outbreak of disease—malaria, typhoid, dysentery, and yellow fever—in both the recruit camps and American bases in Cuba. So devastating were the epidemics that the troops were dubbed "an army of convalescents." When newspaper reports began charging the army with inadequate care for the men and exposed the shocking conditions aboard two hospital transports, there was a call for congressional investigation. Under this pressure Sternberg relented. In newspaper interviews (in contrast to his memos, in which he consistently refused to allow women in any army hospital), he denied that he had ever objected to female nurses working in the United States. He had, Sternberg said, only opposed those who he felt "would be an encumbrance to troops during active operations."[83]

The reversed decision brought an immediate response from Auxiliary No. 3, which in all sent over seven hundred nurses to camps and hospitals during the short-lived conflict. With scarcely an exception, they proved Sternberg's fears wrong. In some cases, such as at Camp Thomas in Georgia, where conditions were distressingly similar to the camps of the reconcentrados, they did really heroic work. Sentimentalists and the nation's poets began to speak of the Red Cross nurse as "angelic" and begged to be allowed to "cast a flower at her feet." More significant were the sober statements about their exceptional work, contained in the reports of disciplined army surgeons. "Our recent experience may justly be held to have shown," read one official document, "that female nurses, properly trained and properly selected, can be duly cared for and are of the greatest value. Those who have been serving under contract in our military hospitals . . . have with scarcity and exception done excellent work."[84]

Like so many of the other confusions of the war period, the problems with Sternberg could have been greatly reduced had someone been in Washington to deal with the government and coordinate relief efforts. But Barton preferred to remain in the field, where her efforts—even if criticized as grand, romantic gestures—seemed to do direct good, and where she would see the action and excitement that so satisfied her spirit.[85]

The tropical fevers that made such inroads on the United States army also took their toll on Barton's staff in Cuba. Barely a fortnight after they began serving in the field hospitals near Siboney, Dr. Lesser and his wife Bettina were stricken with yellow fever; within a week eleven members of the staff had succumbed to the disease. Afraid that her ship would be quarantined (for it was not yet known that yellow fever was carried by mosquitoes), Barton made arrangements for the infected workers to be cared for at a nearby yellow fever hospital. She further decreed that no outsiders be allowed aboard the *State of Texas*, for fear her small group would be further infected.

Barton's decision was controversial. The Red Cross had come to Cuba claiming that the battlefield was not their only domain, that they were there to aid soldiers and civilians in any way they could. To retreat from a disease that was then one of the chief liabilities of tropical warfare was thought by some to show a kind of cowardice not often associated with Barton. Dissension over the decision was strong among her own crew, with George Kennan the most vocal critic. He met with Barton and told her that he believed she was fulfilling the worst predictions of General Sternberg and, further, that her abandonment of the stricken staff members might seriously endanger them.[86] The disagreement finally escalated into a full-scale fight, with Barton treating Kennan as a traitor and silently fuming with a martyrlike air. "The manner in which I expressed my disapproval . . . was hasty and inconsiderate," Kennan later apologized, "and in my anger I may have used expressions that fully justified the withdrawal of your confidence from me and the treatment you subsequently gave me."[87] In spite of this apology he chose to resign from the Red Cross. Anxious that no scandal should arise and unwilling to lose a prestigious officer and charter member, Barton told Kennan she had dismissed his remarks as only a few of the "many hard, belittling and disgraceful things said of me in the last few months," adding that she hoped he would not leave the Red Cross at this critical hour.[88] But Kennan had seen enough to make him immune to even Barton's considerable powers of manipulation. He left the ship a few days later, leaving behind a strongly worded letter which Barton chose to ignore. Not until two years later did she acknowledge the rift between them and formally accept his letter of resignation.[89]

Bickering as well as fear of illness was now rampant among the staff, but an event occurred in early August that helped Barton overcome the general demoralization. As she and Kennan fumed, she ordered that the ship leave Siboney for Santiago. Word had arrived that the strategic city had surrendered to Admiral Sampson a few days earlier, and Barton was hopeful that she would be allowed to land there, renew her connection with Elwell, and utilize the warehouses full of stores that were still in the city. The residents of Santiago were rumored to be starving; Barton, hoping to avoid conflict with the military authorities who shunned her services, proposed that she enter the city to give civilian assistance. Admiral Sampson accepted her offer and went so far as to send boats to escort her through the mouth of the difficult harbor.[90]

A few hours later it became apparent that Sampson meant for the Red Cross ship to lead the victorious procession of naval vessels into the harbor. The entrance had been delayed for several days while the mines that dotted the bay were dismantled, and the arrival of the *State of Texas* had coincided with the hour of entry. Even Barton, used to triumphal tours and standing ovations, was thrilled by the honor of this gesture. As the ship, guidied by a naval pilot, glided through the long strait that led to the city, Barton and her staff stood on the deck, while the "gulls sailed and flapped and dipped" in the late afternoon sun. Overcome with emotion, Barton requested that someone begin the doxology, and after it had been sung, the men struck up "My Country 'Tis of Thee." As they neared the shore they could see the excitement with which the populace was receiving them. "Men, women, and children ran down to the water's edge, waving their hats and handkerchiefs, or brandishing their arms in joyous welcome," recalled George Kennan, "and even old gray-haired and feeble women . . . stood in front of their houses, now gazing at us in half-incredulous amazement, and then crossing themselves devoutly, with bowed heads, as if thanking God that siege and starvation were over and help and food at hand."[91] Another of those present also was affected by the dramatic scene and later wrote of it, with quiet pride, in his memoirs. "Miss Barton was standing on the forward deck," he recalled. "A hundred glasses were on her as she stood queenly and majestic, one of the bravest of the brave, always going where suffering humanity most needed her."[92]

Barton began to distribute bread as soon as the *State of Texas* landed. In the first twenty-four hours she and the tiny group that accompanied her fed over ten thousand people. Dirt and disorder reigned in Santiago, and for the next five weeks the Red Cross remained to establish soup kitchens, clinics, and orphanages. Since the fear of disease was widespread, Barton continued to impose her own quarantine, allowing no one on or off the ship, save those charged with unloading supplies. Distribution was handled by Elwell and local officials. Army officers as well as civilians were presented with supplies, though Barton continued to keep a low profile in her relations with the army. "I did not happen to see any United States quartermaster in Cuba who, in the short space of five days, had unloaded and stored fourteen hundred tons of cargo, given hot soup daily to ten thousand soldiers, and supplied an army of thirty-two thousand men with ten days rations," commented one observer. "It is a record, I think, of which Miss Barton had every reason to be proud."[93]

In spite of her assistance, Red Cross relations with the army remained precarious. Whenever possible she loaned or gave them medicine and food. Once she and her associates were startled to see Colonel Theodore Roosevelt striding purposely toward them. He requested supplies for his wounded and ill men, but when Barton offered to send them, he declined, saying that heavy though they were, he would lug them back himself. "Before we had recovered from our surprise," Barton later recalled, "the incident was closed by the future President of the United States slinging the big sack over his shoulders, striding off, and out of sight through the jungle."[94] Unfortunately, not all officers were as cordial as Roosevelt. One surgeon told her frankly that had he the authority he would send her home, despite the fact that she had just furnished fresh meat and numerous other delicacies to his men.[95] Frequently the army requisitioned her stores; yet the officers consistently refused to allow her to use their equipment or wagons. "The army grasps at everything," she complained to Stevé, "[yet] not even a lighter can be borrowed."[96] Faced with such obstacles, she concentrated on civilian assistance as she had originally set out to do.

Only when she began to see that the Cubans were able to handle their own relief in Santiago did Barton order the ship to move on to Havana, where the suffering was rumored to be even greater.[97] There more difficulties were to beset her. The shipping line that owned the *State of Texas* had recalled the ship, and before leaving for Havana, Barton was forced to transfer staff and supplies to the S.S. *Clinton*, which had been placed at her disposal by President McKinley. On reaching Havana, she encountered another bureaucratic delay. The capital had not yet surrendered, and the Spanish authorities demanded legal documents and clearance papers before allowing the *Clinton* to land. Barton pleaded her case before the governor of Havana, arguing that the workers and goods were neutral under the Treaty of Geneva. Although she was received courteously, a fine of five hundred dollars was nonetheless imposed on the ship, and it was requested that her stores be turned over to the colonial officials for distribution. "Ordinarily, it would not be supposed that Charity must go armed with a cudgel," wrote one Red Cross officer. "But really the present situation would seem to indicate that the Spanish Dons have little sense of appreciation."[98] To Barton the terms were unacceptable, and the unwillingness of the American government to intervene on her behalf was an additional insult. The war was now over. Perceiving that any further work would be accomplished only by continual fighting with the army, she paid her fine and sailed for Tampa.[99]

Inability to successfully enter the port of Havana was the ostensible reason for Clara's return home. But the threat posed by the activities of the New York committees and her critics in the army had become increasingly clear to her, and she was determined to investigate the matter and reassert her control. Outwardly the relations between the CCRC and the several bodies affiliated with the Red Cross were cordial—a happy state of affairs largely attributable to the diplomatic maneuvering of Stevé. He had taken a leave of absence from his job with a major insurance company in order to serve as the chairman of the CCRC, and had spent a frustrating year juggling the various and opposing demands of his willful aunt, several persnickety doctors, the forceful businessmen of the Red Cross Relief Committee, and the United States government. He had done an admirable job but toward the end of the summer relations began to be a bit muddled. The New York Red Cross, heady with their success in so many home camps, had begun to be recognized as the only significant Red Cross in America, and it was clear that they were operating (as were their sister auxiliaries in California, Washington State, Minnesota, and elsewhere) independently of the national association. Stevé had tried to counter this problem by sending field agents from headquarters to oversee relief in several recruit camps, but even he recognized that these were token gestures. At the end of the conflict the American National Red Cross Relief Committee published their own report and began making plans for postwar activities that were clearly divergent from the national body. Anita McGee was also making plans to institutionalize her wartime success. With the hope that her nurses would gain a permanent status within the armed forces, she introduced to Congress an "army nurse bill," which called for employment of females in the military hospitals but made no mention of any affiliation with the Red Cross during wartime. Stevé's attempts alternately to warn his aunt about these developments and to protect her from them, proved unsuccessful.[100]

Isolated, and beset by problems with military officials, Clara began to suspect deviousness and disloyalty in everyone connected with the New York committee. She had never completely understood the arrangement there; as late as October 1898 she was still writing that the committees "have all been a mixture to me, and the explanation given me by Judge Sheldon today is the first tolerably clear comprehension I have had of what committee was which or which committee was what."[101] Toward the end of the war communications began to break down even with Stevé. When two ships chartered by the CCRC, the *Red Cross* and *Moynier,* proved disappointing, she blamed her nephew. When he informed her that her telegrams were often unintelligible, and that he was troubled by the lack of vouchers or other financial records, she was outraged.[102] She charged that Stevé was trying to take over her organization and attempting to direct her operations in Cuba. "I regret exceedingly that I cannot make our movements here conform to your idea of the proper course in New York," she flatly told him. "There are some slight differences in the conditions, which do not quite harmonize, and I am not able to find anyone here who would be equal to doing it."[103] Her suspicions aroused, Barton issued a dictatorial memo entitled "General Order #3," which, among other things, prohibited any doctors or nurses to work under the badge of the Red Cross without her express approval and forbid employees to discuss Red Cross business with anyone outside of her immediate circle.[104] Stevé tried desperately to convince her of the "good will and loyalty which inspired Mr. Wardwell personally, and I believe most of his associates."[105] But there were so many rumors and little snipings directed at her operations in Cuba that she remained unconvinced. "It is really a new experience to me to feel that I am giving such immense and intense concern to people in regard to my ability, my endeavors to do something I am not capable of doing, and the integrity with which I could handle it," she wrote to Stevé with some indignation.[106]

For the most part, she found praise for Red Cross field work, but criticism for what were considered severe omissions in the management of the relief. No one questioned that the Red Cross work at Siboney had been useful; neither did anyone doubt that Barton should have left this field to subordinates and remained in Washington to handle administrative matters. Similar complaints surfaced about her remaining aboard the *State of Texas* during crucial negotiations between the Red Cross and the government. At times the field work had so little direction that one of the nurses who was sent aboard the *Lampass* commented, "there seemed to be no organization. One never knew what would become of one next. All one's service seemed haphazard."[107] Some critics harped on finances, others on Barton's inability to bring full-scale Red Cross operations to the field of battle. Several people charged that Barton had carelessly used untrained personnel, just when feminists and medical professionals were so desperately trying to upgrade the image of female nurses. (This accusation was true: Barton was prone to utilizing every available bit of labor she could find in times of crises and questioning the background and fitness of her workers later. As one of the amateurs who had helped her at Siboney retorted, "It was no time to stand on trained service, and everybody, man or woman, was ready to lend a hand."[108]) Though in all of these cases the volunteers acquitted themselves with considerable service and dignity, their very presence in hospitals was anathema to those who were trying so hard to establish themselves as skilled professionals in the medical field.[109]

Of the many criticisms of her work, the one that hurt Barton the most was the continual reference to her age. She had been sensitive to the subject for nearly fifty years, since her student days in Clinton, where the twelve-year gap in age between her and the rest of the pupils caused her to feel awkward and out of place. As the years advanced, Barton grew ever more self-conscious about the subject. "She could not bear to have anyone think of her as an old lady, and deeply resented any allusion to her age," a friend noted.[110]

As a consequence, she began to give out her birthdate as 1830, chopping away nearly ten years from her real age. Reporters, *Who's Who in America*, even the census taker, were given this figure, though she would disclaim any knowledge of the error when pointedly questioned.[111] As a septuagenarian she insisted on dyeing her hair (she traded recipes for dye with feminists such as Lucy Hall Brown), padding her corsets with tissue paper "to make a nice rounded bust," and using powder, rouge, and eyebrow pencil to enhance her looks. ("Aunt Clara used them skillfully," a great-niece recalled, "and the result was most amazingly good. She looked years younger when she had finished.")[112] The lavenders and grays that society thought appropriate to her station and years were actively shunned; Clara still liked a green dress and a dash of red at the neck. Once, while Barton was shopping with a friend, a young clerk suggested that some cherry red ribbon she had selected might not be the best choice for a lady of her stature. Barton's "dark eyes flashed and her teeth clamped together," remembered an observer, "her wide thin lips opened just sufficiently to allow the sound of her deep vibrant voice to escape as she said, 'Dida, evidently this girl does not know that I wear what I please when I please.'"[113]

Her looks artfully enhanced, she also took pains to appear well and hearty. Afraid that the public would lay her "on the shelf for all time," she roused herself to "make an [sic] public demonstration of living existence even if it kills me."[114] After a daylong outing to Mount Vernon in 1897, she nearly burst into tears when people continually asked her if she were not tired, or if she would like to sit down.[115] Attempts to help her on and off streetcars and wagons posed a similar problem. Stephen Barton, George Pullman, and other young men found themselves in the embarrassing position of having to stand by helplessly while Barton clambered uncertainly onto whatever conveyance was at hand. Once, when two nephews insisted on lifting her onto a trolley car, she turned to them angrily and remarked: "I certainly hope that when I reach the pearly gates I have you two there to hustle me through."[116]

Yet, sadly, as they all recalled, she really did need help. Despite her capacity for work and her own staunch denial, Barton appeared to others as old, and her small stature made her often seem very frail. Great-niece Edith Riccius, who frequently shared a room with Aunt Clara when she visited Massachusetts, thought of her as an eccentric, very elderly lady who gave herself daily sponge baths while "scrooching down by the side of [a basin] in the corner of the room," wore peculiar dark blue nightgowns, and made little puffing noises when she snored. Clara had gotten a little deaf and a little forgetful. It was obvious to everyone but herself that the long days wore her out, and often she would fall asleep in her chair while people spoke to her.[117]

Older in appearance and shorter of energy than she cared to admit, Barton was nonetheless young at heart. She welcomed the dramatic changes in technology of the nineteenth century with unusual equanimity. Gramophones, telephones, and typewriters were early additions to her home and office, and at the first opportunity she took a ride in an automobile, exclaiming at the brisk twenty-five-mile-per-hour pace.[118] Her intellect continued to be more challenged by new ideas and the progressive notions of the times than by memories of the life already lived. Perhaps most significantly, Barton retained her delightful sense of humor, and the most frequent brunt of her jokes was herself. Her niece Edith commented on this several times, as did others who were close to Barton. But Clara herself attests best to this fine attribute in her diary and letters, which she filled with remarks like one written on a rough crossing to Cuba in June 1898. She could not, she noted in her diary, "lift my head from the soppy pillow, even to change it—the pillow I mean. I didn't try to change the head, it wouldn't have been marketable."[119]

Deeply wounded by the whispers and insinuations she felt all around her, Barton retreated to Glen Echo and virtually cut off communication with the outside world. Even to her closest friends she wrote only brief notes or let their letters be answered by her new financial secretary, Charles Cottrell. With fierce determination, she went about housecleaning and set to work on a long overdue account of the services the American Red Cross had performed since 1882. For once, Barton refused to let correspondence or outside demands interfere with her project, and for the next five months she devoted herself entirely to writing.[120]

The book, which came to be entitled *The Red Cross in Peace and War*, was meant as an answer to those who had commented on the dearth of field reports, financial accounts, or even personal reminiscences of Red Cross relief activities. Desperate to defend her activities without seeming to do so, Barton rounded up every available helper, including Julian Hubbell, Joseph Sheldon, and a friendly Civil War veteran named William H. Sears, and set to work. Barton was not altogether sure what the focus of the book should be; she was merely determined to see it published before someone wrote a similar account containing false information.[121] With no framework, a disorganized and desperate group of writers, and an almost unbelievably short schedule, the resultant book resembled, in Clara's words, "a crazy quilt."[122] Official documents appeared with lengthy quotations from Clara's diary; references to finances were included, but no detailed financial accounts. Most of the book was anecdotal; there was virtually no discussion of the theory or methodology of Red Cross work. Half of the seven-hundred-page volume dealt with Cuba, its descriptions so detailed that it is hard to believe Barton's assertions that the haste caused her to "cut short the sentences" she had "hoped to embellish."[123] There was, not surprisingly, no critical discussion of the Red Cross. Lucy Hall and Judge Sheldon both urged her to expose rival groups and defend her name, but Barton was adamantly opposed to sacrificing "the dignity of the book by any indulgence in personalities."[124]

The American Historical Press published the book early in 1899. Barton was not wholly satisfied with it. She recognized that it was disjointed and thought it was too short; possibly it should have been published in two volumes. "You will understand that I do not consider it much of a book," she later told her niece Ida. "It was gotten up quick, for the publisher to try to make money on."[125] Her hopes for financial benefits—always an issue in the impoverished Red Cross—never materialized, however, for the book received little attention from either press or public when it finally appeared.

Clara insulated herself well from the world during the months of writing. Stevé tried desperately to consult with her over the reorganization of the American Red Cross and asked her to oversee the work the California chapter was sustaining in the Philippines. She showed but the slightest concern over these matters and would make decisions only under persistent prodding from her nephew.[126] The one subject she would discuss was the continuance of work in Cuba, about which she had definite ideas.

With the end of hostilities between Spain and the United States, the government had taken over the direction of relief to the island. The military claimed that they were doing all that was needed, but civilians still reported tremendous suffering among the inhabitants. Barton initially believed that the national Red Cross should forego this field, for its small staff was exhausted and its treasury nearly empty. Moreover, the army had made it clear that it intended to handle all Cuban relief, and she feared that her work would be considered an intrusion. As the government officials debated the future of the dazed and hungry Cubans, however, a number of individuals and organizations began offering assistance and collecting money for the islanders. Among these groups was the New York Red Cross, bolstered by their success in the late war. William W. Howard, editor of the *Providence Journal*, used his newspaper as a platform to promote an "industrial relief plan" for Cuba, according to which economic recovery would be fostered by the establishment of sugar mills and other factories. Another group that formed at this time took the imitative name "White Cross" and offered to send medical personnel and supply hospitals. In light of these spontaneous overtures and a report of the desperate conditions written by one of her own agents, Barton felt that the national Red Cross must also offer its services in Cuba. Should another group, especially the New York Red Cross, be accepted over hers, the national organization would completely lose its standing. The American National Red Cross had started the Cuban work before the war, Barton told Stevé, and "the whole world, will look to them rather than the Government to finish the work."[127]

Throughout the early months of 1899 the government negotiated with the various organizations and the army. In March the War Department decided to have the national Red Cross take up the establishment of hospitals and orphanages, while Howard promoted the agricultural and industrial recovery of the country. The situation was not altogether satisfactory to Barton. She disliked having competition on the field and felt that the more important job had been given to Howard. She feared, too, that the editor had "with his influence and wealth and enthusiasm and earnestness so fastened himself upon the President," that her own projects might come under his supervision.[128] Despite her eagerness to embrace all of the Cuban work, however, Barton was not certain how she would support any relief work at all. The organization was so bereft of funds that she once again had to reach into her own pocket, this time expending the small sum she had put away for an unforeseen emergency. (Later in the year she would see the painful necessity of asking the Rochester branch for a loan.) "I do not look for much, if any, assistance for the Cuban work," she told Stevé; "indeed I do not see how it could be expected. The country has been drained for a year and a half *in the name of the national Red Cross* of all that the people felt disposed to give or be able to give."[129]

With her mind preoccupied by the work of "rival" groups and the uncertainties of her financial position, Barton began to design the relief plan for her third mission to Cuba. She did not at first plan to go herself. Hubbell, Cottrell, and Dr. Alexander Kent of the New York Red Cross would join Elwell and a number of Cuban doctors to survey the island and make arrangements for the establishment of clinics, hospitals, and orphanages. The Philadelphia society was also supporting the expedition by contributing large quantities of supplies and several trained nurses. Late in March the group embarked for Cuba, where they were met by two island doctors, Juan B. Sollosso and Julio Carbonell.[130]

They found the situation, especially in the countryside, as horrifying as anything they had yet seen. The island was now an agricultural wasteland. Starvation and disease had decimated the population and left the survivors unable to work. A hundred times daily they were greeted by families such as those described by Carbonell: "horribly bloated, pale as wax, full of vermin, with itch and repulsive ulcers, with chronic hunger and despair reflected on their death-like faces." Destitute children, who ran begging in the streets, were a particular problem.[131]

In small, isolated towns like San Nicholas, Guinis, Jaruca, and Guanajay, they consulted the area's leaders, transformed warehouses into hospitals, and made provision for their care after the departure of the Red Cross. In most cases they were able to leave abundant supplies, and great emphasis was placed on cultivating vegetable gardens where the children themselves could learn skills and raise their own food. "Other field grounds are quarantined when they are able to work them," noted Hubbell proudly, "thus making them largely self-supporting." Notwithstanding the expected frustration in dealing with army and customs officers, more than two thousand children were cared for by the Red Cross.[132]

The work was progressing nicely when Barton decided to take over the supervision of the field. Reports from her subordinates indicated that all was going well, but she could not bear to leave the direction of a field of this magnitude to others. "You know how hard it was for me not to go when you went," she admitted to one of the nurses stationed on the island, "and nearly every week since I have been going, and yet not quite certain of it to say so."[133] It was an ill-advised trip, for the doctors read her arrival as mistrust, and it meant the unnecessary expenditure of precious dollars. Even President McKinley was surprised by the move and commented—much to Clara's horror—that he thought she was certainly due for a furlough.[134] There was little that would dissuade her from going, however, and on May 2 she left Glen Echo to join her staff in Cuba.

In one sense the trip was a kind of triumphal tour around the countryside. Cheers and flowers greeted her arrival everywhere. Sollosso and Hubbell proudly escorted her through the orphanages and hospitals, and she conferred with American and Cuban dignitaries. Photographs show her in black silk and a little flower-bedecked hat, watching grateful orphans perform complicated ring games reminiscent of those her pupils once played, a sweet benevolent smile on her face. Still plucky though nearing her seventy-eighth birthday, she traveled the rutted roads in an old wagon, frequently driven by a driver who was much the worse for rum. "She looked like a very tired old lady, but she kept going," wrote an admiring aide.[135]

An important part of Barton's mission was to turn this good will into a positive future for the Red Cross. Wherever she went she explained the organization and promoted the idea of a Cuban branch of the American national association; "planting seeds," she called it.[136] It was imperative, she advised Charles Schieren, that the Cubans "become, not only the almoners, but the sources of their own charities—to get themselves off the roll of national beggars." During the summer of 1899 she was able to establish a Cuban society under the direction of

Colonel Estes Rathbone, the director-general of the Post Office, and his wife. She believed it to be the most important aspect of her postwar work, especially as it was apparent that the national organization could not much longer sustain relief work in the island.[137]

The picture of Barton, serenely and triumphantly inspecting orphanages throughout Cuba, is at distinct odds with her private woes and fears at this time. More than ever she was feeling threatened by the strong personalities that joined her in the effort to bring assistance to Cuba, and now she saw menace in the very staff of the Red Cross. Throughout the negotiations of early 1899 she had refused any cooperation with the powerful New York Red Cross. There were, as she feared, some grasping and ambitious figures in the state organization, and some who were prone to criticism and gossip. But the vast majority were entirely sincere in the desire to do their best for both Cuba and the Red Cross. "My sole aim and object . . . ," a wealthy New Yorker wrote, "was to assist in putting the Red Cross upon a firm and lasting basis as I have said before. I wish to see it so well organized that when men who will be our successors take charge of it ten, thirty or fifty years hence, they will find it in good working shape."[138] When Stevé tried to convince Barton of this and suggested that they embrace the New Yorkers who had worked so hard by incorporating a few of them into the executive committee of the national body, she began to regard him with suspicion. "It is not a pleasant thing to be compelled to run a tilt and work in competition with your subordinates," she explained in an angry letter. "It is much as I always supposed it would be. When the people got a hold on the Red Cross they would be uncontrollable."[139] Barton was now far too emotionally involved with the situation to see that the interest and active participation of wealthy, influential citizens was exactly what she had campaigned so hard for during the last twenty years. She saw only a plot to usurp her position and her glory, and she recognized there was a rich and well-knit organization that was a reproach to her own skimpy national society.

Her paranoia was greatly exacerbated by the trip to Cuba in the spring of 1899, for it was almost immediately apparent that her staff did not at all appreciate her presence. Hubbell, still smarting from his loss of Mea, believed he had the situation well in hand, and the other doctors felt competent to perform their duties without her close supervision. Charles Cottrell, viewing the situation from the fresh viewpoint of a young man, found a good deal to question in Barton's forty-year-old methods and authoritarian manner; his attempts to modify even slightly the operation of the Red Cross met with sharp reproofs. Feeling boxed in on every side, Barton began to imagine that her staff were plotting against her and saw mischief in such innocent events as a daylong picnic to which she was not invited.[140] Most dangerous of all were the activities of David Cobb, an attorney hired by Stephen Barton to help Clara with the interminable government documents that work in foreign aid entailed. A bright and ambitious young man with a commanding manner and stentorian voice, Cobb was perhaps the one member of the staff who really deserved Barton's suspicions. Desiring to make a name for himself in the Red Cross and viewing Clara as an old lady on the way out, he spent a good deal of energy trying to convince her to run the Red Cross through a committee and to move the offices to New York. When this failed he simply began to take over.[141] A friend who happened to drop by the Red Cross offices when Barton was out was surprised to find Cobb meeting people at the door and giving the impression "that he is, to use the slang expression 'the whole thing.'"[142] Fearful that Cobb might actively rebel against her, Barton, after seven weeks on the island, determined to end the Cuban relief and recall all of the staff. Against the protests of Hubbell, she prepared to hand over their projects to the army and the newly formed Cuban Red Cross, urging her doctors and nurses to complete their work as quickly as possible. She sent Cobb packing and soon after made plans for her own departure for home.[143]

Under the pressures of the situation Barton lost all perspective on the work and the people with whom she was dealing. Even after her decision to abandon work in Cuba she was restless and terrified, expecting any day to find herself the victim of a full-scale mutiny. "Cobb has usurped the power of the organization and is proceeding to conduct it to suit himself," she wrote in panic to Joseph Gardner.

> The great NY com[mittee] take all our money and will of course swallow us. Cobb and his party are a nest of vipers, all taking a hand in the Red Cross.—he with his law knowledge has the advantage—shall we step out and let it go? Let them do with it as they will—I can either resign openly to the people, or quietly to the Directors, and let it all go as it will—I don't care now. . . . We are, I think ruined; there are so many grasping at us, that it is impossible to stand . . . I don't suppose anything can save us or me—The vipers are so poisonous, and sting so deep.
>
> Shall I let them take it?—and turn me out? I don't care much—I am heartbroken, and no wonder.[144]

She let her anguish work itself to the point that she became physically ill in a way she had not known since the early 1870s. Her eyesight grew dim and bronchial attacks began, ones that would trouble her for the remainder of the year.[145] With alarm she noted in her diary her inability to concentrate on her work and the return of the unsettling symptoms: "back hot, felt like breaking down like old days"; and later: "I am not in any reasonable state of mind and may never be again. It may be the end coming."[146] When, after tying up the Cuban work and making some rapid consultations in New York, she was finally able to return to Glen Echo, it was with the hopes that the familiar surroundings would soothe her raw nerves and sore heart.[147]

In contrast to her private anguish, the Cuban campaign was publicly closed amidst cheers and honors for Clara Barton. The Grand Old Army veterans saluted her in September, and huge jewel-encrusted medals arrived from both Spain and Cuba in the closing months of 1899.[148] A glowing tribute that President McKinley had given her in his annual message to Congress the previous December was seconded and expanded by the Senate in a unanimously adopted resolution.[149] Even the army swallowed its pride and acknowledged her contribution: "Miss Clara Barton . . . has performed her onerous duties during the entire war with a devotion and earnestness that merit universal recognition at home and abroad."[150] Barton's soul, as always, basked in the warmth of these kind words, yet in many ways she felt they represented a shallow tribute. Barton had always believed that it would take a war to root the Red Cross firmly in American soil and had anticipated the event for some time. She had foreseen the difficulties, the need for wisdom, loyalty, and patience to accomplish her goals, and had not been without her "apprehensions that they might be insurmountable."[151] Still, she had hoped that the situation would clarify her work and mission; it was with keen disappointment that she saw her efforts fragmented, the organization divided, and the government skeptical about further relations with the Red Cross. She would never blame herself for the problems and believed the words of her critics to have been formed in spite and jealousy. Those who had been entrusted with the assocciation's work had betrayed her trust and sometimes had shown little regard for its noble mission. Thus the work in Cuba closed, "a hard field, full of heartbreaking memories."[152] Much saddened, Barton reflected on her efforts in behalf of the reconcentrados and her prospects for the future: "In the last two years I have given to Cuba all my time, my strength until I have little left of my peace of mind, my friends, much of the hard-earned reputation of a lifetime, and stand literally alone watching the dying embers, with none to speak to and none to speak for me."[153]

seventeen

On June 6, 1900, President William McKinley signed a bill that incorporated the American National Red Cross and gave a measure of protection to its insignia. It had been rather hastily put together in the beleaguered days following the Spanish-American War, when Barton feared that the New York Red Cross or another outside group would take over the nation's relief work, and she had done much of the lobbying for it herself. For six months she wearily traveled the sixteen miles to and from Washington each day, while the legislation went from committee to committee and from Senate to House "in the zig-zag way that bill[s] go."[1] Stevé came down to do his bit, and Judge Sheldon added his legal advice and moral support to that of her friends in Congress. The most forceful argument heard on Capitol Hill was Clara's insistence that the congressmen's praise for her work in the Spanish-American War and their avowed intention of voting her "thanks and a medal" were meaningless if the organization she had founded was allowed to sink into insignificance through lack of proper protection. "To this effort on my part, to bring our government, through its busy legislators to a realizing sense of this obligation . . . ," she told General Joseph Wheeler, "I have given the best thought, effort, and means of nearly ten years of my life; and all will understand, I think, how needless and empty in comparison a vote of thanks and a medal would seem to me, who have striven and waited so long, and must still strive and patiently wait."[2] Heeding the common sense of her plea, Wheeler and others worked to guarantee a tangible tribute to her life's work.

The bill, as passed, was not without its flaws. Commercial lobbyists had also done their work effectively, and the protection of the insignia was consequently incomplete. Only those employing the badge for "fraudulent" uses such as the raising of funds were culpable; businesses were free to advertise with the name or sign as long as they did not claim endorsement by the organization.[3] The

325

inadequacy of this became apparent when one company took the liberty of flaunting a piece of American Red Cross letterhead stationery in their advertisement. This action so angered George Kennan, who thought Barton had authorized the use, that he severed his remaining ties to the organization. In an apologetic letter Barton wrote that she had not approved the advertisement and had found the company's misuse of Red Cross material "repulsive and painful." They could take only cold comfort, she told Kennan, in the knowledge that the use of the insignia was prevalent "not . . . because our organization had done badly, or gained an unsavory name, but because it had *done so well*, and gained a name to be *coveted, even stolen*, if it could be gotten no other way."[4] Powerless to prevent such abuses, she lamented: "I regard the Bill is of very little use."[5]

Barton was also disappointed that the legislators would not give her unlimited authority over the domestic relief of the country. The rise of the White Cross in 1899 had given her efforts toward national legislation a sort of frantic fervor. Because it had the support of the powerful Catholic Church, and apparently the support of Congress as well (a bill to incorporate the White Cross was passed at the same time as her own bill, though it was never signed into law), she feared that such a group could easily eclipse her faltering association. Second Assistant Secretary of State Alvey Adee hastened to reassure her of the unique status of the Red Cross. "Of Course Congress can incorporate as many domestic Cross societies as it pleases, green, blue or any other color of the Spectrum," he wrote soothingly, "but the operations of these variously tinted organizations in international war could have no standing under the Geneva conventions unless they adopted the insignia of the Red Cross which alone is recognized."[6] Barton was not entirely mollified, for she felt insult as well as threat in the sudden recognition of a body that, even if composed of prestigious people, was untried, when her own group had worked so hard to gain a reputation.[7] In the end, like every other group that had bedeviled her, the White Cross faltered and fell.

Because Barton felt a menace in the White Cross legislation, the bill to incorporate the American Red Cross was rapidly drawn; this caused yet another confusion in the resulting congressional act. In their hurry she and Stevé left off a number of the names of the original incorporators of 1881. Correctly surmising that some sensitive natures might take offense at this, she tried to have it corrected but found that it could not be done without an entire rewriting and resubmittal of the bill. After the bill was signed Barton quickly called a meeting to add, at least in the new charter of the organization, the omitted names with the same prominence and prestige as those listed in the bill. "This however, would not satisfy," she noted sadly, "& very sharp and cutting remarks were passed and added indifference shown, if that were possible." Those that complained the loudest, she remarked, were the same members who had failed to give her any help or support during the ten years that the bill had been before Congress.[8]

Despite these bothersome points, Barton was much relieved at the incorporation of the organization. "The end has been reached," she told a jubilant group that had gathered at the Arlington Hotel to celebrate the victory and make plans for the future, "the Red Cross in America is an accomplished fact."[9] The bill required a new set of bylaws; those passed on June 6, 1900, provided for elected officers who were to be responsible to a board of control, also to be elected by the members. With its new status and the publicity of the Spanish-American War, the long-sought men and women of wealth and influence were beginning to take their places in the organization. Ellen Spencer Mussey, a noted lawyer and prominent society woman, was elected a vice-president, as was Brainard H. Warner, whose real estate speculations had brought him an un-paralleled position of influence in the nation's capital. With the Red Cross in such capable and, she believed, friendly hands, Barton hoped that the moment had finally come for her to retire.

She had always maintained that she awaited only the securing of the organization's national position before she would resign. At the end of the business meeting that day she made a graceful speech of thanks to all those had aided her, then added: "I now ask of you my release, that you take up my burden and allow me the few days—nay, years, if that may be—that fall to me. In your many hands the burden will be light that has been heavy on mine. With your united wisdom . . . it will reach the height it *should* reach."[10] In this speech Barton made her most sincere attempt to resign from the presidency. Her work had been to establish the Red Cross and to demonstrate its possibilities; that accomplished, she believed others would bring to it the organizational skills she lacked. Now nearly seventy-nine, Barton knew she needed a rest. The enthusiastic crowd at the Arlington, however, disagreed. Exultant over the passage of the Red Cross bill and desirous of paying their leader a compliment, they ignored her wishes and once more elected her president. Barton was flattered, and she happily convinced herself that one more year, during which she could advise and support the organization, would not be too much. As she floated among the guests at a reception given on the grounds at Glen Echo after the meeting, accepting the congratulations of senators, army generals, and cabinet officers, she became increasingly convinced that her reelection had indeed been in the best interests of the Red Cross.[11]

That summer Barton traveled to Chicago to attend a GAR rally and to visit the Gardners. She was still riding the crest of the wave. To the balm of old friendships were added the attentions of Ellen Spencer Mussey and a secretary, Mary Agnes Coombs, who accompanied her. Clara tired more quickly these days, however; the August heat drained her and she had to rally herself for each public appearance. Though the administrative duties of the Red Cross were now spread among a number of co-workers, her own activities do not seem to have diminished. Even on the long midwestern journey she faithfully kept up her correspondence. When she arrived back in Washington the first week in September she was in high spirits but fatigued and somewhat ill.[12]

There was no time to rest, however, before the Red Cross received a call for assistance that she felt bound to accept. On September 8 and 9, 1900, a hurricane swept across the Gulf of Mexico, heavily damaging Galveston and other portions of the Texas coast. Five to six thousand people were killed, and nearly every home in Galveston was destroyed. Millions of dollars worth of public property, telephone and telegraph wires, boardwalks and hospitals were wiped away. Barton could easily picture the scene as she perused reports that read, "eight thousand homeless," "city in confusion," "government rations and tents inadequate."[13] When the New York World offered to sponsor her and supply her with all funds contributed through it, she hurriedly began packing her relief stores. The collective eyebrows of the board of control might be raised apprehensively at this rush to the front, but the single-minded Barton never hesitated. "It was naturally my work to go to that field which I did," she declared.[14]

The World sent a well-appointed palace car to take Barton to Galveston, and after a roundabout journey, she and her staff of six arrived there on September 15. Dr. Hubbell was sick in Iowa, but Mussey, Coombs, Fred L. Ward (the former treasurer of the CCRC), and Stevé all accompanied her. The New York Red Cross had also sent workers. Barton, wisely remembering the strife of the two previous years, declined to supervise them but offered to share materials and ideas. There was certainly more than enough for all willing hands to do. Barton found the people of Galveston a "dazed and tearless throng, such as Dante might have met in his passage through inferno."[15] The remnants of the city were enveloped in a thick smog, resulting from the enormous piles of burning trash and bodies that dotted the island. Fear of disease and the impossibility of burying the dead in the sodden and shifting earth made it necessary to ignite the remains as soon as they were found. The smell of Galveston became the most vivid memory the relief workers held of that field. "That peculiar smell of burning flesh, so sickening at first," one woman recalled, "became horribly familiar within the next two months, when we lived in it and breathed it, day after day."[16]

Already tired when she left Washington, Barton arrived in Texas so ill that she kept to her bed for several days. She downplayed her weakness as much as she could but was unable to hide her illness completely. Ellen Mussey, who had vehemently protested Barton's decision to go to Galveston, began to strengthen her opinion that the Red Cross president should never have left Washington. Solicitation for Barton's welfare was Mussey's purported reason for advocating her return to headquarters, but others suspected that she did not approve of the older woman's penchant for field work and may have even hoped, as vice-president, to direct the relief herself. Determined to take matters into her own hands, Mussey arranged, while Barton slept, for a private railway car and navy cutter to take the ill woman back to Washington and delegated Stevé—the only other ranking Red Cross officer in Texas—to accompany his aunt. Stevé, fearing a plot to discredit Clara, informed her of Mussey's plan, whereupon she exercised her still formidable powers of command. The next day it was Mrs. Mussey who took the train to Washington.[17]

Barton was careful for the remainder of the mission to appear well and active, though she rarely left her hotel room and directed much of the work from a day bed. She established a local chapter of the Red Cross and put its most energetic members in charge of the day-to-day operations. Each division (clothing, orphans, food, and so on) had a worker from headquarters to advise it and keep track of the finances. The Red Cross established an orphanage, provided temporary shelter for the homeless, and handed round hot soup daily.[18] After just three weeks Barton boasted that the only order in chaotic Galveston was the organization she had brought. "They are running like clock work," she told Philadelphia doctor J. Wilkes O'Neill, "and with a most entire unanimity that could be even hoped for. There is not a discordant element in our entire force or that of the scores of men and women of Galveston who are nobly aiding the work."[19]

Most of the donations to the Red Cross were not money but materials: lumber, clothing, seeds, and bandages. As always, Barton showed an extraordinary ability to stretch the available goods to give the maximum benefit. Cash was saved for those who could not fit into the clothing on hand or who needed transportation to relatives willing to adopt them temporarily. Discarded finery was made over, makeshift homes were built. Even the Sea Islanders, remembering their own misfortune, sent a small sum of money, which Barton gave to the black people of the town. Despite Barton's best efforts, however, some of the goods remained unusable. One shoe salesman sent a box of 144 samples—all for the left foot. A zealous manufacturer boxed up one million Mother Hubbard gowns of sleazy print and skimpy cut, and with no fastenings: "wrappers enough to disfigure every female in Southern Texas." Barton sometimes surmised that the donors of these items felt "that comfortable feeling of lending to the Lord—but it was no use at our end of the line."[20] In all, $120,000 in cash and goods were donated to the Red Cross for Galveston relief. Critics would complain that this was an insignificant sum, amounting to only 2 percent of the total contributions made to Galveston, but J. R. Kemper, a sage city father, later noted that the organization's influence could not be measured solely by the number of donations it collected. Nearly one quarter of all monies received, Kemper estimated, had been sent "due to the appeal of Miss Barton." Once it was known that she was at the field, it was accepted that there was a need and that the money would be wisely spent.[21]

There were no innovations in the field work at Galveston, just a job smoothly and swiftly done. The Texas mainland had also suffered, but the state government and the army directed that relief. Barton's contribution to this area consisted chiefly of the much-publicized distribution of one million strawberry plants to farmers, whose lucrative fall crop had been ruined and who faced years of debt before they could replant their fields.[22] The strawberry distribution was Barton's final act before leaving Texas. Nearly two months had elapsed since her arrival, and she instinctively felt that the time had come when the city could provide for itself. Her staff, suffering from continual exposure to the hideous funeral pyres, had grown "pale and ill," and Barton herself admitted to needing "the help of a steadying hand as I walked to the waiting Pullman on the track."[23] It would be several months before she completely recovered from the exertion at Galveston, yet she revealed her ill health only to her diary, afraid that her fatigue would be used as a pretext to diminish her power. "It is needless to say how weak and out of sorts I was," she wrote at the end of 1900, "and how necessary I found it to keep all people away from me."[24]

Reaction to Barton's two months in Galveston was mixed. The victims that the Red Cross aided had never complained about Barton's services, nor had they attached much importance to her methods; they simply noted that they were effective and unencumbered by worrisome bureaucratic details. Galveston's dazed citizens did not deviate from this general applause. Both the town council and the state disaster relief committee voted a resolution of thanks, and the numerous cards and letters of appreciation sent by grateful individuals formed a touching collective tribute. "Your presence amongst us at this trying time, even without the substantial aid which you have rendered, would be indeed a benediction," the governor of Texas wrote to Barton, "and it has served to inspire our people with energy, self-confidence and self-determination. Nothing I can say or do would adequately compensate you and the Red Cross for your, and its kindly and substantial offices at this time."[25]

The members of the board of control in Washington, however, were not so convinced of Barton's wisdom. Mussey had returned from the field with sharp criticisms, and William J. Flather, who had been elected treasurer, resigned in protest over the handling of fiscal matters. A financial committee was formed to overhaul the confusing scraps of paper that passed for vouchers and to enquire into the reason that all contributions had not been sent directly to the national treasurer and distributed under his supervision. The most serious matter the board was concerned with involved William W. Howard, the energetic newspaper magnate who had become interested in philanthropy during the Spanish-American conflict. Howard was far from an altruist. His business interests in oil and wood had frequently prospered during the disasters he purported to "relieve," since through his philanthropic projects he was able to gain the confidence of the needy and buy land and timber from them at greatly reduced prices.[26] Barton, more anxious to forestall Howard's activities as a rival than curious about his background, had not enquired into his credentials too closely when, shortly after the hurricane, he had offered to use his influence to raise funds for the Red Cross. Neither, however, had the board of control, and Barton had been careful to get their approval before contracting with Howard. As the work had progressed in Galveston, Barton lost contact with Howard. When she finally requested information about the funds he had collected, he refused to give her a direct answer, and Barton was forced to take the matter to the board. Incensed at what they perceived as Barton's mismanagement and afraid that Howard had collected funds under the name of the Red Cross and pocketed the return, the board demanded an explanation. Howard, claiming that he had collected no money and that he had a "special relationship" with Barton, refused to deal with any other Red Cross officers. At length Barton quietly requested him to close his "work," which he did.[27]

Barton was as concerned about the matter as the board of control, but she found their accusatory manner extremely provoking. She tried to remain aloof from the indignity of having her vouchers for two or three dollars questioned, and her only reply to the sharp questioning was that her work "at the field of dying or dead, sick or starving, is not the work of a bank, and cannot be squared by its rules and still be worth maintaining."[28] She let Stevé, who was outraged at the accusations made against Fred L. Ward, whom he knew to be a sincere and competent man, fight her battles before the board. His anger, and an unrestrained speech about Red Cross members "on whom the varnish is not yet dry," unfortunately further divided the body.[29] In the end the board passed a set of resolutions that censured Barton's actions in directly receiving money at Galveston and placed her authority under that of the board of control. "I will not name the Resolutions," she wrote sorrowfully, "they stand there a rebuke to me, an insult that no *man* would take from another man, and which no man would *dare* offer to another man—a superior officer at that." As an added token of protest, every businessman on the board resigned his position.[30]

"I *always had* great respect for mighty forests and giant trees," Barton wrote in an attempt to lightly pass off the situation, "but I never until now, learned the power of a single Board."[31] At heart she was greatly disturbed by their actions. She believed that they intercepted her mail and that their real purpose was to eliminate her entirely from the Red Cross leadership. "Nothing would prevent them from voting me out but the little fear they might have of the disapproval of the public," she confided to her diary.[32] Under the pressure she collapsed into inaction and self-pity. Countless days she recorded that she was too unsettled to work, that she was unappreciated and misunderstood.[33] Her reports to Congress and the board on the Galveston work were turned in late and contained little beyond an essay describing high winds and humble thanks. In a teary farewell letter to Howard she gave vent to her full feelings of persecution. He should forget the American Red Cross as it had been under her direction, she told him; forget all of her aspirations,

> remembering only that a deluded misguided woman once picked it up and carried it awhile on her march of life, sometimes floating out a little—delusively, oftener draggled & mud besmeared, till at length the train of hooting children that had followed, had grown longer and stronger, the few friends also on the march, who sometimes came and walked with her a little grew busy and tired and one by one dropped off, until *one* stands alone.[34]

Throughout the spring of 1901 the financial committee continued to scrutinize every receipt, report, and voucher sent in from Galveston. Their ardent interest in two-dollar receipts for postage stamps was perhaps overly zealous, but they also raised serious questions about expenditures for railway travel, tailor-made clothing for some of the victims, and amusements for the Red Cross volunteers. Barton and Fred L. Ward launched a vigorous defense, but the vouchers were so disorganized, and certain of them so questionable, that even the president's strongest allies were worried and could only plead Barton's reputation against the accusations of the financial committee. "I agree with you that the bills are technically such as should not have been paid by the Red Cross," wrote S. W. Briggs, a staunch Barton supporter, to a Red Cross officer, "but in view of Miss Barton's life work and expenditures it is about the smallest affair that I ever knew." [35] With both sides clinging tenaciously to their opinions, it was well into 1902 before the Galveston financial report was finally accepted.

Among the trio that audited these accounts a leader was emerging. She was Mabel T. Boardman, a forty-one-year-old dynamo with impeccable family background and seemingly endless connections among business and social leaders. Her father, a prominent attorney in Ohio and a principal benefactor of Yale University, had raised his large family to be conscious of their philanthropic responsibilities. Mabel, the oldest daughter, had shown an early proclivity toward humanitarian pursuits. A dignified and impressive woman, she marched through life with an erect carriage and a quick step. There was a kind of brusqueness to her appearance that discouraged too much familiarity. She was said to bear a remarkable likeness to Queen Mary of England, and she treasured the story that when the Duke of Windsor first visited Washington, he caught a glimpse of her at a reception and blurted out, "Good Lord there's Mother." Boardman looked like the figure of the upper class that she was; she reflected its values and prejudices with every bit of her considerable personality. [36]

Boardman's involvement in the American Red Cross had begun in 1900 when she was elected a member under the rules of the new incorporation. Her early association had been inactive but cordial; Barton replied to an "appreciative and genial" letter from Boardman by saying that, although she did not believe they had met, "the tone of your letter won me like an old friend, and when we do meet we will not be strangers." [37] Between 1900 and 1902 Boardman's time was primarily occupied with a crusade to reform the system of customs inspection at United States ports, and she gave only sporadic attention to the Red Cross. Her work on the financial committee changed her focus, for she began to be seriously concerned about the direction the organization was taking. Boardman began studying Red Cross societies in other nations to learn of their activities and official status, and she talked with prominent people in New York and Washington about the problems the American organization had encountered during the Spanish-American War. Mabel Boardman would not emerge as the leader of the opposition until late 1902 (Ellen Mussey was Barton's chief critic until that time), but when she did it would be with a wealth of knowledge about the international treaty, definite ideas about the future of the association, and the backing of the most influential men and women in the nation. [38]

332

Barton had long sought assistance for her organization and was open to—even anxious for—advice. But she had never looked for direction and could barely tolerate criticism. As her actions at Galveston were debated week after week, she began to believe that the new incorporation had been a mistake. Mussey assured her that the board was actually behind her, that they were only "cleaning out the weeds and tares," leaving "a great deal of good wheat standing."[39] After the passage of the chastizing resolutions and the resignations of the members of the board of control, however, Barton no longer trusted Mussey. Her inclination, Clara told Stevé, was to turn the clock "back to the 11th of July last—before any Board had been formed."[40] She realized that this radical step might even have to be approved by Congress, but she saw no other way to retain control over the organization. Under the old bylaws she had been overworked and handicapped by her own limitations, but she had been independent. At eighty she was not about to endure the direction and censure of the newfangled board of control.

Barton made no move to change the structure of the corporation at the June 1901 meeting of the Red Cross. She was, nonetheless, sharply attuned to the growing strength of those who questioned her work. "We do not want to fight to lose," she told Stevé. "They are old politicians, know their power and are in council with each other. We are few and separated."[41] Quick to see an enemy, Barton had actually drawn battle lines before a clear conflict was evident. Her own strongly confrontational attitude would add to the growing belligerence, until, at length, her mistrust was justified.

Throughout the fall of 1901 Barton watched with dismay as her small coterie of followers and the board of control became increasingly alienated. As ever reluctant to publicly defend herself, Barton encouraged others to rally forces for the annual meeting, which was to take place in December 1901. In the fall Barton sent a letter to members, urging them to attend the meeting and to support an important revision of the bylaws. The changes included "the abolition of the Board of Control which has proven oppressive even to cruelty, to the honored founder and head of the American National Red Cross . . . ," and the substitution of a "more simple and democratic form of administration."[42] Barton did not look forward to the encounter, which she feared would be a public embarrassment to her. "I am heavy of heart," she wrote three weeks before the meeting. "I see only bitterness and enmity as the result of it all. I don't know how to play the part I am expected to as the President." With trepidation she prepared her plan for a reorganization and, in case this failed, composed a resignation speech.[43]

She need not have dreaded the meeting so much. The *Washington Post* reported that the tone of the assembly on December 10 was one of complete affirmation for Barton and her policies. Not only was her resignation rejected, but she was unanimously reelected to a three-year term as president. As she had hoped, the board of control was abolished. It was replaced by a board of directors, a slightly larger body with slightly less power. An executive committee of three, again including Mabel Boardman, was appointed with Barton's approval. The "high regard in which she was held," concluded the *Post*, "was clearly shown after the meeting when the members crowded around her and gray haired veterans kissed her hand and thanked her for the work she had done."[44]

In the long run, Barton knew that these bright reports reflected only a surface victory for her supporters. Ten of the fifteen who had opposed her on the board of control were elected directors; Mabel Boardman was on the executive committee and the board; others who had been faithful friends declined to continue to serve as Red Cross officers. Barton's aim had been not just to abolish an institutional body but to rid herself of the "bugs and the worms [which] had got in and were working among the roots of our Red Cross tree."[45] This she had failed to do. Within a few months she would sadly acknowledge that there was "small difference between the present state of things and the former Board of Control; the same parties are in power to deal with, with some important additions to their ranks, with naturally no improvement in good feeling after the events which transpired."[46] More than ever she felt surrounded and incapable of moving out of the net of critical eyes and penurious minds. "There are only four of us . . . ," she told Stevé; "all the others are a clique."[47]

To remove herself from the watchful eyes of the new board of directors, Barton decided to move the operational headquarters of the Red Cross to New York. It was at Stephen E. Barton's insistence that she did this. He believed that since the Red Cross had secured national incorporation Washington influence was unimportant; what was needed was the financial backing of New York businessmen, who had contacts over the entire country. By January 3, 1902 she was established in a new seven-room suite of offices on East 59th Street, with Francis Atwater, the younger brother of long-cherished Dorence, installed as general manager.[48]

There was now an urgent need for Barton to harness some kind of financial resources. The war with Spain had left the Red Cross treasury nearly empty, and Clara's own strained funds had been called upon to secure the passage of the congressional bill. Money had been donated during the Galveston crisis, of course, but operating monies were nonexistent. Congress prodded her to establish local auxiliaries, but there were simply no funds for such a project. The printing of the Galveston report—required under the congressional charter—was paid for out of Barton's own pocket. "Even the national Red Cross cannot work entirely without money or material," Barton complained to Stevé, "although I grant that it comes nearer than any known body in existence." The infighting of the previous year had also taken its toll on the organization. Both income and membership were down, and a number of local chapters, among them the pioneering Rochester, New York, branch, decided to close their doors.[49]

Clara was not adept at fund raising and felt ill at ease in the New York financial world. She had already entrusted the Red Cross name and future to two outsiders: W. W. Howard and Frank Higbee. The latter had promised to raise a fortune by establishing a series of "meetings on New Year's Eve 1900, to herald the turn of the century." His idea was to collect greetings from eminent persons throughout the world and to read them at the meetings. Those present would pay a substantial fee to attend, and the proceeds would go to the Red Cross. Higbee did solicit a number of greetings (at Red Cross expense) from persons as diverse as Mark Twain, Auguste Rodin, Sarah Bernhardt, Thomas Hardy, and Chief Lame Deer of the Sioux Nation. But the meetings were a notable failure, and Barton was forced to pay Higbee a considerable commission, while trying to explain the matter to the board of control.[50] The embarrassments with Higbee and Howard should have made her wary of enthusiastic promoters who did not have a personal stake in her organization, but they did not. Determined to divert the Red Cross from its course of "making bricks without straw," she contracted with a public relations man named Amos Atwell to solicit contributions for a percentage of all that he raised.[51]

The Atwell connection was still strong when Barton moved to New York, by which date he had raised but fifteen hundred dollars and had submitted vouchers for nearly seventy-six hundred. Yet Barton had allowed him to borrow a thousand dollars from her personally, on the good faith that he would use it to become acquainted with potential donors. Seeing virtually no return from Atwell, the board of directors voted to cancel his contract, whereupon he threatened to sue the organization to recover the alleged six thousand dollars in expenses. After many sleepless nights, Barton finally persuaded him, early in 1902, to accept a settlement of the fifteen hundred dollars he had raised and the cancellation of Barton's note. Though she was greatly relieved that the matter had not resulted in a public trial, she observed grimly: "No one loses anything, but me."[52]

The business community was not entirely uninformed of these affairs, and the knowledge did little to encourage them to support the foundering organization. Some form of reorganization was needed, they believed, before they could feel comfortable pledging any large sum. After six months in New York, the balance sheet of the American Red Cross looked precisely as it had at the time of the annual meeting in 1901.

While still in New York, Barton heard news of the Seventh International Red Cross Conference, to be held in St. Petersburg, Russia. She was not anxious to attend the meeting. As usual, she dreaded the long sea voyage and feared that her absence would give the board of directors greater opportunity to usurp her territory. At the same time, she was unwilling to have someone else represent her at the conference; that would imply loss of power and perhaps give rise to rumors of incapacity. These latter considerations made up her mind. In March Barton accepted the secretary of state's appointment and began making plans to attend the May conference.[53]

Representation at the international conference took on symbolic significance for the two factions in the Red Cross. To Barton's dismay, both Mussey and one of Mussey's most active supporters, an attorney named Judith Ellen Foster, wrangled official appointments. With Julian Hubbell incapacitated and Judge Sheldon unwilling to accompany her, Barton searched for an effective companion for the convention. She decided on Benjamin F. Tillinghast, her old ally in Iowa, who accepted with pleasure. At the last minute Mussey had to decline, and Barton moved quicky to fill her spot with another from her camp; Nicholas Senn, an influential army doctor, was her choice.[54] The fifth delegate was Admiral William K. Van Reypen, the retired surgeon general of the navy. (Though he inclined toward the group that was calling for complete reorganization of the American Red Cross, he maintained a dignified silence on the matter.) John Hay, the secretary of state, was a personal friend of the admiral and, as Van Reypen's memoirs attest, begged him to travel to Russia to act as mediator. "There is to be an International Red Cross Congress . . . ," Hay told Van Reypen,

> and I am to appoint the delegates. The American Red Cross is about equally divided into two discordant factions. One headed by Clara Barton and the other by a very aggressive woman. They are worrying the life out of me by their demands that I must appoint the five delegates from the section of the party that they represent. If I should do that it would end the Red Cross in America. . . . I want you to keep peace between those two belligerent women and to see that there are no scandals growing out of the behavior of any of the members of our delegation.[55]

With feelings running this high, the various delegates obviously did not travel together. (In fact they did not associate at all during the conference, stayed in separate hotels, and did not appear together as a whole except at meetings of the congress and occasional entertainments.) As Van Reypen recalled: "At the meetings I always sat between the two antagonistic women, while they both talked to me without looking at each other."[56] Barton and Tillinghast landed in Europe on May 15 and completed their long journey by train, arriving in St. Petersburg a few days before the congress opened on May 29. They found that the rest of the party had already arrived and that luxurious accommodations had been provided for them.[57]

Before the conference even opened the splendid festivities began. "We were simply overwhelmed with invitations to banquets, theaters, garden parties, and concerts," noted Van Reypen.[58] The delegates were driven to Moscow to visit churches and the site of the battle with Napoleon. Both the empress dowager (the mother of the czar) and the czar hosted receptions so sumptuous that they outshone even the entertainments given by the Court of Baden in 1887. The empress dowager, an octogenarian like Barton and shy of the roomful of men, singled Clara out for attention, and the reigning monarchs spoke with flattering familiarity of her work. Among the delegates, she was the only one officially praised and decorated. In memory of her work among the starving peasants a decade earlier, Czar Nicholas II awarded her the Silver Cross of Imperial Russia, that nation's highest civilian honor.[59]

The conference was more notable for the official pomp than for substantive discussions. Barton gave an understated report on the Spanish-American War, stressing not domestic quarrels but the fact that the Treaty of Geneva had been honored by both sides. Announcement of the congressional charter met with prolonged applause. The remainder of the sessions reiterated topics of former conventions: the need for protection of the insignia; new advances in surgical dressing; organizational problems in member countries. Excursions were taken to hospitals and orphanages, and there were a few demonstrations of medical techniques by Russian surgeons. On June 4 the conference was officially closed; by then the numbers of delegates had thinned and the last strains of military music had died down. For Barton it had been a difficult experience, full of nostalgia for a cause she was in danger of losing and tensions between her and the other delegates. Yet it did not fail to inspire her, and she left the conference determined to carry on with her work.[60]

Clara remained in Europe for two more months. It would be her last trip to the Continent, and it was a sentimental one, full of little side trips and moist-eyed reunions. She visited Berlin and mused over the days of Kaiser Wilhelm's greatness. At Strasbourg she relived her first notable civilian relief work, and in Geneva she shed a tear over poor Minna Kupfer's grave. The Grand Duchess Louise urged her to spend a fortnight in Carlsruhe. There Barton moved smilingly among the elite society, was included with the royalty in the formal closing of the parliament, and was accorded all the respect of visiting nobility. The Europeans had no time for criticism of her work and no thought to inquire into the financial arrangements of her services. Barton basked in their esteem and left with the words of the grand duchess ringing in her ears. "Tell them," she said, "in America, how I love you, tell them."[61]

As best she could, Barton stayed clear of the Mussey faction on her return to America, spending most of the fall of 1902 in travel and consultation with friends. She stayed a month in Connecticut listening to the encouragement and advice of Francis Atwater and the Sheldons, and escaped to the New York office whenever she could. With one notable exception she made no public appearances. At the end of September she accepted an invitation of the Spanish-American War veterans to attend their reunion in Detroit, outshining even the personable war hero and president, Theodore Roosevelt. "Everywhere she was recognized," Atwater reported, "and the ovation to this little woman was greater than that given to the Chief executive."[62]

There were no ovations from the board of directors, however, in fact no recognition of her existence. Barton also chose to ignore their work and associated as little as possible with the governing committee of the Red Cross. She was, among other things, extremely annoyed with the board for failing to respond to a disaster that occurred during her absence in Russia. On May 8, Mount Pelée, on the island of Martinique, had erupted, killing forty thousand people. The devastated survivors had been left virtually friendless in their attempts to clear the rubble and restore their normal lives. The board stated that they had no money and no ready staff for such an operation. Barton, who had started on numerous relief missions with fewer resources than those available in 1902, scoffed at this and preferred to view the episode as proof of the incompetence of the board of directors.[63] Her disenchantment grew as she learned of a scheme to supplant her at the annual meeting in December. Boardman and Mussey hoped to force her resignation by admitting a large number of new members whose sympathies lay with those wishing to reorganize. With their votes assured, the group would elect officers and committees dedicated to a new, more businesslike Red Cross.[64]

Barton caught wind of this plan a few weeks before the annual meeting. She took it as a personal attack, speaking strongly of the "hunters that follow and strike and shoot at me" and hastened to form a counterattack.[65] With Stevé, Mrs. Mary Logan, and a few others she drafted a complete revision of the bylaws, giving the president the right of appointment over virtually every committee, abolishing the board of directors, and essentially eliminating any controlling power from the executive committee. She was well aware of the possible consequences of these radical changes; they were, she remarked in her diary, "perhaps not quite wise in view of ugly remarks that may be made."[66] To ensure their passage, Clara contacted all friendly Red Cross members and begged them to attend the meeting or sign their proxy votes over to her. She told them nothing of the sweeping revision she proposed in the organizational structure but informed them instead that she desired "some slight changes" in the bylaws and wished to show a consensus when they passed.[67]

By December 9, the "day of all days to be dreaded," Barton had nearly one hundred proxies in hand. The meeting at the Arlington Hotel proved as divisive as she had feared. The opposition fought every move of Barton's supporters, questioned the use of proxies, and tried to seat the newly elected members (the vast majority of which sided with Mussey and Boardman) for the afternoon election of officers and the vote on the bylaws. At the directors' meeting these questions were settled during a "stormy scene." Although the result was in Barton's favor, the heightened feelings foretold future trouble. For the first time, Mabel Boardman showed herself to be the clear leader of the opposition. Barton was aghast at the way she represented herself, Mussey, and "all the room she could control," and noted that she was "continually on the floor interrupting everyone." Boardman was especially dexterous at capturing the votes of those who remained undecided, but even her skill could not completely manipulate this meeting, which was already packed with Barton's hand-selected proxies. By a narrow margin the revised bylaws were approved, and to cap this triumph Barton was elected president for life. With Stevé and Mary Logan as her vice-presidents, there appeared to be no room for the opposition within the American Red Cross.[68]

Like a victorious general at the end of a long siege, Barton looked back with satisfaction at the year's achievements. "One year ago I had fallen afresh into the hands of my enemies, some known, others to be learned, . . ." she gloated that Christmas.

The fight opened, victory after victory was won through the long hard warring day, till at length night brought *complete victory,* our foes were slain at our feet, we laid down on our arms and slept on the field. The little army of the Lord had conquered, our banner was saved and waved triumphant, we trust forever more. The Red Cross is free and in the hands of its friend.[69]

Clearly convinced that her methods had been justified and her supporters virtually divinely inspired, Barton saw no shame in the methods she had used to assure her victory. Others could not agree. Among the Red Cross members there were a number who believed that this tightly engineered meeting exemplified a lack of integrity in Barton about which they had previously only dared to hint. Even her staunchest supporters worried that if not strictly illegal, neither had the use of proxies been strictly honorable. Achievement of her goals by this Machiavellian method ill-became a woman of Barton's stature.

Boardman and Mussey were not satisfied this time with discreet innuendos about Barton's methods. They now had proof that she meant to rule the American Red Cross in any way she could. Late in December they wrote to President Theodore Roosevelt, who, like all of his predecessors, had the honorary position of chairman of the Red Cross board of advisors. They complained of Barton's highhanded tactics at the December 9 meeting and shared their worry that the new bylaws did not contain enough safeguards against absolute rule by Barton or any other president. Their forceful letter was given additional clout by the signature of the president's sister, Anna Roosevelt Cowles, who was a close friend of Mabel Boardman. Roosevelt had, like many other military men, been puzzled and concerned by the sporadic activity of the American Red Cross during the war in Cuba, and he had little respect for Barton. (He once wrote that he was "by no means favorably impressed by the type of work she did during the Spanish-American War.") Roosevelt had the greatest admiration, however, for Boardman. A few days after the New Year he moved to sever all of the official ties his administration held with the American Red Cross.[70]

Roosevelt's letter, which Barton received on January 3, 1903, was the most crushing missive of her Red Cross career. In it the president accused her of "loose and improper" financial arrangements and censored the "very irregular and arbitrary proceedings" at the meeting on December 9. He requested that his name, and the names of his cabinet officers, be removed from the Red Cross board of advisors, and he hinted that the official connection between the organization and the American government had been completely broken.[71]

Barton's reply, carefully written a few days later, did not change the president's mind. It was an obsequious, almost whining letter, which alternately asserted that her use of proxies had been technically within the bounds of the Red Cross constitution and pleaded for the continuance of the president's favor. She tried to appeal to Roosevelt's sense of tradition and dramatically recounted the organization's history of relief work. "For twenty years this Red Cross work, so small at

339

first—a mere spark," she wrote, "has grown up under our hands until its welcome blaze lighted the footsteps of relief for an entire and direful contest of nations, and of which none better than your honored self know the hardships or the needs."[72] Roosevelt did not choose to reply to this letter. While still reeling from this rebuke, Barton heard that the twenty-three dissatisfied Red Cross members had sent a similar petition to apprise Congress of the situation and to solicit support in the reorganization of the Red Cross.[73]

Mary Logan was delegated to reply to the petition. In her rebuttal she stressed the unfairness of the president's decision, which had been made so hastily that he had waited neither to consult his own advisors nor to hear Barton's side of the story. Logan emphasized Barton's surprise that this band of remonstrants could induce the president "to reject and spurn all counsel or oversight of a treaty, accepted and ratified by the action of his own Department of Government and for twenty years, sanctioned and counseled by his honored predecessors."[74] As the matter became increasingly public, the ruling powers of the Red Cross signaled their displeasure at what they considered gross disloyalty by suspending the membership of the twenty-three signers of the memorial to Congress.[75]

At the outset Boardman and her compatriots appear to have had no animosity toward Barton personally. They were steeped in the spirit of the "progressive era," a reform-minded period of twenty years when everything from orphanages to major corporations was undergoing change. There was a great stress on professionalism during this time, and well-meaning amateurs in social work, medicine, and every other field were being replaced by those with rigorous academic backgrounds. (Ironically, Boardman, who was the chief critic of Barton's self-acquired qualifications, was herself but a glorified amateur.) With or without Clara Barton the remonstrants longed to see "a fine Red Cross Auxiliary in each of our states . . . some regular income, which should come from these auxiliary society dues, and also an emergency fund always on hand."[76] Boardman was ready to contact her wealthy friends to provide an endowment fund, but she found Barton herself an obstacle to the program. George C. Boldt, another member who was anxious to enlarge the organization's purse, had found this to be true a few years earlier and had bluntly told the aged president that when he called on men such as Levi Morton and William E. Dodge, "it was apparent from the first that none of these gentlemen would consider in taking up this work, unless you as president, would resign from active work."[77] Boardman claimed that she could collect pledges she had secured for one million dollars if only Barton would step down. In an extended correspondence with Mary Logan, she urged Barton's friend to promote the idea of a painless retirement. "I know you will use all your influence to have her accept the position of honorary President for life, with an annuity . . . ," Boardman told Logan. "People are continually urging that a complete and rigid investigation be made of Red Cross expenditures and methods . . . but we do not want to have to do this, and will not if Miss Barton in the true interest of the

Red Cross, and in the true interest of her own name and fame, will consent to take the dignified position of Honorary President."[78] Though Logan concurred with Boardman, she was unable to convince Barton to resign.

Boardman blithely termed her suspension from the Red Cross "a slight matter," but it signaled an important change in her campaign to reorganize the Red Cross. No longer did she emphasize only the need for revision of the bylaws (which Barton had agreed to after the memorial to Congress[79]); she now launched a full-scale personal attack on Clara Barton. She sent researchers to North Oxford to inquire into any property Barton might own and to discover the amount of money left to her by her father. She found traces of the old troubles at the Red Cross Park, ferreted out John Morlan, and calmly believed everything he told her. No one's testimony was too scandalous to be disregarded. Those currently estranged from Barton, such as Antoinette Margot, and even Captain James Moore of the ancient feud at Andersonville, were sought out and questioned. Boardman noted down every insinuation about Barton's sexual life, including a wild accusation that she and Henry Wilson had parented three mulatto children, and she used the floor plan at Glen Echo, which showed that Barton and Hubbell had adjoining rooms, as proof of sexual misconduct. Of more serious consequence was Boardman's discovery of the discrepancy in figures between what Barton could actually have spent during the Civil War and the fifteen thousand dollars awarded to her by Congress in 1868. When Boardman's researchers found that the *Official Records of the War of the Rebellion* contained no reference to her work, and that another source, Frank Moore's *Women of the War*, barely mentioned her, Boardman chose to believe that the work of the "Angel of the Battlefield" in that conflict had been, at best, insignificant.[80] The evidence she mustered was such a conglomeration of truth, half-truth, petty remarks, and spiteful rumors that even today it is difficult to untangle the web of accusation she created. But Mabel Boardman believed it all. She came to see Clara Barton as "an adventuress from the beginning and a clever one," and for the rest of her life, she was strangely obsessed with the idea of undermining her predecessor's credibility. When in 1916 a new national headquarters was built in Washington, D.C., she adamantly refused to include even a plaque commemorating the organization's founder. "Her connection with the Red Cross is like a skeleton in the closet upon which the doors have been closed," she remarked.[81]

With the change in Boardman's attitude and the suspension of the remonstrants, the public, and previously unaligned Red Cross members, began openly to take sides in the conflict. "The indefinite suspension of over twenty prominent residents of Washington without a hearing for the offense of calling public attention to the alledged [sic] mismanagement of the funds of the society appears to me so absurd as to lead to the suspicion that there must be something that the Committee is desirous of covering up," wrote one heretofore neutral observer.[82] George Kennan was an early defector from Barton's ranks, though he never openly sided with the other faction. For five years he had argued the need for reorganization, he wrote sadly, but "she evaded, postponed, or put aside all my suggestions, without actually opposing them, and I finally gave it up."[83] Adolphus Solomons was another of the original incorporators to remove his support. Though he once told Barton that his future was "indissolvably connected . . . with the grand old organization, and you as the head of it" and that he would "stand by you and the society *nolens volens!*" he now felt he must work for reorganization.[84] Like Kennan he chose not to openly side with the Boardman faction but worked discreetly on his own, going so far as to write to Gustave Moynier to ask his help in tactfully securing a reorganization of the American Red Cross.[85] Sara A. Spencer, Brainard Warner, and Admiral Van Reypen followed the lead of President Roosevelt and Boardman; even Richard Olney, the organization's attorney and a fellow native of North Oxford, declared the Red Cross "a good corporation to retire from."[86] Most of these people had no wish to harm Barton and hoped that she would resign gracefully, to take her place as the legendary grand old lady of philanthropy.

Mary S. Logan agreed with men such as Richard Olney—on both points. She firmly held that the Red Cross needed system and new blood but even more strongly believed that Barton should in no way be humiliated or forced to retire. She worried about Clara's financial affairs and persisted, against Barton's protests, in promoting a course of action that would "provide handsomely" for Barton. Stevé, of course, joined Logan in defense of his aunt. To the press, Red Cross members, and the Congress, he became the active voice of Clara's defenders, stating that anyone thinking that they would abandon Miss Barton and turn the organization over "to a coterie of society's bright ornaments . . . is deluded, not to say demented."[87] To those who questioned Aunt Clara's mental vigor he had an equally strong reply. "As a matter of fact Miss Barton is as smart as a whip, and fuller of energy than an egg is full of meat. Her retirement at this time would burst the organization wide open. . . . She was never quite so badly needed as she is at this moment."[88] Walter Phillips also remained loyal, and even W. W. Howard broke his long silence with Barton to declare himself "strongly in favor of letting the Red Cross remain as it is. It has done pretty well for twenty years without a large organization. In other hands but yours a large organization would be necessary to existence. While Clara Barton lives, Clara Barton is enough."[89]

"What she feels or thinks or the way her inner life is lived," wrote the Glen Echo housekeeper to Barton's nephew, "I know no more of than you do—perhaps not so much—for I know nothing."[90] Throughout the conflict in the Red Cross Barton kept the outward demeanor of unruffled calm that made her so inscrutable to those around her. Well aware that demoralization was one of her rivals' key weapons, she tuned her public comments to appear cheerful, determined, and balanced, and she made no public protest over the actions of the Boardman faction, choosing to ignore them as she had ignored unruly boys in the classroom. "I have given the dignified silence I felt they deserved," she told one supporter. "I haven't yelped back to the little snapping, barking crowd behind me. There is no doubt but they will try to bite as well as bark but our course will be, to push on so much, and so successful *work* as to bury their attack."[91] The image Barton hoped to project was one of energy and mild, smiling scorn for the people who dared to criticize her. "I work as many hours, walk as many miles, and am not broken by all this succession of seemingly endless attacks . . . ," she jotted down in a memo that was probably meant to become a press release. "I am the same [as] I always have been, and shall probably remain so, while permitted to remain at all."[92]

The criticism had the effect of locking her firmly into a position she would have happily relinquished a few years earlier. In 1900 she could look at her situation objectively and admit that she was the last of a generation and did not fit among the dynamic and professionally trained younger men and women in her field. "I have lacked the knowledge of the newer generations, and done my work badly, and naturally grown discouraged and timid," she once admitted to Stevé.[93] Yet never would she concur with similar words from other mouths. She viewed her tenure as Red Cross president as a vindication of her actions—after the 1902 meeting she suspected that resignation would be capitulation and vowed never to give Boardman that satisfaction: "there is strength and determination enough in me to sit down on the lightening [sic] struck log and declare that I will sit there."[94] Never after 1901 would she admit, either publicly or privately, that there were any valid charges against her; at times she would claim to be astonished by the remonstrants' behavior precisely because they had yet to make an accusation that she could take seriously.

Inwardly, Barton was far from serene: "Who can estimate the pain of a sensitive nature but the possessor?" Clara wrote to a friend from her home town. "I have envied the rhynoceros [sic] his hide many a time."[95] She poured out her true feelings to her diary and to those friends she knew would not judge her. Her correspondence expanded considerably during the conflict, as she reached out for support from relatives, former pupils, old colleagues, and loyal friends. The careful language she reserved for public consumption was absent, and often the letters were surprisingly sharp. Always they reflected Barton's feelings of persecution and despair. She characterized the minority groups as a "crowd of vultures and vampires" whose assertions were but "a sack of wind and lies."[96] That the public and many of her friends had allowed the conflict to happen was an insult she felt keenly. She was abandoned and besieged, her thirty years of service were ignored, and her organization, which she continued to refer to as a child, was to be given "into the hands of a self-appointed body of persons who knew nothing of it, had never done anything for it, and cared only for its possession."[97] To yet another acquaintance she put the matter more dramatically: "Alone, a target on the skirmish line, I wait results."[98]

It was difficult, under the pressures of criticism and her own demoralization, for Barton to be enthusiastic about the routine administration of the Red Cross. "I know nothing now in these days of the old interest I used to feel in the work I was trying to push forward," she complained; "it seems to me now like something I carried and laid down, but cannot quite let go, in some way the straps still hang under it and I cannot quite pull them out, but the confinement which they entail upon me is, I think, all the connection that I feel."[99] Concurrently, she felt intense pressure to carry on the Red Cross work so effectively that no one could doubt her value as president. The task was nearly impossible, since the long-standing financial and organizational difficulties were now compounded by the disharmony between Red Cross members, which made serious inroads into the society's prestige. Barton feared that rival groups would take over the work the Red Cross had once so proudly dominated. Her goal was to build up a nation-wide network that would bring widespread support to her presidency and enough dollars to the Red Cross treasury that Boardman's plan for an endowment would become irrelevant.[100]

Working once more from the offices on East 59th Street, Barton espoused a program that would ultimately prove of lasting benefit to the nation. The cause she backed was "first aid," an educational program that would teach citizens to give basic emergency care to accident victims. The idea was not a new one. St. John's Ambulance Corps in Britain had been promoting such activities for hundreds of years, and Barton had considered connecting first aid to the Red Cross as early as 1884.[101] Her plan was to have first aid supersede the old auxiliary system, which she admitted had not been particularly successful. First aid societies would spring up for a purpose—the teaching of emergency medical techniques—and would charge a small fee for the course. Most of this money would be transferred to the national headquarters. Barton believed the idea would be well received and not only would prop up the old organization by drawing attention away from its problems but would bring in significant revenue. "There is no reason, under the system established, why the Red Cross should not become as rich as Russia and every reason why it should become far more so," she predicted. Cautiously, in the spring of 1903, she inaugurated the program in her home state of Massachusetts.[102]

Eighty years later the first aid branch of the American Red Cross was all Barton had prophesied, but in 1903 it was slow to develop. Attendance at the first classes was small, despite support among firemen and police officers and Barton's persistent efforts to interest the owners of factories in the training. It proved of no immediate financial benefit and a year later was dropped. The idea of first aid limped along, with occasional support from Barton, for another five years until, with the backing of the army, it was reestablished with the Red Cross in 1909.[103]

The collapse of the first aid program left the American Red Cross in dire financial straits. In August Clara noted that the organization did not have enough money to pay its monthly bills, and she decided to use her own funds rather than report this to the executive committee.[104] She had swallowed her pride and written careful letters requesting donations from philanthropists such as John D. Rockefeller and Andrew Carnegie, but they had been answered by curt refusals.

By December, she was forced to add a pitiful note to the annual report to Congress, stating that during 1903 the Red Cross had not received one dollar in revenue and that the executive committee was "compelled to make these reports by its own labor and publish & print them at its own expense."[105]

Barton still believed that the Red Cross could command significant support for its field work, and she began to hope a need would arise that would once more place her group at the center of relief services. Hence she contemplated relief to Macedonia, which was again under Turkish fire, and the next year debated involvement in the Russo-Japanese War.[106] Though uncertain about her mental and physical strength, she had unshakable confidence in her ability to rally the nation to her side. That she still had the power to awe, inspire, and comfort the afflicted by her very presence was shown at the last field to which she was called. In December 1903 typhoid fever broke out in the small community of Butler, Pennsylvania. Newspaper stories gave conflicting reports as to the severity of the epidemic, and on a sudden impulse Barton decided to go and judge the situation for herself. Without waiting to consult the executive committee, she packed her Red Cross stores and went to the field.[107]

Ray D. Hill, a young man staying with Clara at Glen Echo, was at breakfast with her on the morning she announced this intention. He saw in her cool and deliberate movements and the completeness of her packing the skill and excitement that had made her work famous. The whole household was caught up in the historic aspect of the scene. Hill's description of Barton's departure caught the drama of an almost legendary heroine going to her last field:

> She . . . stepped out into the dark, wild night, with her small staff, and a little colored girl went before her with a lantern. As we stood, grouped on the porch, watching her departure, we saw gleaming in the darkness, nothing but the steady bright light of the lantern advancing down the long board walk leading to the car track. And we pictured the light going on and on through the night until it should stop over the stricken town of Butler, and the suffering people there would look upon it as the light of a great soul that had come to them out of the darkness, bringing comfort and healing and the calm spirit that banishes all fear.[108]

Barton's visit to Butler lasted only two days. She found nearly the entire population down with the fever but also saw that the situation had been well handled by state and local charities. She addressed the relief workers in the town hall, cheering and encouraging them with her words. She then distributed a few cases of supplies and left. It was a perfect situation in which to gain maximum publicity with minimal effort. The town made no demands on scanty Red Cross funds, and Barton's rush to the scene gave her and the organization the appearance of vigor. To Judge Sheldon, Barton confided that it had been a "grand stroke in every way. They were just at the point there when they needed a steadying hand, and a more grateful people you cannot find. Everything runs like clockwork there, for us here—it settles all chance of criticism that we were not able to go to a field. . . . We went in the old time way as we always have been—finished our work and came home."[109]

During the course of the infighting Barton made several comments that indicate she believed at least a portion of her troubles were due to her being a woman. She did not think that the recalcitrant members of the American Red Cross would have dared to challenge her authority so directly had she been a man. Throughout her presidency it had been a struggle to keep the attention of the high government officials on whom she had to rely; her ability to penetrate the male bureaucracy at all was due to her Civil War reputation, the backing of the politically powerful GAR, and her impressive manner of speaking. "Mine has not been the kind of work usually given to women to perform," she explained to Richard Olney, "and no man *can* quite comprehend the situation. No man is ever called to do a man's work with only a woman's power and surroundings. How can he comprehend it?"[110] Now she felt at a similar disadvantage with her fellow women. Highly educated and more confident than Barton in the masculine world of business, they moved with advantage in circles that Barton had never been able to enter. From her vantage point—and it was the traditional vantage point of the pioneer—these brash new women ignored her work and took her small successes for granted. She was resentful of this and found it ironic and sad that her removal from the Red Cross would come at the hands of her own sex, for whom she had worked for forty years.[111]

In this she was in complete accord with the leaders of the feminist movement, who, far from gloating over the rivalry, saw the divisions in the Red Cross as a personal attack on one of the grande dames of their cause. Susan B. Anthony sent her hearty support in a flood of affectionate letters, though she strongly hinted at the pleasures of having slipped the administrative reins of the suffrage movement into other hands.[112] To show their loyalty the suffrage leaders singled Clara out for praise, included her in conventions and rallies, and sought her opinion on subjects that ranged from the desirability of lenient divorce laws to the international peace movement. Barton's reaction to the backing of the feminists was a renewed commitment to their activities.

During the hectic years of Cuban work, Barton had declined to take part in their conventions, but now she attended all that she could squeeze into an already tightly packed schedule. In 1902 and 1904 she took hotel rooms in Washington to be nearer the convention activity, attending lectures and receptions given by the DAR, National Council of Women, and the suffrage associations. In February 1904 she gave a reception at Glen Echo for four hundred of the feminists, offering cocoa and anecdotes to those who had endured the freezing trolley ride in order to shake her hand.[113] There were many touching and impressive scenes at these forums, including a standing ovation as Barton delivered a speech on the Red Cross at the 1902 Women's Suffrage Convention and a teary-eyed tribute from Susan B. Anthony on February 17, 1904. Anthony called Barton to the stage, then, with her arm around the Red Cross president's waist, spoke of her long work for the cause of women's rights. That night in her diary Barton jotted down sketchy views of the scene.

> She told the audience that I was at the first suffrage meeting in Washington in 1869, that later I sent out my call to the soldiers to stand by women as I had stood by them— that there were only us left now to stand together at this last meeting tonight. I said a few words and sat down. Miss Anthony spoke *one* minute and came back and we remained together till the close—we both realized that we should never stand together again before a Washington audience.[114]

Affecting as such personal moments were, Barton was most impressed with the fact that these conferences were now so widely accepted and so eagerly attended. In her girlhood she had been barred from speaking out on school reform in her home town because of her sex, and as a lecturer she had faced audiences that were as curious to see a female speaker as they were to hear her words. Now women congregated, debated, presided over meetings, and ran their own organizations without a thought of societal censure. "It was interesting to me to live over the old days," she wrote after one round of well-run meetings,

> when the boy reporter used to sit down with his fresh nibbed pen to watch his chance for ridicule, whenever a 'woman's meeting' was announced to be held in some little hall or out of the way place, and the gusto with which he made up his article and walked out triumphantly in the certainty of gratifying his employers. Now he sits down beside a girl or woman who reports along side of him and all the little good grammar he ever knew is called into play to escape criticism and a reprimand from the speakers who refuse to be ungrammatically quoted, and request ye editor to send better scholarship at least, if he cannot supply better talent.[115]

In the fall of 1903, Clara's time was largely taken up with plans for the annual Red Cross meeting. She again dreaded the event, which would include election of officers, approval of yet another set of bylaws, and discussion of the sensitive proxy issue. "We cannot know how it will result," she wrote fearfully to Enola Gardner that November; "if by any means we carry the meeting it is a great fortune. If we lose it all is lost, and there is no more Red Cross for us."[116] To minimize the potential strife, all of the suspended members were quietly reinstated and invited to the meeting. But at the same time Barton was working to pack the meeting with her proponents. Ignoring the uproar that her use of proxies had caused a year earlier, she again persuaded those who could not come to sign their votes over to her. For those who promised to come and personally pledge their support, she obtained half-price tickets from the railways. Despite this, many of her old friends could not—or would not—attend the meeting. The absence of Stevé and Senator Redfield Proctor was an especial cause of concern.[117]

The meeting, held on December 8, was less eventful than Barton expected. None of the remonstrants appeared, and the new bylaws, which slightly limited her power, were easily passed. There was a spirited debate over the use of proxies, but at length even this was upheld. Barton's presidency for life was reaffirmed, and a resolution, unanimously passed, expressed "confidence in the integrity and capacity of the Executive officers of the society."[118] The new board of trustees was friendly. Boardman and her friends charged that the meeting was irrelevant, since only those loyal to Barton had been present. Clara, however, preferred to view it as a "remarkable manifestation of the loyalty and devotion of the members of the Society."[119] The one jarring note was a proposal that Red Cross procedures from the time of the Johnstown flood be investigated by an impartial body. To fend off the appearance of an indictment, Barton's group took the offensive and themselves offered to let the books be scanned and the officers questioned. A committee, led by Senator Proctor, was appointed, but no official charges or specific accusations were made.[120]

As if anticipating disgrace, Barton kept away from public appearances and even declined invitations from close personal friends at this time. She was correct in assuming that the investigation would center around her: "when they name the 'Red Cross' they *mean* only *me*."[121] She had dismissed the idea of actively refuting the charges or shielding herself: it would be undignified and appear defensive. At the same time, she feared that no one would stand up for her defense. "No one comes to me, and I would not go to anyone uncalled," she complained. "I know of no one who will say a word to the committees."[122] Her friends were not so inactive as she thought, however. Francis Atwater had begun publishing the *Red Cross Bulletin* in 1903, which contained little but laudatory comments about the association's president. The same year a pamphlet entitled *The Red Cross: Some Facts Concerning Clara Barton's Work* was edited by Joseph Sheldon and widely circulated. It contained brief descriptions of her achievements in war and at scenes of disaster, and a list of her decorations and commendations. With mild exaggeration it portrayed her as the confidante of presidents and the friend of kings. Yet, it was difficult for Clara to acknowledge these efforts. As always when under siege, she viewed herself as essentially alone.[123]

The avowed purpose of the investigating committee was to produce "harmony" between the opposing factions of the Red Cross through an objective arbitration of the points in dispute. Clara had little faith in the outcome. She gloomily expected that the committee would try to placate both sides by declaring that each group was to some degree correct, that it was "neither so *bad* as it might be, nor so good, that while we haven't done badly enough in our past work to be entirely condemned, still it was not so well, and properly done as to render complaints of the aggrieved party groundless—Consequently, we should all be good children and not disagree anymore."[124] The early acts of the investigating committee, however, certainly were not geared to produce cordial relations. For three months they set no date for a hearing: cold looks and petty criticism characterized this time of "unformed committees, confusion, obstruction, disgrace

348

and distress."[125] Each side tried to line up supporters and evidence. With President Roosevelt behind her rival, Barton found that she had very little real influence in the capital any more. She and Stevé had badly misjudged the importance of the men in Washington when they had proposed moving the headquarters to New York. Now, when a push or a prod from a well-placed government official would have meant a great deal, she was without allies in that quarter. Sensing the futility of eleventh-hour lobbying, Barton chose to reinforce the ties that had never been broken. Julian Hubbell, the Gardners, Joseph Sheldon, and Mary Logan stood staunchly by her, and the GAR sent messages containing the "assurance of approval and loyal friendship."[126] It was Stevé that she leaned on most for encouragement and hard work, and as the investigation neared, she urged him to place the full weight of his resources behind her in the fight. "They have muttered, threatened and stormed a long time," she told him, "but now they are on the step and their hands are on the knob. . . . We either hold and win, or yield and lose, and Stevé, it is you and I, just you and I, that can turn the scale, and settle it all, forever."[127]

With charges as yet unspecified, rumors were rampant. The words "malfeasance" and "incapacity" were casually bandied about, as were insinuations of fraud and the misappropriation of funds. Of the many real and imagined charges, the latter was both most cruel and most unfair. When Barton shocked Admiral Van Reypen in St. Petersburg by patting her pocket and declaring "this is the treasury of the Red Cross," she was referring to the source of withdrawals, not deposits.[128] She had been casual in her accounting of exact debits and credits, but she knew that the organization had taken far more from her than it had ever contributed to her income. Her anxiety all along had been to be "a little relieved from the costs of the work of the Red Cross" to which she had long donated an office, supplies, and her own valuable time.[129] In 1900 she estimated she had spent nearly seventy-six thousand dollars to build up the Red Cross over the years, exclusive of her services.[130] Whatever pecuniary advantages she held because of the Red Cross presidency—including the privilege of living at the headquarters in Glen Echo—they were minuscule compared to the sacrifices she had made for its continuance.

Barton's critics were not simply unwilling to acknowledge her contribution to the organization; they accused her of extravagant living and entertaining on Red Cross funds as well. To those who knew Clara and had shared her hospitality at Glen Echo, this charge was so absurd that it was almost laughable, for Barton had kept the frugal habits she acquired early in life. She rose at dawn, filling the dimly lighted morning with housework before settling down to breakfast and her business activities; neighbors recalled that they could neither get up early enough nor retire late enough to find Miss Barton in bed. Her meals were spartan; she seemed to subsist largely on cheese, apples, and whole-grain mush, though she provided a more lavish table to guests. At eighty-three she still took an active part in household matters and rejoiced that she was capable of doing so. She occasionally employed servants, but she had the same trouble with them that she had with all subordinates and preferred to do as much of the work herself as possible. After six weeks of stifling summer weather, during which she fixed a broken stove, dusted, washed and ironed the laundry for a household of twelve, and cooked innumerable meals, she felt nothing but satisfaction in the hard labor. "I am so thankful—so grateful that I *can* do it—and am not a helpless invalid to be waited on," Barton wrote in her diary.[131]

Instead of taking to her bed, she waited on those around her, taking in friends and relatives who were ill or homeless. Between 1900 and 1904, over a dozen such refugees made their way to Glen Echo and Barton's ministrations.[132] She warned the new arrivals of her simple life and begged them to consider well before they joined her household, lest they find it "distasteful and . . . tire of it, and get to find a weary disgust and then come to wonder how I could endure it."[133] Her house had muslin, not plaster, covering the bare boards, and it always retained the look of a warehouse. There were only occasional embellishments in the way of furnishings. She considered it vain and extravagant to buy new clothes when old ones could be mended or altered, and her diaries reveal a constant round of darning, ripping, hemming, and refitting. When one portion of a dress wore out, she replaced it with a piece similar in color, but she did not balk at patches, sleeves, or collars that did not match. Great-niece Edith Riccius remembered one such outfit made of three terrible shades of green, which combined the styles of several generations and was finished off around the bottom with a six-inch "strip of the most awful old motheaten beaver fur." "The poor old dear," wrote Edith, "was dressed like Mrs. Astor's plush horse, but she was pleased and proud of the dress for had she not, in good, old New England fashion, utilized the odds and ends of material she had on hand and wasted nothing?"[134]

Eccentric she might be, and parsimonious to a fault, but to accuse Clara Barton of material self-indulgence or extravagant entertaining was to show a sad lack of familiarity with her fundamental character.

"At last, the war is upon us," Clara wrote to Stevé on March 13, 1904.[135] The committee had been chosen (it consisted of Redfield Proctor, Michigan congressman J. Alden Smith, and a General Ainsworth, a noncommittal member of the American Red Cross) and hearings had begun. The remonstrants' charges, which centered on financial irregularities, were surprisingly mild, considering Mabel Boardman's earlier assertion that she did not want peace and that if "she could not have it as she wanted it, she would ruin the Red Cross and build up a new one herself."[136] Boardman and her followers complained that no financial reports had been submitted following the field work of the 1880s, that funds had gone directly to Barton without being first recorded by the organization's treasurer, and that similar lax procedures had been used at Johnstown, in Armenia, and again at Galveston. They placed a great deal of emphasis on the transaction involving the Red Cross Park in Indiana, accusing Barton of appropriating property to herself that should have been donated to the association, failing to produce proper financial records, and using funds donated for Russian famine relief to enhance the property.[137] When closely pressed, the remonstrants were careful not to accuse the Red Cross president of willful wrongdoing. "We do not charge that anybody has been guilty of malfeasance . . . ," stated one of their lawyers, "but we do think that there has been a great deal of carelessness." Barton was given two weeks to reply to the charges in writing before witnesses would be called.[138]

Joseph Sheldon, Stevé, and her lawyer, L. A. Stebbins, helped Barton to prepare the reply. They took the lawyer's approach of answering only the specific questions presented, though Barton also prepared a lengthy narrative of the association's field work. (She was so pleased with the report that she later had it published under the title A History of the Red Cross: Glimpses of Field Work.[139]) Stebbins and Sheldon carefully noted that during disaster relief there was frequently no time to send out detailed financial records, but that vouchers and receipts had always been available to those interested in the matter. Moreover, the secretaries of state had not wished to be encumbered by these reports and had trusted Barton's discretion in such matters. At Galveston, noted Stebbins, the entire relief party had acted under the advice of Ellen Mussey, now a key opponent, who had not only approved their plans but failed to complain of the expenditures until the money had been spent and accounted for—an assertion that was backed up by the minutes of the board of control.[140] Barton punctuated these comments by reiterating her belief that monies should be accepted directly at the scene of disaster and that the provision for this, written into the controversial bylaws of 1902, was the "result of thought and liberal justice and not carelessness or dishonesty."[141] They defended Clara's handling of the Red Cross Park on the grounds that it had been a personal gift to Barton for Red Cross use, that it had been donated at a time when the organization could not itself hold title to property, and that it was therefore logical to give title to her. It was also asserted that all actions concerning the park had been discussed at length with the executive committee. To avoid embarrassment to the Gardners, nothing was said of the entanglements that had evolved over the adjoining lands or the unclear titles to the tract.[142]

Once the charges were known, Barton's spirits lifted. She believed the hated investigation would vindicate her, and she refused all polite proposals that she retire and save herself any further ignominy. "It would seem that there is yet truth enough left in the world to meet these issues of lies and overcome them," she wrote on the day that her reply was sent to Senator Proctor.[143] Her only concern was the great interest of the press, which at various times she considered a nuisance, a blessing, or a reason to sue for libel. She disapproved of the journalists' desire to ferret out the details of any unpleasant story—especially if it were connected with her—and to create their own story if none appeared by itself. For the most part the press had remained friendly during the years of Red Cross infighting and had roundly admonished those making "petty attacks" on the distinguished Miss Barton. (The notable early exception was the New York Herald Tribune, which sided with the board of control, declaring that the Red Cross was a "discredited and decaying institution" that needed to be "broken completely and irrevocably with its ruinous past."[144]) After the annual meeting of 1902, Barton could not tolerate even stories that tried to be unbiased by presenting both sides of the case. She refused to give any personal interviews, fearing that her words would be twisted or her age and anxiety revealed. With bitterness she wrote that "since the annual meeting of 1902 all the scrill of the Press has been passed over me like the filth of a sewer." By the third week of the hearings, though newspaper accounts had been comparatively mild, she consulted her lawyer about the possibility of suing for defamation of character.[145]

Her advisors urged her not to attempt too much at this time. Since September she had been complaining of a urinary disorder, which she believed was caused by anxiety, and she was far from well and strong.[146] They stopped her attempts to optimistically plan new projects for the organization and agreed with her opinion that it would be best to leave all appearances before the committee to her lawyers. But during this brief interlude, when she believed her name would be easily cleared and her position restored, she was uniformly cheerful. When Joseph Gardner warned her that she was hardly in a position to take on the dissenting members, the government, and the press, she wrote airily that they could "do no worse than they have done. . . . They have gone down to 'bed rock' with me, Joseph: They have probed the *grit* of my nature; & it will stand their drills." With a light heart, she looked forward to an early conclusion of the investigation and the restoration of her beloved child.[147]

But on April 26 Barton's confidence was badly shaken by the appearance of John Morlan in the Senate caucus room where the investigating committee was meeting. Of the many people Boardman's researchers had interviewed during the course of their investigation, Morlan was the only one willing to personally speak out against Barton. His motives for doing so still remain unclear. Morlan testified that Barton had slyly managed the purchase of the Red Cross Park out of funds donated to the victims of the Johnstown flood and Russian famine, intending it as a quiet home for herself, and that he had carried out the purchase, using several different names and banks. He then asserted that the Gardners' "princely gift" was a cover for these actions. He also stated that Barton had tried to raise a fund of five hundred dollars in Johnstown to build a house on the Indiana land. Morlan hinted that he had documents and letters to back up his assertions and agreed to reappear before the committee on May 3.[148]

Morlan's testimony was false, but the defense was put in a difficult position by the friendship between Barton and the Gardners. If she told the real story, including the Gardners' hopes of making money from their gift and their negligence in telling her of the encumbrances on the land, she would not only be accused of mismanagement but her valued friendship with Joseph and Enola would be threatened. She thus refused to have her diary for 1895, which detailed the whole sorry case and which would have instantly exposed Morlan, admitted as evidence and also refused to testify herself. Stebbins and Stevé sought out Morlan, who appeared in a haughty mood, broadly hinting that he might not be opposed to taking money in return for silence.[149] When Stebbins had questioned Barton closely about the content of any letters she had written to her former staff member, she had looked him "straight in the eye" and begged him to read for himself from her letterbooks. Satisfied that Barton had nothing to hide, Stebbins badgered and bullied Morlan and threatened to take him straight to Senator Proctor if he did not produce the letters he claimed to have. At Stebbins's prompting, Proctor informed Morlan that he must bring the letters to the hearing on May 3.[150]

By now, Barton was keeping herself aloof from the whole investigation. Morlan's appearance had caused her to write that she had lost hope and would resign rather than drag on the investigation any longer. Yet she felt no rancor toward this man who had taken advantage of her so many times. She was sorry that there had been threats and harsh words between Stebbins and Morlan. "I would rather let him go," she wrote. "I have no hardness towards him, he is as he is, and cannot help it, he has great kindness in his nature, he was dear to me, and I loved and trusted him."[151] There was little hope of keeping the matter quiet, however, since someone was leaking verbatim transcripts of the hearings to the major newspapers. Thus, with Stevé, Julian Hubbell, the Gardners, and other old associates, Barton made plans for the majority of Red Cross officers to resign in a group and for authority to be transferred to Vice-President Mary Logan. She noted the similarity in composition between this gathering and the one that had met when expectations were so high in the summer of 1900. The faces were the same, the tone quite different: "The one seemed a marriage feast, the other a funeral." Two days later, in anticipation of more trouble with Morlan, she ended her diary entry with the short but pregnant phrase: "I have written my last official signature."[152]

But Morlan did not appear at the next day's hearing. He was, perhaps, scared away by Stebbins's threats or the knowledge that he had perjured himself. Senator Proctor was livid when he found that Morlan had fled and that none of the remonstrants could produce the evidence on which they had so confidently made their accusations. In a flurry, he pronounced the investigation the "most outrageous proceeding that has ever come under my observation. All the charges against Miss Barton are found false. She is completely exonerated." Proctor asked that Morlan's testimony be stricken from the record and immediately closed the investigation.[153]

For a fleeting moment Barton considered continuing as Red Cross president. Now, completely vindicated, she still would sometimes dream of leading the association to an unassailable position within American society. But at heart she knew the dispute that had led to the investigation had not been settled by Senator Proctor's forthright adjournment. At some point the questioning would begin again, and she would be caught up in fresh accusations and new investigations. Not wishing to be left "hanging between Heaven and Earth," Barton decided to resign from the Red Cross presidency and to sever all ties with the association. She declined to accept either honorary position or annuity and requested only that her vindication be announced through the Associated Press.[154]

Barton presented her resignation to the American Red Cross executive committee on May 14, 1904. She faced this, the saddest moment of her life, with the same courage that had sustained her before the guns at Antietam and among the male delegates of the world at numerous international conventions. In a low, tense voice, she thanked all who had supported and aided her, and pledged her willingness to help continue the work of the Red Cross. Though a number of the committee thought Barton's decision was wrong—Mary Logan, for example, worried that the trials of the preceding two years "had upset her mentally," argued that this moment of triumph was hardly the time to consider a move that might carry the look of defeat—the resignation was accepted.[155]

Since 1900 Barton had hoped to ease out of her role with the Red Cross, but she had left neither gradually nor gracefully, and this abruptness, as well as the fact that inevitably she was handing her organization to parties that seemed hostile, tinged her resignation with deep sorrow. Thus, at the end of the meeting, benumbed and confused, anxious about the future, and feeling desperately alone, she rode home to Glen Echo on the streetcar. There she began to ponder the events of the preceding months and to face the uncertain days ahead.[156]

eighteen

In the weeks following her resignation from the Red Cross, Clara Barton frequently grieved over the estrangement as if it were the loss of a child. Like a young adult who abruptly cut the ties to his mother's apron strings and independently denounced her tastes and habits, the organization had drifted forever beyond her control. It was the personal rejection that hurt her, Barton told one acquaintance, for she had long believed the Red Cross was ready to make its own way in the world. But after so many years of nurturing the infant body, it was difficult to watch another set of eyes beam fondly on its achievements and to see both her own hopes for its future and her sage parental advice ignored. "I didn't think it needed a stepmother," she sadly wrote.[1]

During the summer of 1904, anxiety about her future accompanied Clara's heartbreak. The interim organization, to which she had agreed in May, consisted of a twelve-member ruling committee, of whom four were from her chosen executive committee, four were remonstrants, and four were selected by the president. Mary Logan had succeeded her as the chief executive. In June, however, the annual meeting was held, and the body came completely under the control of Mabel Boardman and her friends. They spoke strongly of obtaining a new congressional charter and of continuing the investigation into Barton's expenditures.[2] Tired and sick at heart, Barton felt she could not face another probe into her conduct and sorrowfully mused over the hostility of those who opposed her; "the discontents have what they craved, and I believe *all* that they desired, only that *I* still continue to exist. They would like a first class funeral and all go as *mourners.*"[3] She tried to recruit the old faithfuls to make a stand on her behalf at the annual meeting in December but found them as beaten down as she was and disposed to think that the less said about the preceding year's events the better.[4] Finally, however, a number of Boardman's supporters called an end to the hearings. "I was associated with [Miss Barton] for many years," B. F. Warner told

Mabel Boardman, "and notwithstanding the peculiarities she developed in the latter part of her life, know that during a long period of her career she rendered service that was very valuable in relief work."[5] Pressure such as this, and the skilled diplomacy of Senator Proctor, forced Boardman to withdraw her plans for continued investigation.

The new management of the Red Cross, led by President William Van Reypen, kept after Barton in other ways. They were interested in the property she had acquired during her presidency and began to make claims for its transfer to the organization. The lots on Kalorama Heights, which had been purchased in 1890, were their initial concern. The property was funded chiefly with monies left over from relief work at Johnstown, but Barton had personally contributed one-third of the purchase price. The new officers of the Red Cross were incensed that Barton held the title, though she maintained this was so because the Red Cross could not at that time of purchase legally hold property. In June 1904 Van Reypen demanded the return of the land, and Clara, afraid more of scandal, acceded to it without receiving compensation. She neatly foiled the group in their attempt to claim the Red Cross Park, however, for that had been given to her personally, and she simply deeded it back to the Gardners. She feared, however, that the Red Cross would try to retake the property at Glen Echo as well; throughout the summer she dreaded this action, which would leave her homeless.[6]

Barton's fear was justified, for Van Reypen noted in his memoirs that he "knew of her house in Glen Echo . . . but we did not see our way clear to getting possession."[7] The title to the land was hazy at best, though the house, built with lumber donated for Red Cross disaster work, seemed clearly to belong to the organization. The Baltzleys had donated the property to the Red Cross, but through the years Clara had personally financed their projects and extended the original acreage. A number of confusing deeds listed her as the owner; others were held jointly by her and Hubbell and still others by Hubbell alone.[8] The situation was so uncertain that Barton began to make hurried preparations to leave Glen Echo, though she had little idea where to go. Only when it became clear that the adverse publicity resulting from a forceable removal of Barton would greatly injure the image of the new Red Cross did Boardman's followers reluctantly decide to allow the aging humanitarian to remain on at Glen Echo.[9]

They did not, however, relent in their demands for the records of the Red Cross, still in Barton's possession, or the contents of the house. There was no clear delineation between Barton's papers, desks, or supplies and those purchased for official uses; in all aspects of her life, public and private elements were hopelessly enmeshed. There had been no Red Cross operating fund, and Barton had provided most of the cash used to supply the office. Yet the organization could also validly claim that her expenditures had been a voluntary donation, which, once made, could not be rescinded. Clara tried to be accommodating to the new Red Cross secretary, who called to inquire about office furnishings, but she could not help feeling that most of the requests were unjustified. "The new Red Cross has no more right to or concern with, the present contents of that house, than it has with my wearing apparel," she declared hotly, "although I believe the ladies claim *that*."[10] Papers proved an even greater problem. Fond letters to nieces and nephews, cagy little notes between Barton and Hubbell, and directions to her personal bankers were interspersed with the official correspondence of the organization in letterbooks; checks for household items and new clothing followed receipts for Red Cross supplies in bank statements; official diaries contained the most intimate remarks. Barton frantically sorted through the voluminous records, and even as she sent box after box to the new headquarters, she feared the hostile members would come to claim the remainder. She retained as much as she could, to the great annoyance of Van Reypen, who proclaimed the papers she did release to be "a mass of rubbish that should long ago have been consigned to the waste basket." He and Boardman believed that Barton hoarded the bulk of the papers because they contained "evidence of her peculations." To them it was clear proof that during Barton's presidency "there was no accountability, order, or system anywhere."[11]

Under these pressures, and with disgrace still on her mind, Barton went through a serious emotional upheaval that summer. "The world looks very dark to me . . . ," she wrote. "I need advice and protection but have no way of obtaining them."[12] Escape was, as always, her initial desire. At the first hint of investigation she had written to a friend in California inquiring about the possibilities of living in Mexico; as tensions heightened in July 1904 she wildly sought friends who would accompany her there. She hoped that she could work once again by establishing a Mexican Red Cross—for that country had not yet signed the Treaty of Geneva—and that she would receive the acclaim that seemed to follow her on all foreign tours. "The government which I thought I loved, and loyally tried to serve," she bitterly noted, "has shut every door in my face and stared at me insultingly through the windows. What wonder I want to leave?"[13] But though the impulse to leave "was almost stronger than the ties of life," she gradually accepted the idea of a quiet retirement in the United States.[14] Friends such as Lucy Hall Brown and her husband, who came to stay with her during that difficult summer, gently dissuaded her by pointing out the harsh life she would have to undertake at age eighty-three. The encouragement she received at various GAR functions helped her to believe that she was still admired in her own country, and the favorable reviews of her book, A *Story of the Red Cross*, softened her angry feelings.[15]

"The First Aid is all that in any way reconciles me to the fact that I did not leave the country on the receipt of President Roosevelt's letter," Barton wrote in 1907.[16] Once the flurry of sorting papers and calming emotions had subsided, she was faced with the frightening prospect of retirement from public life. Clara had never coped well with inactivity; in many ways she had created her career to fill her time usefully and fend off depression. Soon after she dropped her plan to escape to Mexico she began to look around for meaningful work in her own

357

country. By late 1905 she could write with pleasure to her friends that "another work reaches out its hands to me and I have taken them."[17]

Barton had, of course, advocated the concept of first aid several years earlier in a desperate attempt to broaden the scope of the Red Cross. There were pragmatic reasons for its promotion then, but she also had a strong personal belief in the importance of teaching practical nursing skills to the American people. "It is a deplorable weakness of a great people," she would tell a newspaper reporter, "that they do not know how, in an emergency, to care for the injured."[18] The new leaders of the Red Cross had chosen not to continue a first aid program, a decision of which Barton strongly disapproved. When Edward Howe, who had helped her to establish the first aid auxiliaries in 1902–3, approached her with the idea of forming a separate organization to teach first aid techniques, she was delighted to offer her support.

Barton was, nonetheless, reluctant to take too prominent a role in the proposed society. Her confidence was so low that she believed her association with the burgeoning group would be detrimental to them and humiliating to her, and she balked at Howe's proposal that she accept the presidency of the organization. "I am now living out the results of forming an organization and *heading* it *personally*," she told Howe firmly, "and would not be willing to repeat the venture, even twenty-five years younger."[19] As friends urged her to reconsider, arguing that it would add interest to her life and that she had an obligation to help establish first aid classes, Barton flashed out with a statement reflecting the depth of her bitterness. "They tell me I 'owe it to the world and to my country,'" she retorted. "I fail in my ingratitude to see on what grounds *I* more than others am in debt to either. I have always given, the best I had, and all there was of me, to both my country and my people. It seems to me the returns do not place me under life obligations."[20] Only when Howe assured her that it was the unanimous desire of everyone involved that she head the organization and changed the title to "honorary president" did Barton reluctantly accept.[21]

The National First Aid Association of America, established in April 1905, differed little from the first aid program that had been established in 1902. Its nominal central establishment left the formation of classes and hiring of qualified teachers up to the local agencies, but it supervised activities and disseminated information. Barton and Howe hoped eventually to see classes offered in every town and ambulance brigades attached to each fire station and large factory. The group also developed the original "first aid kits," which contained not only the familiar bandages, splints, and iodine, but all of the ingredients needed to concoct an emergency mustard plaster. Rather than compete for attention in the ever-growing turmoil of Washington, their headquarters were established in Boston where there would be no "strings left out for politics, or Congress to pull."[22]

For the next five years Barton would work with the National First Aid Association in a role that gave her freedom and pleasure. She left the functional operations completely to the small staff, preferring to support the organization financially and by allowing generous use of her name for publicity purposes. She began to believe (and history would bear her out) that first aid would "permeate more homes, penetrate more hearts," and help more persons than ever the Red Cross could, and that emergency preparedness would come to constitute the most effective part of disaster relief. "What was the years of work in the fields of the old Civil War but First Aid . . . ?" she queried. "What were Johnstown, the Sea Islands, Armenia, Galveston but First Aid? And what was the secret of the seemingly marvelous relief performed by so few workers? Simply that our little band had learned its lesson and knew what and how to do it."[23] She talked energetically to railroad executives, school associations, and church leaders of the need for each family, and every company, to have trained individuals prepared to cope with accidents or sudden illness. Once she arrived by canoe at a summer camp to stress the importance of these principles to high school students. One reporter who interviewed her found her zeal infectious and wrote in amazement that despite her long history, her talk was "not of the past, but of the future. . . . The enthusiasm of youth shone from her face as she described what she hoped to accomplish."[24] Fired again by her old humanitarian ideals, Barton tried to establish an international first aid board; when the response was lackluster she accepted it gracefully and promoted her plan in America only. "When the . . . man in overalls can administer scientific treatment to his maimed fellow workman, stricken at his side, and hold him in life till help can come . . . ," she declared, "when the little lad of ten and twelve shall know how to rescue his playmate in the accidents of childhood . . . when this and many times more shall be the common knowledge of the people, it ought to make them safer, better off and happier."[25]

Barton's duties with the National First Aid Association were light enough to allow her time, in 1904 and 1905, to think of writing an autobiography. Since the days of the Civil War she had been approached by publishers and journalists who wished her to leave a record of her remarkable career. She had always side-stepped these requests, rather archly stating that she intended to go "on creating new matter rather than rehearsing the past."[26] As time passed, however, Barton herself noted that she ought to tell her version of the often controversial events with which she had been involved. *The Red Cross in Peace and War* had been a memoir of sorts, but she was dissatisfied with it, feeling that it was incomplete and disorganized. Despite her protests, Barton had never completely rejected the idea of writing her life story, and thus she had refused to let any other author be her official biographer. She had hoarded her vast records, saved every letter, and carefully preserved newspaper clippings, menus, speeches, and trinkets, but she would not allow anyone to use them. "While I *live*, the record of my life is my *own*," she told one would-be biographer. "It is my *capital*, if I choose to use it, and its appropriation by others for mercenary purposes is theft."²⁷ With her finances low, time on her hands, and a desire to defend her career, Barton gave serious consideration to the writing of an autobiography.²⁸

When she finally began, during the winter of 1904–5, she found the task more difficult than she had imagined. She began at the beginning, tracing the life of her parents and the confused, frightened days of her childhood. She did not wish to discuss anything unpleasant or too personal, and for that reason she omitted the tempestuous relations of her mother and father and the violent insanity of her sister Dolly. The result was a cheery and shallow view of her precarious childhood, with only an occasional glimpse of the insecurities that had affected her through life. After a few weeks of effort she gave up the manuscript in hopes that at another time the muse would hover nearer, or more benevolently.

For two years the book lay untouched in Barton's safety deposit box, but the idea of recording her recollections still surfaced from time to time. She put a minimum of actual effort into the work during her years of retirement, yet the thought of completing it, and the pressure to do so, were with her continually. She recorded scarcely a day in her diary without referring to the guilt and dissatisfaction she felt in leaving the final words on her life unspoken.

In order to gain some peace for her writing and to be closer to the First Aid headquarters in Boston, Barton purchased a house in North Oxford in 1905. It was a splendid old mansion, a significant step up from the little clapboard house down the road where she had been born. It was large and airy, a colonial relic with fourteen rooms and a good-sized garden. She took little trouble in furnishing it but felt comfortable there, as she did in the "hallowed old town" of her earliest associations. Should the Red Cross suddenly make a claim on the Glen Echo house, Barton now had an alternative. Furthermore, during the sultry summer months it was pleasant to retreat to the cooler New England town and "tramp the byeways [sic], [to] look at the old tumbled down houses and cellar holes" wherein lay so many of her memories. For nearly every summer that remained to her, Barton could be found among the shady, elm-lined streets of North Oxford.²⁹

Hot weather was not Clara's only incentive for leaving Glen Echo. The little community had changed since the idealistic days when the Baltzley brothers had seen it as a haven of intellectual pursuit and gracious living. It was now seedy and overgrown with weeds, built up with little shacks and houses instead of the stately mansions once anticipated. The Chautauqua had been sold to an entrepreneur named Shaw, a man with a piscine face and glinty eye, who promptly expanded the amusement park. He no longer respected the wide buffer the Baltzleys had kept between Barton's home and the pleasure grounds; indeed, he built a new roller coaster entirely around her front yard. Though Clara lightheartedly told friends that "Glen Echo now, is a kind of Coney Island. It has all the embellishments," she was worried about Shaw's motives.³⁰ Unpleasant, too, were the frequent incidents of drinking and crime in the neighborhood.[31] Several times burglars broke into her home. Barton's nephew has left a wonderful picture of his aunt on one of these occasions. Startled by a sound in the middle of the night, she began creeping stealthily around the house in her long blue nightgown, with nightcap fastened securely under her chin and a toy pistol in her hand. She succeeded in catching the burglar and throwing him out, after which she calmly retired, with the toy pistol under her pillow.[32]

Autumn, winter, and spring were not so aggravating as summer, however. In addition, Glen Echo was the closest thing to a home that Barton had ever had, and she was reluctant to leave the place for more than one season of the year. She and dour, shallow little Dr. Hubbell settled into a subdued domesticity there, bereft of servants and keeping company chiefly with Baba the horse, Jersey the cow, and the doctor's pet goats. Barton continued to take in whatever friends or relatives were in need of help and to show astonishing energy in her household activities. At eighty-five she still worked until midnight on her correspondence after a day of shoveling snow or raking leaves, and in April of 1906 she even undertook to paint the entire house.[33] She and Hubbell had planted an overabundance of fruit trees and bushes, and consequently many of the autumn months were spent "picking in despair," or canning plums, making jellies, and bottling grape juice.[34] She liked to refer to herself as a "dairymaid," and many of the neighbors recalled Barton, clad in a calico dress with several medals pinned to her chest, carrying milk pails back from the barn.[35] When a journalist expressed her surprise at finding the great lady, dressed in a faded sunbonnet and old knitted shawl fastened with a huge royal jewel, on her hands and knees mending a sidewalk, Barton mildly replied, "Well my child, I should be very much ashamed if, after the life of hard work I have had, I had not learned how to wield a hammer." Reflecting on this later, the reporter decided that it was a fitting role for the renowned humanitarian after all. It seemed, she wrote, "to epitomize her whole life, a life of mending broken things—broken bodies, broken lives—her face always hidden from the world but bent upon the work needing her, and the great jewel of sympathy shining in her heart."[36]

The reporters who braved the long trolley ride to Glen Echo found Barton willing to discuss nearly any subject save the Red Cross controversy of 1904 or her opinion of the present organization. She had decided not to speak publicly on the matter when the infighting began, and she kept this pledge for the remainder of her life. But for an occasional request for records and a perfunctory inclusion of her among the incorporators on a new congressional charter in 1905, the Red Cross ignored Barton. To the best of her ability she tried to reciprocate, but here and there, in little slips and private asides, she showed her deep hurt and continuing interest in the organization.

Initially, when friends pressed her for a reaction to the new policies of the American Red Cross—which included an effort to establish local auxiliaries and to create an endowment fund at the expense of disaster relief—Barton tried to look aloof and disdainful. "Of the official doings I know nothing," she told one friend, "and might almost say care less."[37] As time went on, she formulated several explanations for her loss of the Red Cross and often answered inquiries by parroting these conciliatory, yet self-interested, views. She would never concede that Boardman had had any justification for her complaints; instead the Red Cross had been "stolen" by wealthy and powerful people, who saw in it a successful organization they wished to control: "Our little plant grew tall and strong, and its flowers and fruit were too great a temptation."[38] If the Red Cross had come to their attention it was because Barton had brought it to a peak of public recognition; if it was successful under its new officers it was because she had laid an unshakable foundation. Only ingratitude and spite would hold its leaders back. "In their way the Red Cross should become a great, popular and powerful organization," she told a friend and reporter. "How can it help becoming so? They are the Head of the nation—abundant, wealthy and took a cause with twenty years growth, with never a tarnish on it but what themselves put there."[39]

Barton's disinterested posture belied the close watch she kept on the reorganized body. Her papers contain mountains of newspaper clippings about Red Cross work after 1904, and diary entries reveal a detailed knowledge of its activities. She was sorry to see the organization become embroiled in politics (Mabel Boardman kept close ties with Presidents Roosevelt and Taft) and criticized the continual fund raising: "the Red Cross, since its adoption had developed into a most arrant *beggar*," she remarked. "I have not noticed much, if any, real *work* that it has done, but it surely begs busily in all directions, and upon all occasions."[40] She could not help taking some satisfaction in the mixed reactions received by Red Cross workers who labored at the San Francisco earthquake of 1906, recalling their criticism of her own relief efforts. (When Dr. Lucy Hall Brown visited the scene and wrote a detailed account of a number of Red Cross bunglings, Barton had the letter copied and circulated to her old friends.[41] Her greatest criticism centered on the leaders' reluctance to move quickly to the scene of disaster. When the Red Cross refused aid to the victims of a cyclone in Mississippi, she wrote that she believed they would "not find it to their taste to do these rough things," then added sarcastically, "They are taking care that the *money* of the people is not used in an 'unbusinesslike manner.' This then is 'businesslike' suffering—."[42]

But in spite of her criticism Barton could not quite relinquish her fondness for the organization. She was hurt that the body ignored her and prejudiced new members against her—"ignorant of every fact, simply enemies by transmission."[43] So strong were her maternal feelings that despite her humiliation she sincerely wished the best for the Red Cross. For twenty years she had struggled to ensure that it survived after her retirement, and in the long run she could only hope that it would thrive. "It *must* grow," Barton eventually conceded; "I want it to, it is *my* planting. I should rejoice the crop no matter who harvests it."[44]

Nowhere did the distress of Barton's expulsion from the Red Cross surface more clearly than in the intense interest she showed in spiritualism during the last five years of her retirement. She had always been keenly sensitive to the intangible elements in her life; she felt mood strongly and in her mind gave substance to many shadowy events that others would have labeled coincidence. Her interest in the supernatural increased with the 1904 visit of Sam Barton, who brought a Ouija board with him. Like Sam, Clara took seriously the cryptic messages spelled out on the board. She believed that Dolly, her mother, and several old friends were speaking comfort to her, and she linked the mystery to her religious beliefs. "Of the *meaning* of these phenomina [sic] I know nothing;—That they do exist is beyond doubt. I see no harm in Them. If they are one proof to a doubting world of the fact of immortality, it would seem to be well."[45]

Within a year Barton had expanded her fascination with the occult to include regular visits to a spiritualistic medium named Mrs. Warneke, who showed a shrewd understanding of Barton's emotional needs. While Clara settled into an overstuffed chair in the darkened parlor, Warneke conjured up images of past presidents, family members, and old admirers. The constant theme of their messages was to praise Barton's excellent work, to tell her that history would laud her and forget Mabel Boardman, and to extol her to finish the autobiography, which would vindicate her before the world. With complete sincerity Barton recorded conversations with Abraham Lincoln, Kaiser Wilhelm I, and General Grant, all directed toward consoling her and justifying her actions. These are sad diary entries, indicative as they are of a heart sorely in need of reinforcement and praise. For the remainder of her life, she and Julian Hubbell would consult Warneke for practical advice and pretty compliments. Under the medium's influence Hubbell would eventually give away his entire inheritance and the house at Glen Echo.[46]

Barton's deepening belief in spiritual forces and the unexplained powers of the human mind also led her to an active interest in Christian Science. She first became intrigued when the Universalist minister in North Oxford converted to the controversial religion. He explained to her Mary Baker Eddy's thirty years of charismatic teaching, the history of the church, its emphasis on positive thought and wholesome living, its doctrine of self-healing. Barton herself then read the literature of the church, saw that Mrs. Eddy formed many of her ideas while in a trance, and began to identify strongly with Eddy's followers.[47]

It was natural that Barton should come to revere Mary Baker Eddy, for in numerous ways their lives paralleled one another. Eddy had been born in New Hampshire a few months before Barton and, like the famed humanitarian, she was an afterthought—the youngest by a number of years in an already established family. Unstable emotions and poor health plagued her, and, like Barton, she spent many of the middle years of her life a depressed invalid. She had been cured by the common sense and warm atmosphere of a sanitarium run by Dr. Phineas Quimby of Portland, Maine, a place not unlike the Jackson Sanitarium in Dansville. Quimby's theories of "natural healing," expanded to include the intervention of God and a complicated set of beliefs about positive and negative forces in the world, came to make up Eddy's creed. By the 1880s she had written her major work, *Science and Health*, and had, largely through the force of her own personality, securely established the Christian Science church in the United States.[48] Barton was fascinated by this woman, who had been able to build up a religion despite great prejudice and ridicule, and saw her work as one that promoted health and peace in the world. More than once she spoke of Eddy as "the greatest woman of all," and at the church leader's death in 1910 she would write in sorrow, "There is no such person left, no such mind, no such ability."[49]

As time went on and she met more of Eddy's followers, Barton was greatly impressed with their intellect, optimism, and forbearance. "I find among them, and constantly coming into their ranks, the most thoughtful and intelligent people in the country . . . ," she wrote in admiration, adding that she believed the group followed Jesus' example of kindness "more closely than I have ever seen it in any denomination of Christians."[50] She saw hope for the aches and pains of the world—which she agreed were generally self-created—in the creed and took to recommending it to all who came within her reach. Depressed nieces and ailing acquaintances were given tracts and newspaper articles with the admonition to "read and re-read and you will find a new life, peace, and happiness and health." Barton eagerly sent for books and pamphlets on the subject and kept up an enthusiastic correspondence with those willing to discuss her views.[51]

Yet she shied away from completely embracing the faith. Barton had never been "what the world denominates a church woman," had not even joined the Universalist church of her father in North Oxford, and would not now relinquish her independence to an organized body.[52] Her personal faith was just that—an intimate belief in the justice and omniscience of God—and she had found it neither comforting nor enriching to share her spirituality in a communal sense. Barton also confessed to a certain mystification about a number of the religion's more esoteric doctrines and once said that though she understood the letter of the arguments, she could not feel them spiritually.[53] When chided by a friend for her evangelical tendencies, Barton retreated still more. "I was not especially advocating 'Christian Science,'" she maintained. "I do not belong to its vast number of followers. I simply look on . . . and try to find why I should have anything *against* or for them."[54] Until her death she kept the position of highly interested bystander, preferring to integrate certain elements of Christian Science into her private theology rather than to become an active participant in the church.

In 1907, at the insistence of her spiritual mentors, Barton again took up the task of completing her memoirs. Overwhelmed by the monumental work a full-scale autobiography would involve, she decided to publish the first chapter as a separate book, a sort of appetizer for those interested in a more complete description of her career. *The Story of My Childhood*, as it came to be called, would be the first in a series of "little books," small in size and low in price, designed for popular consumption. After a few weeks of editing, the book was published by Francis Atwater's Journal Publishing Company.[55] Reviewers found it delightful, if insubstantial. A "tantalizing scrap of autobiography," one critic called it. Another criticized Barton for wasting the opportunity to write a "great human document" but admitted he had found the volume "crisp bright & summary." Sales, even at fifty cents a copy, were indifferent, but Barton was pleased that the press had given the little book the type of attention often reserved for significant memoirs.[56]

Under the stimulus of this modest success, she began work on the next volume a few months later. Anecdotal, cheerful, and uncritical it chronicled her life from the days of teaching in North Oxford to her departure from Bordentown in 1853. Barton spent most of the fall of 1908 at her old roll-top desk, poring over letters and diaries and recording incidents forgotten for half a century. This second book was painfully written, and though she finished the sequel, she never published it, feeling after all that it was of little merit and that there would be few financial rewards. Early in November she decided to abandon her autobiographical project. "The more I would write the poorer I would be," was her final comment on the work, "and no one will lay down a novel to read this humdrum trash."[57]

Barton was also distracted from her writing by pressing problems within the National First Aid Association. Though handicapped by financial difficulties (Barton supplied a large portion of its small income), the movement had established classes and ambulance brigades in two-thirds of the states and had begun to influence the safety policies of conservative manufacturing firms, as well as schools, churches, and community leagues. Indeed, Barton proclaimed that the "mystery to me is how so few, accomplish so much, with so little means."[58] Her own contribution had gradually shrunk to an occasional newspaper interview and an appearance at the annual meeting each June. Still, the organization looked to her for advice and support and made few policy shifts without at least a perfunctory nod from their honorary president. Now, in 1908, they faced a serious challenge from the American Red Cross. Ignored by this body until they had attained their little success, their work was suddenly coveted by Red Cross directors, who cited Barton's own activities of 1902–3 as justification for claiming them. The administrators of the First Aid Association wanted to fight any attempt of the larger organization to appropriate their methods, but Barton, who was all too aware of the enormous political power supporting the Red Cross, counseled them to avoid litigation. She personally felt panic at the idea of any further conflict with her hard-nosed opponents, but she also recognized that in the long run the effort would be useless. "I can see nothing in it," she wrote as the maneuvering continued a year later. "Nothing can be done with the Red Cross as a competitor."[59] The Red Cross action served to reinforce her belief that Boardman simply waited until others established a successful program, then co-opted it for herself. In 1909, with the backing of the War Department, first aid training became an integral part of the American Red Cross. Soon afterward, the National First Aid Association of America quietly disbanded.[60]

The years during which Barton worked on her autobiography and wrestled with the dilemma of the First Aid Association were intensely private ones for her. She still felt protective of herself after the long exposure to public criticism and preferred the familiarity and comparative anonymity of Glen Echo and North Oxford to a more prominent role. She even shunned contact with many of her oldest friends, owing to a feeling of lingering humiliation and fear of public embarrassment for those who knew her, which she expressed in 1909: "I have strongly endeavored to keep myself so retired and aloof from my friends as not to draw attention to them, lest some harm might result from the observance of friendly relations."[61] Barton gave only two interviews during the last four years of her life. Both were to young female reporters who traveled to her retreat to find a retiring but sweetly gracious older woman, ready to regale them with stories. (Her foreign medals and royal jewels, which she kept constantly by her side in a dilapidated wicker satchel, were her favorite topic of discussion.)[62] Barton occasionally took mild pleasure in seeing her name listed as one of the "World's Greatest Women," or "Greatest Living Humanitarian," but the accolades did not touch her in any meaningful way.[63] "*What matters the praise of the world?*" she wrote emphatically in her journal, "*and what matter after we leave it especially? How hollow is that thing called fame.*"[64]

Barton's self-enforced loneliness was made more poignant by the death of good friends and respected associates. Mary Livermore and Dorence Atwater died in 1905, and in the next few years Clara and the world would lose Henri Dunant, Lucy Hall Brown, Samuel Barton, Nicholas Senn, Mary Baker Eddy, and George Pullman. The death of Mark Twain in 1910 affected her greatly, though she had never met him. "All the country is poorer. . . ," she declared. "There are losses which may be *filled* in some way, but *never made up.*"[65] Julian Hubbell, the Gardners, Stevé, Ida Riccius, and the Grand Duchess Louise still remained to her, but her own generation had gone. Increasingly she felt like a survivor in an alien world. "One scarcely can think on *which side* to place a friend at first thought," she mused. "This world begins to seem poor to us who have known and had them so long."[66]

Only two groups could consistently coax Barton into a public appearance: the feminists and the gray-haired members of the GAR. For the latter group she still held a special love and loyalty. The young reporter who talked to Clara in 1910 noted with some amusement that she continued to refer to the aging veterans as "her boys," calling her relationship with them "the deepest sentiment of her life." "Her eyes first flash, and then grow blurred with tears as she speaks of them, and the joy it is to meet them each year at the annual reunion."[67] Between 1904 and 1911 she attended camp reunions in Iowa, Minnesota, Saratoga, New York, Indiana, and, of course, Boston and Worcester. On Memorial Day and the

Fourth of July, Barton stood proudly with the soldiers to salute the dead or unveil a statue. Illness did not keep her from these rallies, and even when her voice grew too faint to speak for more than a few minutes, she would rise to address the veterans. The warm camaraderie, the flash of swords and the proudly worn uniforms, the ringing of cheers that were "very old timey to say the least," were the source of her greatest strength and inspiration.[68] To the end she believed in the rejuvenation of two veterans clasping hands, and one of her last poems was dedicated to this spirit:

> Ye have met to remember, may ye ever thus meet.
> So long as two comrades can rise to their feet;
> May their withered hands join, and clear to the last
> May they live o'er again the great deeds of the past,
> Till summoned in victory, honor and love,
> To stand in the ranks that are waiting above,
> And on the cleared vision God's glory shall burst
> Reunited in Heaven, the old 21st.[69]

Barton was received with equal enthusiasm at the women's rights conventions she attended. Now considered one of the pioneers of the movement, her appearance was a signal event at any suffrage rally or feminist convention. In 1905 Barton traveled to Boston for a meeting of the New England Woman Suffrage Association, which included an emotional reunion between Julia Ward Howe and Susan B. Anthony. Years later a newspaperman could still remember vividly how she had "appeared upon the platform and the three, introduced to the audience as 'all that was left of the Old Guard,' received a notable ovation."[70] The following year the scene was to be repeated in Baltimore, at a meeting of the National Woman Suffrage Association. Susan B. Anthony was, however, too weak to appear on stage; only Barton and Howe were there to speak of the past and lend continuity to the cause. Before an audience of thousands, Clara gave the opening remarks to the convention and paid tribute to her old friend Anthony. She charged the enthusiastic delegates to take heart from the hardships of their predecessors and to work on through disappointment or ridicule. "I recall a suffrage meeting years ago," Barton told the audience in a voice termed "delightfully distinct," "where the chairman fled at the last moment, fearing the opposition of the audience. We were referred to as old crows—Mary Livermore, Lucy Stone, and myself. We did not know how the gathering was going to receive us. But when Mary Livermore faced the meeting there was silence and throughout we had a respectful hearing." After this speech, a banquet was held in honor of Barton and her colleagues.[71]

The congress in Baltimore was the last major suffrage convention Barton would attend, but this was by no means indicative of a waning commitment to the elevation of women. Indeed, she showed a notable interest in and loyalty to her sex for the remainder of her life. The last survivor of her generation, she wrote lengthy tributes to Howe and Anthony at their deaths. She believed that they had contributed to the advancement not only of women, but of the society as a whole, that they should be heroines of the nation, not just of their own sex. "A few days ago someone said in my presence that every women in the world should stand with bared head before Susan B. Anthony," she wrote shortly after the death of her friend.

> Before I had time to think I said "And every man as well." I would not retract the words. I believe her work is more for the welfare of man than for that of woman herself. Man is trying to carry the burdens of the world alone. When he has the efficient help of woman he should be glad, and he will be. Just now it is new and strange, and men cannot comprehend what it would mean. But when such help comes, and men are used to it, they will be grateful for it. The change is not far away. This country is to know woman suffrage, and it will be a glad and proud day when it comes.[72]

Though she could not always admire the tactics of those who fought for women—"Huge hats, dangerous hatpins, Hobble and Harem skirts and some moves of the suffragists are hard to defend when assaulted"—Barton had tremendous faith in the examples of the past and the exceptional abilities of the present leaders.[73] She found it easy to nominate eight women to the Hall of Fame when she was asked; her difficulty was in limiting the list to Harriet Beecher Stowe, Lucretia Mott, Lucy Stone Blackwell, Frances Dana Gage, Mary A. Bickerdyke, Abigail Adams, Dorothea Dix, and Maria Mitchell.[74] She applauded Mary Logan's attempt to compile a history of American women. "From the storm lashed decks of the Mayflower . . . to the present hour; woman has stood like a rock for the welfare and the glory of the history of the country, and one might well add . . . unwritten, unrewarded, and almost unrecognized," she wrote.[75] As for the future, Barton had nothing but optimism. She believed that the elevation of women would improve everything from the longevity of men to the conduct of the United States Senate, and that their employment prospects and civil rights would rapidly increase.[76] Only a lingering bitterness over the part women had played in her removal from the Red Cross kept her from feeling unqualified enthusiasm for the stronger role women were playing in the society. "I only regret," she remarked, on hearing of the great London suffrage parade of 1911, "that the course of women toward me personally has been so hard, as to take the sweet from the triumph I should so much enjoy."[77]

Attendance at conventions and encampments took its toll on Barton, in spite of her efforts to limit the engagements. In part this was due to the heavy demands placed on her at these gatherings. It was impossible for her to slip quietly into a meeting or to be simply an interested observer. Always she was called on to speak, to attend receptions, or to take part in some ceremonial function. As

Barton noted in her diary in 1906, few people realized the strain caused by such public engagements. "All these people are pushing for *entertainments* and none can see the real work and cost that rests on me, nor raise a finger to help me on with it," she complained, "but all want the benefit of the name I have earned in just such struggles all my life."[78] Her only hope was to turn down invitations outright, for she found the appearances consistently demanded more than she had to give.

Public appearances tired her, but to a large degree the fatigue Barton suffered was the result of her own stubborn insistence on self-sufficiency. She frequently traveled alone to the meetings—at eighty-eight she undertook a thousand-mile journey to Chicago to attend a social science conference by herself—and always vigorously refused help with luggage, assistance on and off the train, or any other gesture she felt would reflect on her independence. At home she strictly maintained her onerous regimen. A reporter noted that even after an illness Clara was "as impatient of coddling as she has always been. She insisted on being up at the break of day, as she had always been; on attending her usual duties, taking complete charge of her room, writing through much of the day, reading through much of the night, as she had always done."[79] She did just as she chose in matters of sleep and diet—not always to her benefit. One little girl, taken by her mother to meet the great lady, was shocked to see her nibbling on some cheese at three o'clock in the afternoon instead of sitting down to a proper dinner. Told quickly that Miss Barton ate "what she pleased, when she pleased," the child noted, "This seemed to me to be very tangible evidence of greatness."[80] Barton fiercely resented anything that hampered her and took pains to conceal any fatigue from those with whom she was staying. As a result, her trips generally ended with a bout of bronchitis or acute exhaustion. After a day of hand shaking and polite greetings during an especially arduous trip in 1910, Barton jotted this note: "*pulse all out of time*—just a wreck. But it was a glorious day, and none knew how *I* made it."[81] Yet, when a close associate urged her to rest, she snapped, "How can you insult one so young as I by asking them to rest in the middle of the afternoon? Are you in your right mind to ask *me* to rest?"[82]

She greatly resented the physical changes brought on by the years. Overall her health remained good, but she could not halt the plague of little infirmities. Her hair fell out, often she felt dizzy or faint, and there were days when her eyesight failed her. She remained mentally vigorous to the end, but her once perfect letters now sometimes contained errors of syntax or spelling, and occasionally she forgot to mail important letters or First Aid diplomas.[83] On her eighty-sixth birthday she confessed that there was "a lack of coordination between the brain and limbs" which she feared would increase. "I do not know how to reach or avoid it."[84] Eventually she had to relinquish the cherished correspondence that had kept her overworked but in close touch with the friends of a lifetime. Only the grand duchess, Stevé, and a few others received letters in the last two years of her life.

Barton tried to appear young and fought to stave off the interest of the press in what she called the "eternal attack of the ninetieth birthday,"[85] but old age had its compensations. She felt less pressed to accomplish her goals, and many of the days drifted by in a kind of dreamy haze. "It is scarcely worth the while to attempt to keep these days in turn—one is so like the other," she recorded.[86] For perhaps the first time in her life she was at ease mentally. Financially secure, with a glorious lifework behind her, and released from the pressure of excelling in a professional world not wholly accepting of women, she was at last at peace with herself. Resentments vanished, and remarkably, generally pleasant memories remained. In a reflective vein she wrote in her diary of the visit of professional associates on Independence Day, 1911. "It seemed very like the old days—and yet I would not change back. If they must be lived I am devoutly thankful they are past. I would prefer my present physical weakness rather than the unrest of those days, in strength to bear them. In fact I do not see where I got the strength to live them through."[87]

Barton suffered a spinal injury late in 1908, which kept her in bed on and off for nearly a year. She believed herself recovered enough by the spring of 1910 to make the lone trip to Chicago, but on her return home she felt her old antagonist, bronchitis, returning. She spent the summer alone in North Oxford, fending off a crippling cough and shooing away reporters. She attributed her fretful nights to bulky food and limited herself to Dr. Jackson's prescription of corn and rye mush, taken only once or twice daily. Despite this dubious diet, Barton gained strength and in the fall summoned the energy to return to Glen Echo. She arrived to find the house in a dreadful mess—Dr. Hubbell's housekeeping having improved not at all in his years with her—and undertook to clean it herself. Throughout the fall she worked on, accomplishing remarkable amounts with the little strength she possessed.[88]

In January 1911, while still weak and overworked, Clara heard the news of Ida Riccius's unexpected death. Emotional trauma and physical illness had always been linked for her, and as Dr. Hubbell observed, "the shock was too much for the weakened strength—the heart fluttered and nearly stopped." For several months Barton lay gravely ill of pneumonia. She refused medication during her illness and was often too drowsy or weak to eat; twice she lay near death.[89] Yet when the doctor told her that she had but one chance to live, she briskly told him: "I will take that chance."[90]

By spring she could sit up and look in wonder at the drawers full of letters and greetings that had poured in at the news of her illness. With her precarious hold on life she managed to retain her sense of humor. When just able to write she told a friend that she was "*locally* recovered, and call myself well, but the strength must, I sometimes think, be coming by freight, and got sidetracked somewhere, and I am forbidden to write letters. I am stealing this, out of sight of my keepers."[91] Her "keepers" also could not prevent her from trying to garden or sweep her room, activities she continued, though she admitted that she lost strength and felt faint if she moved.[92] Worried that the summer heat and noise of Glen Echo would worsen her condition, Barton let Stevé—against Hubbell's express orders—persuade her to travel to North Oxford in July 1911.[93]

Hubbell was incensed to find that Clara had arrived to an empty house, with no one to help her and no provisions. "You left her there *alone*," he wrote angrily to Stevé, "a weak sick woman—the great *Clara Barton*—the *Treasure* of the Nation."[94] But Clara needed little in these days. Her mind was preoccupied with setting her affairs in order. She contacted the caretaker of the North Oxford cemetery to provide for care of her family plot after her death and designed a Barton monument with an inscription for herself. She had already deeded the Glen Echo property to Dr. Hubbell, both in recognition of his lifelong services and as a guard against claims by the American Red Cross. Now she began to consider the distribution of her other property and the obligations she must fulfill before departing this life. Guests were surprised and saddened to find her dwelling, for the first time, on her own demise. The Reverend Percy Epler, who would preside at her funeral and become her first biographer, felt he was holding an "audience of death," her words were so "stately and measured." "She seemed already adjusted to a place beyond the mortal," he wrote. "Her playful, buoyant spirit was gone. The dignity of last things charged the atmosphere."[95] When Hubbell arrived in North Oxford, he too found her changed and hastened to take her back to Glen Echo where he could supervise her recovery.

She never really regained her old vigor, however. As she celebrated her ninetieth birthday, the press noted her fierce independence and quoted her secret for longevity—"low fare, hard work." Yet the pieces dwelt on the past, not the future. Barton felt restless and disturbed, and she fostered her weakness by insisting on a diet of raw eggs, buttermilk, and gruel, and these in minute amounts.[96] In January 1912, she succumbed again to pneumonia, this time with a body too battered to fight it effectively. Convinced that this illness was his aunt's last, Stevé insisted on a doctor and enough medication to "make her as *comfortable* as possible." When the doctor offered morphine, her nephew did not balk, though Hubbell bitterly opposed it and believed afterward that the drug had killed his heroine.[97]

For the next several months Barton hung between life and death, in a state of drugged semiconsciousness. Occasionally she rallied enough to read a little—she was still "educating" herself with the classics—or to sit up in the old walnut bed that filled her Glen Echo chamber. Bit by bit she penned the last letter of her life. "They tell me I am changing worlds," she wrote to the grand duchess, "and one of my last thoughts and wishes is to tell you of my unchanging love and devotion to you."[98] At other lucid moments Stevé talked to her of her funeral and helped her to write her will. Hubbell would claim that Stevé unduly influenced the sick, comatose woman to leave her holdings to him; "In her feeble exhausted state too tired to think, to tired to talk, she nodded assent." Whatever her state, she signed the document with a shaky hand and slumped into unconsciousness.[99]

On April 10 she suddenly awoke and told Dr. Hubbell of a dream she had had. She was again on the battlefield, wading through blood, watching agonized men braving the most hideous wounds. "I crept round once more, trying to give them at least a drink of water to cool their parched lips, and I heard them at last speak of mother and wives and sweethearts, but never a murmur or complaint. Then I woke to hear myself groan because I have a stupid pain in my back, thats all. Here on a good bed, with every attention. I am ashamed that I murmur."[100] She again slipped away from him, and for two more days the poor devoted doctor hovered frantically over her. At last, at nine o'clock on the morning of April 12, she again opened her eyes and spoke to Stevé, Hubbell, and her attending physician, Dr. Pratt. They hoped for words of inspiration and contentment; instead they heard the last murmuring of a great but troubled and restless spirit. "Let me go, let me go," she cried, and in that instant she was gone.[101]

abbreviations

These abbreviations are used throughout the Notes.

AAS   Clara Barton Papers, American Antiquarian Society, Worcester, Mass.

ANRC   American National Red Cross, Washington, D.C.

B-DU   Clarissa Harlowe Barton Papers, Manuscript Department, Duke University Library, Durham, N.C.

CB   Clara Barton

CBJ   Clara Barton Journal

CB-LC   Clara Barton Papers, Manuscript Division, Library of Congress, Washington, D.C.

CBNHS   Clara Barton National Historic Site, Glen Echo, Md.

CMJ   Charles Mason Journal

D-DU   Mary Norton Papers, Dalton Collection, Manuscript Department, Duke University Library, Durham, N.C.

DAB   Johnson, Allen, and Dumas Malone, eds. *Dictionary of American Biography*. New York: Charles Scribner's Sons, 1931–36.

E-WRHS   Elwell Papers, Western Reserve Historical Society, Cleveland, Ohio

HL   Barton Papers, Huntington Library, San Marino, Calif.

GPJ   Journal of George Pullman

Jack MS   Collection of Dr. A. J. Jack, typescript in Hightstown Memorial Library, Hightstown, N.J.

K-LC   George Kennan Papers, Library of Congress, Washington, D.C.

373

LC   Library of Congress, Washington, D.C.

MHS   Minnesota Historical Society, St. Paul, Minn.

NARS   National Archives and Records Service, Washington, D.C.

O-LC   Robert Ogden Papers, Library of Congress, Washington, D.C.

RARC NARS   Records of the American Red Cross, Record Group 200, National Ar-
            chives and Records Service, Washington, D.C.

SBJ   Journal of Stephen E. Barton

SSC   Clara Barton Papers, Sophia Smith Collection, Smith College Ar-
            chives, Northampton, Mass.

notes

Chapter 1

1. Saidee F. Riccius, "Memories of Our Aunt Clara," in William Conklin, ed., *Clara Barton and Dansville* (Dansville, N.Y.: F. A. Owen Publishing Co., 1966), pp. 542–43; and statement of Elvira Stone in "The Clara Barton Home," *Church Messenger*, May 7, 1896, clipping, CB-LC.

2. For a lengthy description of the novel, see William E. Barton, *The Life of Clara Barton* (Boston: Houghton Mifflin Co., 1922), 1:6–7.

3. Stone, in "Clara Barton Home."

4. See CB to Elvira Stone, November 29, 1898, CB-LC; Riccius, "Memories of Our Aunt Clara," in Conklin, ed., *Dansville*, pp. 542–43; and CB, *The Story of My Childhood* (Meriden, Conn.: Journal Publishing Co., 1907), p. 13.

5. "Sayings of Clara Barton," in CB, *Childhood*, p. 165.

6. Vital statistics for the Barton family are found in George F. Daniels, *History of the Town of Oxford Massachusetts* (Oxford: privately published, 1892), p. 391; also CB, *Childhood*, p. 16.

7. Jeremiah Spofford, *Historical and Statistical Gazetteer of Massachusetts* (Newburyport: Charles Whipple, 1828), pp. 264–65; and Daniels, *History of Oxford*.

8. William E. Barton, "The Barton Family of Oxford, Massachusetts," *The New England Historical and Genealogical Register* 85 (October 1930): 405; and W. E. Barton, *Life*, 1:9, 12–13.

9. Mary deWitt Freeland, *The Records of Oxford Massachusetts* (Albany: Munseries Sons, 1894), pp. 225, 235–36; and Daniels, *History of Oxford*, p. 210.

10. Daniels, *History of Oxford*, pp. 390–91; and untitled genealogical sketch of CB's family, n.d., AAS; also Joyce Butler Hughes to author, May 17, 1979; and Clara Barton Gilbert to author, September 9, 1979, in possession of the author.

11. CB to Bernard Vassall, November 22, 1890, AAS.

12. Untitled genealogical sketch, n.d., AAS; and Hannah Moore Barton diary in James C. North, *The History of Augusta* (Augusta, Maine: Clapp and North, 1870), p. 297.

13. See CB, *Childhood*, pp. 20–21 (quotation p. 20); also CB to Mrs. B. C. Whitney, July 18, 1901, CB-LC.

14. Daniels, *History of Oxford*, pp. 270–80; untitled genealogical sketch, n.d., AAS; CB, *Childhood*, p. 21; P. M. Harwood to CB, February 10, 1902, CB-LC; CB to Walter Phillips, April 12, 1904, CB-LC; and CB to Harriet Austin, n.d. [March 1880], in Conklin, ed., *Dansville*, p. 75.

15. CB to Stephen E. Barton, March 8, 1903, CB-LC.

16. Bill of Jacob Bone to Stephen Barton, April 3, 1839, CB-LC; and account of Stephen Barton, 1823 and 1825, Creggan and Dudley Store Records, AAS.

17. The Clara Barton birthplace in North Oxford, Mass. still contains a small chair, desk, and other pieces made by Stephen Barton.

18. Ernest Cassara, ed., *Universalism in America* (Boston: Beacon Press, 1971), pp. 53–56, 182, 247–48; CB to Jennie S. M. Vinten, October 6, 1904, CB-LC; J. B. Holmes to CB, February 20, 1899, CB-LC; Daniels, *History of Oxford*, p. 76; and quotation CB lecture to First Universalist Church of Minneapolis, n.d., typescript, CB-LC.

19. Daniels, *History of Oxford*, p. 223.

20. Thomas Lamb to CB, December 12, 1876, CB-LC.

21. Untitled genealogical sketch, n.d., AAS; and CB to Hiram Moffitt, August 3, 1879, in Conklin, ed., *Dansville*, pp. 109–10.

22. Antislavery petitions to the House of Representatives, Legislative Records, Record Group 46, NARS.

23. CB, address at May Festival for Women's Suffrage, n.d., CB-LC.

24. CB to Dr. Edward Foote, draft answers to "Questions of Invalids," n.d. [c. 1876], SSC.

25. Edith Riccius King, "Tales told by Ida Barton Riccius about her Grandmother Sarah Stone Barton," October 20, 1934, CB-LC.

26. Ibid.

27. Ibid.

28. CB to Moffitt, August 3, 1879, in Conklin, ed., *Dansville*, pp. 109–10; Bernard Barton Vassall, "Genealogy of the Barton Family," n.d., CB-LC; Edith Riccius King, "Childhood Memories," October 20, 1934, CB-LC; school papers of Dolly Barton, March 21, 1821, CB-LC; CB, *Childhood*, p. 17; untitled genealogical sketch, n.d., AAS; CBJ, November 2, 1869, B-DU; and quotation CB to Ida Riccius, October 2, 1906, AAS.

29. CB to Foote, draft answers, n.d. [c. 1876], SSC; King, "Childhood Memories," October 20, 1934, CB-LC; statement of Joyce Barton Hughes, September 1975, notes at CBNHS. Dolly's modified rocking chair is preserved at the Clara Barton birthplace, North Oxford, Mass.

30. CB to Moffitt, August 3, 1879, in Conklin, ed., *Dansville*, pp. 109–10.

31. CB to Foote, draft answers, n.d. [c. 1876], SSC.

32. CB, *Childhood*, p. 76.

33. Untitled genealogical sketch, n.d., AAS; and CBJ, March 16, 1852, CB-LC.

34. Untitled genealogical sketch, n.d., AAS.

35. Daniels, *History of Oxford*, p. 210; and Lucien Burleigh to CB, May 14, 1838, CB-LC.

36. Samuel Willis to CB, July 23, 1903, CB-LC; untitled genealogical sketch, n.d., AAS; and Daniels, *History of Oxford*, pp. 270–80.

37. CB, *Childhood*, p. 18.

38. Daniels, *History of Oxford*, p. 391; and David Barton's untitled poetry, CB-LC.

39. CB, *Childhood*, p. 19.

40. Ibid., pp. 19, 80.

41. Burleigh to CB, May 14, 1838, CB-LC.

42. CB, *Childhood*, p. 80.

43. Receipt of Stephen Barton from Nicholas Academy, Clara Barton birthplace, North Oxford, Mass.

44. CB, *Childhood*, pp. 17, 76; and CB to Moffitt, August 3, 1879, in Conklin, ed., *Dansville*, pp. 109–10.

45. CB, *Childhood*, pp. 76, 89.

46. CBJ, n.d. [1907], CB-LC; and CBJ, January 8, 1882, typescript, AAS.

47. CB, *Childhood*, p. 16.

48. Ibid., p. 23.

49. Ibid., pp. 22, 25, 29, 106.

50. Ibid., p. 45.

51. Barton mentions several times in her autobiography that she lisped, though she does not define it as a speech impediment. She overcame the handicap in her adulthood. Observers noted, however, that she always spoke with her mouth held in an unusually rigid manner. Her great-nieces believed that she had an extra row of upper teeth behind her normal ones. Such a malformation would certainly have caused difficulties in speech. See CB, *Childhood*, pp. 21, 42, 43. Also King, "Childhood Memories," October 20, 1934, CB-LC.

52. CB to Jennie S. Vinten, October 6, 1904, CB-LC; and CB, *Childhood*, p. 111.

53. CB to Henry Wilson, January 27, 1863, AAS; and CB to Moffitt, August 3, 1879, in Conklin, ed., *Dansville*, pp. 109–10.

54. CB, *Childhood*, p. 111.

55. Ibid., pp. 18, 27, 29–30. Lucy Larcom, a chronicler of early New England, acknowledged that she started school at two and a half and that this was an accepted practice. Lucy Larcom, *A New England Girlhood* (Boston: Houghton Mifflin Co., 1924), p. 44.

56. Daniels, *History of Oxford*, p. 103; and Richard Cecil Stone, *Life Incidents of Home, School, and Church* (St. Louis: Southwestern Book and Publishing Co., 1874); and CB, *Childhood*, pp. 28, 64, 65, 72.

57. CB, *Childhood*, p. 32.

58. CB copybook, c. 1830, CB-LC. See also Bernard Wishy, *The Child and the Republic* (Philadelphia: University of Pennsylvania Press, 1968), pp. 74–78.

59. CB, *Childhood*, pp. 96–97; and letters of Lucien Burleigh to CB, April–May 1838, CB-LC.

60. CB, *Childhood*, pp. 97–98.

61. Ibid., p. 18.

62. See Barbara Welter, "The Cult of True Womanhood, 1820–1860," in Michael Gordon, ed., *The American Family in Socio-Historic Perspective* (New York: St. Martin's Press, 1978).

63. CB, *Childhood*, p. 45.

64. Ibid., pp. 41–47.

65. Ibid., p. 95; and Stone, quoted in "Clara Barton Home."

66. CBJ, April 23, 1907, CB-LC.

67. CB, *Childhood*, p. 21.

68. CB, miscellaneous notes on life, n.d., CB-LC.

69. CB, *Childhood*, pp. 90–93.

70. Ibid., p. 94. For lack of dolls in childhood, see CB to Margaret Besland, December 27, 1898, CB-LC.

71. CB, *Childhood*, pp. 47–49; untitled genealogical sketch, n.d., AAS; and CB to Johnny Stafford, n.d., [February 15, 1901], CB-LC.

72. CB, *Childhood*, p. 56.

73. Ibid., pp. 55–57 (quotation p. 55).

74. Ibid., p. 58.

75. CB to Joseph and Enola Gardner, March 13, 1883, CB-LC; and CB to Mary L. Tower, December 1, 1892, RARC NARS.

76. CB, *Childhood*, p. 73.

77. Ibid., pp. 58–61. The Bartons' method of punishment was not uncommon, especially in New England, with its long Calvinist tradition. See Wishy, *Child and Republic*, p. 46; also CB, *Childhood*, p. 62; and CB to Henry Wilson, January 27, 1863, typescript, AAS.

78. CB, "A Child's Party," MS story, n.d. [c. 1901], CB-LC.

79. CB to Gardners, March 13, 1883, CB-LC; CB to Elvira Stone, May 3, 1895, and November 29, 1898, both CB letterbook, CB-LC.

80. Mrs. E. M. Yannimore to CB, May 31, 1903, CB-LC; CB to Annie Wittenmeyer, April 3, 1891, CB-LC; and CB, *Childhood*, p. 70.

81. Larcom, *New England Girlhood*, p. 9.

82. CB to Mr. Ridgely, August 25, 1903, CB-LC; and Wishy, *Child and Republic*, p. 78.

83. CB, *Childhood*, pp. 51–52.

84. Ibid., pp. 77–86.

85. Ibid., pp. 87–88.

86. Ibid., pp. 101–4 (quotation p. 104).

87. Nella Garman to Saidee Riccius, November 10, 1921; Yannimore to CB, May 31, 1903; and Thomas Lamb to CB, December 12, 1876, all CB-LC.

88. Lamb to CB, December 31, 1876, CB-LC.

89. Welter, "Cult of True Womanhood," pp. 320–22.

90. CB, *Childhood*, pp. 98–99; and CB to Foote, draft answers, n.d. [c. 1876], SSC.

91. Beverly Wright Smith, "Clara Barton Had Relatives in Maine, Still Living in Vienna," *Lewiston Maine Journal*, November 5, 1960, copy in AAS.

92. CB, *Childhood*, pp. 89–93, 123.

93. CB to Ida Riccius, November 30, 1879, AAS.

94. CB, *Childhood*, pp. 110–11.

95. Frederick N. Binder, *The Age of the Common School, 1830–1865* (New York: Wiley, 1974); and Orson Squire Fowler and L. N. Fowler, *Fowler's Practical Phrenology* (Boston: Saxton and Pierce, 1836).

96. CB, *Childhood*, pp. 112–15.

Chapter 2

1. W. E. Barton, *Life*, 1:56; statement of Fanny Vassall, July 17, 1917, AAS; and CB, *The Story of My Childhood* (Meriden, Conn.: Journal Publishing Co., 1907), p. 114.

2. Julian B. Hubbell, "Some Personal Traits of Miss Clara Barton," unpublished MS, n.d., CBNHS.

3. See CB to Grace Donahue, March 23, 1900; CB, untitled MS sequel to *Childhood*, October 12, 1908; CB, teaching certificate, 1839; Lucien Burleigh wrote of her upcoming teaching on May 14, 1838, all CB-LC.

4. CB, *Childhood*, p. 119.

5. Ibid., pp. 114–16.

6. Elvira Stone, quoted in "The Clara Barton Home," *Church Messenger*, May 7, 1896, clipping, CB-LC.

7. CB, *Childhood*, pp. 117–18.

8. Former pupil quoted in CB to Mrs. J. H. Balcom, January 20, 1911, CB-LC.

9. CB, *Childhood*, p. 119.

10. Ibid., pp. 119–20.

11. CB, MS sequel to *Childhood*, October 12, 1908, CB-LC.

12. Ibid.; and Charlton, Massachusetts, School Records, MS Ledger, AAS.

13. CB, MS sequel to *Childhood*, October 12, 1908, CB-LC.

14. Ibid.; and *Centennial History of the Town of Millbury Massachusetts* (Millbury, 1915), p. 333.

15. CB, *Childhood*, pp. 17–18, 38; and George F. Daniels, *History of the Town of Oxford Massachusetts* (Oxford: privately published, 1892), pp. 99, 100, 276, 374.

16. Burleigh to CB, May 14, 1838, CB-LC.

17. Stone, quoted in "Clara Barton Home."

18. CB to Robert Hale, August 16, 1876, CB-LC.

19. CB, MS sequel to *Childhood*, October 12, 1908, CB-LC.

20. Ibid.

21. Mrs. John Balcom to CB, April 7, 1910, CBNHS; and CB to Alfred T. Osmond, February 1, 1902, CB-LC.

22. CB, *Childhood*, pp. 120–23.

23. Ibid., p. 122.

24. CB to Elsie Barton Holway, March 8, 1900, CB-LC.

25. CB, *Childhood*, p. 122; and MS autograph album, 1838, ANRC.

26. L. T. Bacon to CB, n.d. [late 1830s], CB-LC.

27. Notes on a conversation between Stephen E. Barton, Jr., Herman Riccius, and Saidee Riccius, July 8, 1917; and statement of Fanny Childs Vassall, both AAS.

28. Bacon to CB, n.d. [late 1830s], CB-LC.

29. L. T. Bacon to CB, n.d. [second letter, late 1830s], CB-LC.

30. Notes on Barton and Riccius conversation, July 8, 1917, AAS; and CBJ, April 18–24, 1849 (quotation April 21), CB-LC.

31. Notes on Barton and Riccius conversation, July 8, 1917, AAS.

32. CB, MS sequel to *Childhood*, October 12, 1908, CB-LC.

33. Frances Childs Vassall quoted in W. E. Barton, *Life* 1:83–84.

34. CB to Bernard Vassall, n.d. ("Schoolroom, Wednesday Morning"), CB-LC.

35. Vassall quoted in W. E. Barton, *Life* 1:83–84.

36. L. A. Stebbins, "An Unpublished Chapter in the History of the American National Red Cross," April 6, 1942, CB-LC.

37. See, for example, CBJ, February 2, 5, 17, 20, March 7, 13, 1852, and September 10, 1897 to January 29, 1898, all CB-LC.

38. CB, MS sequel to *Childhood*, October 12, 1908, CB-LC.

39. CB to Samuel Rich Barton, October 25, 1850, HL.

40. CBJ, March 17, 1849, CB-LC.

41. CB to Samuel Rich Barton, October 25, 1850, HL.

42. CB scrapbook, c. 1830–45, CB-LC.

43. CBJ, February 24, 1849, CB-LC.

44. CB, MS sequel to *Childhood,* October 12, 1908, CB-LC; and Daniels, *History of Oxford,* pp. 210, 391.

45. CB to O. M. Vinton, October 6, 1904, CB-LC.

46. CB quoted in speech given by Saidee F. Riccius, 1921, copy in CB-LC.

47. See Lucien Burleigh to CB, May 15, 1838; and John Andrews to CB, September 16, 1843, both CB-LC.

48. CB quoted in Charles Sumner Young, *Clara Barton: A Centenary Tribute* (Boston: Gorham Press, 1922), p. 372.

49. CB, MS sequel to *Childhood,* October 12, 1908, CB-LC; and School Report of Millbury School Committee, 1844–45, Miscellaneous Millbury Massachusetts Papers, AAS.

50. CB, MS sequel to *Childhood,* October 12, 1908, CB-LC.

51. Ibid.; and Daniels, *History of Oxford,* p. 98.

52. CB, MS sequel to *Childhood,* October 12, 1908, CB-LC.

53. CB, MS sequel to *Childhood,* October 12, 1908; and CB to Leonard Richardson, March 27, 1850, both CB-LC.

54. CB, MS sequel to *Childhood,* October 12, 1908, CB-LC.

55. Ibid.

56. Ibid.

57. Lucien Burleigh to CB, May 24, 1838, CB-LC.

58. CBJ, May 19, 1849, CB-LC.

59. Ibid., February 19, 1849.

60. CB to Richardson, March 27, 1850, copy in CB-LC.

61. CB, MS sequel to *Childhood,* October 12, 1908, CB-LC.

Chapter 3

1. CB, untitled MS sequel to *The Story of My Childhood,* October 12, 1908, CB-LC.

2. CB to Leonard Richardson, March 27, 1850, copy in CB-LC.

3. CB to Samuel Rich Barton, October 25, 1850, HL.

4. CB, MS sequel to *Childhood,* October 12, 1908, CB-LC.

5. CBJ, notes in back of 1849 volume, CB-LC.

6. CB, MS sequel to *Childhood,* October 12, 1908, CB-LC.

7. See ibid.; and Helen Nelson Rudd, "A Century of Schools in Clinton" (Clinton, N.Y.: Clinton Historical Society, 1964), p. 10, in Universalist Papers, Andover-Harvard Theological Seminary, Cambridge, Mass.

8. "Catalogue of the Officers and Students of Clinton Liberal Institute, Clinton, Oneida County, N.Y., for 1850–51" (Utica: D. C. Grove, 1851), p. 22.

9. *Seventh Decennial Census of the United States* (1850), Oneida County, N.Y., NARS; "Catalogue of Clinton Liberal Institute," pp. 5–18; and Uriah Clark, *Life Sketches of Rev. George Henry Clark* (Boston: Abel Thompkins, 1852).

10. CB, MS sequel to *Childhood,* October 12, 1908, CB-LC.

11. Ibid.

12. "Catalogue of Clinton Liberal Institute," pp. 21–22.

13. CB, MS sequel to *Childhood,* October 12, 1908, CB-LC.

14. "Catalogue of Clinton Liberal Institute," pp. 21–22.

15. CB, MS sequel to *Childhood,* October 12, 1908, CB-LC.

16. Ibid.; and *Seventh Decennial Census,* Oneida County.

17. CB, MS sequel to *Childhood,* October 12, 1908, CB-LC; and unidentified former classmate of CB, quoted in article appearing in the *Hampshire Gazette* (Northampton, Mass.), May 1, 1866.

18. "Reminiscences of Miss Clara Barton," n.d., Austin Craig and Family Papers, MHS.

19. CB, MS sequel to *Childhood,* October 12, 1908, CB-LC.

20. Unidentified classmate, *Hampshire Gazette,* May 1, 1866.

21. Statement of Fanny Childs Vassall, July 8, 1917, AAS.

22. CB, MS sequel to *Childhood,* October 12, 1908; and CB to Abby Barker Sheldon, December 23, 1899, both CB-LC.

23. CB to Sheldon, December 23, 1899, CB-LC.

24. CB to Samuel Rich Barton, May 7, 1851, CB-LC.

25. Unidentified classmate, *Hampshire Gazette,* May 1, 1866.

26. CB to Samuel Rich Barton, June 7, 1851, HL.

27. Ibid.

28. "Reminiscences of Miss Clara Barton," n.d., Austin Craig and Family Papers, MHS.

29. CB, MS sequel to *Childhood,* October 12, 1908, CB-LC; and unidentified classmate, *Hampshire Gazette,* May 1, 1866.

30. Ibid.

31. Notes on a conversation between Stephen E. Barton, Jr., Herman Riccius, and Saidee Riccius, July 8, 1917, AAS.

32. Massachusetts Vol. 96, p. 335, R. G. Dun and Company Collection, Baker Library, Harvard University Graduate School of Business Administration, Boston, Mass.

33. Stephen Barton, Jr., to CB, July 1851, CB-LC.

34. Ibid.; and CB to Richardson, March 27, 1850, CB-LC.

35. Stephen Barton, Jr., to CB, July 1851, CB-LC.

36. CB, MS sequel to *Childhood,* October 12, 1908, CB-LC.

37. Unpublished interview between CB and Leonora Halsted, July 29, 1890, CB-LC.

Chapter 4

1. Unpublished interview between CB and Leonora Halsted, July 29, 1890, CB-LC; and CB, untitled MS sequel to *The Story of My Childhood,* October 12, 1908, CB-LC.

2. CB-Halsted interview, July 29, 1890, CB-LC.

3. CB, MS sequel to *Childhood,* October 12, 1908, CB-LC.

4. CB to Mary Norton, n.d. [c. 1878], D-DU.

5. CB, MS sequel to *Childhood,* October 12, 1908, CB-LC.

6. CB to Bernard Vassall, n.d. ("Schoolroom, Wednesday Morning"), CB-LC.

7. CB-Halsted interview, July 29, 1890, CB-LC.

8. Eleanor Burnside to CB, January 10, 1901, CB-LC.

9. CB to Bernard Vassall, n.d. [c. 1851], CB-LC.

10. CB, MS sequel to *Childhood,* October 12, 1908; and CBJ, November 30, 1851, both CB-LC.

11. CB to Bernard Vassall, October 19, 1851, CB-LC.

12. Description of Hightstown in Maurice P. Sherman, Jr., "Clara Barton in Hights-

town, 1851–52: The Forgotten Chapter in the Life of a Humanitarian," unpublished research paper for Villanova University, 1971–72, p. 5, copy courtesy of the author; and *Agricultural Census of the United States, Mercer County, New Jersey, 1850, East Windsor Township*, p. 661, copy in New Jersey Room, Rutgers University, New Brunswick, N.J.

13. CB, MS sequel to *Childhood*, October 12, 1908; and CB to Vassall, October 19, 1851, both CB-LC.

14. CB to Vassall, October 19, 1851, CB-LC.

15. Abel C. Thomas, *Century of Universalism* (Philadelphia: J. Faganana Sons, 1872), pp. 2–10; Evan Morrison Woodward and John Hageman, *History of Burlington and Mercer Counties, New Jersey with Biographical Sketches of Many of their Pioneers and Prominent Men* (Philadelphia: Evart and Peck, 1883), pp. 758–59; *Seventh Decennial Census of the United States* (1850), Mercer County, New Jersey, NARS; and CB, MS sequel to *Childhood*, October 12, 1908, CB-LC.

16. CB to Bernard Vassall, November 30, 1851, CB-LC.

17. Ibid.; CB to Vassall, October 19, 1851, CB-LC; CB to Bernard Vassall, March 26, 1852, CB-LC.

18. CB to Wycoff Norton, December 26, 1880, quoted in Dorothea Reynolds, "The Clara Barton House at Hightstown," n.d., copy in Hightstown Memorial Library, Hightstown, N.J.

19. CB to Sarah Vassall, n.d. [1851], CB-LC.

20. Note of Sally Vassall on CB to Bernard Vassall, July 21, 1852, CB-LC.

21. CB, MS sequel to *Childhood*, October 12, 1908, CB-LC.

22. CBJ, October 23, 1851; and Hart W. Bodine, untitled article in the *New York Daily Tribune*, August 21, 1898, clipping, both CB-LC.

23. CB, MS sequel to *Childhood*, October 12, 1908; and Bodine article, *New York Daily Tribune*, August 21, 1898, clipping, both CB-LC.

24. CB to Leonard Richardson, March 27, 1850, CB-LC; and quotation of Mrs. Shumway Davis in Percy Epler, *The Life of Clara Barton* (New York: Macmillan, 1915), p. 18.

25. Bodine article, *New York Daily Tribune*, August 21, 1898, clipping, CB-LC.

26. CB to Bernard Vassall, January 29, 1852, CB-LC.

27. CB to Vassall, November 30, 1851, CB-LC.

28. Bodine article, *New York Daily Tribune*, August 21, 1898, clipping, CB-LC.

29. CB to Bernard Vassall, November 31, 1851, CB-LC.

30. Ibid.; and CB, MS sequel to *Childhood*, October 12, 1908, CB-LC.

31. CBJ, March 18, 1852, CB-LC.

32. CB, MS sequel to *Childhood*, October 12, 1908, CB-LC.

33. Bodine article, *New York Daily Tribune*, August 21, 1898, clipping, CB-LC.

34. CB to Vassall, November 30, 1851, CB-LC.

35. CBJ, March 31, 1852, CB-LC.

36. Ibid., February 18 and April 17, 1852; CB to Bernard Vassall, January 21, March 16, 1852, and n.d. [1852], CB-LC; statement of Fanny Childs Vassall, July 17, 1917, AAS; and James Norton to Bernard Vassall, March 16, 1852, CB-LC.

37. CB to Bernard Vassall, December 31, 1851, CB-LC.

38. Ibid.; and, for example, CBJ, February 2, 3, 5, 17, 20, March 7, 13, 1852, CB-LC. For CB walking to school in rubber boots, see Bodine article, *New York Daily Tribune*, August 21, 1898, clipping, CB-LC.

39. Norton to Vassall, March 16, 1852, CB-LC.

40. CBJ, February 12, 1852, and March 19, 1852, CB-LC.

41. Ibid., March 31, 1852.

42. Ibid., March 24, April 3 and 20, 1852.

43. Ibid., March 11 and 16, 1852.

44. Ibid., March 11, 16, and 31, 1852.

45. Ibid., March 11, 1852.

46. Ibid., March 24, 1852.

47. CB to Bernard Vassall, n.d., CB-LC.

48. CBJ, March 11, 24, 31, 1852, CB-LC.

49. Ibid., April 29, 1852; and CB to Bernard Vassall, March 15, 1852, CB-LC.

50. CBJ, March 31, 1852, CB-LC.

51. Ibid., April 20 and May 25, 1852; and CB, MS sequel to Childhood, October 12, 1908, CB-LC.

52. John D. Magee, Bordentown 1682–1876, an Illustrated History of a Colonial Town (Bordentown, N.J.: Bordentown Register, 1932); CB to Bernard Vassall, January 24, 1852, CB-LC; CBJ, March 31, 1852, CB-LC; and CB-Halsted interview, July 29, 1890, CB-LC.

53. CBJ, May 25, 1852, CB-LC.

54. "Report of the State Superintendent of Public Schools of New Jersey for the Year 1852," copy in LC; and Roscoe L. West, Elementary Education in New Jersey: A History (Princeton: D. Van Nostrand Co., 1964), pp. 30–42.

55. CB, MS sequel to Childhood, October 12, 1908; and CB-Halsted interview, July 29, 1890, both CB-LC.

56. Ibid.; and "Report of State Superintendent 1852."

57. CB, MS sequel to Childhood, October 12, 1908, CB-LC.

58. Ibid.

59. CB to Bernard Vassall, June 17, 1852, CB-LC.

60. Peter Suydam quoted in ibid.; and CB, MS sequel to Childhood, October 12, 1908, CB-LC.

61. Teaching contract of CB quoted in Edith Blitz, "Clara Barton Made Pupils Out of Hoodlums," April 16, 1970, copy in Bordentown Public Library, Bordentown, N.J.; and CB, MS sequel to Childhood, October 12, 1908, CB-LC.

62. CB, MS sequel to Childhood, October 12, 1908; and CB, quoted in CB-Halsted interview, July 29, 1890, both CB-LC.

63. CB, MS sequel to Childhood, October 12, 1908, CB-LC.

64. CB to Mary Norton, July 16, 1852, D-DU.

65. Ibid.

66. CB, MS sequel to Childhood, October 12, 1908, CB-LC.

67. Ibid.

68. George Ferguson to CB, March 11, 1878, CB-LC.

69. Fanny Childs Vassall, "To the Friends at Bordentown," n.d. [1924], AAS.

70. CB, MS sequel to Childhood, October 12, 1908; and CB-Halsted interview, July 29, 1890, both CB-LC.

71. CB to Vassall, June 17, 1852; Stephen Barton to CB, February 24, 1854, CB-LC.

72. Statement of Fanny Childs Vassall in William E. Barton, The Life of Clara Barton (Boston: Houghton Mifflin Co., 1922), 1:66; CB to Vassall, June 17, 1852, CB-LC; and Seventh Decennial Census, Mercer County.

73. CB to Vassall, n.d. ("Schoolroom, Wednesday Morning"), CB-LC.

74. "Report of State Superintendent 1852," pp. 39–40.

75. "Report of the State Superintendent of Public Schools of New Jersey for the Year 1853," p. 31, copy in LC.

76. Ibid.; and CB, MS sequel to *Childhood*, October 12, 1908, CB-LC.

77. George Ferguson quoted in Epler, *Life*, p. 21; and CB, poem written to Bernard Vassall, n.d. [March 1853], CB-LC.

78. CB, MS sequel to *Childhood*, October 12, 1908, CB-LC; and "Report of State Superintendent 1853," p. 31, copy in LC.

79. West, *Elementary Education*, p. 28; Stephen Barton to CB, December 12, 1853, CB-LC; and CB, MS sequel to *Childhood*, October 12, 1908, CB-LC.

80. Woodward and Hageman, *History of Burlington and Mercer Counties*, p. 486; and CB to Frank Clinton, April 19, 1854, AAS.

81. "Report of State Superintendent 1853," p. 31; and Stephen Barton to CB, March 19, 1854, CB-LC.

82. E[llen] H. Bartine to CB, March 11, 1878, CB-LC.

83. George Ferguson to CB, March 11, 1878, CB-LC.

84. Undated newspaper clipping [1854], *Bordentown Register*, CB-LC.

85. CB, MS sequel to *Childhood*, October 12, 1908; and CB-Halsted interview, July 29, 1890, both CB-LC.

86. Undated clipping [1854], *Bordentown Register*, CB-LC.

87. Stephen Barton to CB, February 21, 1854, CB-LC.

88. Stephen Barton to CB, September 1, 1853, CB-LC; and Stephen Barton to CB, December 12, 18, and 25, 1853, CB-LC.

89. Stephen Barton to CB, February 2, 1854, CB-LC.

90. Stephen Barton to CB, February 21, 1854, CB-LC.

Chapter 5

1. Unpublished interview between CB and Leonora Halsted, July 29, 1890, CB-LC; and CB, "Scutari," undated lecture, typescript, AAS.

2. Margaret Leech, *Reveille in Washington* (New York: Harper Brothers, 1941), pp. 5–13; and Constance McLaughlin Green, *Washington, A History of the Capital, 1800–1950* (Princeton: Princeton University Press, 1962), pp. 178–230.

3. CB-Halsted interview, July 29, 1890; and CB to Kate Field, February 11, 1893, both CB-LC.

4. Stephen Barton to CB, May 3, 1854; and untitled clipping, *Bordentown Register*, n.d., both CB-LC.

5. CB to Julia Barton, March 3, 1857, in William E. Barton, *The Life of Clara Barton* (Boston: Houghton Mifflin Co., 1922), 1:95.

6. Charles Mason Remey, "Life and Letters of Judge Charles Mason," unpublished MS, 1932, copy in Remey Papers, LC.

7. Statement of Mary Mason Remey in ibid.

8. CB-Halsted interview, July 29, 1890, CB-LC.

9. CB to Frank Clinton, July 17, 1854, typescript, AAS.

10. Ibid.; also Leila Sellers, "Commissioner Charles Mason and Clara Barton," *Journal of the Patent Office Society* 22, no. 11 (November 1940): 803–6; Remey, "Life of Charles Mason," p. 278, Remey Papers, LC; and *Phelps' Washington Described* (Washington, D.C., 1857).

11. Sellers, "Charles Mason and Clara Barton," pp. 804–8.

12. CB-Halsted interview, July 29, 1890, CB-LC; CB to Clinton, July 17, 1854, AAS; S. T. Shugert to Robert McClelland, July 9, 1855, in Records of the Secretary of the Interior, Record Group 48, NARS; and *Register of Officers and Agents, Civil, Military, and Naval, in the Service of the United States* (Washington D.C.: ADP Nicholson and Son, 1855).

13. CB to Clinton, July 17, 1854; quotation CB to Frank Clinton, October 4, 1854, typescript, both AAS.

14. CB to Clinton, October 4, 1854, AAS.

15. Stephen Barton to CB, March 4, 1855, CB-LC.

16. L. P. Brockett, *Women's Work in the Civil War: A Record of Heroism, Patriotism, and Patience* (Philadelphia: Zeigler, McCurdy and Co., 1967), pp. 179–83.

17. CMJ, May and June, 1855, Remey Papers, LC.

18. Shugert to McClelland, July 9, 1855, RG 48, NARS.

19. Sellers, "Charles Mason and Clara Barton," p. 820.

20. S. T. Shugert to Robert McClelland, August 30, 1855, Miscellaneous Letters File, Interior Department Records, Record Group 48, NARS.

21. CMJ, October 14, 1855, Remey Papers, LC.

22. Stephen Barton to CB, September 28, 1855, CB-LC.

23. Alexander DeWitt to Robert McClelland, September 22, 1855, Miscellaneous Letters File, Interior Department Records, Record Group 48, NARS.

24. Robert McClelland to Alexander DeWitt, September 27, 1855, Outgoing Correspondence of the Secretary of Interior, Record Group 48, NARS.

25. For further information about the early employment of women in the government, see Cindy S. Arar, "'To Barter Their Souls for Gold': Female Clerks in Federal Government Offices, 1862–1890," *Journal of American History* 67, no. 4 (March 1981): 835–53.

26. Sellers, "Charles Mason and Clara Barton," pp. 819–21.

27. CB-Halsted interview, July 29, 1890, CB-LC.

28. CMJ, November 3, 1855, Remey Papers, LC.

29. Ibid., December 6, 1856; CB-Halsted interview, July 29, 1890, CB-LC; and Sellers, "Charles Mason and Clara Barton," p. 821.

30. William C. Langdon to William Woodward, April 4, 1855, William C. Langdon Papers, LC.

31. CB-Halsted interview, July 29, 1890, CB-LC.

32. Barton evidently told this story to numerous people. For one account, see Cora Bacon Foster, *Clara Barton, Humanitarian* (Washington, D.C.: Columbia Historical Society, 1918), pp. 7–8.

33. CB-Halsted interview, July 29, 1890, CB-LC.

34. CB to ?, letter fragment, c. 1856, AAS.

35. CB to Julia Barton, September 6, 1857, CB-LC.

36. Unsigned affidavit of accusations against Clara Barton, n.d.; and statements of Dr. Mary Walker, n.d. [1903], both RARC NARS.

37. CB to Julia Barton, September 6, 1857, CB-LC.

38. CB to Bernard Vassall, May 7 or 8, 1857, CB-LC; and CB to Stephen Barton, Sr., July 12, 1857, typescript, AAS.

39. CB to Julia Barton, September 6, 1857, CB-LC.

40. Stephen Barton to CB, April 25, 1855, CB-LC.

41. CB to Stephen Barton, Sr., June 26, 1857, typescript, AAS.

42. CB to Julia Barton, March 3, 1857, in W. E. Barton, *Life* 1:94.

43. CB to Bernard Vassall, April 13, 1857; Jesse Jarrett to Alfred Bronn, February 9 and September 10, 1856; and Stephen Barton to CB, February 25, 1855, all CB-LC.

44. Irving Vassall to Bernard Vassall, May 30, 1857, CB-LC.

45. CB to Bernard Vassall, May 10, 1857, CB-LC.

46. Irving Vassall to Stephen Barton, Sr., February 3, 1857, CB-LC.

47. CB quoted in Percy Epler, *The Life of Clara Barton* (New York: Macmillan, 1915), p. 27.

48. CB to Julia Barton, March 3, 1857, in W. E. Barton, *Life* 1:94–95.

49. CB to Julia Barton, November 2, 1856, in W. E. Barton, *Life* 1:99.

50. CMJ, June 27, 1857, Remey Papers, LC.

51. CB to Bernard Vassall, May 10, 1857, CB-LC.

52. CB to Bernard Vassall, June 16, 1857, typescript, AAS.

53. CB to Stephen Barton, Sr., July 12, 1857, typescript, AAS; and CB to Stephen Barton, Sr., June 26, 1857, typescript, CB-LC.

54. CB to Stephen Barton, June 26, 1857, CB-LC; and CB to Julia Barton, September 6, 1857, in W. E. Barton, *Life* 1:96–98.

55. Sellers, "Charles Mason and Clara Barton," pp. 824–25.

56. CB to Julia Barton, September 6, 1857, in W. E. Barton, *Life* 1:96–98.

57. CB-Halsted interview, July 29, 1890; and CB to Elvira Stone, October 23, 1857, both CB-LC.

58. CB to Stone, October 23, 1857; and CB to Bernard Vassall, December 14, 1857, both CB-LC.

59. Stephen Barton to David Barton, December 23, 1857, CB-LC; and Thomas E. Parramore, "The Bartons of Bartonsville," *The North Carolina Historical Review* 51, no. 1 (January 1974): 23–26.

60. CBJ, February 5, 1859, CB-LC; and CB to Mary Norton, March 8, 1859, D-DU.

61. Ibid.

62. CB to Norton, March 8, 1859, D-DU; and CBJ, January–February 1859, CB-LC.

63. See letters of Irving Vassall to CB and Bernard Vassall, 1857–62, CB-LC; and CBJ, 1859, CB-LC. Quotation CB to Norton, March 8, 1859, D-DU.

64. CB to Elvira Stone, March 11, 1859, CB-LC.

65. CBJ, February 1, 3, 1859, CB-LC.

66. CB to Stone, March 11, 1859, CB-LC.

67. See CBJ, June 23, July 7 and 14, 1859, CB-LC; quotation CBJ, August 14, 1859, CB-LC.

68. CBJ, February 2, March 2, April–May, 1859, CB-LC; and CB to Mary Norton, April 3, 1859, D-DU.

69. CBJ, June 15, 1859, CB-LC; CB to Bernard Vassall, January 17, 1860, CB-LC; and CB to Frank Clinton, January 2, 1860, typescript, AAS.

70. CBJ, January–August and February 24, 1859; CB to Elvira Stone, December 10, 1858; and CB to Bernard Vassall, February 3, 1860, all CB-LC.

71. CBJ, July 30, 1859; quotation CB to Irving Vassall, August 21, 1859, both CB-LC.

72. CB to Bernard Vassall, August 4, 1859, CB-LC.

73. Ibid.

74. CBJ, September 12–18 and 26, 1859, CB-LC.

75. "Reminiscences of Miss Marion C. Sloan," unpublished MS, n.d., Marion Louisa Sloan Papers, MHS.

76. Untitled newspaper clipping, n.d., CB-LC, II, 57; "Personal Recollections of Clara Barton," *Housekeepers Weekly*, April 10, 1892, CB-LC; and CBJ, miscellaneous travel notes in back of diary, 1859, and December 11, 1859, CB-LC.

77. CB to Bernard Vassall, August 21, 1859, CB-LC.

78. CB to Bernard Vassall, January 17, 1860, CB-LC.

79. Ibid.

80. CB to Bernard Vassall, February 21, 1860, CB-LC.

81. CB to Bernard Vassall, January 17, February 7 and 10, 1860, CB-LC.

82. CB to Bernard Vassall, January 26, 1860, CB-LC.

83. CB to Bernard Vassall, January 26, 1860, CB-LC.

84. Ibid.

85. CB to Bernard Vassall, February 3 and 13, March 7, and April 4, 1860; quotation CB to Bernard Vassall, March 6, 1860, all CB-LC.

86. CB to Bernard Vassall, February 13, 1860, CB-LC.

87. Ibid.

88. CB to Bernard Vassall, April 4, 1860, CB-LC.

89. Ibid.

90. CB to Bernard Vassall, April 9, 1860, CB-LC.

91. CB to Bernard Vassall, February 7, 1860, CB-LC; and deed between Clara Barton and Stephen Barton, May 24, 1860, Worcester County Deed Book, Liber 626, p. 401, Worcester County Courthouse, Worcester, Mass.

92. CB to Bernard Vassall, April 22, 1860, CB-LC.

93. CB to Elvira Stone, June 14, 1860; quotation CB to Bernard Vassall, June 17, 1860, both CB-LC.

94. Barton's copy of O. S. Fowler and L. N. Fowler's *New Illustrated Self-Instructor in Phrenology and Physiology*, with L. N. Fowler's notes, is in CB-LC.

95. CB to Bernard Vassall, June 17, 1860, CB-LC.

96. Ibid.

97. Ibid.

98. CB to Bernard Vassall, July 28, 1860, CB-LC.

Chapter 6

1. CB to Bernard Vassall, August 9, 1860, CB-LC.

2. CB to Elvira Stone, February 7, 1861; and "Clara Barton First Woman Given U.S. Job," *Rochester Democrat and Chronicle* (N.Y.), May 16, 1940, both CB-LC.

3. Leila Sellers, "Commissioner Charles Mason and Clara Barton," *Journal of the Patent Office Society* 22, no. 11 (November 1940): 825.

4. *Register of Officers and Agents, Civil, Military, and Naval, in the Service of the United States* (Washington, D.C.: ADP Nicholson and Son, 1861), p. 87; and *Phelps' Washington Described* (Washington, D.C., 1857), p. 104.

5. Henry Adams, *The Education of Henry Adams* (Boston: Houghton Mifflin Co., 1961), p. 99.

6. Margaret Leech, *Reveille in Washington* (New York: Harper Brothers, 1941), pp. 33–45.

7. CB to Elvira Stone, January 21, 1861, CB-LC.

8. Robert E. Lee to Custis Lee, December 14, 1860, quoted in Douglas Southall Freeman, *R. E. Lee* (New York: Charles Scribner's Sons, 1934), 1:416.

9. CB to "My dear Cousin," April 14, 1861, AAS.

10. CB to Annie Childs, March 5, 1861, in William E. Barton, *The Life of Clara Barton* (Houghton Mifflin Co., 1922), 1:104–6; and Leech, *Reveille*, p. 43.

11. CB to Stone, February 7, 1861, CB-LC.

12. Ibid.

13. CB to Elvira Stone, March 29, 1861, CB-LC.

14. CB to Elvira Stone, April 7, 1861, CB-LC.

15. Senator George Hoar quoted in Allen Johnson and Dumas Malone, *DAB*, s.v. "Wilson, Henry."

16. Royston Betts, "An Exposition of D. P. Holloway's Management of the Affairs of the Patent Office," January 1863, copy in LC.

17. CB to Stone, March 29, 1861, CB-LC.

18. CB to Elvira Stone, February 20, 1861, CB-LC.

19. CB to Stone, April 7, 1861, CB-LC.

20. Quotation in L. P. Brockett, *Women's Work in the Civil War; A Record of Heroism, Patriotism, and Patience* (Philadelphia: Zeigler, McCurdy and Co., 1967), p. 113.

21. CB to Elvira Stone, February 2, 1861, CB-LC.

22. Ibid.; and CB to Stone, February 7, 1861, CB-LC.

23. For theater parties, see CB to Stone, January 21 and February 15, 1861, CB-LC. R. O. Sidney's attentions are discussed in CB to Stone, April 7 and May 15, 1861, CB-LC.

24. Unidentified acquaintance quoted in Brockett, *Women's Work*, pp. 114–15.

25. For more detail on the incidents in Baltimore, see Charles B. Clark, "Baltimore and the Attack on the Sixth Massachusetts Regiment, April 19, 1861," *Maryland Historical Magazine* 56, no. 1 (March 1961): 39–71; Mathew Page Andrews, "Passage of the Sixth Massachusetts Regiment Through Baltimore, April 19, 1861," *Maryland Historical Magazine* 14, no. 1 (March 1919): 60–75; and Leech, *Reveille*, pp. 63–65.

26. Ibid.

27. CB, "Work and Incidents of Army Life," MS lecture on the Civil War, n.d. [c. 1866], CB-LC.

28. Interview with CB in the *National Repository* 5, no. 2 (February 1879): 159.

29. "Clara Barton and the International Red Cross Association," unpublished article, n.d. [c. 1890], typescript with notations in CB's hand; and CB to B. W. Childs, April 25, 1861, both CB-LC.

30. CB to Childs, April 25, 1861, CB-LC.

31. CB quoted in W. E.. Barton, *Life* 1:102.

32. Draft of letter from CB to J. W. Denny, n.d. [spring 1862], CB-LC.

33. Statement of CB, c. 1886, in Percy Epler, *The Life of Clara Barton* (New York: Macmillan, 1915), p. 32.

34. CB to "My Darling Cousin," December 24, 1861, CB-LC.

35. "Reminiscences of Mary Josephine Mason," vol. 8, 8, 157, Remey Papers, LC; and CB to Stephen Barton, May 19, 1861, CB-LC.

36. CB to Bernard Vassall, May 29, 1861; quotation CB to Mrs. Miller, December 16, 1861, both CB-LC.

37. "The Story of the Lifelong Friendship of Clara Barton and Elvira Stone," *Worcester Telegram*, December 22, 1935.

38. Fanny Childs Vassall quoted in W. E. Barton, *Life*, 1:121–22.

39. CB to Stephen Barton, May 19, 1861, CB-LC.

40. CB to Elvira Stone, December 26, 1861, CB-LC.

41. CB to Stephen Barton (draft), July 22, 1861, CB-LC.

42. CB, "Work and Incidents," n.d. [c. 1866], CB-LC.

43. CB to Miller, December 16, 1861, CB-LC.

44. "To the Ladies and Friends of the Soldiers," *Worcester Daily Spy*, September 17, 1861.

45. CB to Miller, December 16, 1861, CB-LC.

46. CB to Mary Norton, September 26, 1862, D-DU.

47. Brockett, *Women's Work*, p. 115; and "Barton and the Red Cross," n.d. [c. 1890], typescript, CB-LC.

48. CB to Elvira Stone, quoted in Ishbel Ross, *Angel of the Battlefield: The Life of Clara Barton* (New York: Harper and Row, 1956), p. 30.

49. Brockett, *Women's Work*, pp. 279–83 (quotation on p. 281); and diary of Mary Josephine Mason, March 27, 1863, typescript, Remey Papers, LC.

50. Brockett, *Women's Work*, p. 280.

51. CB to General Q. A. Gillmore, September 18, 1863, Records of the U.S. Army Command, Record Group 393, NARS.

52. "Clara Barton," *National Repository*, undated newspaper clipping, CB-LC.

53. Maria H. Grafton to CB, September 8, 1902, CB-LC.

54. "Clara Barton First Woman," *Rochester Democrat and Chronicle*, May 16, 1940, CB-LC; Betts, "Exposition"; and CB to Fanny Childs, January 7, 1862, CB-LC.

55. Betts, "Exposition"; and CB to Fanny Childs, January 7, 1862, CB-LC.

56. CB to Denny (draft), n.d. [spring 1862]; and CB to John A. Andrew, March 20, 1862, both CB-LC.

57. CB to Sarah Vassall, December 29, 1860; "oak and iron" quotation in CB to Andrew, March 20, 1862, both CB-LC.

58. Samuel Barton to CB, June 18, 1862 [1861], CB-LC.

59. CB to Andrew, March 20, 1862, CB-LC.

60. Death notice of Captain Stephen Barton, *Christian Freeman*, April 18, 1862.

61. CB to Gillmore, September 18, 1863, RG 393, NARS.

62. CB to Leander Poor, March 27, 1862, CB-LC.

63. *Worcester Evening Transcript*, April 14, 1862; CBJ, March 25, 1862, CB-LC.

64. CB to Gillmore, September 18, 1863, RG 393, NARS.

65. CB to Denny (draft), n.d. [spring 1862], CB-LC.

66. See Ann Douglas Wood, "The War Within a War: Women Nurses in the Union Army," *Civil War History* 18, no. 3 (1972): 197–212; and Agatha Young, *The Women and the Crisis; Women of the North in the Civil War* (New York: McDowell, Obolensky, 1959), p. 60.

67. CB to Andrew, March 20, 1862, CB-LC.

68. John A. Andrew to CB, March 24, 1862, CB-LC.

69. See letters of CB to Leander Poor and Irving Vassall, April–May, 1862, CB-LC.

70. Irving Vassall to CB, April 13, 1862, CB-LC.

71. CB to Leander Poor, May 2, 1862, CB-LC.

72. CB to Fanny Childs, January 7, 1862, CB-LC.

73. CB to Denny (draft), n.d. [spring 1862], CB-LC.

74. CB to Poor, May 2, 1862, CB-LC.

75. CB to Elvira Stone, June 9, 1861; and CB to Childs, January 7, 1862, both CB-LC.

Chapter 7

1. "Clara Barton and the International Red Cross Association," unpublished article, n.d. [c. 1890], typescript with notations in CB's hand, CB-LC.

2. See Mathew Brady's portrait of CB taken a few years later, in photographic collection of NARS.

3. "Barton and the Red Cross," n.d. [c. 1890], typescript, CB-LC.

4. Ibid.; and orders of William Hammond, D. H. Rucker, R. C. Wood, and James S. Wadsworth, July 11, 1862, in Correspondence of the Surgeon General, Record Group 112, NARS (quotation in orders of D. H. Rucker).

5. CBJ, July 18–23, 1862; and CB to Leander Poor, August 2, 1862, both CB-LC.

6. CBJ, August 1–5, 1862, CB-LC.

7. CB, "Work and Incidents of Army Life," MS lecture on the Civil War, n.d. [c. 1866], CB-LC.

8. CB to Julia Barton, June 26, 1862, AAS; and CB quoted in William E. Barton, *The Life of Clara Barton* (Boston: Houghton Mifflin Co., 1922), 1:129.

9. CB to Poor, August 2, 1862, CB-LC.

10. CBJ, August 11–13, 1862; CB to "My own darling Cousin," August 12, 1862; "A Missionary Fallen," undated newspaper clipping in CB scrapbook; and "Cornelius M. Welles," undated clipping in CB scrapbook, all CB-LC.

11. CB to the Ladies of the Soldiers Relief Society of Hightstown, August 19, 1862, printed in *Bordentown Register*, September 12, 1862; and CBJ, August 14, 1862, both CB-LC.

12. James Dunn to wife, quoted in undated newspaper clipping, CB-LC.

13. CB to Ladies of Hightstown, in *Bordentown Register*, September 12, 1862, CB-LC.

14. "Massachusetts Women at Cedar Mountain," undated clipping in CB scrapbook; and CB to Ladies of Hightstown, in *Bordentown Register*, September 12, 1862, both CB-LC.

15. CB, "Work and Incidents," MS lecture, n.d. [c. 1866], CB-LC.

16. CB to "My Dear Old Time Friend," August 14, 1862, printed in undated newspaper clipping, CB scrapbook, CB-LC.

17. Ibid.

18. "Massachusetts Women," n.d., clipping in CB scrapbook, CB-LC.

19. CB, "Work and Incidents," MS lecture, n.d. [c. 1866]; and CBJ, August 15, 1862, both CB-LC.

20. CB to "My Dear Old Time Friend," printed in undated newspaper clipping., CB scrapbook, CB-LC. CB claimed she wrote this literary letter on August 14, 1862, at the time that she also claimed she was working consistently without time for sleep or food.

21. Ibid.

22. CB to Julia Barton, n.d. [c. August 1862], AAS; CB to Ladies of Hightstown, in *Bordentown Register*, September 12, 1862, CB-LC.

23. CB to D. P. Holloway, December 11, 1863, copy in CBJ, 1863, CB-LC.

24. Jane Pardee to "sister," March 7, 1859, in Gertrude K. Johnston, ed., *Dear Pa, And So It Goes* (Harrisburg: Business Service Co., 1971), p. 111.

25. CBJ, August 30, 1862, CB-LC.

26. Statement of Fanny Childs Vassall, in W. E. Barton, *Life* 1:221; and Ross, *Angel*, p. 35.

27. CB to "Dear Brother and Sister," August 31, 1862; and CB to Elvira Stone, August 31, 1862, both CB-LC.

28. CB, "Work and Incidents," MS lecture, n.d. [c. 1866], CB-LC.

29. Louis C. Duncan, *The Medical Department of the United States Army in the Civil War* (Washington, D.C.: Department of Defense, n.d.), p. 34.

30. CB, "Work and Incidents," MS lecture, n.d. [c. 1866], CB-LC.

31. Alonzo Quint of the Second Massachusetts, quoted in Duncan, *Medical Department*, p. 34.

32. CB, "Work and Incidents," MS lecture, n.d. [c. 1866], CB-LC.

33. Ibid.

34. Ibid.

35. CB to Stone, August 31, 1862; and CB, "Work and Incidents," MS lecture, n.d. [c. 1866], CB-LC.

36. Dunn to wife, undated clipping, CB-LC.

37. Duncan, *Medical Department*, pp. 34–46; Horace H. Cunningham, *Field Medical Services at the Battle of Manassas* (Athens, Ga.: University of Georgia Press, 1968), pp. 49–76; and "Medicine and the Civil War," catalogue of exhibit at National Library of Medicine, Bethesda, Md., 1973.

38. See CBJ, 1862, CB-LC; CB, untitled MS war lecture, [c.. 1868], CB-LC; also CB to Mary Norton, September 4, 1862, D-DU.

39. CB to "dear friends," September 4, 1862, typescript, CB-LC.

40. CB, "Work and Incidents", MS lecture, n.d. [c. 1866], CB-LC.

41. CB to Norton, September 4, 1862, D-DU.

42. CB, "Work and Incidents," MS lecture, n.d. [c. 1866], CB-LC.

43. CB to "dear friends," September 7, 1862, CB-LC.

44. CB to Norton, September 4, 1862, D-DU.

45. Emmeline Machen to Arthur Machen, September 2, 1861 [1862], Machen Papers, LC.

46. CB, "Work and Incidents," MS lecture, n.d. [c. 1866], CB-LC.

47. Ibid.; and CB to "dear friends," September 4, 1862, CB-LC.

48. CB to Norton, September 4, 1862, D-DU.

49. Jane Pardee to "sister," March 7, 1859, in Johnston, ed., *Dear Pa*, p. 111.

50. CB quoted in W. E. Barton, *Life* 1:129.

51. Leander Poor to Elvira Stone, September 3, 1862, CB-LC.

52. "Barton and the Red Cross," n.d. [c. 1890], typescript, CB-LC.

53. CB, "The Women Who Went to the Field," 1891, typescript, CB-LC.

54. CB to "dear friends," September 4, 1862, CB-LC.

55. "Barton and the Red Cross," n.d. [c. 1890], typescript, CB-LC.

56. CB to Ladies of the Soldiers' Friend Society of Hightstown, N.J., February 14, 1863, newspaper clipping in CB scrapbook, CB-LC.

57. CB, "Work and Incidents," MS lecture, n.d. [c. 1866], CB-LC.

58. Ibid.

59. "Barton and the Red Cross," n.d. [c. 1890], typescript, CB-LC.

60. Ibid.; and CB, "Work and Incidents," MS lecture, n.d. [c. 1866], CB-LC.

61. CB, "Work and Incidents," MS lecture, n.d. [c. 1866], CB-LC; and John M. Sanderson, "A Report on the Activities of Clara Barton at the Battle of Antietam," September 17, 1862, unpublished MS for the National Park Service, 1973, copy in CBNHS.

62. Duncan, *Medical Department*, p. 13; CB, "Work and Incidents," MS lecture, n.d.

[c. 1866], CB-LC; and "Barton and the Red Cross," n.d. [c. 1890], typescript, CB-LC.

63. C. M. Welles to Bretheren [sic], September 22, 1862, in "Missionary Labors on the Battlefield," undated clipping in CB scrapbook, CB-LC.

64. Oliver Wendell Holmes, "My Hunt After the Captain," *Atlantic Monthly* 10, no. 12 (December 1862): 743–44.

65. Quotation CB, "Work and Incidents," MS lecture, n.d. [c. 1866], CB-LC; also F. H. Harwood, "An Army Surgeon's Story," *St. Louis Illustrated Magazine* 24, no. 150 (April 1883): 137–50.

66. Harwood, "Army Surgeon's Story," p. 136.

67. CB, "Work and Incidents," MS lecture, n.d. [c. 1866], CB-LC; Dunn to wife, undated clipping, CB-LC; and "Clara Barton's Light," *Pittsburgh Christian Union*, July 4, 1896.

68. "Evolution of the Field Hospital," in Duncan, *Medical Department*, pp. 8–13; William Hammond to Edmund Stanton, September 7, 1862, in Duncan, *Medical Department*, p. 13; and Margaret Leech, *Reveille in Washington* (New York: Harper Brothers, 1941), pp. 216–17.

69. For Sanitary Commission information, see Katharine Prescott Wormely, *The United States Sanitary Commission* (New York: Little Brown and Co., 1863); William Q. Maxwell, *Lincoln's Fifth Wheel* (New York: Longmans, Green, and Co., 1956); and Leech, *Reveille*, p. 217.

70. *United States Christian Commission: First Annual Report* (Philadelphia, 1863), p. 50.

71. Leech, *Reveille*, pp. 209–11; and R. H. Bremer, "Philanthropic Rivalries in the Civil War," *Social Casework* 49, no. 1 (January 1968): 60.

72. L. P. Brockett, *Women's Work in the Civil War: A Record of Heroism, Patriotism, and Patience* (Philadelphia: Zeigler, McCurdy and Co., 1967), p. 176.

73. CB, "Women Who Went to the Field," 1891, typescript, CB-LC.

74. CB quoted in W. E. Barton, *Life* 1:280.

75. Dr. Henry Bellows to the Ladies of Worcester, in the *Worcester Daily Spy*, August 15, 1861.

76. CBJ, quoted in Blanche Colton Williams, *Clara Barton: Daughter of Destiny* (Philadelphia: J. B. Lippincott Co., 1941), p. 168.

77. CB, "Wilderness," MS lecture, n.d. [c. 1866–68], CB-LC.

78. Walt Whitman quoted in Justin Kaplan, *Walt Whitman: A Life* (New York: Simon and Schuster, 1980), p. 280.

79. CB quoted in W. E. Barton, *Life* 1:287.

80. CBJ, December 7, 1863, and August 6, 1864, CB-LC.

81. Ibid., August 6, 1864.

82. Welles to Bretheren [sic], September 22, 1862, in "Missionary Labors," undated clipping in CB scrapbook, CB-LC.

83. "Barton and the Red Cross," n.d. [c. 1890], typescript, CB-LC.

84. Ibid.; and Leander Poor to Samuel Rich Barton, August 23, 1863, HL.

85. Asst. Adj. General John P. Sherburne to CB, October 25, 1862, CB-LC.

86. CB to ?, December 3, 1862, quoted in Percy Epler, *The Life of Clara Barton* (New York: Macmillan, 1915), p. 65.

87. James Madison Stone, *Personal Recollections of the Civil War* (Boston: privately printed, 1918), p. 96.

88. CBJ, n.d., quoted in Epler, *Life*, p. 64.

89. Bruce Catton, *Glory Road* (New York: Doubleday and Co., 1952), p. 16.

90. CB, "Address to the German Soldiers and Brothers in Arms at Milwaukee, Wisconsin," n.d., CB-LC.

91. CB to Thaddeus Meighan, June 24, 1863, CB-LC.

92. CB to General Q. A. Gillmore, September 18, 1863, Records of the U.S. Army Command, Record Group 393, NARS.

93. CBJ quoted in Epler, *Life*, p. 64.

94. CB, "Work and Incidents," MS lecture, n.d. [c. 1866], CB-LC.

95. "Barton and the Red Cross," n.d. [c. 1890], typescript, CB-LC.

96. CB, untitled lecture, c. 1867, CB-LC; for further information on the self-satisfaction of women relief workers, see Ann Douglas Wood, "The War Within a War: Women Nurses in the Union Army," *Civil War History* 18, no. 3 (1972): 197–212.

97. CB to ?, December 3, 1862, in Epler, *Life*, p. 65.

98. Samuel Barton to "My dear Cousin," December 3, 1862, CB-LC.

99. Ibid.; C. M. Welles to Bretheren [sic], December 14, 1862, printed in "Letters from Bro. Welles," clipping in CB scrapbook, CB-LC; and Catton, *Glory Road*, p. 31.

100. Draft of letter from CB to Mr. Z. Brown & Co., December 8, 1862, CB-LC.

101. CB to Elvira Stone, December 12, 1862, CB-LC.

102. CB, untitled lecture, c. 1867, CB-LC.

103. Walt Whitman, *The Wound Dresser* (New York: Bodley Press, 1949), p. 37.

104. C. M. Welles to Bretheren [sic], December 27, 1862, printed in "Letters from Bro. Welles," clipping in CB scrapbook, CB-LC.

105. Hart Bodine to CB, January 11, 1863; and CB, untitled lecture, c. 1867, CB-LC.

106. Bruce Catton, *Never Call Retreat* (New York: Doubleday and Co., 1965), pp. 23–24; and "Barton and the Red Cross," n.d. [c. 1890], typescript, CB-LC.

107. Colonel Shotwell quoted in Douglas Southall Freeman, *R. E. Lee* (New York: Charles Scribner's Sons, 1934), 2:470–71.

108. Whitman, *Wound Dresser*, p. 46.

109. Dr. Watson quoted in "Change Wrought in an Old Virginia Mansion,—the Ravages of War," clipping in CB-LC.

110. CB, untitled lecture, c. 1867, CB-LC; and CB to Margaret Hamilton, n.d. [c. 1903], quoted in Epler, *Life*, p. 74.

111. CB to Annie Childs, May 28, 1863, CB-LC.

Chapter 8

1. CB to Mary Norton, January 19, 1863, Jack MS.

2. CB to Annie Childs, May 28, 1863, CB-LC.

3. CB to Norton, January 19, 1863, Jack MS.

4. CB to Mary Norton, February 12, 1863, Jack MS.

5. "Clara Barton and the International Red Cross Association," unpublished article, n.d. [c. 1890], typescript with notations in CB's hand, CB-LC.

6. CB to Mary Norton, December 12, 1863, D-DU.

7. CB, untitled lecture, c. 1867, CB-LC.

8. Ibid.

9. CB to Henry Wilson, February 22, 1863; and draft of letter from CB to Henry Wilson, January 12, 1863, both CB-LC.

10. Quotation CB to Henry Wilson, January 27, 1863, CB-LC; and CB to David Barton, February 6, 1863, CB-LC; also CB to "Cousin," February 20, 1863, AAS.

11. Stephen Emory Barton quoted in Percy Epler, *The Life of Clara Barton* (New York: Macmillan, 1915), p. 86.

12. CBJ, April 1–7, 1863 (quotation April 7), CB-LC.

13. For further information about the Sea Islands experiments, see Willie Lee Rose, *Rehearsal for Reconstruction* (New York: Vintage Books, 1967).

14. CBJ, April 11, 1863, CB-LC.

15. CB to Elvira Stone, July 24, 1863, CB-LC.

16. CB to Mary Norton, June 26, 1863, Jack MS.

17. CBJ, April 17–18, May 19, June 19, 1863, CB-LC.

18. CB to Annie Childs, May 19, 1863, AAS.

19. CB to Mary Norton, April 16, 1863, Jack MS.

20. Ibid.

21. CBJ, April 13 and 23, 1863, CB-LC.

22. Ibid., April 13 and 18, and May 10, 1863.

23. CB to Mary Norton, July 3, 1863, Jack MS.

24. CBJ, May 11, 1863, CB-LC.

25. Charles Nordruff, "Two Weeks at Port Royal," *Harper's New Monthly Magazine* 27, no. 157 (June 1863), p. 113.

26. John J. Elwell to CB, June 23, 1876, CB-LC.

27. CBJ, April 30, 1863, CB-LC.

28. Ibid., May 17 and 22, 1863; CB to Stephen E. Barton, June 19, 1863, CB-LC; and Ishbel Ross, *Angel of the Battlefield: The Life of Clara Barton* (New York: Harper and Row, 1956), p. 64.

29. John Elwell to CB, May 9, 1863, and October 27, 1863, both SSC. Several dozen other notes from him are in this collection.

30. Elwell quoted Barton several times with this phrase. See Ross, *Angel*, p. 134; and John J. Elwell to CB, May 24, 1884, CB-LC.

31. CB to Dr. Edward Foote, draft answers to "Questions to Invalids," n.d., SSC.

32. Elwell quoted in Ellen Henle, "Against the Fearful Odds," draft Ph.D. thesis, Case Western Reserve University, 1976, pp. 28–29.

33. "Birdie" to John Elwell, n.d. [May 1863], E-WRHS.

34. Elwell to CB, May 9, 1863, SSC.

35. Ibid.

36. "Birdie" to Elwell, n.d. [May 1863], E-WRHS.

37. John Elwell to CB, May 19, 1863, SSC.

38. An excellent summary of this battle is in Bruce Catton, *Never Call Retreat* (New York: Doubleday and Co., 1965), pp. 217–24.

39. Leander Poor to Elvira Stone, July 8, 1863, CB-LC; John Elwell to CB, August 23, 1898, CB-LC; and Ross, *Angel*, p. 61.

40. "The Fort Wagner Charge," *The Summit County Beacon* (Ohio) June 30, 1886, copy in CB-LC.

41. CB to Elvira Stone, July 11, 1863, CB-LC; and statement of John J. Elwell in William E. Barton, *The Life of Clara Barton* (Boston: Houghton Mifflin Co., 1922), 1:251–52.

42. "What Clara Barton Did for Humanity During the War," *New York Daily Graphic*, December 12, 1884; and "Letter from Mrs. Gage," July 28, 1863, newspaper clipping in CB scrapbook, both CB-LC.

43. CBJ quoted in Ross, *Angel*, p. 63.

44. Catton, *Never Call Retreat*, pp. 224–26.

45. CB to Lieutenant Ritchie, July 14, 1863; and CB, "Charleston," MS lecture, n.d. [c. 1866–68], both CB-LC.

46. Samuel T. Lamb to CB, August 13, 1863; ? to "my dear Colonel," September 7, 1863; and James F. Hall to CB, November 15, 1863, all CB-LC.

47. CB to Annie Childs, October 27, 1863, CB-LC.

48. Leander Poor to Elvira Stone, August 21, 1863, CB-LC.

49. General C. M. Smith to CB, September 14, 1863, Records of the U.S. Army Command, Record Group 393, NARS.

50. CB to General Q. Gillmore, September 18, 1863, Records of the U.S. Army Command, Record Group 393, NARS.

51. CB to "My dearest Colonel," September 7, 1863, CB-LC.

52. Ibid.; and Rose, *Rehearsal*, p. 66.

53. CBJ, December 5, 1863, CB-LC.

54. Edward T. James, ed., *Notable American Women, 1607–1950* (Cambridge: Belknap Press, 1971), 2:2–4.

55. CB, untitled MS sequel to *The Story of My Childhood*, October 12, 1908, CB-LC.

56. CBJ, May 4, 1863, CB-LC.

57. Frances D. Gage to CB, September 6, 1864, CB-LC.

58. CB to Mary Norton, November 15, 1863, Jack MS.

59. CBJ, April 15, 1863, CB-LC.

60. CB to Drs. Brown and Drier, March 13, 1864, CB-LC. See also CB to "My Most esteemed and dear friend," July 5, 1864, CB-LC.

61. CB to Frances D. Gage, May 11, 1864, in CBJ, 1864, CB-LC.

62. Poem from Frances D. Gage to CB, n.d. [1863], CB-LC.

63. Frances D. Gage, "Impromptu" to CB, May 28, 1863, CB-LC.

64. CBJ, December 5, 1863, CB-LC.

65. See "A Servant of God Called Home," *The American Baptist*, n.d.; and "Cornelius M. Welles," n.d., both CB scrapbook, CB-LC.

66. CB to Norton, November 15, 1863, Jack MS.

67. CBJ, December 10, 1863, CB-LC.

68. CB to D. P. Holloway, December 11, 1863, in CBJ, 1863, CB-LC.

69. CBJ, December 26, 1863, CB-LC.

70. Ibid., December 15 and 23, 1863.

71. "Mrs. Gage and My Heart," January 1864, typescript, AAS.

72. CBJ, February 14, 1864, CB-LC.

73. Ibid., March 17, 1864 (quotation April 6, 1864).

74. Ibid., March 3 and April 1, 1864.

75. Ibid., March 25 and April 8, 1864.

76. CB to Henry Wilson, April 7, 1864, copy in CBJ, April 7, 1864, CB-LC.

77. CBJ, April 8, 1864.

78. Ibid., April 19, 1864.

79. CB to Frances D. Gage, May 1, 1864, in CBJ, 1864, CB-LC.

80. Dr. Alfred Hitchcock to E. B. Hayward, and H. A. Goodrich to A. P. Kimball, May 25, 1864, quoted in "From the Battlefields," *Filchburg Sentinal*, May 27, 1864, copy in CB scrapbook, CB-LC.

81. CB, miscellaneous notes on Fredericksburg, n.d. [1864], CB-LC.

82. CB, "Wilderness," MS lecture, n.d. [c. 1866–68], CB-LC.

83. CB, miscellaneous notes on Fredericksburg.

84. CB, "Wilderness," MS lecture, n.d. [c. 1866–68], CB-LC.

85. Ibid.

86. CB, "To the Clergy and Soldier's Friends," May 16, 1864, copy in CB-LC.

87. Honora Connors to CB, February 15, 1897, CB-LC.

88. CB to Mr. Baldwin, May 30, 1864, in CBJ, 1864, CB-LC.

89. CB to Mrs. Allen, May 30, 1864; quotation CB to Baldwin, May 30, 1864, both CB-LC.

90. Henry Wilson to Benjamin F. Butler, June 20, 1864, in Jesse Ames Marshall, ed., *Private and Official Correspondence of General Benjamin F. Butler* (privately printed, 1917), p. 423.

91. CBJ, June 23, 1864, CB-LC.

92. For more on Butler, see Margaret Leech, *Reveille in Washington* (New York: Harper Brothers, 1941), pp. 433–34.

93. Official records for the Army of the James, Butler's personal and official correspondence, Records of the U.S. Army Command, papers of the secretary of war (all in NARS), and Miss Dix's correspondence have all been searched for any hint of such an appointment.

94. Register of the Sick and Wounded, July–December, 1864, Flying Hospital, Tenth Army Corps, Record Group 94, NARS; and CBJ, January 1, 1865, CB-LC.

95. John G. Perry to ?, June 27, 1864, in Martha Derby Perry, ed., *Letters from a Surgeon of the Civil War* (Boston: Little Brown and Co., 1906), p. 208.

96. CB to William Ferguson, July 1, 1864, printed in "A Graphic and Excellent Letter from Clara Barton," *New York Evening Express*, n.d., clipping in CB scrapbook, CB-LC.

97. Ibid.; and CB to Frances Childs Vassall, September 3, 1864, in W. E. Barton, *Life* 1:286–89.

98. CB to the Soldiers' Aid Society, July 20, 1864, in "Letter from Miss Clara Barton," *Worcester Daily Spy*, n.d., clipping in CB scrapbook, CB-LC.

99. CBJ, July 3, 1864, CB-LC.

100. Jane Stuart Woolsey, *Hospital Days* (New York: D. Van Nostrand, 1870), p. 41.

101. CBJ, August 3, 1864, CB-LC; and Adelaide Smith, *Reminiscences of an Army Nurse During the Civil War* (New York: Greaves Publishing Co., 1911), p. 80–83, 90.

102. Records of the Tenth Army Corps, RG 94, NARS; and CB to Elvira Stone, October 30, 1864, CB-LC.

103. CB to Elvira Stone, October 30, 1864, CB-LC.

104. CB to Eliza Golay, March 5, 1865, in Epler, *Life*, p. 102.

105. CB to Ferguson, July 1, 1864, in CB scrapbook, CB-LC.

106. Ibid.

107. Thomas E. Parramore, "The Bartons of Bartonsville," *The North Carolina Historical Review* 51, no. 1 (January 1974): 28–29, 36; and Samuel Rich Barton to Elizabeth Barton, October 9, 1864, HL.

108. Statement of Stephen E. Barton to Lt. Col. O. L. Mann, March 6, 1865; and Joel R. Griffin to CB, August 1865, both Samuel R. Barton Papers, DU.

109. Stephen Barton to Benjamin Butler, November 19, 1864, CB-LC.

110. Statement of Stephen Barton to Mann, March 6, 1865; and statement of Brackney T. Spiers and I. D. Van, December 27, 1865, both Samuel R. Barton Papers, DU.

111. Samuel Barton to Elizabeth Barton, October 9, 1864, HL.

112. Parramore, "Bartons of Bartonsville," p. 36.

113. Statement of CB, n.d., [March 1865], CB-LC.

114. Stephen Barton to Ada Ida Emory and Mary Barton, December 11, 1864, CB-LC.

115. Samuel Barton to Elizabeth Barton, October 9, 1864, HL.

116. CBJ, October 12, 1864, and January 14, 1865, CB-LC; and Parramore, "Bartons of Bartonsville," p. 37.

117. CBJ, January 28, March 4 and 6, 1865, CB-LC.

118. Ibid., February 13 and 17, 1865.

119. Ibid., February 20, 26, 27, 28, 1865; quotation March 1, 1865.

120. Ibid., January 27 and 31, February 1 and 13, March 10–18, 1865.

121. Ibid., April 9, 1865; and *Report of William A. Dale, the Surgeon General of Massachusetts* (Boston: Wright and Potter, 1866), p. 24.

122. CBJ, January 1, 1866, CB-LC.

123. Ibid., March 12, 1865; and W. E. Barton, *Life* 1:305.

Chapter 9

1. Abraham Lincoln to "Friends of Missing Persons," March 11, 1865, in Ishbel Ross, *Angel of the Battlefield: The Life of Clara Barton* (New York: Harper and Row, 1956), p. 86.

2. L. P. Brockett, *Women's Work in the Civil War: A Record of Heroism, Patriotism, and Patience* (Philadelphia: Zeigler, McCurdy and Co., 1967), p. 128.

3. Ibid., pp. 128–29.

4. Figures supplied by the Navy and Old Army Division, NARS.

5. William E. Barton, *The Life of Clara Barton* (Boston: Houghton Mifflin Co., 1922), 1:306–7; and untitled article, *The Globe*, February 16, 1866, clipping, CB-LC.

6. Newspaper clipping, n.d., in CBJ, 1865, CB-LC.

7. Draft of letter from CB to "My always good friend," n.d. [c. 1866], CB-LC.

8. "J. H. H." to CB, October 16, 1865; and CB to "J. H. H.", n.d., quoted in W. E. Barton, *Life* 1:312–13.

9. CB to Elvira Stone, June 17, 1865, CB-LC.

10. CB to the People of the United States, n.d. [1865], CB-LC.

11. CB to Captain C. K. Smith, n.d. [July 1865], CB-LC.

12. CB to "My Always good friend," n.d. [c. 1865], CB-LC.

13. CB to Abraham Lincoln, February 28, 1865, CB-LC.

14. CB to Andrew Johnson, May 31, 1865, CB-LC; T. S. Burns to CB, June 24, 1865, CB-LC; and W. E. Barton, *Life* 1:306.

15. CB, "Petition to the Masonic Fraternity in the United States," May 15, 1865; CB to Henry Wilson, April 29, 1865; and CB to the People of the United States, n.d. [c. 1865], all CB-LC.

16. Dorence Atwater to CB, June 22, 1865; and "Statement of Dorence Atwater Concerning the Larceny of the Andersonville Prison Records," n.d. [September or October 1865], both CB-LC.

17. Ibid.; and "Proceedings of Court Martial Against Dorence Atwater," September 1, 1865, Records of the Provost Marshall, Record Group 154, NARS.

18. Untitled notes in CB's handwriting, n.d., CB-LC; and E. M. Stanton to Montgomery Meigs, June 30, 1865, Consolidated Correspondence of the Quartermaster General, Record Group 92, NARS.

19. CB to Edmund M. Stanton, n.d. [c. September 1865]; and CBJ, July 12, 1865, both CB-LC.

20. CBJ, July 21 and 22, 1865, CB-LC.

21. Ibid., July 12, 1865.

22. Ibid., July 18, 1865; and J. M. Moore to Montgomery Meigs, July 16 and July 30, 1865, both in Consolidated Correspondence of the Quartermaster General, RG 92, NARS.

23. CB to Mr. Brown, August 7, 1865, CB-LC.

24. CB to Edmund Stanton, n.d. [September 1865], CB-LC; "Report of the Secretary of War to Congress on the Graves of Union Prisoners at Andersonville: Report of Captain Moore," (Washington, D.C.: Government Printing Office, 1865), pp. 263–66. For more information on Andersonville Prison, see MacKinlay Cantor, Andersonville (Franklin Center, Pa.: Franklin Library, 1970); Ovid L. Futch, History of Andersonville Prison (Gainesville: University of Florida Press, 1968); and Eugene Forbes, Diary of a Soldier and a Prisoner of War in Rebel Prisons (Trenton: Murphy and Bechtel, 1865).

25. CB to Stanton, n.d. [September 1865]; and CBJ, July 26, 1865, both CB-LC.

26. CB, MS lecture on Andersonville, n.d. [1866–68], typescript, CB-LC.

27. CBJ, July 25, 1865, CB-LC.

28. CB, untitled poem, August 1865, typescript, CB-LC.

29. See "Copies of Forged Letters Published while We were in Andersonville," n.d., CB-LC.

30. See Moore to Meigs, July 16 and July 30, 1865, RG 92, NARS; and "Report of Secretary of War."

31. CB to Stanton, n.d. [September 1865], CB-LC.

32. CBJ, July 12 and August 11, 1865, CB-LC.

33. Ibid., August 5–8, 1865.

34. Receipt for loan of items to the Howellsville Loan Exposition, n.d. [c. 1878], CB-LC.

35. CBJ, July 26, 31, August 5, 6, 13, 1865 (quotation August 13), CB-LC; and CB to Ira Moore Barton, July 3, 1863, Ira Moore Barton Papers, American Antiquarian Society, Worcester, Mass.

36. CBJ, August 17, 1865, CB-LC.

37. Ibid., August 18–23, 1865.

38. Ibid, July 13 and August 14, 1865; and "Statement of Dorence Atwater," n.d. [September or October 1865], CB-LC.

39. For details of the prison's Civil War operations, see Margaret Leech, Reveille in Washington (New York: Harper Brothers, 1941), pp. 148–58.

40. "Proceedings of Court Martial Against Atwater," September 1, 1865; and Samuel Breck to George S. Goddard, January 22, 1913, both RG 154, NARS.

41. "Proceedings of Court Martial Against Atwater," RG 154, NARS; and CBJ, September 9, October 6, 1865, and June 25, 1866, CB-LC.

42. CB to Henry Wilson, December 19, 1865, CB-LC.

43. CBJ, November 10, 1865, CB-LC.

44. Ibid., November 11 and December 21, 1865.

45. Quotation ibid., September 19, 1865; and CB to Benjamin F. Butler, October 3, 1865, CB-LC.

46. CBJ, October 4, 1865; and General E. D. Townsend to CB, December 8, 1865, both CB-LC.

47. CB to Henry Wilson, October 27, 1865; and CBJ, October 25, 1865, both CB-LC.

48. CBJ, December 1–8, 1865; and CB to Benjamin Butler, December 1, 1865, both CB-LC.

49. Frances D. Gage, "Relics of Andersonville," *New York Independent*, January 25, 1866.

50. CBJ, October 26 and December 17, 1865, CB-LC.

51. Ibid., December 25, 1865.

52. Ibid., January 5, 1866.

53. Frances D. Gage to CB, December 28, 1880, quoted in Henle, "Against the Fearful Odds," draft Ph.D. Thesis, Case Western Reserve University, 1976, p. 38.

54. CBJ, January 1, 1866, CB-LC.

55. Gage, "Relics of Andersonville," *New York Independent*, January 25, 1866; and Frances D. Gage, "Petition to the Senators and Representatives of the Thirty-Ninth Congress," n.d. [February 1866], copy in CB-LC.

56. Testimony of CB before the Joint Committee on Reconstruction, February 21, 1866, House of Representatives Record No. 30, pt. 3, pp. 102–3. For evidence of public disapproval of the testimony of women, see Eleanor Flexner, *Century of Struggle* (New York: Atheneum, 1974), pp. 58–60.

57. Conversation between Saidee Riccius and Fanny Childs Vassall, n.d. [c. 1916], AAS.

58. "Nice Thing for Clara," *Boston Post*, March 12, 1866.

59. "House of Representatives," *New York Daily Tribune*, March 9, 1866.

60. CB ledger, March 15 and April 15, 1866, CB-LC.

61. CB to Mrs. [Fanny Childs] Vassall, December 29, 1865, typescript, CB-LC.

62. CB to Elvira Stone, April 1, 1866, CB-LC.

63. Gage, "Relics of Andersonville," *New York Independent*, January 25, 1866; and CB to Elvira Stone, April 1, 1866, CB-LC.

64. CB ledger, October through December 1866, CB-LC.

65. "Miss Barton's Lecture," *Jersey City Evening Journal*, April 3, 1868.

66. See CB, MS lectures, 1866–68, CB-LC.

67. "Miss Barton's Lecture," *Jersey City Evening Journal*, April 3, 1868.

68. "Miss Clara Barton's Lecture," *Syracuse Daily Standard*, November 27, 1867.

69. CBJ, January 13, 20, and March 1, 1867, CB-LC.

70. CB quoted in Ross, *Angel*, p. 99; and CB to General A. C. Voris, September 12, 1867, CB copybook, CB-LC.

71. Appointment book of Dorence Atwater and CB, CB-LC.

72. CB to Henry Cross, October 3, 1866, in CB copybook, ANRC.

73. CB to Mrs. Curtis, January 20, 1867; and CB to E. S. Brown, July 13, 1867, CB copybook, ANRC.

74. CB ledger for November 1866, CB-LC.

75. CBJ, January 13, 1867, CB-LC.

76. Ibid., January 25, 1867.

77. A description of this incident is found in W. E. Barton, *Life* 1:205.

78. "GAR," *The Mercury*, January 16, 1868; and CB, MS lecture on woman suffrage, n.d. [c. 1869], CB-LC.

79. Ibid.

80. CB, "The Women Who Went to the Field," 1891, typescript, CB-LC.

81. "Clara Barton," *The Revolution*, March 26 and April 2, 1868; Susan B. Anthony to CB, April 29, 1869, CB-LC.

82. CB, MS lecture on woman suffrage, n.d. [c. 1869], CB-LC.

83. William Conklin, ed., *Clara Barton and Dansville*, (Dansville, N.Y.: F. A. Owen Publishing Co., 1966), pp. 430–31.

84. Ibid.; Notes for suffrage speech in CBJ, January 8–22, 1868, CB-LC; and Flexner, *Century of Struggle*, pp. 142–52.

85. Flexner, *Century of Struggle*, pp. 142–52.

86. CB, MS lecture on universal suffrage, n.d., CB-LC.

87. I am indebted to Ellen Henle for first suggesting Griffing's contribution to me. Edward T. James, ed., *Notable American Women, 1607–1950* (Cambridge: Belknap Press, 1971), 2:92–94; and CBJ, November 5 and December 24, 1868, CB-LC.

88. John Hitz to CB, October 19, 1880; quotation CBJ, October 20, 1868, both CB-LC.

89. CB to Elizabeth Cady Stanton and Susan B. Anthony, May 11, 1869, in "Annual Meeting of the American Equal Rights Association," *The Revolution*, May 20, 1869.

90. CBJ, December 30, 1868, CB-LC.

91. Ibid., November 11, 1868, and prescription enclosed in same.

92. F. J. Homer to CB, September 25, 1911, quoted in W. E. Barton, *Life* 1:313–14; and CB, "Report to Congress on the Office of Correspondence with the Friends of the Missing Men of the United States Army," February 1867, CB-LC.

Chapter 10

1. United States passport issued to CB, 1869, CB-LC; and CB to Mary Norton, May 21, 1869, D-DU.

2. CB quoted in Percy Epler, *The Life of Clara Barton* (New York: Macmillan, 1915), p. 123.

3. CB to John Hitz, September 25, 1869, CB-LC.

4. CBJ, November 1, 1869, B-DU.

5. CBJ, January 1, 1870, CB-LC.

6. CBJ, November 11–24 and December 25, 1869, B-DU.

7. See ibid., September–December 1869; photograph of Appia in CB, *The Red Cross in Peace and War* (Washington, D.C.: American Historical Press, 1899), p. 16; and CB, MS lecture on the Franco-Prussian War, n.d. [post 1882], typescript, CB-LC.

8. See Violet Kelway Libby, *Henry Dunant, Prophet of Peace* (New York: Pageant Press, 1964), pp. 1–72; and Jean Henri Dunant, *Un Souvenir de Solferino* (Geneva: Cassell, 1974).

9. Dunant, *Un Souvenir*, pp. 35 and 57.

10. Libby, *Dunant*, chaps. 18–20; and CB, *Peace and War*, pp. 57–58.

11. For a copy of the original Treaty of Geneva, see CB, *Peace and War*, pp. 57–59.

12. CB, lecture on Franco-Prussian War, n.d. [post 1882], typescript, CB-LC.

13. CBJ, January 1, 1870, CB-LC; CBJ, December 24, 1869, B-DU; and Ishbel Ross, *Angel of the Battlefield: The Life of Clara Barton* (New York: Harper and Row, 1956), p. 104.

14. Abby Sheldon to CB, January 19, 1870, CB-LC.

15. CBJ, January 1, 1870, CB-LC; Ross, *Angel*, p. 104; and Abby Sheldon to CB, March 4, 1870, CB-LC.

16. CB to David Barton, May 30, 1870, AAS.

17. CBJ, December 31, 1869, B-DU; see also CB to General E. Whitaker, January 3, 1870, CB-LC.

18. CBJ, July 10, 1870, CB-LC.

19. Michael Howard, *The Franco-Prussian War* (London: Rupert Hall Davis, 1961), pp. 1–40.

20. CB to Editor, *Soldiers Record*, August 5, 1870, clipping, CB-LC; and CBJ, July 28 and 30, 1870, CB-LC.

21. CB, lecture on Franco-Prussian War, n.d. [post 1882], typescript, CB-LC.

22. Ibid.

23. CBJ quoted in Blanche Colton Williams, *Clara Barton: Daughter of Destiny* (Philadelphia: J. B. Lippincott Co., 1941), p. 178.

24. Quotation CB, lecture on Franco-Prussian War, n.d. [post 1882], typescript, CB-LC; also Elizabeth S. Kite, "Antoinette Margot and Clara Barton," *Records of the American Catholic Historical Society* 55, no. 1 (March 1944): 31–33.

25. CB, lecture on Franco-Prussian War, n.d. [post 1882], typescript, CB-LC.

26. CBJ, August 26, 1870, CB-LC.

27. Ibid.

28. "Story from Mlle. Margot," January 11, 1916, RARC NARS; and CB to Editor of the *Grand Army Journal*, September 5, 1870, CB-LC. For another example, see CB to Grand Duchess Louise, June 26, 1872, CB-LC.

29. "Story from Mlle. Margot," January 11, 1916, RARC NARS.

30. CBJ, August 31, 1870, CB-LC; and Henle, "Against the Fearful Odds," draft Ph.D. Thesis, Case Western Reserve University, 1976, p. 52.

31. Henle, "Against the Fearful Odds," p. 52; "The Hospitals of Germany," unidentified clipping in CB scrapbook, CB-LC.

32. Henle, "Against the Fearful Odds," p. 52; CBJ, September 21, 1870, CB-LC; and certificate from the Badischer Frauen-Verein, October 10, 1870, CB-LC.

33. CB, lecture on Franco-Prussian War, n.d. [post 1882], typescript; and CBJ, October 2, 1870, both CB-LC.

34. CBJ, October 3, 1870, CB-LC.

35. CB, lecture on Franco-Prussian War, n.d. [post 1882], typescript; broadside of the Comité de Secours Strasbourgeois, n.d. [c. 1870]; and quotation CB, rough notes on a lecture on Strasbourg, n.d., all CB-LC.

36. Howard, *Franco-Prussian War*, pp. 272–75; and CB, notes on Strasbourg, n.d., CB-LC.

37. CB to M. Bergman, January 3, 1879, CB-LC.

38. CBJ, October 8 and 17–19, 1870; and CB, lecture on Franco-Prussian War, n.d. [post 1882], typescript, both CB-LC.

39. CB quoted in Ross, *Angel*, p. 15; and Hannah Zimmerman to CB, April 24 and May 1, 1871, both CB-LC.

40. CBJ, October 18, 1870, CB-LC.

41. Ibid., October 17 and November 14, 1870.

42. Antoinette Margot to "Mr. Editor," May 3, 1871; "The Strasbourg Picture," statement of Marion Balcom Howe, March 1939; and Antoinette Margot to "Editor of the Tribune," April 23, 1871, clipping in CB scrapbook, all CB-LC.

43. Antoinette Margot, "The Three Stitches," quoted in Williams, *Daughter of Destiny*, pp. 184–87.

44. Anna Zimmerman, "Clara Barton and the Women of Strasbourg," unpublished MS, December 23, 1872, typescript, CBNHS.

45. CB to Annie Childs, August 20, 1871, CB-LC; and Louise of Baden in "Blarter des Badischens Frauen Vereins," April 25, 1912, copy in RARC NARS.

46. CBJ, December 9, 10, 1870, CB-LC.

47. Ibid., December 1, 1870.

48. CB to Count Otto von Bismarck, December 9, 1870, CB-LC. For other fund-raising work, see CBJ, October 8, 12, 19, 31, 1870, CB-LC.

49. Draft of letter from CB to Benjamin Moran, May 1871, CB-LC.

50. Press releases in CB's handwriting, n.d. [c. 1870–71]; also Margot to "Editor of the Tribune," April 23, 1871; and Anna Zimmerman statement, December 23, 1872, CB letterbook, all CB-LC.

51. CBJ, June 3, 1871, CB-LC.

52. CB to M. Bergman, n.d. [1870]; and CB to Moran, May 1871, both CB-LC.

53. MS records of Strasbourg relief work, January–June 1871, CB-LC.

54. CB to Sally Vassall, n.d. [December 1870], AAS.

55. CB to Fanny Vassall, December 25, 1870, AAS.

56. CBJ, December 1870, CB-LC.

57. CB to Josephine Griffing, December 22, 1870, typescript, AAS.

58. CB to Edmund Dwight, October 23, 1871, CB-LC.

59. "Clara Barton," The Revolution, November 25, 1871.

60. CBJ, March 6, 1861, CB-LC; and Sally Vassall to CB, January 26, 1871, CB-LC; also Williams, Daughter of Destiny, p. 187.

61. CB to Elvira Stone, November 7, 1871, CB-LC.

62. CB, draft of a letter to "my fellow countrymen," n.d. [1871], CB-LC.

63. Quotation CB to Sally Vassall, January 31, 1872, AAS; CBJ, March–April, 1871; and CB to Stone, November 7, 1871, both CB-LC.

64. CBJ, June 1, 1871, CB-LC; and Howard, Franco-Prussian War, pp. 325–27.

65. "How Miss Barton Was Protected," The New Voice, December 29, 1898.

66. "The Red Cross of Europe and America," unidentified clipping, May 1904, CB-LC; Elihu B. Washburne, Recollections of a Minister to France (New York: Charles Scribner's Sons, 1887), 2:147–55; and CB quoted in Epler, Life, p. 165.

67. See Louis Appia to CB, December 12, 1870, CB-LC; and Edward Crane, quoted in Proceedings of the Fifth Annual Meeting of the Association of Military Surgeons of the United States (Cincinnati: Earhart and Richardson, 1896), p. 101.

68. Washburne, Recollections 2:131; Adolph Hepner, America's Aid to Germany in 1870–71 (St. Louis: privately printed, 1905), p. 145; Ross, Angel, p. 117; and "Story from Mlle. Margot," January 11, 1916, RARC NARS.

69. CB to Fanny Vassall, September 18, 1871, AAS.

70. "Story from Mlle. Margot," January 11, 1916, RARC NARS.

71. CBJ, August 13, 15, and 20, 1871, CB-LC.

72. Ibid., September 1 to October 15, 1871; and CB to Edmund Dwight, October 23, 1871, CB-LC.

73. Howard, Franco-Prussian War, pp. 287–92, 448; and CB to Dwight, October 23, 1871, CB-LC.

74. Quotation CB to Dwight, October 23, 1871. Also CBJ, October 23, 1871, CB-LC; receipts for monies given in Belfort and Besançon, CB-LC; and "Story from Mlle. Margot," January 11, 1916, RARC NARS.

75. CBJ, November 2, 1871, CB-LC.

76. CB to Stone, November 7, 1871, CB-LC.

77. Antoinette Margot to "Madame," n.d. [1871], CB-LC; CBJ, December 1–18, 1871, CB-LC; and "Story from Mlle. Margot," January 11, 1916, RARC NARS.

78. CB to Sally Vassall, January 31, 1872, AAS.

79. William E. Barton, *The Life of Clara Barton* (Boston: Houghton Mifflin Co., 1922), 2:55, 64; and CBJ, January–February 1872, CB-LC.

80. CB to Sally Vassall, January 31, 1872, AAS.

81. CB to Josephine Griffing, June 17, 1871, CB-LC.

82. CBJ, August 29, 1870, CB-LC.

83. CB to Fanny Vassall, September 18, 1871, AAS.

84. Quotation in CB to Griffing, June 17, 1871, CB-LC; CB to Sally Vassall, September 17, 1871, CB-LC; and CB to Josephine Griffing, December 22, 1870, typescript, AAS.

85. CBJ, March–April 1872, CB-LC.

86. CB to Sally Vassall, September 19, 1872, AAS.

87. CBJ, June 5 and 21, and July 19, 1872, CB-LC; and Ross, *Angel*, p. 121.

88. Abby Barker Sheldon to CB, July 29, 1872, CB-LC; and Ross, *Angel*, p. 123.

89. CBJ, September 1–22, 1872 (quotation September 22), CB-LC.

90. Ibid., December 24, 1872.

91. CB to Mamie Barton, n.d. [winter 1873], typescript, CB-LC.

92. CB, untitled poem, 1873, typescript, AAS.

93. Fanny Vassall to CB, April 10, 1873, CB-LC; and CB to Sally Vassall, April 6, 1873, AAS.

94. CB to Sally Vassall, April 6, 1873, AAS.

95. "Clara Barton," *National Repository* 5, no. 2 (February 1879).

96. CBJ, September 7–30, 1873, CB-LC; CB to Sally Vassall, September 13, 1873, AAS; and Joseph Sheldon to Bernard Vassall, July 9, 1873, AAS.

97. CB, "Have Ye Room?" quoted in W. E. Barton, *Life* 2:85–87.

Chapter 11

1. Mary Norton to CB, April 9, 1874, CB-LC.

2. J. K. H. Willcox to CB, October 25, 1875, and April 27, 1884, CB-LC; and untitled item in *Women's Journal*, October 27, 1873.

3. CB to Sally Vassall, March 6 and 30, 1874, AAS.

4. CB to Sally Vassall, n.d. [c. December 1873]; and conversation between Saidee Riccius and Fanny Childs Vassall, both AAS.

5. CB to Polly ?, n.d. [c. February 1874] quoted in Percy Epler, *The Life of Clara Barton* (New York: Macmillan, 1915), pp. 221–22; CB to Sally Vassall, April 2, 1874, and May ?, 1874, both AAS.

6. CB to Sally Vassall, May 15, 1874, AAS.

7. Ibid.

8. CB quoted in Epler, *Life*, p. 212.

9. CB to Dr. Edward Foote, draft answers to "Questions to Invalids," n.d. [c. 1876], SSC.

10. Bernard Vassall to CB, April 19, 1874. See also Abby Sheldon to CB, May 15, 1874; and Sally Vassall to CB, March 28, 1874, all CB-LC.

11. CB to Foote, n.d., SSC.

12. Ibid.

13. CB quoted in Epler, *Life*, p. 212.

14. CB to J. N. Bradley, July 27, 1877, quoted in William Conklin, ed., *Clara Barton and Dansville*, (Dansville, N.Y.: F. A. Owen Publishing Co., 1966), p. 51.

15. CB to Samuel Barton, May 24, 1878, in CB letterbook, CB-LC; Mary E. Gage to CB, November 26, 1874, CB-LC; and CB to J. J. Elwell, January 23, 1876, E-WRHS.

16. CB, address on James Caleb Jackson, 1880, in William D. Conklin, comp., "The Jackson Health Resort," 1971, typescript, National Library of Medicine, Bethesda, Md.

17. Abby Sheldon to CB, n.d. [c. June 1874]; and Minna Kupfer to CB, July 31, 1874, both CB-LC.

18. Minna Kupfer to Mamie Barton, October 21, 1874; quotation CB to Mamie Barton, n.d. [c. 1875], both in Epler, *Life*, p. 213; and CB to Foote, draft answers, n.d. [c. 1876], SSC.

19. Most of the sympathetic letters are to be found in CB-LC.

20. CB to Mrs. Southmayd, May 20, 1884, CB-LC.

21. J. Westfall to CB, November 17, 1875, CB-LC.

22. CB to Sally Vassall, March 6, 1874, AAS.

23. CB to Robert Hale, July 2, 1875; and CB account book, October 1874–December 1875, both CB-LC.

24. CB to Peter Balcom, September 27, 1875, AAS.

25. Marion Balcom Howe to Edith Riccius King, December 8, 1935, AAS.

26. CB to Fanny Vassall, July 11, 1873, AAS.

27. CB to Hale, July 2, 1875, CB-LC; CB account book, 1874–75, CB-LC; and CB to Foote, draft answers, n.d. [c. 1876], SSC.

28. CB to Foote, draft answers, n.d. [c. 1876], SSC.

29. Address on Jackson in Conklin, comp., "Jackson Health Resort," 1971, typescript, National Library of Medicine; and letters of Harriet Austin and James C. Jackson to CB, January 1876, CB-LC.

30. CBJ, March 16, 1876, CB-LC.

31. Ibid., March 16 through April 10, 1876; James C. Jackson to CB, May 12, 1876, CB-LC; and CB, Farewell Address, in Conklin, ed., *Dansville*, pp. 25 and 38.

32. For a complete history of Dansville, see A. O. Bunnell, *Dansville: Historical, Biographical, Descriptive* (Dansville: Instructor Publishing Co., 1902).

33. Ibid., pp. 178 and 249; and A. O. Bunnell quoted in Conklin, ed., *Dansville*, p. 81.

34. Ibid.

35. Gerald Carson, "Bloomers and Breadcrumbs," *New York History* 38, no. 3 (July 1957): 298; and Ellen Reeve Brodt, "Dansville and the Water Cure in 1872," *Dansville Breeze*, March 7 and 14, 1950.

36. Brodt, "Dansville in 1872,"

37. Conklin, ed., *Dansville*, p. 429; and CB to Elvira Stone, July 15, 1876, CB-LC.

38. CB quoted in Conklin, ed., *Dansville*, p. 44.

39. Carson, "Bloomers and Breadcrumbs," pp. 300–303.

40. Menu for Christmas dinner, 1883, in Conklin, ed., *Dansville*, p. 58.

41. CB to Elvira Stone, July 15, 1876, CB-LC.

42. CB to ?, n.d. [1876], quoted in Epler, *Life*, p. 216.

43. See, for example, CB to Mamie Barton, July 21, 1876, quoted in Epler, *Life*, pp. 216–17.

44. CB quoted in Conklin, ed., *Dansville*, pp. 44–45.

45. CB to Grand Duchess Louise, May 19, 1877, CB letterbook, CB-LC.

46. CB to Stone, July 15, 1876, CB-LC.

47. Blanche Colton Williams, *Clara Barton: Daughter of Destiny* (Philadelphia: J. B. Lippincott Co., 1941), pp. 225–26.

48. CB to Dr. L. H. Thompson, December 31, 1876; and letters of Mary Weeks to CB, February 1877–September 1881, both CB-LC.

49. Conklin, ed., *Dansville*, pp. 76–77; Carson, "Bloomers and Breadcrumbs," p. 297; letters of Harriet Austin to CB, n.d. [1876], September 21, 1876, October 23, 1877, and "Saturday before . . . Christmas," CB-LC; and quotation in CB on Harriet Austin, speech read at Woman Suffrage Convention, January 16, 1893, CB-LC.

50. Benjamin Tillinghast, untitled MS sketch of CB, n.d., CB-LC.

51. CBJ, January 1, 1877, CB-LC.

52. Conklin, ed., *Dansville*, pp. 129–30.

53. "Ovation to Miss Barton," *Dansville Advertiser*, June 7, 1877.

54. CBJ, January 1, 1877, CB-LC.

55. CB to Mary Norton, March 6, 1886, D-DU.

56. CBJ, January 8, 1877, CB-LC.

57. CB to Edmund Dwight and P. T. Jackson, April 24, July 5 and 26, 1876, and March 16, 1877, all CB-LC.

58. CB to Robert Hale, August 16, 1876, quoted in William E. Barton, *The Life of Clara Barton* (Boston: Houghton Mifflin Co., 1922), 1:87.

59. Ibid.; Robert Hale to CB, September 30, 1876, and February 3, 1877, CB-LC; and S. Gleason to CB, July 15, 1876, CB-LC.

60. CB to Theodore Pfau, April 17, 1877, CB-LC.

61. CB, autobiographical sketch for Susan B. Anthony and Elizabeth Cady Stanton, *History of Woman Suffrage* (New York: Fowler and Wells, 1881–82), draft copy, September 1876, CB-LC; and CB to Susan B. Anthony, September 23, 1876, quoted in Conklin, ed., *Dansville*, pp. 95–96.

62. CB to Ida B. Riccius, May 18, 1890, AAS.

63. CB to "Mr. Brooks," n.d. [c. 1876], CB letterbook, CB-LC.

64. CB to Edmund Dwight, July 31, 1877, CB-LC.

65. CB to Samuel Barton, May 24, 1878, in CB letterbook, CB-LC.

Chapter 12

1. CB to Theodore Pfau, CB letterbook, April 19, 1877, CB-LC.

2. CB to J. J. Elwell, October 25, 1876; and CB to the Grand Duchess Louise, May 19, 1877, CB letterbook, both CB-LC.

3. CB to Louis Appia, May 17, 1877, CB letterbook, CB-LC.

4. Ibid.

5. Louis Appia to CB, June 14, 1877, typescript, AAS; and Louis Appia to CB, July 5, 1877, CB-LC.

6. Gustave Moynier to CB, June 20, 1877, CB-LC.

7. CB to Appia, May 17, 1877, CB-LC.

8. CB to Grand Duchess [Louise], May 19, 1877, CB-LC; and CB to Harriett Austin, n.d. [c. July 1877] in William Conklin, ed., *Clara Barton and Dansville*, (Dansville, N.Y.: F. A. Owen Publishing Co., 1966), p. 61.

9. CB to Louis Appia, July 1, 1876 [1877], CB-LC.

10. William Seward to George C. Fogg, July 13, 1864, Records of the Secretary of State, Switzerland Dispatches, Record Group 59, NARS; and Gustave R. Gaeddert, "The History of the American National Red Cross," unpublished MS, n.d., 1:44–46, 2:2–3, ANRC.

11. Gaeddert, "American Red Cross," n.d., 2:4, ANRC.

12. I. W. Knusel to George Harrington, May 16, 1866; George Harrington to I. W. Knusel, May 19, 1866, Record Group 59, both NARS. C. Bethany to William Seward, March 14, 1868; quotation William Seward to C. Bethany, March 31, 1868, both Diplomatic Correspondence, Pt. 1, 1868, pp. 455–56, NARS.

13. Seward quoted in Gaeddert, "American Red Cross," n.d., 2:2–3, ANRC; also Foster Rhea Dulles, The American Red Cross: A History (New York: Harper Brothers, 1950), p. 10.

14. Dulles, American Red Cross, pp. 10–11.

15. CB quoted in Gaeddert, "American Red Cross," n.d., 2:10–11, ANRC.

16. Appia to CB, June 14, 1877, AAS.

17. CB to Appia, May 17, 1877, CB-LC.

18. CB to Louis Appia, July 1, 1877, in Conklin, ed., Dansville, p. 206.

19. Jonathan Defrees to CB, September 18, 1877, CB-LC.

20. CB to General E. W. Whitaker, July 21, 1877, in Conklin, ed., Dansville, pp. 208–9.

21. CB to David Barton, May 13, 1877, AAS.

22. George Kennan to "mother," February 18, 1880, K-LC.

23. CB to Louis Appia, January 14, 1878, CB letterbook, CB-LC.

24. Ibid.; and CBJ, January 1, 1878, CB-LC.

25. CBJ, January 3, 1878, CB-LC.

26. Ibid.; Gaeddert, "American Red Cross," n.d., 2:14, ANRC; and CB to Edmund Dwight, January 1878, CB-LC.

27. CBJ, January 17, 1878, CB-LC.

28. CB to Appia, January 14, 1878, CB-LC.

29. Ibid.; and quotation in Ishbel Ross, Angel of the Battlefield: The Life of Clara Barton (New York: Harper and Row, 1956), p. 133.

30. CBJ, January 20, 1878, CB-LC.

31. Ibid., January 17, 1878; and CB to Dwight, January 1878, CB-LC.

32. CB to Dwight, January 1878, CB-LC.

33. CB to Harriet Austin, February 9 and March 1, 1878 (quotation March 1), in Conklin, ed., Dansville, pp. 67 and 69.

34. CBJ, March 8, 1878, CB-LC.

35. CB to Theodore Pfau, April 10, 1878; CB to Samuel Barton, May 24, 1878, CB letterbook; and CBJ, June 7–14, 1878, all CB-LC. Also CB to Harriet Austin, March 1, 1878, and CB to James C. Jackson, May 16, 1877, both in Conklin, ed., Dansville, pp. 49, 69, 90.

36. CBJ, June 14, 1878, CB-LC.

37. Ibid., June–July 1878.

38. Ibid., July 4, 1878; and Frances D. Gage to CB, February 5, 1877, and January 12, 1878, all CB-LC.

39. Frances D. Gage to CB, December 5, 1878, CB-LC.

40. CBJ, August 27, 1878, CB-LC; and CB to Mary Norton, December 11, 1878, D-DU.

41. CB to Mary Norton, December 16, 1879, D-DU. See also Mary Norton to CB, September 22, 1878, CB-LC.

42. CBJ, October 8, 10, 21, 1878, CB-LC.

43. CB, "The Red Cross of the Geneva Convention: What It Is," 1878, in William E. Barton, *The Life of Clara Barton* (Boston: Houghton Mifflin Co., 1922), 2:139–43 (quotation p. 142).

44. See excerpt from Jean Henri Dunant, *Un Souvenir de Solferino* (Geneva: Cassell, 1974), in Conklin, ed., *Dansville*, p. 220.

45. CB to Edmund Dwight, September 7, 1878, in Conklin, ed., *Dansville*, p. 221.

46. CB, "The Red Cross," in W. E. Barton, *Life* 2:143.

47. Rutherford B. Hayes to William Evarts, January 4, 1879, card enclosed from Charles Devin, CB-LC.

48. CB quoted in Ross, *Angel*, p. 133.

49. Senate Resolution No. 67, February 1879, copy in CB-LC; and Conklin, ed., *Dansville*, p. 222.

50. CB to Mary Norton, August 27, 1879, D-DU.

51. CB to Gustav Bergman, January 15, 1878; in Conklin, ed., *Dansville*, p. 215, also p. 108.

52. CB to Ida Riccius, November 3, 1879, AAS.

53. David Barton to Ida and Adolph Riccius, June 13, 1880, typescript, AAS.

54. Ibid.; and CB to Norton, December 11, 1878, D-DU.

55. Anna Preston to CB, December 7, 1880, CB-LC.

56. A. O. Bunnell quoted in Conklin, ed., *Dansville*, p. 118.

57. Lillian F. Lewis, "A Neighbor's Impressions of Clara Barton," in Conklin, ed., *Dansville*, p. 134.

58. CB to Mrs. Kent, February 17, 1881; in Conklin, ed., *Dansville*, p. 223.

59. Statement of Myrtis Barton Butler, September 21, 1941, in Conklin, ed., *Dansville*, p. 116.

60. Conklin, ed., *Dansville*, pp. 372–73.

61. See Julian Hubbell to CB, October 4, 1882, CB-LC.

62. Quotation in Susan B. Anthony to CB, September 19, 1876; also July 4, 1878; J. H. K. Willcox to CB, January 7, 1877, and December 25, 1880; Lucy Stone to CB, January 16, 1881, all CB-LC.

63. J. H. K. Willcox to CB, August 8, 1881, CB-LC.

64. CBJ, January 8, 1878, CB-LC.

65. CB, Decoration Day Address, 1879, in Conklin, ed., *Dansville*, p. 174.

66. Conklin, ed., *Dansville*, pp. 453–54.

67. CB to Ida Barton, April 22, 1877, AAS; Mary G. Davenport to CB, July 31, 1876, CB-LC; and CB to Dr. L. H. Thompson, December 31, 1876, CB-LC.

68. CB to Lucy Stone, January 21, 1881, typescript, AAS.

69. Victor Rosewater, *History of Cooperative Newsgathering in the United States* (New York: D. Appleton and Co., 1930), pp. 157, 171; and *DAB*, s.v. "Phillips, Walter Polk."

70. "The Red Cross," *Yonkers Gazette*, July 26, 1879.

71. Elizabeth Churchill, "The Red Cross and Clara Barton," *Providence Daily Journal*, December 16, 1878; see also "Letter from Buckeye," *Toledo Blade*, December 29, 1877, January 5, 1878, copies in CB-LC.

72. "The Red Cross," *Yonkers Gazette,* July 26, 1879.

73. Mary R. Dearing, *Veteran in Politics* (Baton Rouge: Louisiana State University Press, 1952), pp. 87–88.

74. Ibid., pp. 96, 268.

75. See, for example, William Haskill to CB, January 27, 1875, CB-LC; Charles Harding to CB, September 11, 1879, CB-LC; J. W. Neighbor to CB, June 16, 1879, CB-LC; "Message to the Veterans," *Fall River Daily News* (Mass.), October 21, 1875; quotation George S. Ball to CB, August 13, 1880, CB-LC.

76. CB to Major Seth Hedges, June 10, 1881, CB-LC.

77. *DAB,* s.v. "Logan, John Alexander"; also Mrs. J. A. Logan, "Clara Barton," 1913, CB-LC; Conklin, ed., *Dansville,* pp. 169–75, 189–90; and "Not Forgotten," *Women's Word,* July 1877.

78. CB quoted in Conklin, ed., *Dansville,* p. 456.

79. CB to James A. Garfield, February 16, 1881, James A. Garfield Papers, LC. For a similar note Barton wrote to Omar D. Conger, see Conklin, ed., *Dansville,* pp. 460–61.

80. W. E. Barton, *Life* 2:149.

81. Ibid.; Foster Rhea Dulles, *Prelude to World Power* (New York: Macmillan Co., 1965), p. 40; and *DAB,* s.v. "Blaine, James Gillespie." See also Milton Plesur, *America's Outward Thrust: Approaches to Foreign Affairs, 1865–1890* (DeKalb: Northern Illinois University Press, 1971); and Matthew Josephson, *The Politicos* (New York: Harcourt Brace Jovanovich, 1963).

82. SBJ, April 11, 1881, typescript, AAS.

83. Ibid., April 12, 1881; "Miss Barton and Abraham Lincoln's Son," *Providence Journal,* n.d., quoted in Conklin, ed., *Dansville,* p. 186; and W. E. Barton, *Life* 2:151.

84. Stephen E. Barton to Harriet Austin, March 16, 1881, ANRC; and SBJ, April 12, 1881, AAS.

85. Harriet Austin to CB, March 21, 1881, CB-LC.

86. CB to Louis Appia, March 17, 1881, typescript, RARC NARS.

87. Letters between Moynier and Blaine are quoted in W. E. Barton, *Life* 2:153–54.

88. Samuel Ramsey to CB, May 1, 1881, CB-LC; and Dulles, *American Red Cross,* p. 15.

89. Gaeddert, "American Red Cross," n.d., 2:22, ANRC; Mrs. Peter De Graw quoted in Ross, *Angel,* p. 137; and statement of Mrs. H. V. Boynton, July 24, 1916, in *Memorial to Clara Barton* (Hearing before the Committee on Library, House Resolution 16606) (Washington, D.C.: Government Printing Office, 1916), p. 8.

90. See CB to Grand Duchess Louise, March 20, 1881, CB copybook, CB-LC; Henle, "Against the Fearful Odds," draft Ph.D. Thesis, Case Western Reserve University, 1976; and W. E. Barton, *Life* 2:159.

91. Dulles, *American Red Cross,* pp. 15–16; CB to James G. Blaine, May 27, 1881, and to Walker Blaine, August 29, 1881, both in Conklin, ed., *Dansville,* p. 253; and *DAB,* s.v. "Blaine, James Gillespie."

92. See, for example, John Dulwell to CB, June 10, 1881; and Arabella Simmott to CB, n.d. [June 1881], both CB-LC.

93. CB to General S. D. Sturgis, June 10, 1881, in Conklin, ed., *Dansville,* p. 240, also p. 269; and Ramsey to CB, May 1, 1881, CB-LC.

94. CB to Stephen E. Barton, n.d. [June 1881], CB-LC; and W. E. Barton, *Life* 2:159.

95. CB to Gustave Moynier, August 17, 1881, in Conklin, ed., *Dansville,* p. 252.

96. Gaeddert, "American Red Cross," n.d., 2:20, ANRC; and W. E. Barton, *Life* 2:172–74.

97. For Atwater and Shepard information, see CB to James C. Jackson, May 16, 1877, in Conklin, ed., *Dansville*, p. 49; and Fanny Atwater to CB, March 10, 1876, CB-LC; quotation "The Women's National Relief Association," *The Alpha* 6, no. 10 (June 1, 1881): 3–4.

98. Hannah Shepard, letter to the editor of the *Philadelphia Evening Telegraph*, November 14, 1882 [1881], copy in CB's hand, CB-LC.

99. Conklin, ed., *Dansville*, pp. 243–47; and CBJ, quoted in W. E. Barton, *Life* 2:176.

100. "Red Cross: A Move in the Right Direction," *Dansville Advertiser*, August 25, 1881; Susan B. Anthony to CB, September 20, 1881, CB-LC. Detailed information on the opening of these chapters can be found in Conklin, ed., *Dansville*, pp. 344–64.

101. See Stewart H. Holbrook, *Burning an Empire* (New York: Macmillan Co., 1943), pp. 102–7; Broadside, "Michigan's Terrible Calamity; A Cry for Help," September 13, 1881, CB-LC; quotation CB to William Lawrence, September 18, 1881, in Conklin, ed., *Dansville*, p. 376.

102. Conklin, ed., *Dansville*, pp. 360–61 (quotation p. 360); "Relief of the Suffering," *Rochester Democrat and Chronicle*, October 18, 1881; and CB, *The Red Cross in Peace and War* (Washington, D.C.: American Historical Press, 1899), p. 108.

103. CB to Lawrence, October 18, 1881, in Conklin, ed., *Dansville*, p. 376.

104. "Relief of the Suffering," *Rochester Democrat*, October 18, 1881.

105. CB, Report on Michigan Fire Relief, October 1881, CB-LC.

106. Julian B. Hubbell to CB, October 6, 1881, in Conklin, ed., *Dansville*, p. 381.

107. "Relief of the Suffering," *Rochester Democrat*, October 18, 1881.

108. Julian B. Hubbell to CB, October 9, 1881, CB-LC; and Hubbell to CB, October 6, 1881, in Conklin, ed., *Dansville*, p. 381.

109. CBJ, October 13, 1881, CB-LC.

110. CB to Edmund Dwight, n.d. [December 1881], copy in CB-LC.

111. Arthur quoted in "The Red Cross," broadside of newspaper excerpts, December 18, 1881, CB-LC.

112. CBJ, January 16, 18, and 31, and February 8, 1882, typescript, AAS.

113. Ibid., January 31, 1882; and CB to Walter Phillips, November 15, 1881, CB-LC.

114. CBJ, January 13 and 25, and February 27, 1882 (quotation January 19, 1882), AAS.

115. Ibid., February 6, 1882.

116. Ibid., February 25, 1882.

117. Ibid., March 10 and 16, 1882.

118. ? Mullet, article written for the *New York Sun*, January 10, 1905, typescript, CB-LC.

119. CBJ, June 8, 1907, CB-LC.

Chapter 13

1. Baroness von Mentizinger for the Grand Duchess Louise to CB, October 5, 1882, CB-LC.

2. Henry Bellows quoted in Annie M. Russell, "Famous Worcester People—Clara Barton," *Light*, July 19, 1890.

3. E. R. Hanson, *Our Women Workers* (Chicago: The Star and Covenant Office, 1882), p. 369.

4. *Washington Evening Star*, November 3, 1881, quoted in William Conklin, ed., *Clara Barton and Dansville* (Dansville, N.Y.: F. A. Owen Publishing Co., 1966), p. 268; and Elvira Stone to CB, January 18, 1881, CB-LC.

5. GPJ, 1897, CB-LC; and J. L. Jackson to John Morlan, June 5, 1898, RARC NARS.

6. CB to George B. Ferguson, November 18, 1882, CB letterbook, CB-LC.

7. Percy Epler, *The Life of Clara Barton* (New York: Macmillan, 1915), p. viii.

8. CB to Ida Riccius, May 18, 1890, AAS.

9. CB to Edward Seve, November 30, 1881, CB-LC.

10. CBJ, January 15, 1882, typescript, AAS.

11. CB to Ida Riccius, October 29, 1890, AAS.

12. CB to F. R. Southmayd, November 8, 1882, CB letterbook, CB-LC.

13. CB to David Barton, December 25, 1886, AAS.

14. CB to Baroness von Mentizinger, n.d. [c. November 1882], CB letterbook, CB-LC.

15. CB to Clara Knittle, March 15, 1883, CB-LC.

16. CB to Benjamin Butler, March 26, 1883, CB-LC.

17. CB to Brown Brothers Bank, December 8, 1882, CB letterbook, CB-LC.

18. CBJ, April 3, 1882, CB-LC.

19. Ibid., April 7, 1882; and "The Red Cross," *Dansville Advertiser*, April 13, 1882.

20. CBJ, April 7, 1882; CB to David Barton, July 31, 1882, typescript; draft of letter from George W. Childs to ?, n.d. [spring 1882]; and Senate Resolution No. 73, May 26, 1882, all CB-LC.

21. "Clara Barton's Testimony," *The Woman's Journal*, April 1, 1882; and broadside of American Red Cross, n.d. [spring 1882], CB-LC.

22. Gustave Moynier to CB, March 24, 1882, CB-LC.

23. CB to David Barton, July 31, 1882, typescript; and "The American National Red Cross," broadside, 1882, both CB-LC.

24. See, for example, "The Geneva Treaty," *Meridan Sunday Times* (Conn.), April 23, 1882.

25. "Social Incidents," clipping from unidentified Washington, D.C., newspaper, n.d. [March 1882], CB-LC.

26. Moynier to CB, March 24, 1882, CB-LC.

27. Frances D. Gage to CB, December 26, 1882; and Walter K. Phillips to CB, November 23, 1882, both CB-LC.

28. CBJ, April 10, 1882, CB-LC.

29. Ibid., April 4, 1882.

30. Moynier to CB, March 24, 1882, CB-LC.

31. CB to Stephen Barton, April 26, 1882, CB-LC.

32. CB to Gustave Moynier, August 11, 1882, typescript, RARC NARS.

33. Deed between CB, Edward Whitaker, and John Sherman, November 9, 1878, CB-LC. A photograph of the house is in CB, *The Red Cross in Peace and War* (Washington, D.C.: American Historical Press, 1899), p. 21.

34. "The American National Red Cross," broadside, 1882, CB-LC.

35. Draft of position paper by American Association of the Red Cross, May 1882, CB-LC.

36. J. B. Hubbell to CB, May 22, 1882, CB-LC.

37. Benjamin Butler to CB, January 8, 1883, CB-LC.

38. J. L. Jackson to John Morlan, June 5, 1898, RARC NARS.

39. Julian B. Hubbell, notes for a sketch on CB, June 21 and 29, 1893, CB-LC.

40. CBJ, February 27, 1883, CB-LC.

41. George Kennan to Mary Weeks Burnett, May 21, 1882, CB letterbook; G. E. Gordon to CB, March 26, 1883; and quotation CB to F. R. Southmayd, February 25, 1883, CB letterbook, all CB-LC.

42. CB, miscellaneous notes on Mississippi River floods, March 10, 1882, typescript, RARC NARS.

43. Julian B. Hubbell to CB, April 24 and 30, 1882, CB-LC.

44. Julian B. Hubbell to CB, May 30, 1882; and Hiram Sibly to Dr. E. M. Moore, May 29, 1882, both CB-LC.

45. Hubbell to CB, April 24 and 30, 1882, CB-LC.

46. Ibid.; and William Oliver to F. R. Southmayd, April 30, 1883; "Aid for Tornado Sufferers," New Orleans Times Democrat, May 2, 1883; and "The Red Cross," undated clipping, all CB-LC.

47. Julian B. Hubbell to CB, February 28, March 1, and March 7, 1883; and George Kennan to CB, March 30, 1883, all CB-LC.

48. Hubbell to CB, February 28, 1883, CB-LC.

49. CB to F. R. Southmayd, February 20, 1883; CB to D. R. McKee, February 18, 1883, CB letterbook; Hubbell to CB, March 7, 1883; and quotation CB to Hamilton Fish, March 4, 1883, CB letterbook, all CB-LC.

50. F. R. Southmayd to CB, October 10 and 21, 1882; Julian B. Hubbell to CB, September 23, 1882; quotation CB to F. R. Southmayd, November 8, 1882, CB letterbook, all CB-LC.

51. Hubbell to CB, February 28, March 1, and March 7, 1883; and Julian Hubbell to CB, May 14, 1882, all CB-LC.

52. CBJ, January 1–10, 1883; and Benjamin Butler to CB, January 8, 1883, both CB-LC.

53. DAB, s.v. "Butler, Benjamin Franklin"; Estelle B. Freedman, Their Sister's Keepers (Ann Arbor: University of Michigan Press, 1981), pp. 72–75; and "The Best Woman's Prison," New York Times, November 8, 1895.

54. CBJ, January 17, 1883; quotation CB to Dr. A. Van Derver, July 18, 1882, both CB-LC.

55. CB to Benjamin Butler, April 17, 1870, CB letterbook, CB-LC.

56. CBJ, January 31 to February 5, 1883; and CB to Benjamin F. Butler, February 3, 1883, CB letterbook, both CB-LC.

57. A. C. Stockin to CB, February 9, 1883, CB-LC.

58. CBJ, March 26 and 27, 1883, CB-LC.

59. Stephen E. Barton to CB, February 20, 1883; and T. E. Major to CB, April 11, 1883, both CB-LC.

60. CBJ, April 6–8, 1883 (quotation April 7), CB-LC.

61. Ibid., May 1, 1883; and Eliza Mosher quoted in Freedman, Sister's Keepers, p. 67.

62. "The Best Woman's Prison," New York Times, November 8, 1895; Freedman, Sister's Keepers, p. 68; CBJ, May 4, 1883, CB-LC; and "Miss Barton's Charge," Boston Herald, May 3, 1883.

63. Freedman, Sister's Keepers, pp. 23–58; Dorothea L. Dix, Remarks on Prisons and Prison Discipline in the United States (Philadelphia: Joseph Kite and Co., 1845), pp. 8–11, 25; Blake McKelvey, American Prisons: A Study in American Social History Prior to 1915

(Montclair, N.J.: Patterson Smith, 1968), pp. 57–68, 79. Barton quoted in *Sixth Annual Report of the Commissioners of Prisons on the Reformatory Prison for Women* (Boston: Wright and Potter Printing Co., 1884), p. 47.

64. *Eleventh Annual Report of the Commissioners of Prisons of Massachusetts* (Boston: Rand Avery and Co., 1882); Josephine P. Holland, "The Reformatory Prison for Women at Sherborn, Massachusetts," *The Golden Rule*, November 24, 1883; and "The Best Female Prison," *New York Times*, November 15, 1895.

65. CB to Mary Norton, August 5, 1883, D-DU.

66. CB quoted in Epler, *Life*, p. 240.

67. *Sixth Annual Report*, p. 10.

68. E. M. Mosher, "Health of Criminal Women," *Boston Medical and Surgical Journal*, October 5, 1882.

69. *Eleventh Annual Report*, pp. 7–12, 16–18.

70. *Sixth Annual Report*, pp. 47–48.

71. CB to D. K. Carter, October 25, 1887, CB-LC.

72. *Sixth Annual Report*, pp. 47–58; *Eleventh Annual Report*; and Freedman, *Sister's Keepers*, p. 91.

73. CB to Norton, August 5, 1883, D-DU; Julian B. Hubbell to John Van Voris, October 17, 1883, CB letterbook; and quotation CB lecture to the International Prison Congress, July 1886, all CB-LC.

74. Lucy Hall Brown quoted in "The Best Woman's Prison," *New York Times*, November 8, 1895; CB to H. S. Olcott, July 20, 1901, CB-LC; and notes on a conversation between Stephen E. Barton, Jr., Herman Riccius, and Saidee Riccius, July 8, 1917, AAS.

75. Sarah K. Bolton, "Clara Barton," *The Golden Rule*, April 28, 1892; letters of inmates to CB, June to December 1883; E. M. Babcock, D. B. Fox, and Effie A. Owenden to CB, June 29, 1883 and CB to same, June 30, 1883, all CB-LC. For examples of CB taking up a legal case, see CB to Benjamin Butler, June 14, June 15, and December ?, 1883, all CB-LC.

76. CB to Edmund Dwight, February 8, 1884, CB-LC.

77. CB, lecture to the International Prison Conference, July 1886, CB-LC.

78. CBJ, May 29, 1883, CB-LC; and "Clara Barton," *Woman's Journal*, July 31, 1886.

79. Note in CBJ, n.d. [1883]; and CB to Charles H. Allen, June 18, 1883, both CB-LC.

80. CB to Allen, June 18, 1883; Henrietta Wolcott to CB, November 15, 1883, both CB-LC; and "Clara Barton," *Framingham Gazette*, January 4, 1884.

81. Lucy M. Hall to CB, June 3 and 5, 1883, CB-LC.

82. For Butler's comments on CB, see "Butler Let Loose," *Boston Herald*, October 11, 1883. Quotation in CB to Daniel H. Rucker, November 14, 1883, CB-LC.

83. CB, draft of letter to "My dear Child" [Dr. Lucy Hall], n.d. [c. November 1883], CB-LC.

84. Ibid.

85. CB to Benjamin Butler, November 3 and 15, 1883, CB-LC; and Blanche Colton Williams, *Clara Barton: Daughter of Destiny* (Philadelphia: J. B. Lippincott Co., 1941), p. 281.

86. CB to Mrs. Canfield, September 30, 1883, CB letterbook, CB-LC; and "Clara Barton," *Woman's Journal*, July 31, 1886.

87. "The Woman's Congress," *Chicago Inter-Ocean*, October 17, 18, 19, 1883; and "Woman's Kingdom," *Chicago Tribune*, October 18, 20, 1883.

88. CB to Butler, November 3 and 15, 1883, CB-LC.

89. CB, lecture to the International Prison Congress, July 1886; and CB to Dwight, February 8, 1884, both CB-LC.

90. CB, lecture to the International Prison Congress, July 1886, CB-LC.

Chapter 14

1. CB to W. S. Paxton, May 12, 1883, CB letterbook, CB-LC.

2. Ellen Johnson to CB, June 30, 1883; and Benjamin Butler to CB, June 30, 1883, both CB-LC.

3. Kate Fox to CB, n.d. [c. December 1883], CB-LC.

4. See John Silver Hughes to CB, October 8, 1884; Gustave Moynier to CB, February 9 and 10, 1884; Mary M. North to CB, April 16, 1884; and Edward W. Allison to CB, December 30, 1884, all CB-LC. For Barton's relief at getting back, see CB quoted in Ishbel Ross, *Angel of the Battlefield: The Life of Clara Barton* (New York: Harper and Row, 1956), p. 154.

5. *Woman's Journal*, February 23, 1884.

6. CB, *The Red Cross in Peace and War* (Washington, D.C.: American Historical Press, 1899), p. 116; Gustave R. Gaeddert, "The History of the American National Red Cross," unpublished manuscript, n.d., 2:64, ANRC; and "Scenes Along the River When It Was at the High Point," *Chicago Inter-Ocean*, February 21, 1884.

7. Gaeddert, "American Red Cross," n.d., 2:64, ANRC; and CB to Rev. E. Frank Howe, February 22, 1884, CB letterbook, CB-LC.

8. Percy Epler, *The Life of Clara Barton* (New York: Macmillan, 1915), p. 242; and Gaeddert, "American Red Cross," n.d., 2:66, ANRC.

9. CB, notes for untitled article for *New York Sun*, January 10, 1908, CB-LC.

10. Ruth Riley, "Clara Barton's Visit to Flooded Smithfield, Kentucky in 1884," unpublished interview, 1936, RARC NARS.

11. Quotation in Epler, *Life*, pp. 244–45.

12. CB, *Peace and War*, p. 117.

13. P. De Graw to CB, May 23, 1887, CB-LC.

14. "Red Cross Association," *Evansville Courier*, March 18, 1884.

15. *St. Louis Democrat* quoted in CB, *Peace and War*, p. 120.

16. "Red Cross," *Chicago Inter-Ocean*, March 22, 1884.

17. CB to Joseph Sheldon, December 22, 1884, CB letterbook, CB-LC.

18. CB, *Peace and War*, pp. 131–33.

19. Ibid., p. 117; and Clyde E. Buckingham, *Clara Barton, A Broad Humanity* (Alexandria, Va.: privately published, 1980), p. 152.

20. CB to A. S. Solomons, May 24, 1884, ANRC.

21. CBJ, March 26–April 2, 1884, CB-LC; and CB, *Peace and War*, p. 120.

22. CB, *Peace and War*, pp. 121–22; "Red Cross," *Chicago Inter-Ocean*, March 22, 1884; and CBJ, April 17–18, 1884, CB-LC.

23. Andrew Leslie to "My dear Doctor," April 18, 1884, CBNHS.

24. CB to Bernard Moulton, February 17, 1884, CB letterbook, CB-LC.

25. CB, *Peace and War*, p. 122; CB to Walter Phillips, April 24, 1884, CB letterbook, CB-LC.

26. CB to Solomons, May 24, 1884, ANRC.

27. Quotation CB, *Peace and War*, pp. 122–23; and Mahala Chaddock to Annie Childs, April 15, 1884, AAS.

28. Ibid.; and "Red Cross," *Chicago Inter-Ocean*, March 22, 1884.

29. Leslie to "My dear Doctor," April 18, 1884, CBNHS.

30. CB to Solomons, May 24, 1884, ANRC.

31. Mahala Chaddock to Julian Hubbell, May 8, 1884, CB-LC.

32. "Minutes of the Regular Meeting of the American Association of the Red Cross," June 19, 1884, CB-LC.

33. Chaddock to Hubbell, May 8, 1884, CB-LC.

34. CB, *Peace and War*, p. 126.

35. CB to A. S. Solomons, May 7, 1884, CB letterbook, CB-LC.

36. CB to A. Wakeman, May 7, 1884; and CB to Gustave Moynier, June 7, 1884, both CB letterbook, CB-LC.

37. CB to Omar D. Conger, July 29, 1884, CB-LC.

38. Epler, *Life*, p. 245; meeting of the executive committee of the Red Cross, July 1884, CB-LC; Joseph Sheldon to CB, August 13, 1884, CB-LC; "Maz" to CB, August 1, 1884, CB-LC; copy of letter from Joseph Sheldon to U. G. Durham, July 7, 1885, CB-LC; and Minnie Golay to CB, August 7, 1884, CB-LC.

39. "Troisième Conference Internationale des Sociétés de la Croix Rouge, Genève, 1–6 Septembre, 1884—Programme," CB-LC; and "The Red Cross," *New York Tribune*, September 27, 1884.

40. "Society of the Red Cross," *Boston Herald*, September 30, 1884; and "Texte des Voeux et Resolutions Adoptés par la Troisième Conférence Internationale des Sociétés de la Croix-Rouge," n.d., copy in CB-LC.

41. "The Red Cross," *New York Tribune*, September 27, 1884.

42. Bernard H. Conn, "Adolphus S. Solomons," October 1957, typescript, American Jewish Archives, Hebrew Union College, Cincinnati, Ohio.

43. "Clara Barton," *New York Daily Graphic*, November 21, 1884.

44. "Texte des Voeux et Resolutions," n.d., copy in CB-LC.

45. Joseph Sheldon to Julian B. Hubbell, October 13, 1884, CB-LC.

46. "The Red Cross," *New York Tribune*, September 27, 1884.

47. CB to Grand Duchess Louise, September 23, 1884, RARC NARS.

48. Antoinette Margot to J. R. Wilcox, n.d., [c. September 1884], copy in CB letterbook, CB-LC.

49. "Clara Barton," *New York Daily Graphic*, November 21, 1884.

50. CB to Louise, September 23, 1884, RARC NARS.

51. CB to Harriet Austin, February 22, 1885; CB to Mary Gage, April 23, 1885, both CB letterbook, CB-LC.

52. CB to Julian Hubbell, December 17, 1884; and untitled clipping, *New Orleans Times Democrat*, May 2, 1885, CB-LC.

53. CB to Mr. Saunders, April 12, 1885, CB letterbook, CB-LC.

54. "Red Cross Celebration at New Orleans Exposition," May 5, 1885, press release in CB's hand, CB-LC.

55. CB to M. Margot, May 26, 1885; CB to Mr. and Mrs. Johnson, June 8, 1885, both CB-LC.

56. CB to Mary Norton, March 6, 1885, D-DU; CB, untitled speech to GAR post, n.d. [1885], CB letterbook, CB-LC; and William Conklin, ed., *Clara Barton and Dansville* (Dansville, N.Y.: F. A. Owen Publishing Co., 1966), pp. 471–72.

57. See letters of John Hitz to CB, and CB to D. K. Carter, October 1887, CB-LC; Thomas David Williams, *The Story of Antoinette Margot* (Baltimore: John Murphy Co.,

1931), pp. 130–35; Elizabeth S. Kite, "Antoinette Margot and Clara Barton," *Records of the American Catholic Historical Society* 55, no. 1 (March 1944): 42–47; quotation William E. Barton, *The Life of Clara Barton* (Boston: Houghton Mifflin Co., 1922), 2:262.

58. Sarah M., Mary E., and Joseph B. Gage to CB, November 11, 1884; and CB to Mary Gage, April 23, 1885, both CB letterbook, CB-LC.

59. Deed between CB, Stephen E. Barton, and David Barton, April 20, 1881, Worcester County Deed Book, Liber 1094, pp. 60–61, Worcester County Courthouse, Worcester, Mass.; CB to David Barton, December 25, 1886, AAS; and Charles Rawson to Julian B. Hubbell, September 26, 1884, CB-LC.

60. Julia Barton to CB, December 13, 1883, CB-LC.

61. CB to Stephen E. Barton, March 20, 1888, CB-LC.

62. CB to Baroness von Mentizinger, November 17, 1888, CB letterbook, CB-LC.

63. CB to David Barton, December 25, 1886, AAS; and CB to Officers and Ladies of the National Relief Corps, October 6, 1886, CB letterbook, CB-LC.

64. CB, lecture on the twenty-fifth anniversary of the organization of the GAR, n.d. [c. 1890], CB-LC.

65. CB to David Barton, December 25, 1886, AAS; CB to Mr. and Mrs. J. G. Lemmon, February ?, 1888, CB letterbook, CB-LC; and CB to Mary Elizabeth Almon, March 27, 1891, CB-LC.

66. Gaeddert, "American Red Cross," n.d., 2:76, ANRC.

67. Ibid.; CB to Mr. Manning, October 4, 1886, CB letterbook, CB-LC; and Epler, *Life*, p. 248.

68. "The Texas Drought Sufferers," *Galveston News*, January 21, 1887; and CB, *Peace and War*, pp. 136–37.

69. CB, *Peace and War*, pp. 138–40; quotation CB to Fanny Vassall, February 3, 1887, AAS.

70. CB, *Peace and War*, p. 137.

71. Quotation John Hitz to CB, February 2, 1887, CB-LC; and Gaeddert, "American Red Cross," n.d., 2:77–79, ANRC.

72. John Hitz to CB, January 20, 1887, CB-LC; and "Help the Drouth Region," *Dallas Morning News*, February 12, 1887.

73. CB to "Editors of Newspapers," n.d. [1887], CB letterbook, CB-LC; and CB, *Peace and War*, p. 139.

74. CB to Judge H. L. Bartholomew, April 21, 1887, CB letterbook, CB-LC.

75. CBJ, February 15, 1887, CB-LC.

76. CB to Judge Fleming and Mr. Conrad, April 17, 1887, CB letterbook, CB-LC.

77. CB to Mr. Doumus, March 8, 1887; CB to General A. H. Belo, April 17, 1887; and CB to Bartholomew, April 21, 1887, all CB letterbook, CB-LC.

78. CB to President and Recording Secretary of Philadelphia Red Cross, April 27, 1887, CB letterbook, CB-LC.

79. Julian B. Hubbell to Stephen E. Barton, June 10, 1887; and CB to the People of Washington, n.d. [c. June 1887], both CB letterbook, CB-LC.

80. Julian B. Hubbell to Professor Gladwin, June 9, 1887, CB letterbook, CB-LC.

81. CB, *Peace and War*, pp. 147–48; and Gaeddert, "American Red Cross," n.d., 2:82–83, ANRC.

82. CB to the United and Associated Presses, March 1888, CB letterbook, CB-LC.

83. CB, *Peace and War*, p. 146.

84. CB to Robert Princhard, March 6, 1888, CB letterbook, CB-LC.

85. CB to Philadelphia Red Cross, March 6, 1888, CB letterbook, CB-LC; and CB, *Peace and War*, p. 146.

86. CB to the Chairman and Committee of Relief of Mt. Vernon, n.d. [c. March 1888], CB letterbook, CB-LC.

87. CB, address given before the Philadelphia Charity Organization Society, November 1886, CB letterbook; also CB to William Hayes Ward, May 2, 1891, both CB-LC.

88. Buckingham, *Clara Barton*, p. 157; quotation *Evansville Daily Journal* (Ind.), April 3, 1884.

89. CB quoted in Buckingham, *Clara Barton*, p. 158.

90. *Evansville Daily Courier* quoted in Gaeddert, "American Red Cross," n.d., 2, ANRC.

91. CB, Address for Annual Meeting of Congregational Clergymen, June 19, 1888, CB-LC.

92. CB to S. Jane Trueblood, May 10, 1884, CB letterbook, CB-LC.

93. Roy Lubrove, *The Professional Altruists* (Cambridge: Harvard University Press, 1965); and James Leiby, *A History of Social Welfare and Social Work in the United States* (New York: Columbia University Press, 1978).

94. CB to Anna Barton Bigelow, August 1887, ANRC.

95. Ibid.; and Grand Duchess Louise to CB, June 8, 1887, photocopy, RARC NARS.

96. CB, "Fourth International Conference of the Red Cross at Carlsruhe," September 1887, CB letterbook, CB-LC.

97. Report on the Fourth International Red Cross Conference (Senate document No. 231), August 10, 1888; and Lucy M. Hall, "De Temporibus et Moribus," *Vassar Miscellany* 17, no. 3 (December 1882): 99.

98. CB, unpublished article written for *New York Herald*, July 26, 1888; and Lucy M. Hall to CB, October 30, 1887, both CB-LC.

99. Louise to CB, June 8, 1887, RARC NARS; Julian B. Hubbell to Colonel John McElroy, October 12, 1887, CB letterbook, CB-LC; and Epler, *Life*, pp. 251–55.

100. CB to Mr. Chute, January 2, 1890, ANRC.

101. CB to Kate Gannett Wells, November 27, 1885, CB letterbook, CB-LC.

102. CB to Alice Stone Blackwell, February 25, 1885, CB letterbook, CB-LC; and Eleanor Flexner, *Century of Struggle* (New York: Atheneum, 1974), pp. 175–77.

103. CB to Susan B. Anthony, March 4, 1887, CB letterbook, CB-LC.

104. CB, "The Crown" (written for the Women's International Congress), March 1888, CB-LC.

105. CB to Cousin Lucy, March 14, 1885, CB letterbook, CB-LC.

106. CB, response to breakfast invitation at Delmonicos, n.d., CB-LC.

107. CB to Herbert Barton, November 3, 1888, CB letterbook, CB-LC.

108. CB to Alma E. Richardson, April 8, 1888, CB letterbook, CB-LC.

109. CB to Wells, November 27, 1885, CB-LC.

110. "Miss Clara Barton on Women's Rights," *Boston Commonwealth*, July 7, 1888.

111. CB, *Peace and War*, pp. 147–48; and Portia Kernodle, *The Red Cross Nurse in Action, 1882–1948* (New York: Harper Brothers, 1949), pp. 9–11.

112. CB to F. R. Southmayd, October 19, 1883, CB letterbook, CB-LC.

113. CB, *Peace and War*, p. 148.

114. F. R. Southmayd to CB, September 26, 1888, CB-LC; and Southmayd quoted in Kernodle, *Red Cross Nurse*, p. 9.

115. Kernodle, *Red Cross Nurse*, p. 9; "Too High Toned," *St. Louis Post Dispatch*, Sep-

tember 23, 1888; "Drunken Red Cross Nurses," *New York World*, September 16, 1888; and "The Trouble at Jacksonville," *New York World*, September 23, 1888.

116. Kernodle, *Red Cross Nurse*, p. 10.

117. CB, *Peace and War*, pp. 150–54.

118. CB to Mr. and Mrs. Richard J. Hinton, July 12, 1889, CB letterbook, CB-LC.

119. Ibid.

120. CB to William Panwart, October 2, 1888, CB letterbook, CB-LC; and Minutes of the Association of the American Red Cross, May 4, 1893, typescript, RARC NARS.

121. CB to B. W. Bernard, October 8, 1888, CB letterbook, CB-LC.

122. Minutes of American Red Cross, May 4, 1893, typescript, RARC NARS.

123. Julian B. Hubbell to "Cousin," October 24, 1888, CB-LC.

124. Julian B. Hubbell to J. Wilkes O'Neill, March 17, 1888, CB letterbook, CB-LC; F. L. Krieger to CB, November 8, 1889, CB-LC; quotation CB to Richard Chute, January 2, 1890, typescript, RARC NARS; draft of act of Congress to protect Red Cross insignia, n.d. [1888], CB-LC.

125. CB to Dr. Dalles, June 25, 1889, CB letterbook; and CB to Lydia A. Scott, May 1, 1887, both CB-LC.

126. In-house memo relating to Red Cross trademark, August 2, 1946, RARC NARS.

127. CB, notes on Carlsruhe, 1887, CB-LC.

128. CB to Stephen E. Barton, July 5, 1888, CB-LC.

129. CB to John Hoyt, January 19, 1886, CB letterbook, CB-LC.

130. CB to Stephen E. Barton, July 19, 1886, CB letterbook, CB-LC.

131. CB to Lizzie Tittle, November 22, 1889, CB-LC; and CB to Ida Riccius, February 13, 1884, AAS.

132. CBJ, May 17, 1885, CB-LC.

133. CB to Enola Gardner, January 24, 1889, CB letterbook, CB-LC.

134. Gaeddert, "American Red Cross," n.d., 2:87, ANRC; and David G. McCullough, *The Johnstown Flood* (New York: Simon and Schuster, 1968).

135. Nettie Louise White to General W. H. Sears, November 6, 1916, typescript, RARC NARS.

136. CB, "Remarks Made at Williard Hotel," November 2, 1889, CB letterbook, CB-LC.

137. CB, *Peace and War*, p. 159.

138. "Flood Just Part of Little Known Tale Behind Johnstown Woes," *Washington Evening Star*, May 30, 1939; and note from *New York Tribune*, June 5, 1887, clipping in RARC NARS.

139. "Flood Just Part of Tale," *Washington Evening Star*, May 30, 1939.

140. CB to Elizabeth B. Roe, October 16, 1889, CB letterbook, CB-LC; and CB, *Peace and War*, p. 159.

141. Gaeddert, "American Red Cross," n.d., 2:87, ANRC; "Red Cross Consolidation," *Pittsburgh Dispatch*, June 17, 1889; and CB to "My precious sister Emilie," June 24, 1889, CB letterbook, CB-LC.

142. CB to Robert Hunt Lyman, June 22, 1889, CB letterbook, CB-LC.

143. Gaeddert, "American Red Cross," n.d., 2:90, ANRC.

144. CB to Ellen C. Platt, July 4, 1889, CB letterbook, CB-LC.

145. Richard J. Hinton, untitled article on Red Cross at Johnstown, n.d., CB-LC; and CB, *Peace and War*, p. 164.

146. Ellen Henle, "Against the Fearful Odds," draft Ph.D. Thesis, Case Western Re-

serve University, 1976, p. 87; "Arrival of Relief Goods," *Chicago Inter-Ocean*, June 7, 1889; and CB to General John B. Dennis, July 12, 1889, ANRC.

147. CB to Stephen E. Barton, August 22, 1889, CB-LC.

148. Ibid.

149. CB to Peter De Graw, August 15, 1889, CB letterbook, CB-LC.

150. CB to Mary Barton, October 15, 1889, CB letterbook, CB-LC.

151. Governor Beaver quoted in CB, *Peace and War*, p. 169.

152. "Miss Clara Barton," *Johnstown Democrat*, October 17, 1889.

153. "Farewell to Miss Barton," *Johnstown Daily Tribune*, October 23, 1889.

Chapter 15

1. For correspondence pertaining to the aftermath of Johnstown, see CB letterbook, CB-LC.

2. Cortlandt Whitehead to CB, December 11, 1889, CB-LC; and CB, *The Red Cross in Peace and War* (Washington, D.C.: American Historical Press, 1899), p. 168.

3. CB to Dr. [Julian] Hubbell, December 18, 1889, CB-LC.

4. CB to Delia Robbins, January 17, 1891, CB letterbook, CB-LC.

5. CB to Stephen E. Barton, March 26, 1891, CB letterbook, CB-LC; and Edwin Baltzley, *Glen Echo on the Potomac, The Washington Rhine* (privately published, 1891); quotation CB to Delia Robbins, April 22, 1891, CB letterbook, CB-LC.

6. CB to Delia Robbins, June 7, 1891, CB letterbook, CB-LC.

7. CB to Stephen E. Barton, April 8, 1893, CB-LC.

8. CB to Ida Riccius, December 13, 1890 [1891], CB letterbook, CB-LC.

9. CB to William Windom, June 21, 1890, CB letterbook; CB to Walter Phillips, February 24, 1890, CB letterbook; and Brief for Senate Committee on Foreign Relations on Red Cross Bill, 1892, all CB-LC.

10. CB to Mary Elizabeth Almon, July 4, 1890, CB letterbook; and Joseph Sheldon to CB, July 17, 1890, both CB-LC.

11. CB to Joseph Sheldon, February 5, 1890, CB letterbook, CB-LC.

12. CB to Joseph Gardner, May 6, 1890; and minutes of meeting of American National Red Cross, May 1891, both CB letterbook; also Constitution of American National Red Cross, n.d. [1892], all CB-LC.

13. CB to N. P. Elliot, June 20, 1890, CB letterbook, CB-LC.

14. "The Red Cross Donation," *Washington Post*, November 1, 1892.

15. CB to Edwin Lee Brown, February 5, 1890; CB to J. B. Bremer, February 2, 1890; and CB to editor of *Courier Journal*, April 6, 1890, all CB-LC; and Gustave R. Gaeddert, "The History of the American National Red Cross," unpublished MS, n.d., 2:101, ANRC.

16. CB to J. B. Vinet, August 19, 1892, CB letterbook, CB-LC.

17. CB to John Morlan, March 13, 1893, RARC NARS.

18. CB, *Peace and War*, p. 175; Gaeddert, "American Red Cross," n.d., 2:114, ANRC; and quotation in Merle Curti, *American Philanthropy Abroad* (New Brunswick, N.J.: Rutgers University Press, 1963), p. 99.

19. Curti, *American Philanthropy*, pp. 100–109.

20. Clyde E. Buckingham, *Clara Barton, A Broad Humanity* (Alexandria, Va.: privately published, 1980), p. 167; and Gaeddert, "American Red Cross," n.d., 2: 112, ANRC.

21. CB, miscellaneous notes on Russian famine, n.d. [1892], CB-LC.

22. Curti, *American Philanthropy*, pp. 103–5; and Alice French, "An Appeal to the People of Iowa," newspaper clipping, December 19, 1891, CB-LC.

23. "Terrible State of Affairs," *Davenport Democrat*, December 23, 1891; "The Awful Truth," undated clipping, CB-LC; and Alexander Johnson to CB, February 22, 1892, CB-LC.

24. See Curti, *American Philanthropy*, pp. 103–5, 119.

25. CB to L. G. Jeffrey, August 12, 1892, CB letterbook, CB-LC.

26. Curti, *American Philanthropy*, p. 114; letters of B. F. Tillinghast to CB, CB-LC; and quotation, Robert Ogden to Governor [John] Hoyt, February 17, 1892, CB-LC.

27. Curti, *American Philanthropy*, p. 117; and CB, *Peace and War*, pp. 184–96.

28. Ibid.

29. Robert Ogden to Spencer Trask, December 31, 1895, O-LC.

30. Buckingham, *Clara Barton*, p. 167; "A Woman Commissioner," *New York World*, April 29, 1892; "Mrs. M. Louise Thomas Home," *New York World*, November 2, 1892; and CB to E. Louise Demorest, August 6, 1892, CB letterbook, CB-LC.

31. Myrtis Wilmot Barton, "Clara Barton and the Red Cross," 1896, typescript, CB-LC; and photograph of house in CB, *Peace and War*, p. 22.

32. Myrtis Wilmot Barton, "CB and the Red Cross," 1896, typescript, CB-LC.

33. CB to Marietta Holley, May 29, 1895, CB letterbook, CB-LC.

34. See Constance McLaughlin Green, *Washington, A History of the Capital, 1800–1950* (Princeton: Princeton University Press, 1962), pp. 77–100; and George Kennan Papers, LC.

35. CB to Edith Riccius, March 12, 1889, AAS.

36. CB to Delia Robbins, April 14, 1893, CB letterbook, CB-LC; and CB to John Morlan, March 18, 1893, RARC NARS.

37. CB to Gustave Moynier, April 26, 1893; quotation CB to Lizzie Tittle, February 7, 1893, CB letterbook, both CB-LC.

38. "An Interesting Reception," *Baltimore American*, February 25, 1893; "Red Cross Association," *Washington Evening News*, February 25, 1893; CB to Mary Elizabeth Almon, March 8, 1893, CB letterbook, CB-LC; quotation CB to Francis J. Dyer, March 13, 1893, CB letterbook, CB-LC.

39. Julian B. Hubbell to B. F. Tillinghast, March 2, 1893, CB letterbook, CB-LC.

40. Joseph Gardner to CB, February 10, 1893, CB-LC.

41. Buckingham, *Clara Barton*, p. 199. For a picture of Joseph and Enola Gardner, see CB, *Peace and War*, p. 55.

42. Copy of deed in Buckingham, *Clara Barton*, p. 206.

43. CB to Joseph Gardner, March 18, 1893, CB-LC; and CB to Mary Elizabeth Almon, quoted in Buckingham, *Clara Barton*, p. 217, also pp. 212–13.

44. CB to John Morlan, February 5, 1893, RARC NARS.

45. Buckingham, *Clara Barton*, p. 225.

46. Ibid., p. 220.

47. CBJ, July 4, 1893, CB-LC.

48. CB to Stephen E. Barton, August 6, 1893, CB letterbook, CB-LC.

49. CB to Joseph and Enola Gardner, April 10, 1893, CB letterbook, CB-LC.

50. CB to John Morlan, August 23, 1893, RARC NARS.

51. CBJ, July 18, 1893, CB-LC.

52. Gaeddert, "American Red Cross," n.d., 2:93–95, ANRC.

53. CB, *Peace and War*, p. 201.

54. CB, "Explanation of the System of Work Adopted by the Red Cross in the Sea Islands," n.d., CB-LC.

55. CB to William E. Stowe, October 4, 1893, CB letterbook, CB-LC.

56. CB quoted in Joel Chandler Harris, "The Sea Islands' Hurricane: The Relief," *Scribner's Magazine* 15, no. 3 (March 1894): 272.

57. CB to J. J. Elwell, July 5, 1894, CB letterbook, CB-LC.

58. CB, *The Story of the Red Cross: Glimpses of Field Work* (New York: D. Appleton Co., 1904), p. 80.

59. CB, unfinished letter, n.d. [c. 1894], CB-LC.

60. CB to Charles Hebard, January 3, 1893 [1894], CB-LC.

61. CBJ, October 1, 1893, CB-LC.

62. Harris, "Sea Islands' Hurricane," p. 271; and CB, *Glimpses of Field Work*, pp. 79–84.

63. CB, *Glimpses of Field Work*, p. 78; and CB, *Peace and War*, pp. 224–25.

64. CB, *Peace and War*, pp. 254–58.

65. Harris, "Sea Islands' Hurricane," p. 347.

66. CB, "John Morlan," n.d. [c. 1902], CB-LC; and J. L. Jackson to John Morlan, June 5, 1898, RARC NARS.

67. CB to John Morlan, August 17, 1894, RARC NARS.

68. Jackson to Morlan, June 5, 1898, RARC NARS.

69. "Report of Shipping Room, Medical Surgical and Sanitary Departments," n.d. [c. 1894], CB-LC; and Gaeddert, "American Red Cross," n.d., 2:98, ANRC.

70. CB to Hebard, January 3, 1893 [1894], CB-LC.

71. CBJ, November 28, 1893, CB-LC; Julian B. Hubbell to B. F. Tillinghast, May 13, 1894, Red Cross letterbook, RARC NARS.

72. Buckingham, *Clara Barton*, p. 240.

73. CB, *Glimpses of Field Work*, p. 92.

74. George Pullman to Annie T. Belcher, May 20, 1894, Red Cross letterbook, RARC NARS; and Julian B. Hubbell, "Some Personal Traits of Miss Clara Barton," unpublished MS, n.d., CBNHS.

75. CB, *Peace and War*, p. 197.

76. Ibid., p. 168.

77. See CB to Julian B. Hubbell, June 21, 1894, CB letterbook, CB-LC; "Letter by Committee to the Press," n.d., Red Cross letterbook, RARC NARS; and "Cursing the Red Cross!" *Columbia Daily Register* (S.C.), May 25, 1894.

78. George Kennan to Mrs. Parker, July 8, 1892, CB-LC.

79. James L. Barton to Talcott Williams, January 20, 1896, O-LC.

80. Gustave Moynier to CB, September 24, 1890, CB-LC.

81. Sophia Wells Royce Williams, "Miss Clara Barton and the Red Cross," *The Review of Reviews* 9, no. 50 (March 1894): 315.

82. John Morlan to Mabel Boardman, August 23, 1903, RARC NARS.

83. CB, "John Morlan," n.d. [c. 1902], CB-LC.

84. Buckingham, *Clara Barton*, p. 207; and Robert Ogden to Spencer Trask, December 31, 1895, O-LC.

85. Daniel Boyles to Robert Ogden, January 3, 1896, O-LC.

86. Williams, "Clara Barton and Red Cross," p. 315.

87. CBJ, September 1, 1896, CB-LC.

88. CB to George M. Pullman, August 25, 1895, CB letterbook; also Kennan to Parker, July 8, 1892, both CB-LC.

89. CB to Elwell, July 5, 1894, CB letterbook, CB-LC.

90. CB quoted in Buckingham, *Clara Barton*, p. 208.

91. Minutes of meeting of the American National Red Cross, January 26, 1895, CB-LC.

92. CB to Peter De Graw, August 14, 1893, CB letterbook, CB-LC.

93. Members of the American National Red Cross to Gustave Moynier, December 14, 1892, copy in CB-LC.

94. See "Injustice to Miss Barton," *Augusta Chronicle* (Ga.), April 30, 1894.

95. CB to Edwin Lee Brown, February 5, 1890, CB letterbook, CB-LC.

96. CB to Myrtis Barton, n.d. [c. 1895], CB-LC.

97. CB to Annie Wittenmeyer, October 11, 1890, CB letterbook; CB to Edmund Dwight, December 14, 1890; CB to "My poor dear sick friend," May 28, 1892; CB to Samuel Barton, March 25, 1894, typescript; and GPJ, February 9, 1896, all CB-LC.

98. CB to Mary Elizabeth Almon, n.d. [c. 1893], CB letterbook, CB-LC; and Williams, *Daughter of Destiny*, pp. 319–20.

99. See CBJ, 1893, CB-LC.

100. CB to Stephen E. Barton, March 26, 1891, CB letterbook, CB-LC.

101. CB to Leonora Halsted, September 11, 1891 [1892], CB-LC.

102. Mrs. Stephen E. Barton to Saidee Riccius, August 1918, typescript, AAS.

103. CB to John Morlan, August 17, 1894, RARC NARS.

104. See, for example, CB letterbook, July–August 1894, CB-LC.

105. "Presentation of Grand Army Post to Clara Barton," March 12, 1894, typescript, CB-LC.

106. Mary Desha to CB, November 6, 1890, CB-LC; GPJ, September 16 and 17, 1895, CB-LC; "Decoration Day," n.d. [May 1894], Red Cross letterbook, RARC NARS; and "Clara Barton to Guests," *New York Times*, September 23, 1892.

107. CB to Mrs. F. E. Russell, January 5, 1891, CB letterbook, CB-LC.

108. CB, "If Women Came to Congress What Would Be the Result?" October 16, 1895, CB letterbook, CB-LC.

109. Sarah J. Elliot to CB, June 6, 1890, CB-LC. For more information about Barton's feminist activities at this time, see Susan B. Anthony to CB, July 28, 1890; May Wright Sewell to CB, September 30, 1890; CB, "Harriet Austin," January 1893; CB to May Wright Sewell, April 20, 1893; CB to Bernard Vassall, May 27, 1893; CB, "Tribute to Elizabeth Cady Stanton," November 12, 1875; and GPJ, October 5–8, 1895, all CB-LC.

110. CB to Isabella Candle, February 7, 1893, CB letterbook; and, "The Women Who Went to the Field," 1891, typescript, both CB-LC.

111. Foster Rhea Dulles, *The American Red Cross: A History* (New York: Harper Brothers, 1950), p. 25.

112. Draft of letter from CB to Gustave Moynier, March 11, 1895, CB-LC.

113. Ibid.

114. Buckingham, *Clara Barton*, p. 252.

115. Copy of letter from John Morlan to CB, August 4, 1894, RARC NARS.

116. CB to John Morlan, August 17, 1894, RARC NARS.

117. CBJ, January 18–20, 1895, typescript, CB-LC.

118. Stephen E. Barton to W. B. Scofield, August 19, 1916, RARC NARS; and CBJ, January 20, 1895, CB-LC.

119. CBJ, January 20, 1895, CB-LC.

120. Ibid., January 21, 1895.

121. GPJ, October 21–29, 1895, CB-LC.

122. CBJ, January 10, 1896, CB-LC.

123. Lord Kross, *The Ottoman Centuries: The Rise and Fall of the Turkish Empire* (New York: Morrow Quill Paperbacks, 1977), pp. 554–63; Gaeddert, "American Red Cross," n.d., 2:118, ANRC; and Curti, *American Philanthropy*, pp. 119–20.

124. Curti, *American Philanthropy*, pp. 120–22; CB, *Peace and War*, p. 329; and CB, *Glimpses of Field Work*, pp. 94–95.

125. GPJ, December 14, 1895, CB-LC.

126. CB, *Glimpses of Field Work*, p. 97; quotation CB to Mrs. George Kennan, December 27, 1895, CB letterbook, CB-LC.

127. Robert Ogden to Spencer Trask, December 31, 1895, O-LC.

128. CBJ, January 9, 1896, CB-LC.

129. Ibid., January 22, 1896; and CB, *Glimpses of Field Work*, p. 97.

130. Dulles, *American Red Cross*, p. 37.

131. See GPJ, January–February 1896, CB-LC; CB to Stephen Barton, February 25, 1896, CB-LC; and Gaeddert, "American Red Cross," n.d., 2:122, ANRC.

132. CB, *Peace and War*, pp. 278–80, quotation p. 280.

133. Gaeddert, "American Red Cross," n.d., 2:123, ANRC.

134. Ibid.; and L. W. Bacon to Robert Ogden, January 28, 1896, O-LC.

135. Dr. Caleb Frank Gates quoted in Curti, *American Philanthropy*, p. 129; also CB, *Glimpses of Field Work*, p. 107; and CB, *Peace and War*, p. 295.

136. CB, *Glimpses of Field Work*, pp. 109–10.

137. Dr. Ira Harris quoted in CB, *Peace and War*, p. 353.

138. Ibid., pp. 294–95 and 354–55; and CB, *Glimpses of Field Work*, pp. 102–6.

139. CB to Leonora Halsted, April 29, 1896, CB-LC; and CB, *Peace and War*, pp. 305–7.

140. See CBJ, March 14–18, 1896, CB-LC.

141. H[alip] Bogigian to J. Ellen Foster, May 1, 1903, RARC NARS.

142. CB, private notes on Turkey, n.d. [1896], CB-LC.

143. CB, *Peace and War*, p. 285; see also Stephen E. Barton to CB, April 7 and May 27, 1896, CB-LC.

144. CB, *Peace and War*, p. 289.

145. CB to Lizzie Barton, May 13, 1896, typescript, CB-LC.

146. CBJ, June 5, 1896, CB-LC.

147. CB to Lizzie Barton, May 13, 1896, CB-LC.

148. CBJ, September 1, 1896, CB-LC.

149. Dr. Ira Harris quoted in Buckingham, *Clara Barton*, p. 261.

150. Program of reception for CB, October 8, 1896, CB-LC.

151. Williams, *Daughter of Destiny*, pp. 341–42.

Chapter 16

1. Thomas A. Bailey and David M. Kennedy, eds., *The American Pageant* (Boston: D.C. Heath Co., 1956), pp. 615–16; and Margaret Leech, *In the Days of McKinley* (New York: Harper Brothers, 1959), pp. 161–62.

2. Editorial in *New York Tribune*, January 10, 1897.

3. CB to Annie A. Williamson, May 28, 1897, CB-LC; and "Clara Barton's Name," *Washington Post,* June 14, 1897.

4. GPJ, June 14–July 14, 1897, CB-LC.

5. Elizabeth B. Pryor, "Clara Barton National Historic Site: Report on the Historic Grounds 1891–1912," March 1977, National Park Service, CBNHS, p. 5.

6. CB to Mrs. Johnson, May 8, 1897. See also CBJ, February 1897; and GPJ, February 26, 1897, both CB-LC.

7. CB to Ida B. Riccius, May 8, 1897, CB-LC.

8. See Charles H. Snell, "Clara Barton National Historic Site: Report on the Historic Structure," National Park Service, 1976.

9. Pictures of the house interior are found in CB, *The Red Cross in Peace and War* (Washington, D.C.: American Historical Press, 1899), p. 144. See also Percy Epler, *The Life of Clara Barton* (New York: Macmillan, 1915), pp. 364–65; and William E. Barton, *The Life of Clara Barton* (Boston: Houghton Mifflin Co., 1922), 2:308–9.

10. Julian B. Hubbell, "Some Personal Traits of Miss Clara Barton," unpublished MS, n.d., CBNHS.

11. CB to Dr. Monae Lesser, November 28, 1897, CB-LC.

12. CBJ, September 11, October 4, 1897, CB-LC; CB to Countess de Brazza, August 27, 1897, CB-LC; CB to Lucy Hall, August 28, 1897, CB-LC; and CB to A. O. Bunnell, October 9, 1897, in "International Red Cross," *Dansville Advertiser,* October 14, 1897.

13. Merle Curti, *American Philanthropy Abroad* (New Brunswick, N.J.: Rutgers University Press, 1963), p. 199; CB to President of the United States, July 9, 1897, CB-LC; CB to William Sulzer, January 10, 1898, CB-LC; and CBJ, June 23, 1897, CB-LC.

14. CBJ, June 21–23 and July 12, 1897 (quotation June 21), CB-LC.

15. Ibid., June 14, 1897.

16. Ibid., November 30, 1897; and CB to Dupuy de Lôme, November 30, 1897, CB-LC.

17. CB to Lesser, November 28, 1897, CB-LC.

18. CB to "My dear Anna," December 18, 1896, CB-LC.

19. Ibid. A rare photograph of Pullman is found in Laura Doolittle, "Clara Barton and the Red Cross," *The Commercial Traveler's Home Magazine* 4, no. 4 (April 1895): 523.

20. See CBJ, January 1–May 1, 1897, also September 16, 1897–January 29, 1898, CB-LC.

21. Ibid., June 10–July 15, 1893, quotation November 30, 1897, CB-LC.

22. Stephen E. Barton to CB, July 18, 1897, CB-LC.

23. Julian B. Hubbell to Stephen E. Barton, December 4, 1897, CB-LC.

24. CBJ, January 15, 1898, CB-LC.

25. "George Pullman's Wife Sues," unidentified clipping in CB scrapbook, n.d.; and CBJ, December 7 and 22, 1897, both CB-LC.

26. CBJ, January 15, 1898, CB-LC.

27. Ibid., July 11, 1897.

28. Ellen Spencer Mussey to CB, April 30, 1898; and CB to Royal Pullman, December 9, 1897, both CB-LC.

29. CB, *Peace and War,* p. 519; and Alvey A. Adee to CB, January 1, 1898, CB-LC.

30. Broadsides from John Sherman, Secretary of State, and Cuban Central Relief Committee, January 8 and February 10, 1898, CB-LC.

31. Louis Klopsch to CB, January 31, 1898; and Stephen E. Barton to William R. Day, February 1, 1898, both CB-LC.

32. CB, *Peace and War*, pp. 519–20; CBJ, January 20–29, 1898, CB-LC; and Letter of Introduction from William McKinley, February 4, 1898, CB-LC.

33. CB quoted in Foster Rhea Dulles, *The American Red Cross: A History* (New York: Harper Brothers, 1950), p. 44; and CB to Stephen E. Barton, February 11, 1898, RARC NARS.

34. CB, *The Story of the Red Cross: Glimpses of Field Work* (New York: D. Appleton Co., 1904), pp. 115–16.

35. CB to B. F. Tillinghast, February 16, 1898, RARC NARS.

36. CB quoted in W. E. Barton, *Life* 2:284.

37. CB to Stephen E. Barton, February 16, 1898, RARC NARS; and Curti, *American Philanthropy*, p. 202.

38. CB, *Peace and War*, pp. 519, 527–31 (quotation p. 529); and Gustave R. Gaeddert, "The History of the American National Red Cross," unpublished MS, 2:139, ANRC.

39. CB, *Peace and War*, pp. 531–32; and Redfield Proctor, "The Condition of Cuba: It Is Not Peace, Nor Is It War" (Washington, D.C.: Government Printing Office, 1898).

40. Proctor, "Condition of Cuba," pp. 9–10.

41. Fitzhugh Lee to William R. Day, March 1, 1898, copy in CB-LC.

42. Charles M. Pepper, *Lifework of Louis Klopsch: Romance of a Modern Knight of Mercy* (New York: Christian Herald, 1910), frontispiece.

43. Stephen E. Baraton to CB, February 18, 1898, copy in CB-LC.

44. Pepper, *Louis Klopsch*, pp. 117–18; and Curti, *American Philanthropy*, p. 203.

45. CB to Stephen E. Barton, April 14, 1898, CB-LC.

46. "Quarrel Impending," *New York Herald*, March 26, 1898.

47. See "Says Miss Barton Will Be Upheld," *New York Herald*, March 25, 1898.

48. "Red Cross Gives Up Cuban Work," *New York Herald*, March 24, 1898.

49. Curti, *American Philanthropy*, pp. 203–4; and Stephen E. Barton to M. H. Bright, March 29, 1898, copy in CB-LC.

50. Bailey and Kennedy, eds., *American Pageant*, p. 618.

51. CB, *Peace and War*, pp. 549–50.

52. See extracts of CB to Stephen E. Barton, April 30, 1898; and CBJ, April and May 1898 (quotation April 30), all CB-LC.

53. CB to Stephen E. Barton, May 21, 1898; also CBJ, May 2, 1898, both CB-LC.

54. Stephen E. Barton to CB, May 9, 1898, copy in CB-LC.

55. CB to Stephen E. Barton, May 21, 1898, CB-LC.

56. CB to Stephen E. Barton, May 10, 1898; and CBJ, May 8 and 9, 1898, all CB-LC.

57. CB to Stephen Barton, May 21, 1898, CB-LC.

58. CBJ, May 11, 1898, CB-LC.

59. *Proceedings of the 5th Annual Meeting of the Association of Military Surgeons of the United States* (Cincinnati: Earhart and Richardson, 1896), pp. 98–99.

60. Ibid., p. 339.

61. "Memoirs of Admiral [William] Van Reypen," unpublished MS, n.d., in possession of Mrs. Edward A. C. Russell, Landrum, S.C.

62. Gaeddert, "American Red Cross," n.d., 2:49–50, 161–65, ANRC; CB, *Peace and War*, pp. 425–69; and *Report of American National Red Cross Relief Committee Reports, May 1898–March 1899* (New York: Knickerbocker Press, 1900).

63. CB to William T. Wardwell, May 21, 1898, CB-LC.

64. CB to Malina Cleaver Faville, May 19, 1898, CB-LC.

65. George Kennan to William Wardwell, June 3, 1898; and George Kennan to Charles Schieren, June 18, 1898, both CB-LC.

66. CBJ, June 22, 1898, CBNHS; and CB, *Peace and War*, p. 557.

67. Ibid.; and George Kennan, *Campaigning in Cuba* (Port Washington, N.Y.: Kennikat Press, 1971), p. 84.

68. CB, *Peace and War*, p. 557.

69. CB, *Glimpses of Field Work*, pp. 128–29.

70. Joseph Gardner to Stephen E. Barton, May 17, 1898, CB-LC; and Kennan, *Campaigning in Cuba*, pp. 132–33.

71. CB to Sir Vincent K. Barrington, August 24, 1898, CB-LC.

72. CBJ quoted in CB, *Glimpses of Field Work*, p. 131.

73. Kennan, *Campaigning in Cuba*, p. 84; and CB, *Peace and War*, p. 558.

74. CB, *Glimpses of Field Work*, pp. 126–27.

75. Ibid., pp. 126–31; CB to Barrington, August 24, 1898, CB-LC; and Report of A. Monae Lesser, *Relief Committee Reports*, pp. 174–209.

76. Julian B. Hubbell to Sarah B. Earle, September 28, 1898, CB-LC.

77. CB, *Glimpses of Field Work*, p. 130.

78. CB to Theodore Kruger, May 9, 1898, CB-LC.

79. CB to Marion E. Balcom, June 23, 1898, CB-LC.

80. Report of A. Monae Lesser, *Relief Committee Reports*, p. 201.

81. Portia Kernodle, *The Red Cross Nurse in Action, 1882–1948* (New York: Harper Brothers, 1949), pp. 22–23; and Gaeddert, "American Red Cross," n.d., 2:145–48, ANRC.

82. George M. Sternberg to B. H. Warner, July 15, 1898, Records of the Surgeon General's Office, Record Group 112, NARS; Kernodle, *Red Cross Nurse*, pp. 18–19; Gaeddert, "American Red Cross," n.d., 2:146, ANRC.

83. "Defines His Position," *Washington Times*, August 30, 1898; Gaeddert, "American Red Cross," n.d., 2:146, ANRC.

84. Dulles, *American Red Cross*, pp. 53–55.

85. Lavinia K. Dock, Sarah Elizabeth Pickett, Clara D. Noyes, Fannie F. Clement, Elizabeth G. Fox, Anna R. Van Meter, *History of American Red Cross Nursing* (New York: Macmillan, 1922), p. 36; and Kernodle, *Red Cross Nurse*, p. 28.

86. George Kennan to CB, August 4, 1898, K-LC.

87. Ibid.

88. CB to George Kennan, August 1, 1898, K-LC.

89. Kennan to CB, August 4, 1898; George Kennan to Mrs. Kennan, July 13, 1898; and draft of letter from George Kennan to CB, May 17, 1900, all K-LC.

90. CB, *Peace and War*, pp. 573–76.

91. Ibid., pp. 576–77; quotation Kennan, *Campaigning in Cuba*, p. 159.

92. Henry M. Lathrop, *Under the Red Cross Flag* (New York: F. B. Warner, 1898), p. 153.

93. Kennan, *Campaigning in Cuba*, pp. 170, 174, 188–91 (quotation p. 191).

94. CB quoted in Epler, *Life*, p. 300.

95. CB, *Peace and War*, pp. 569–70.

96. CB to Stephen E. Barton, August 3, 1898, CB-LC.

97. CB, *Peace and War*, pp. 626, 629.

98. L. H. Goudy to Stephen E. Barton, September 17, 1898, CB-LC.

99. CB, *Peace and War*, pp. 629–30; and CBJ, August 30, 1898, CBNHS.

100. See letters of Stephen E. Barton relating to Red Cross work in Cuba, CB-LC.

101. CB to Stephen E. Barton, October 3, 1898, CB-LC.

102. Stephen E. Barton to CB, July 20 and 30, 1898, CB-LC.

103. CB to Stephen E. Barton, August 11, 1898, CB-LC.

104. General Order No. 3, n.d. [August 1898], CB-LC.

105. Stephen E. Barton to CB, August 23, 1898, CB-LC.

106. CB to Stephen E. Barton, August 6, 1898, CB-LC.

107. Dock et al., *Red Cross Nursing*, p. 34.

108. Janet Jennings quoted in CB, *Glimpses of Field Work*, p. 141.

109. Kernodle, *Red Cross Nurse*, p. 21; Dulles, *American Red Cross*, p. 53.

110. Edith Riccius King, "Reminiscences of Great Aunt Clara Barton," 1938, CB-LC.

111. See "The Century's Heroines," *Omaha Bee*, July 18, 1892; "One of the World's Heroines," *Newburgh Journal* (New York), May 13, 1894; CB, autobiographical sketch for *Who's Who in America*, 1898, CB-LC; and *Twelfth Decennial Census of the United States* (1900), Montgomery County, Md., NARS.

112. King, "Reminiscences," 1938; and Lucy Hall Brown to CB, n.d. [July 1898], both CB-LC.

113. King, "Reminiscences," 1938, CB-LC.

114. CBJ, December 21, 1897, CB-LC.

115. Ibid., June 14, 1897.

116. Conversation with Herman and Saidee Riccius, 1919, typescript, AAS; and King, "Reminiscences," 1938, CB-LC.

117. King, "Reminiscences," 1938, CB-LC; and "Mrs. Thomas Home Again," *New York Recorder*, November 1, 1892.

118. See Ishbel Ross, *Angel of the Battlefield: The Life of Clara Barton* (New York: Harper and Row, 1956), p. 264; and Blanche Colton Williams, *Clara Barton: Daughter of Destiny* (Philadelphia: J. B. Lippincott Co., 1941), p. 433.

119. King, "Reminiscences," 1938; and CBJ, June 22, 1898, both CB-LC.

120. See CBJ, September–December 1898, CBNHS; and CB to Stephen E. Barton, September–December 1898, CB-LC.

121. CB to Mrs. J. G. Lemmon, March 28, 1899, CB-LC.

122. CB to Joseph Gardner, November 7, 1898, CB-LC.

123. Ibid.

124. CBJ, October 30, 1898, CBNHS; and CB to A. K. Keller, December 31, 1898, CB-LC.

125. CB to Ida B. Riccius, January 26, 1901, AAS; also CB to Joseph Sheldon, March 17, 1899, CB-LC.

126. Stephen E. Barton to CB, February 8, 1899, CB-LC.

127. See CB to Fannie B. Ward, April 15, 1899; CB to Dr. Alexander Kent, March 14, 1899; Stephen E. Barton to CB, November 14, 1898; and Stephen E. Barton to Louise M. Gordon, November 5, 1898, all CB-LC. Quotation Charles H. Cottrell to Stephen E. Barton, October 14, 1898, CB-LC.

128. CB to Ward, April 15, 1899, CB-LC.

129. CB to Stephen E. Barton, March 30, 1899; also CB to Dr. E. M. Moore, October 14, 1899, both CB-LC.

130. CB to Dr. Alexander Kent, March 14, 1899, CB-LC.

131. Julio Carbonell, "Labors of the Red Cross in Cuba," 1899, CBNHS.

132. Julian B. Hubbell, "Report . . . of His Work During Its Commencement in the Month of April & Its Better Progress in May," 1899, CB-LC.

133. CB to Fanny B. Ward, April 25, 1899, CB-LC.

134. Dulles, *American Red Cross*, p. 60.

135. Albert LeGendre, "Clara Barton & I in Cuba," March 16, 1956, RARC NARS; and Carbonell, "Labors of the Red Cross," 1899, CBNHS.

136. LeGendre, "Barton & I in Cuba," March 16, 1956, RARC NARS.

137. CB to Charles A. Schieren, November 7, 1899, CB-LC.

138. John Joy Edison to George C. Boldt, April 13, 1899, CB-LC.

139. See CB to Stephen E. Barton, February 22, 1899; Joseph Sheldon to CB, April 24, 1899; and quotation CB to Stephen E. Barton, February 9, 1899, all CB-LC.

140. CBJ, June 4, 1899, CB-LC.

141. David Cobb to Stephen E. Barton, February 21, 1899, CB-LC.

142. Ellen Spencer Mussey to Stephen E. Barton, March 25, 1899, CB-LC.

143. CBJ, June 12, 28, July 5, 12, 1899, CB-LC.

144. CB to Joseph and Enola Gardner, July 10, 1899, CB-LC.

145. CB to Elizabeth Sheldon Tillinghast, April 4, 1899; and CB to Edwin D. Mead, November 3, 1899; also CBJ, September 18–23, 1899, all CB-LC.

146. CBJ, June 10 and 19, 1899, CB-LC.

147. Ibid., September 9 and 14, 1899.

148. Ibid., September 7, 1899; and medals in CB-LC.

149. The words of both the president and the Congress are printed in W. E. Barton, *Life* 2:293.

150. Nicholas Senn, *War Correspondence (Hispano-American War) Letters from Dr. Nicholas Senn* (Chicago: American Medical Association Press, 1899), p. 117.

151. CB to Martha Williamson, June 23, 1898, CB-LC.

152. CB, *Glimpses of Field Work*, p. 161.

153. CB to Julio Carbonell, October 20, 1899, CB-LC.

Chapter 17

1. CBJ, December 12, 1900, CB-LC.

2. CB to Joseph Wheeler, December 13, 1898, CB-LC.

3. See *Congressional Record* 33, no. 55 (February 21, 1900): 2111–12; and CB to W. H. Todhunter, February 15, 1902, CB-LC.

4. See CBJ, April 8, 9, 1901, CB-LC; advertisement for Clara Barton cigars, n.d., CB-LC; and quotation CB to George Kennan, May 26, 1900, K-LC.

5. CBJ, December 12, 1900, CB-LC.

6. *Congressional Record* 33, no. 55 (February 21, 1900): 2111–12; and Alvey Adee to CB, October 26, 1899, CB-LC.

7. See CB to George Cortelyou, December 10, 1899, CB-LC.

8. CBJ, December 12, 1900, CB-LC.

9. Stephen E. Barton, "Clara Barton and the Red Cross," *The Home Journal*, July 19, 1900.

10. CB to Stephen E. Barton, January 20, 1901; quotation "Report of the President to the Committee," July 10, 1900, both CB-LC.

11. Ibid.; and Stephen Barton, "Clara Barton and the Red Cross."

12. Mary Agnes Coombs, "Report on Galveston," n.d. [c. 1901], CB-LC.

13. Stephen E. Barton to J. F. Diehl, N. J. Scully and F. G. Meara, September 21, 1900, CB-LC; and Gustave R. Gaeddert, "The History of the American National Red Cross," unpublished MS, n.d., 2:102–5, ANRC.

14. CBJ, December 12, 1900, CB-LC.

15. Gaeddert, "American Red Cross," n.d., 2:107, ANRC; quotation CB, *The Story of the Red Cross: Glimpses of Field Work* (New York: D. Appleton Co., 1904), p. 171.

16. Fanny L. Ward quoted in CB, *Glimpses of Field Work*, p. 174.

17. Coombs, "Report on Galveston," n.d. [c. 1901]; and CBJ, December 12, 1900, both CB-LC.

18. Coombs, "Report on Galveston," n.d. [c. 1901], CB-LC; and "Clara Barton at Galveston," *Red Cross Bulletin* 1, no. 2 (October 15, 1900).

19. CB to J. Wilkes O'Neill, October 7, 1900, copy in CB-LC.

20. CB, *Glimpses of Field Work*, pp. 182–84.

21. Foster Rhea Dulles, *The American Red Cross: A History* (New York: Harper Brothers, 1950), p. 34; Clyde Buckingham, *Clara Barton; A Broad Humanity* (Alexandria, Va., privately published, 1980), pp. 297–98.

22. CB, "Report of Red Cross Relief at Galveston," n.d. [c. December 1900], CB-LC.

23. CB, *Glimpses of Field Work*, p. 197.

24. CBJ, December 12, 1900, CB-LC.

25. Joseph D. Sayers to CB, October 6, 1900; see also Members of the Governor's Committee to CB, March 5, 1901, both CB-LC.

26. See, for example, W. W. Howard to CB, June 28, 1901, CB-LC.

27. See Gaeddert, "American Red Cross," n.d., 2:187–90, ANRC; CB to Fred L. Ward, February 4, 1901, copy in CB-LC; Minutes of the Board of Control, March 9, 1901, copy in CB-LC; and CB to W. W. Howard, February 18, 1901, copy in CB-LC.

28. CB quoted in Dulles, *American Red Cross*, p. 66.

29. Stephen E. Barton quoted in Gaeddert, "American Red Cross," n.d., 2:190, ANRC.

30. Minutes of the Board of Control, January 12, 1901, RARC NARS; CB to W. W. Howard, January 5, 1901; and CBJ, April 2, 1901, all CB-LC.

31. CB to E. R. Ridgely, February 18, 1901, CB-LC.

32. CBJ, February 3, 1901; and CB to Stephen E. Barton, January 20, 1901, both CB-LC.

33. See, for example, CBJ, January 16 and 30, 1901, CB-LC.

34. CB to William W. Howard, January 5, 1901, CB-LC.

35. "Statement of Miss Barton and Mrs. Ward respecting disputed Galveston Vouchers," March 22, 1902; quotation S. W. Briggs to Mary A. Logan, January 31, 1902, both CB-LC.

36. Dulles, *American Red Cross*, p. 68; and Edward T. James, ed., *Notable American Women, 1607–1950* (Cambridge: Belknap Press, 1971), 1:183–86.

37. CB to Mabel Boardman, June 21, 1900, ANRC.

38. See Mabel Boardman Papers, 1900–1902, LC.

39. Ellen Spencer Mussey to CB, October 23, 1900, CB-LC.

40. CB to Stephen E. Barton, May 26, 1901, CB-LC.

41. Ibid.

42. ? to Officers of the American Red Cross, n.d. [c. fall 1901], CB-LC.

43. CBJ, November 17, 1901, CB-LC.

44. Gaeddert, "American Red Cross," n.d., 2:194–95, ANRC; Dulles, *American Red Cross*, p. 67; and "Miss Barton Re-Elected," *Washington Post*, December 12, 1901.

45. Gaeddert, "American Red Cross," n.d., 2:195, ANRC; and CB to Ida Riccius, January 3, 1902, CB-LC.

46. CB to Richard Olney, March 22, 1902, Richard Olney Papers, LC.

47. CB quoted in Dulles, *American Red Cross*, p. 67.

48. CB to Ida Riccius, January 3, 1902; CB to Stephen E. Barton, January 13, 1901; and CB to Sarah B. Earle, January 3, 1902, all CB-LC.

49. Quotation CB to Stephen E. Barton, March 1, 1900, CB-LC; CBJ, February 13 and March 22, 1901, CB-LC; and Gaeddert, "American Red Cross," n.d., vol. 2, ANRC.

50. Frank Higbee to CB, November 19, 1900; J. Ellen Foster to CB, January 29, 1901; List of Greetings for meetings, December 31, 1900; and quotation CB to William Jarvis, May 11, 1901, all CB-LC.

51. CB to Ida C. Wilsey, February 2, 1900; and "Statement of Amos M. Atwell, Relative to the Work Accomplished By Him and His Agents Under Contract with The American Red Cross," n.d. [c. 1904], both CB-LC.

52. CBJ, April 17, 1901, CB-LC.

53. CB to Admiral W. K. Van Reypen, March 29, 1902, CB-LC.

54. See correspondence between B. F. Tillinghast and CB, and Nicholas Senn and CB, March–April 1902, CB-LC.

55. "Memoirs of Admiral [William] Van Reypen," unpublished MS, n.d., in possession of Mrs. Edward A. C. Russell, Landrum, S.C.

56. Ibid.

57. CBJ, May 6, 1902, CB-LC.

58. "Memoirs of Van Reypen," unpublished MS, n.d.

59. CB to Ida Barton Riccius, June 14, 1902, AAS; and B. F. Tillinghast to Mrs. John A. Logan, n..d., copy in CBJ, June 17, 1902, CB-LC.

60. CB, "Report of the Seventh International Conference of the Red Cross," 1902, copy in ANRC; CB, "Remarks of the President of the American Red Cross," n.d. [1902], CB-LC; CBJ, June 4, 1902, CB-LC; and CB to James Boomer, August 31, 1902, CB-LC.

61. CBJ, June 4–August 6, 1902 (quotation July 10), CB-LC.

62. Francis Atwater, *Memoirs of Francis Atwater* (Meriden, Conn.: Horton Printing Co., 1922), p. 272; and CBJ, September 22, 23, 1902, CB-LC.

63. William E. Barton, *The Life of Clara Barton* (Boston: Houghton Mifflin Co., 1922), 2:297.

64. CBJ, November 9 and 14, 1902, CB-LC.

65. Ibid., November 15, 1902.

66. Ibid., November 10, 23, 1902 (quotation November 10).

67. Gaeddert, "American Red Cross," n.d., 2:205, ANRC.

68. Ibid.; and CBJ, December 9, 1902, CB-LC.

69. CBJ, December 25, 1902, CB-LC.

70. Gaeddert, "American Red Cross," n.d., 2:206–7, ANRC; Dulles, *American Red Cross*, p. 71; and Theodore Roosevelt to Mary S. Logan, June 26, 1916, Theodore Roosevelt Papers, LC.

71. Theodore Roosevelt to CB, January 2, 1903, Roosevelt Papers, LC.

72. CB to Theodore Roosevelt, n.d. [c. January 1903], copy in CB-LC.

73. Gaeddert, "American Red Cross," n.d., 2:211, ANRC; and Dulles, *American Red Cross*, p. 72.

74. Mary S. Logan to George B. Cortelyou, January 19, 1903; and CB to Stephen E. Barton, January 21, 1903, both CB-LC.

75. Letters of suspension are in CB-LC; see also Dulles, *American Red Cross*, p. 72.

76. Mabel Boardman to Mary S. Logan, July 11, 1902, copy in AAS.

77. George C. Boldt to CB, February 17, 1900, copy in CB-LC.

78. Mabel Boardman to Mary S. Logan, February 20, 1903, copy in K-LC; also "Red Cross Troubles," *Washington Star*, March 28, 1903.

79. Gaeddert, "American Red Cross," n.d., 2:214, ANRC; Walter J. Kehr to CB, February 7, 1903, CB-LC; and "Memorial of Walter Phillips and Others to Congress," March 31, 1903, CB-LC.

80. "Charges Made Against the Late Clara Barton by Miss Mabel T. Boardman," September 2, 1916; and files of Red Cross investigation, both RARC NARS. Ten years earlier Barton had explained her absence from Moore by saying that she was "simply terrified by all that threatened notoriety and scrupulously withheld everything 'damaging his book' by its having to appear without me." CB to John H. Frozee, July 16, 1893, CB-LC; and "Notes on Mabel Boardman," by Saidee Riccius, n.d., AAS.

81. Dulles, *American Red Cross*, pp. 69–70, 79–80; and Mrs. John A. Logan to A. L. Stebbins, July 11, 1916, RARC NARS.

82. H. B. Brown to Mabel Boardman, April 12, 1903, Boardman Papers, LC.

83. George Kennan to William T. Wardwell, November 19, 1898; and George Kennan to Walter Phillips, March 27, 1903, both K-LC.

84. Solomons quoted in Abram Vassen Goodman, "Adolphus S. Solomons and Clara Barton: A Forgotten Chapter in the Early Years of the American Red Cross," *American Jewish Historical Quarterly* 59, no. 3 (March 1970): 334.

85. Adolphus Solomons to Gustave Moynier, January 27, 1903, quoted in Cyrus Adler, "Adolphus S. Solomons and the Red Cross," *Publications of the American Jewish Historical Society*, no. 33 (1934): 223.

86. CB to Stephen E. Barton, January 21, 1903, CB-LC.

87. "Red Cross Troubles," *Washington Star*, March 28, 1903; Mary S. Logan to James H. Wilson, May 6, 1903, CB-LC; quotation Stephen E. Barton to Samuel Bowler, March 24, 1903, CB-LC.

88. Stephen E. Barton to Bowler, March 24, 1903, CB-LC.

89. William W. Howard to CB, December 28, 1901 [1902], CB-LC.

90. Mary A. Hines to Herman Riccius, February 6, 1904, CB-LC.

91. CB to Janet Jennings, n.d. [c. March 1903], CB-LC.

92. CB, miscellaneous notes, May 3, 1903, CB-LC.

93. CB to Stephen E. Barton, January 2, 1900, CB-LC.

94. CB to Mary S. Logan, December 12, 1903, quoted in Ishbel Ross, *Angel of the Battlefield: The Life of Clara Barton* (New York: Harper and Row, 1956), p. 244.

95. CB to Lillie Frazier, July 13, 1903, CB-LC.

96. CB to "Mr. Conklin," March 17, 1904; and CB to Richard Olney, February 21, 1903, both CB-LC.

97. CB to Stephen E. Barton, January 21, 1903, CB-LC.

98. CB to "Mrs. Charles," February 24, 1903, CB-LC.

99. CB to Leonora Halsted, March 14, 1902, CB-LC.

100. CB to S. W. Briggs, March 21, 1903, CB-LC.

101. See W. Alexander Johnson to CB, March 29, 1884, CB-LC.

102. See CB to Susan B. Anthony, July 17, 1903; CB to Richard H. Broadhead, January 9, 1904; CB, "Report on First Aid," n.d. [c. 1903]; and quotation CB to B. F. Tillinghast, June 7, 1903, all CB-LC.

103. Buckingham, *Clara Barton*, p. 305.

104. CBJ, August 15, 19, 1903, ANRC.

105. See CB to John D. Rockefeller, December 22, 1903, CB-LC; Jas. Bentham to Mary S. Logan, December 18, 1902, CB-LC; CB to Andrew Carnegie, December 22, 1902, CB-LC; quotation CBJ, December 31, 1903, ANRC.

106. CBJ, October 28, November 2, 1903; and CB to "Mrs. Howe," March 2, 1904, both CB-LC.

107. CB to the Secretary and Officers of the American National Red Cross, December 11, 1903; CB, "Statement of Conditions in Butler," December 18, 1903, both CB-LC.

108. Ray D. Hill, "Clara Barton and Her Methods," n.d. [c. 1920], copy in CB-LC.

109. CB, "Statement of Conditions," December 18, 1903, CB-LC; Richard Broadhead to CB, December 20, 1903, CB-LC; CBJ, December 13, 1903, ANRC; and quotation CB to Joseph Sheldon, December 20, 1903, copy in CB-LC.

110. See CBJ, April 2, 1901; CB to Howard, February 18, 1901; also CB to Richard Olney, December 3, 1903, all CB-LC.

111. See CBJ, July 11 and 14, 1897, CB-LC.

112. Letters of Susan B. Anthony to CB, February–July 1903, CB-LC.

113. CB to Clarence W. Barton, February 24, 1902, CB-LC; "Washington Notes," *Woman's Journal*, February 20, 1904; CBJ, February 15, 1904, ANRC. See also CB to Susan B. Anthony and to May Wright Sewell, both March 30, 1899, CB-LC.

114. CBJ, February 17, 1904, ANRC.

115. CB to J. L. Harbour, March 11, 1902, CB-LC.

116. CBJ, November 1903, ANRC; and CB to Enola Gardner, November 23, 1903, CB-LC.

117. Ibid.

118. Minutes of the Annual Meeting of the American Red Cross, December 8, 1903; and CB to Gustave Moynier, April 4, 1904, both CB-LC.

119. CB to Moynier, April 4, 1904; CB to Mary Logan, January 4, 1904, both CB-LC.

120. Minutes of Annual Meeting, December 8, 1903, CB-LC.

121. CB to Mrs. Donald McLean, January 15, 1904, photocopy, ANRC.

122. CB to Harriette Reed, January 30, 1904, CB-LC.

123. See, for example, Joseph Sheldon, ed., *Red Cross Bulletin* 1, no. 2 (April 7, 1903); and *The Red Cross: Some Facts Concerning Clara Barton's Work* (Bridgeport, Conn., 1903).

124. CB to Reed, January 30, 1904, CB-LC.

125. CB, miscellaneous notes, 1904, typescript, AAS.

126. CBJ, January 1, 1904, ANRC.

127. CB to Stephen E. Barton, February 1904, quoted in Ross, *Angel*, p. 252.

128. "Memoirs of Van Reypen," unpublished MS, n.d.

129. See, for example, CB to George C. Boldt, March 3, 1899, CB-LC.

130. "Expenditures of the American National Red Cross," n.d. [July 1900], CB-LC.

131. See CBJ, July 14–August 26, 1901, CB-LC; and Percy Epler, *The Life of Clara Barton* (New York: Macmillan, 1915), p. 373.

132. For example, CBJ, June 14, 1901, CB-LC; and CBJ, November 25, 1903, ANRC.

133. CB to W. H. Sears, April 4, 1902, CB-LC.

134. Edith Riccius King, "Reminiscences of Great Aunt Clara Barton," 1938, CB-LC.

135. CB to Stephen E. Barton, March 13, 1904, CB-LC.

136. CBJ, March 28, 1904, ANRC.

137. Gaeddert, "American Red Cross," n.d., 2:221–23, ANRC.

138. L. A. Stebbins, "Sketch of the Investigation into the Affairs of the American National Red Cross, and the Administration thereof by Miss Clara Barton in the Spring of 1904," n.d., CB-LC.

139. CB to Leonora Halsted, May 10, 1904, CB-LC.

140. Gaeddert, "American Red Cross," n.d., 2:224–25, ANRC; and Stebbins, "Sketch of the Investigation," n.d., CB-LC.

141. CB quoted in Gaeddert, "American Red Cross," n.d., 2:199, ANRC; and Minutes of Board of Control, January 12, 1901, RARC NARS.

142. See also "Reply of Red Cross," *Washington Post*, March 31, 1904.

143. See CB to Editor, *Washington Post*, March 28, 1904; and CB to Samuel Jarvis, March 30, 1904, both CB-LC.

144. See, for example, CB to Emily D. Martin, December 14, 1897, CB-LC; CBJ, August 15, 1903, ANRC; quotation Dulles, *American Red Cross*, p. 75.

145. Quotation CBJ, December 31, 1903; see also April 10, 1904, both ANRC.

146. Ibid., September 6–8, 1903.

147. CB to Joseph Gardner, April 22, 1904, CB-LC.

148. Gaeddert, "American Red Cross," n.d., 2:232–33, ANRC; and John Morlan to Anna Roosevelt Cowles, n.d. [c. October 1903], RARC NARS.

149. Ibid.; and John Morlan to Mary A. Hines, April 27, 1904, quoted in *Washington Post*, May 4, 1904.

150. Gaeddert, "American Red Cross," n.d., 2:235, ANRC.

151. CBJ, April 26, May 2, 1904, ANRC.

152. Ibid., May 1 and 3, 1904.

153. L. A. Stebbins, "An Unpublished Chapter in the History of the American National Red Cross," unpublished MS, pp. 18–19, ANRC.

154. CBJ, May 4–10, 1904, ANRC; and CB, "Miscellaneous Notes," 1904, AAS.

155. CBJ, May 14, 1904, ANRC; and Mrs. John A. Logan quoted in Gaeddert, "American Red Cross," n.d., 2:243, ANRC.

156. CBJ, May 14 and July 6, 1904, ANRC.

Chapter 18

1. CB to Edward Howe, November 20, 1904; see also CB to Mrs. J. G. Lemmon, March 1, 1901, both CB-LC.

2. "Red Cross Inquiry," *Washington Star*, May 16, 1904; and "Accuses Miss Barton," *Hartford Covenant* (Conn.), June 13, 1904.

3. CB to Leonora Halsted, July 12, 1904, CB-LC.

4. CB to Stephen E. Barton, November 20, 1904; and Joseph Sheldon to Isabella Hinton, January 24, 1905, both CB-LC.

5. B. F. Warner quoted in Foster Rhea Dulles, *The American Red Cross: A History* (New York: Harper Brothers, 1950), p. 75.

6. "Belongs to the Red Cross," *Washington Post*, June 3, 1904; and "Memoirs of Admiral [William] Van Reypen," unpublished MS, n.d., in possession of Mrs. Edward A. C. Russell, Landrum, S.C.

7. "Memoirs of Admiral Van Reypen," unpublished MS, n.d.

8. Montgomery County Maryland Land Records, Liber JA 42, p. 473; and Liber 184, p. 423, Montgomery County Courthouse, Rockville, Md.; also CBJ, June 12, 17, 29, 1897, CB-LC; and Julian B. Hubbell to CB, March 17, 1903, CB-LC.

9. See CBJ, May–June 1904, ANRC.

10. CB to L. A. Stebbins, October 8, 1904, CB-LC; also CBJ, June 22, 1904, ANRC.

11. "Memoirs of Van Reypen," unpublished MS, n.d.

12. CB to "dear friends," July 14, 1904, CB-LC.

13. CB to Charles Sumner Young, January 13, 1904, and April 1909, quoted in Percy Epler, The Life of Clara Barton (New York: Macmillan, 1915), pp. 336 and 339; and "Clara Barton Martyr Revealed by Letters," Los Angeles Examiner, April 28, 1912.

14. CBJ, April 21, 1907, CB-LC.

15. CB to "beloved friend," June 22, 1904; CB to Lucy Hall and R. G. Brown, October 4, 1904; letters of condolence and book reviews, CB scrapbook, all CB-LC; and "Clara Barton Martyr," Los Angeles Examiner, April 28, 1912.

16. CBJ, April 21, 1907, CB-LC.

17. CB Christmas greeting, 1905, CB-LC.

18. CB quoted in untitled newspaper clipping, Washington Times, April 20, 1905, CB-LC.

19. CB to Edward Howe, July 11 and 15, 1904, CB-LC.

20. CB to Janet Jennings, June 14, 1905, CB-LC.

21. CB to Edward Howe, November 26, 1904, and February 13, 1905, CB-LC.

22. Charter of National First Aid Association of America, April 1905, CB-LC; "Funds Needed for First Aid, Says Clara Barton," Boston American, August 6, 1905; CB, speech given at first annual meeting of the First Aid Association, quoted in Boston Evening Transcript, June 7, 1906; and quotation CB to Leonora Halsted, February 11, 1907, CB-LC.

23. "First Aid Her Task," Worcester Telegram, August 13, 1905; also CB to Leonora Halsted, April 2, 1906, CB-LC.

24. Ibid.; and "Clara Barton is Vigorous at 84," Worcester Evening Gazette, January 18, 1906.

25. CB to Halsted, April 2, 1906, CB-LC.

26. CB to John S. Cameron, February 3, 1906, CB-LC.

27. Ibid.

28. See, for example, CB to Lizzie Tittle, July 12, 1895, typescript; CB to Francis Atwater, August 3, 1901; and CB to Leonora Halsted, May 18, 1904, all CB-LC.

29. "Clara Barton's Oxford Home," Boston Globe, January 28, 1906; "Clara Barton is Vigorous," Worcester Evening Gazette, January 18, 1906; and quotations CB to J. B. Holman, March 3, 1906, CB-LC.

30. "End of Glen Echo," unidentified newspaper clipping, n.d., CB scrapbook; copy of an article for the New York Sun, January 10, 1908; and CB to Enola and Joseph Gardner, July 27, 1907, all CB-LC.

31. CBJ, April 2, 1906, CB-LC.

32. Recollections of Walter Harold Riccius quoted in William Conklin, ed., Clara Barton and Dansville (Dansville, N.Y.: F. A. Owen Publishing Co., 1966), pp. 531–36.

33. CBJ, March 12, 18, April 7, 20–21, 1906, and October 22, 1907; CB to Leonora Halsted, February 22, 1906; and CB to Stephen E. Barton, March 4, 1908, all CB-LC.

34. CB to "My dear sister Harriette," July 26, 1901, CB-LC.

35. CB to Marion Bullock, October 8, 1907, CB-LC; and Edith Brownell, "A Glimpse of Clara Barton at Home," unpublished MS, n.d., CBNHS.
36. Brownell, "A Glimpse of Clara Barton," unpublished MS, n.d., CBNHS.
37. CB to "my beloved friend," June 22, 1904, CB-LC.
38. CB to Octavia Dix Fanning, May 23, 1906, CB-LC.
39. CB to Halsted, April 2, 1906, CB-LC.
40. CBJ, September 29, 1910, ANRC; and CB to Frances Dyer, January 16, 1907, CB-LC.
41. CBJ, May 28, 1906; and Lucy Hall Brown to CB, n.d. [1906], both CB-LC.
42. CBJ, March 9, 1906, CB-LC.
43. CB to Charles Sumner Young, April 1909, copy in CBNHS.
44. CB to Halsted, April 2, 1906, CB-LC.
45. CB to Charles Barton, October [November] 7, 1904, CB-LC.
46. See, for example, CBJ, January 31, March 22, April 23, July 10, 1907; and CB to Grand Duchess Louise, October 27, 1907, all CB-LC.
47. William E. Barton, The Life of Clara Barton (Boston: Houghton Mifflin Co., 1922), 2:318; and CB to Frances Barton, December 24, 1908, CB-LC.
48. Edward T. James, ed., Notable American Women, 1607–1950 (Cambridge: Belknap Press, 1971), 1:551–60.
49. CB to Janet Jennings, September 1, 1907, CB-LC.
50. CB to Francis Bolton, December 24, 1906, CB-LC; CB to Lucia Griffin, December 1, 1906, CB-LC; quotation CB to Helen Thompson, September 22, 1907, CBNHS.
51. CB to Mamie Barton Stafford, December 1, 1906, typescript; also CBJ, March 7, 1908, both CB-LC.
52. CB to A. W. Terrill, April 2, 1911, CB-LC.
53. Percy Epler, The Life of Clara Barton (New York: Macmillan, 1915), p. 412.
54. CB to Thompson, September 22, 1907, CBNHS.
55. CBJ, April 6, 1907; and CB to E. M. Rothman, October 21, 1907, both CB-LC.
56. Excerpts from reviews of CB's The Story of My Childhood, n.d. [1908]; and untitled review in New York Evening Mail, August 19, 1907, both CB-LC.
57. CBJ, October 12–November 9, 1908 (quotation November 9), CB-LC.
58. CB to Leonora Halsted, February 11, 1907, CB-LC; also CB Christmas greeting, 1909, CBNHS.
59. CBJ, April 20, 1910, ANRC; see also CBJ, August 16, 1910, and March 23 and 24, 1908; and CB to the Gardners, July 27, 1907, all CB-LC.
60. Dulles, American Red Cross, pp. 97–98.
61. CB to General Whitaker, April 17, 1909, CB-LC.
62. Brownell, "A Glimpse of Clara Barton," unpublished MS, n.d., CBNHS.
63. See, for example, "The World's Famous Women," Detroit News, April 4, 1905.
64. CBJ, February 6, 1907, CB-LC.
65. Ibid., April 24, 1910, ANRC.
66. Ibid., January 5, 1911, CB-LC.
67. Brownell, "A Glimpse of Clara Barton," unpublished MS, n.d., CBNHS.
68. CB to Mrs. Walker, October 7, 1904, CB-LC; CB to Jennings, June 14, 1905, CB-LC; CBJ, February 18, 1906, January 1, 5, July 4, 1907, CB-LC; CB to Halsted, Feb-

ruary 11, 1907, CB-LC; CBJ, May 30, September 21, 1908, CB-LC; CBJ, August 23, 1910, ANRC; and quotation CBJ, January 1, 1907, CB-LC.

69. CB, untitled poem, n.d. [c. 1909], CB-LC.

70. "Clara Barton at 90," *New York Sun*, December 31, 1911.

71. "At Work for Suffrage," *Baltimore Sun*, February 8, 1906; also "Women Suffragists out in Full Force," *Cincinnati Tribune*, February 8, 1906; "Favorite Guest," *Rochester Herald*, February 11, 1906; and CBJ, February 7, 1906, CB-LC.

72. CB quoted in Ida Husted Harper, "The Life and Work of Clara Barton," *North American Review* 195, no. 5 (May 1912): 701–2.

73. CBJ, March 21, 1911, CB-LC.

74. CB to the editor of the *New York World*, March 21, 1910, copy in CB-LC.

75. CB to Mary S. Logan, June 16, 1911, CB-LC.

76. CBJ, March 3, 1907, February 3, 1908; and CB to Stephen E. Barton, March 4, 1908, all CB-LC.

77. CBJ, July 10, 1911, CB-LC.

78. Ibid., June 16, 1906.

79. "Clara Barton Ninety Years Old Today," *Philadelphia Press*, December 24, 1911.

80. Frances Bolton, "Clara Barton," address to Association of Universalist Women, June 1940, CB-LC.

81. CBJ, May 3, 1910, ANRC.

82. Epler, *Life*, p. 393.

83. CBJ, January 2, 1907, and January 31, 1908, CB-LC; CB to Herbert Barton, March 7, 1909, CB-LC; and Lloyd Tenny, "When I Knew Clara Barton," unpublished MS, 1941, CBNHS.

84. CBJ, December 25, 1907, CB-LC.

85. CB quoted in Epler, *Life*, p. 423.

86. CBJ, February 18, 1906, CB-LC.

87. Ibid., July 4, 1911.

88. Ibid., June 3–November 3, 1910, ANRC; and CB to Grand Duchess Louise, December 20, 1909, typescript, RARC NARS.

89. Quotation Julian B. Hubbell to Mrs. Schoppe, February 20, 1911, typescript; also CB to Leonora Halsted, June 19, 1911, both CB-LC.

90. Epler, *Life*, p. 425.

91. CB to Charles B. Rice, April 24, 1911, typescript, RARC NARS.

92. CBJ, April 27, May 6, 1911, CB-LC.

93. CB to Stephen E. Barton, May 24, 1911, CB-LC; and CB to Harriette Reed, April 1911, quoted in Epler, *Life*, p. 426.

94. Julian B. Hubbell to Stephen E. Barton, December 26, 1913, CB-LC.

95. Epler, *Life*, p. 429.

96. CBJ, November 11, 1911; and CB to Stephen Barton, May 24, 1911, both CB-LC.

97. Julian B. Hubbell to Stephen E. Barton, December [January] 10, 1913, CB-LC.

98. CB to the Grand Duchess Louise, February 26, 1912, CB-LC.

99. Hubbell to S. Barton, December [January] 10, 1913, CB-LC.

100. CB quoted in Epler, *Life*, p. 433.

101. Ibid., p. 434; and W. E. Barton, *Life* 2:374.

index

Porter, J. Y., 255–56
Porter, Julia Ann. *See* Barton, Julia Ann Porter
Potomac Corps, 285–86
Potter, Henry C., 290
Prairie cure, 67–69, 71
Press, coverage of Clara Barton, 148–49, 234–35, 239, 256, 261, 351–52
Prison reform, 222–30
Proctor, Redfield, 304, 346–48, 350, 353, 356
Pullman, George, 277, 281, 282–85, 290–91, 298–302, 318, 366
Pullman, Royal H., 302

Quimby, Phineas, 363

Ramsey, Samuel, 35, 61, 182, 204
Rathbone, Estes, 322
Red Cross: American society, formation of, 187–93, 195–97, 201–11; Armenian relief work, 289–95; Conferences, 238–40, 251–52, 299, 335–37; Congressional bills concerning, 265, 287–88, 316, 325–27; criticisms and investigations of, 280–83, 294–95, 316–19, 330–35, 340–43, 348–53; Cuban relief work, 296–97, 299–300, 302–05; disaster relief work, US, 207–09, 219–21, 232–37, 245–49, 255–63, 274–79, 297, 328–30, 345; first aid branch, 344, 358–59; Franco-Prussian War, 159–71; funding of, 215–16, 265, 280–83, 330–35, 344–45, 349–53; headquarters, 217–18, 263–64, 270–71, 298, 334, 341; hotels, 260–61, 263; incorporation of, 325–27; insignia, 157, 251, 257, 265, 287–88, 308, 325–26; International Committee, 156–57, 187–92, 202–04, 216–18, 233, 238–40, 251–53, 280; local chapters, 207, 218–21, 232, 247, 255, 257, 260–61, 266–67, 270, 280, 308, 315–16, 334; official recognition of, 216; philosophy of, 221–22, 249–51; press coverage of, 199–200, 209, 234–35, 239, 256, 261, 351–52; promotion of, 244–45, 261; publications, 266, 348, 351; resignation of Clara Barton, 353–57; rival societies, 206–07, 216–17, 300, 319–21, 326; Russian famine (1891), 267–70; Spanish-American War, 296–97, 299–300, 302–20, 319–24; structure and reorganization of, 218–21, 258, 265–66, 308, 319, 333–34, 338, 340–43
Red Cross in Peace and War, The, 318, 359–60

Red Cross Park, Bedford, IN, 272–75, 288–89, 350–51, 356
Riccius, Edith (great-niece), 318, 350
Riccius, Ida Barton (niece), 185, 366, 370
Robbins, Delia (cousin), 264
Rockefeller, John D., 344
Roosevelt, Theodore, 306, 314, 337, 339–40, 342, 349, 357, 362
Rough Riders, 309
Rucker, Daniel H., 87–88, 92, 97
Russian Famine Committee of the United States, 267
Russo-Turkish War, 187–88, 191

Saarbrücken, 160, 168
Sampson, William T., 306, 313
San Francisco, CA, 245
Sanitary Commission, 92, 100–02, 110, 119, 123–25, 136, 168, 189–90, 219
Santiago, Cuba, 313–15
Saracen, Mrs. Fischer, 161
Saunders, James, 206
Schieren, Charles, 302, 321
Schiff, Jacob, 288, 308
Science and Health, 364
Sea Islands, SC, 111–12, 275–79, 281, 297, 329
Sears, William H., 319
Senn, Nicholas, 336, 366
Seward, Frederick W., 193
Seward, William, 189–90, 193, 202
Shekafet, second order of, 295
Sheldon, Abby, 172–73, 177, 195, 222
Sheldon, Joseph, 145, 177, 195, 209, 222, 238–40, 265, 306, 319, 324, 347–49, 351
Shepard, Hannah, 194, 196, 198, 200, 206–07, 209–10, 216–17
Sherborn, MA, 222–32, 249
Sheridan, Phil, 201
Sherman, William T., 101, 103
Shugert, Samuel T., 58–59, 73
Siboney, Cuba, 309–13
Sidney, R. O., 77
Silver Cross of Imperial Russia, 336
Simpson, Lovett, 14
Sixth Massachusetts Regiment, 78
Slavery, 63, 88, 121, 142
Smith, Adelaide, 129
Smith, J. Alden, 350
Sollosso, Juan B., 320–21
Solomons, Adolphus S., 204–05, 237–39, 342
Sorosis, 253–54

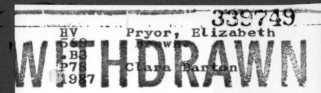

DATE			
		JUN 0 9 2005	
		OCT 1 8 2007	
		MAR 0 1 201	
		MAR 1 5 2011	
		APR 0 4 2011	

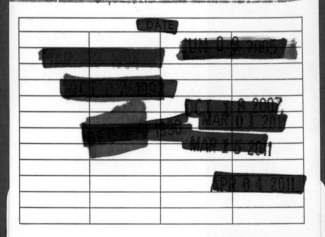